Nutrition, Health and Athletic Performance

Special Issue Editors

Kelly Pritchett
Enette Larson Meyer

MDPI • Basel • Beijing • Wuhan • Barcelona • Belgrade

MDPI

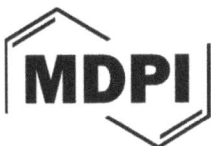

Special Issue Editors

Kelly Pritchett
Central Washington University
USA

Enette Larson Meyer
University of Wyoming
USA

Editorial Office
MDPI AG
St. Alban-Anlage 66
Basel, Switzerland

This edition is a reprint of the Special Issue published online in the open access journal *Nutrients* (ISSN 2072-6643) from 2016–2017 (available at: http://www.mdpi.com/journal/nutrients/special_issues/nutrition_health_athletic_performance).

For citation purposes, cite each article independently as indicated on the article page online and as indicated below:

Author 1; Author 2. Article title. *Journal Name.* **Year.** *Article number,* page range.

First Edition 2017

ISBN 978-3-03842-626-4 (Pbk)
ISBN 978-3-03842-627-1 (PDF)

Table of Contents

About the Special Issue Editors

Kelly Pritchett is an Assistant Professor in Nutrition and Exercise Science at Central Washington University. As a board-certified specialist in sports dietetics, she has consulted with elite and collegiate athletes as well as active individuals. Pritchett is the fact sheet editor and a member of the leadership committee of the Academy's Sports, Cardiovascular and Wellness Nutrition dietetic practice group. She is an active member of the American College of Sports Medicine and has authored research articles for scientific journals and presented at regional and national conferences. Her research interests include post-exercise nutrition for recovery, vitamin D status and nutrition needs of athletes with a spinal cord injury. Pritchett is a graduate of the University of Alabama, where she also earned a doctorate.

Enette Larson Meyer, is a Professor in Human Nutrition and Director of the Nutrition & Exercise Laboratory at the University of Wyoming, USA. Prof. Meyer's overall research interests center on the health and performance of active individuals, particularly women, at all stages of the lifecycle and at all levels of performance - from the casual exerciser to the elite athlete. Prof. Meyer is particularly interested in Vitamin D and Iodine metabolism and the impact of deficiency of these nutrients in athletes and active populations.

Preface to "Nutrition, Health and Athletic Performance"

Optimal nutrition is fundamental for enhancing training, recovery and performance in sport. Research has aimed to determine the efficacy of appropriate intake of nutrients, fluids, and supplements and their role in exercise performance. The purpose of this Special book issue entitled "Nutrition, Health, and Athletic Performance is to highlight recent applied research examining aspects of sports nutrition and exercise performance in human subjects.

Manuscript submissions of original research, meta-analyses, or reviews of the scientific literature, which targets nutritional strategies to benefit performance and health are included in this issue. The .....#... chapters in this book cover a wide spectrum of hot topics in the performance nutrition world. We hope that the chapters will provide scientific basis for which future investigations can be based upon. Futhermore, we hope that this issue provides new recommendations and insights for practitioners (sports dietitians, sports medicine physicians, strenght coaches, athletic trainers, and other members of the sports medicine team), coaches, athletes, and scientists in the field of sports nutrition.

Kelly Pritchett and Enette Larson Meyer

Special Issue Editors

nutrients

MDPI

Article

Protein-Pacing from Food or Supplementation Improves Physical Performance in Overweight Men and Women: The PRISE 2 Study

Paul J. Arciero [1,*], Rohan C. Edmonds [1], Kanokwan Bunsawat [2], Christopher L. Gentile [3], Caitlin Ketcham [1], Christopher Darin [1], Mariale Renna [1], Qian Zheng [1], Jun Zhu Zhang [1] and Michael J. Ormsbee [4,5]

1   Human Nutrition and Metabolism Laboratory, Department of Health and Exercise Sciences, Skidmore College, Saratoga Springs, NY 12866, USA; redmonds@skidmore.edu (R.C.E.); cketcham@skidmore.edu (C.K.); cdarin@skidmore.edu (C.D.); mariale.p.renna@gmail.com (M.R.); qzheng1@skidmore.edu (Q.Z.); junzhu.zhang@gmail.com (J.Z.Z.)
2   Integrative Physiology Laboratory, Department of Kinesiology and Nutrition, University of Illinois at Chicago, Chicago, IL 60612, USA; bunsawa2@uic.edu
3   Department of Food Science and Human Nutrition, Colorado State University, Fort Collins, CO 80523, USA; christoper.gentile@colostate.edu
4   Florida State University, Institute of Sports Sciences & Medicine, Department of Nutrition, Food and Exercise Sciences, Tallahassee, FL 32304, USA; mormsbee@fsu.edu
5   Discipline of Biokinetics, Exercise, and Leisure Studies, University of KwaZulu-Natal, Durban 4041, South Africa
*   Correspondence: parciero@skidmore.edu; Tel.: +1-518-580-5366

Received: 6 April 2016; Accepted: 5 May 2016; Published: 11 May 2016

Abstract: We recently reported that protein-pacing (P; six meals/day @ 1.4 g/kg body weight (BW), three of which included whey protein (WP) supplementation) combined with a multi-mode fitness program consisting of resistance, interval sprint, stretching, and endurance exercise training (RISE) improves body composition in overweight individuals. The purpose of this study was to extend these findings and determine whether protein-pacing with only food protein (FP) is comparable to WP supplementation during RISE training on physical performance outcomes in overweight/obese individuals. Thirty weight-matched volunteers were prescribed RISE training and a P diet derived from either whey protein supplementation (WP, $n = 15$) or food protein sources (FP, $n = 15$) for 16 weeks. Twenty-one participants completed the intervention (WP, $n = 9$; FP, $n = 12$). Measures of body composition and physical performance were significantly improved in both groups ($p < 0.05$), with no effect of protein source. Likewise, markers of cardiometabolic disease risk (e.g., LDL (low-density lipoprotein) cholesterol, glucose, insulin, adiponectin, systolic blood pressure) were significantly improved ($p < 0.05$) to a similar extent in both groups. These results demonstrate that both whey protein and food protein sources combined with multimodal RISE training are equally effective at improving physical performance and cardiometabolic health in obese individuals.

Keywords: protein-pacing; physical performance; cardiometabolic-risk; PRISE exercise training

1. Introduction

Although it is well-accepted that increased protein intake and physical activity are likely effective strategies to combat the rise in obesity [1], there is a paucity of well-controlled lifestyle interventions. Indeed, there is less data available on lifestyle interventions combining increased protein intake above the recommended dietary allowance (RDA) and exercise training in overweight populations that quantify changes in fitness-related performance outcomes such as muscular strength and endurance, flexibility, and balance.

Increasing protein intake above recommended levels has been shown to enhance protein synthesis, postprandial thermogenesis, lean body mass, satiety, and cardiometabolic health [2,3]. We recently demonstrated that, compared to current recommendations (three meals/day and 0.8 g/kg BW/day), a protein-pacing diet (five to six meals/day; three of which were whey protein supplemented and >0.3 g/kg BW/meal; >1.4 g/kg BW/day) elicited greater improvements in body composition and thermic effect of feeding, during both energy balance and deficit in overweight adults [4].

In recent years, increasing attention has been given to healthy lifestyle routines that combine multiple fitness components into one training program or can be delivered with the support of computer-based technologies [5,6]. Indeed, several studies have reported training programs that combine resistance and endurance exercises are more effective at improving body composition and reducing metabolic disease risk than either training modality alone [7–9]. In addition to traditional resistance and endurance exercise, nonconventional modalities such as yoga, tai chi, pilates, and interval sprint training have become increasingly popular among the general public [10–12].

In light of this popularity of both protein-pacing (P) and combined exercise training, we recently compared the effectiveness of P (six meals/day, three meals/day of which were whey protein) combined with either traditional resistance training or a regimen that included resistance exercise, interval sprint exercise, stretching (yoga, pilates), and endurance exercise (RISE training), and found that PRISE (protein-pacing, resistance, interval, stretching, endurance training) resulted in greater reductions in body weight, total and abdominal (including visceral) fat mass, as well as greater gains in percent lean mass [13]. Collectively, these data provide experimental evidence that a whey supplemented protein-pacing diet (WP) combined with a multi-mode fitness program (RISE) results in greater cardio-metabolic health benefits than other training and dietary regimens, a finding supported by others [14]. Whether this diet-exercise (PRISE) combination also favorably improves indices of fitness-related performance outcomes in this obese/overweight population was a major focus of the current study.

Of practical relevance is whether the source of protein supplementation (whey protein supplemented *vs.* food protein sources only) influences metabolic and physical performance outcomes. Some [15,16], but not all [17], studies have reported that whey protein is more effective at improving body composition and disease risk than other protein sources (e.g., soy, pea, casein). Most intervention studies [18], including those from our own laboratory [4,13,19,20], have primarily used powdered or ready-to-drink whey protein supplements, and few data exist comparing the effects of whey protein supplementation to protein derived from a variety of whole food sources (animal and plant). This gap in the literature limits the general application of existing data as well as a preference among some individuals to consume whole foods rather than protein supplements [21].

With this background, the primary purpose of the present study was to compare the effects of a protein-pacing diet consisting of either whey protein supplementation (WP; consumed as three of the six daily meals) or protein-rich food sources (FP; consumed for all six daily meals) combined with RISE training on fitness-related performance outcomes, as well as cardiometabolic and body composition measures. Given the previously documented benefits of whey protein compared to other protein sources, it is hypothesized that the WP will elicit more favorable changes in performance, cardiometabolic, and body composition outcomes than FP. It is important to note that only protein was adjusted whereas fat and carbohydrate intake were not intentionally modified.

2. Materials and Methods

2.1. Participants

A total of 125 individuals from the surrounding Saratoga Springs, NY, USA community responded to flyers and newspaper advertisements and were screened for participation. Of the 71 volunteers who met eligibility criteria, 30 middle aged (50 ± 8 years) men and women started the study (Figure 1).

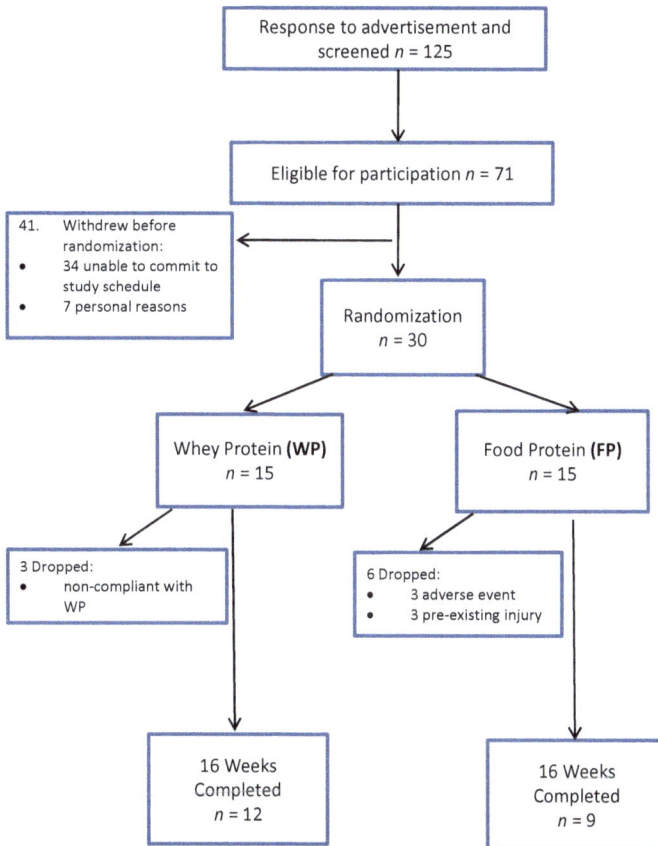

```
          ┌─────────────────────────────┐
          │ Response to advertisement and│
          │     screened n = 125         │
          └─────────────────────────────┘
                        │
          ┌─────────────────────────────┐
          │ Eligible for participation n = 71│
          └─────────────────────────────┘
```

41. Withdrew before randomization:
   - 34 unable to commit to study schedule
   - 7 personal reasons

Randomization
n = 30

Whey Protein **(WP)**
n = 15

Food Protein **(FP)**
n = 15

3 Dropped:
- non-compliant with WP

6 Dropped:
- 3 adverse event
- 3 pre-existing injury

16 Weeks Completed
n = 12

16 Weeks Completed
n = 9

Figure 1. CONSORT (Consolidated Standards of Reporting Trials) flow chart of participants during the study intervention.

All participants were nonsmokers; overweight (body mass index, BMI; 25–29.9 kg/m^2) or obese (BMI > 30.0 kg/m^2); sedentary (<30 min, two days/week of structured physical activity); weight stable ±2 kg for at least six months prior to beginning the study); and absent of overt cardiovascular or metabolic diseases (e.g., type 2 diabetes, thyroid disease) as assessed by a medical history and physical examination. All procedures were approved by the Skidmore College Institutional Review Board Committee. The nature, benefits, and risks were explained to the volunteers and their written informed consent was obtained prior to participation. This trial was registered at clinicaltrials.gov as NCT02594228.

2.2. Experimental Design

Participants were randomized to one of two nutritional intervention groups for the 16-week study (Figure 1): (1) combined exercise training (RISE) and food protein (FP, $n = 15$) or (2) RISE and whey protein (WP, $n = 15$). Both groups were asked to consume five to six small meals each day containing ~20–25 g of a high quality protein source (Supplementary Materials Table S1). Of note, we purposefully did not include a RISE only control group because we were interested in specifically comparing the source of higher protein consumption given the well-established increased dietary protein needs during exercise training [22]. All testing procedures were measured at baseline and following the 16 week intervention period. Participants in the FP group consumed protein only from high quality food sources for each of the meals. The WP group replaced the food protein of three meals on exercise days and two meals on non-exercise days with 20–25 g of whey protein supplement (Classic Whey; Optimum Nutrition). For all meals, participants were provided with a menu of foods from which to choose. Examples included milk, Greek yogurt, eggs, lean meats, fish, poultry, and specific plant sources, including legumes, nuts, and seeds. The number of recommended daily calories to consume was estimated to match the caloric requirements of each individual as measured by resting metabolic rate and measured/estimated physical activity level but was *ad libitum*, and not energy-restricted. Both groups followed the same protocol in terms of the timing of meals: all meals were evenly spaced throughout the day and one meal was consumed within one hour of waking in the morning and another two hours prior to bed. On exercise days, both groups consumed a protein meal (20–25 g) within 60 min after completion of exercise. For WP, they were required to consume this meal as 20–25 g of whey protein giving them a total of three servings of whey on exercise days. For FP, this required a protein-rich food meal of 20–25 g. On non-exercise days, both groups consumed similar amounts of total protein at each of their six meals per day.

2.3. Exercise Training

All subjects in both groups participated in the same multiple exercise training regimen as described previously [13]. Briefly, the training program consisted of four specific types of exercise: (1) resistance training; (2) interval sprints; (3) stretching/yoga/pilates; and (4) endurance exercise (RISE training; Supplementary Materials Table S2). Subjects underwent four exercise sessions/week, and the sessions rotated through the four types of exercise, such that each of the four exercises was performed one day/week. To familiarize participants with the individual exercises and to ensure compliance, all training sessions were performed in the Skidmore College Sports Center under the supervision of at least two members of the research team.

Specific details of the four types of exercises that comprise the RISE training have been previously published [10]. Briefly, the resistance (R) training sessions were completed within 60 min and consisted of a dynamic warm-up, footwork and agility, lower and upper body resistance, and core exercises performed at a resistance to induce muscular fatigue in 10–15 repetitions and for two to three sets. A 30 s recovery was provided between sets and a 60 s recovery was allowed between different exercises. The sprint interval (I) training sessions were completed within 40 min and consisted of 5–10 sets of 30–60 s of all-out exercise interspersed with 2–4 min of rest after each exercise. Participants were allowed to perform the sprints using any mode of exercise (treadmill, elliptical machine, stationary bikes, swimming, snowshoeing, cycling, rollerblading, *etc.*). The stretching/yoga/pilates regimen was based on traditional yoga poses with modern elements of pilates training for a total body stretching, flexibility, and strengthening workout. All sessions were completed within 60 min and were led by a certified yoga instructor (PJA). Finally, endurance exercise training was performed for 60 min or longer at a moderate pace (60% of maximal effort). Participants were allowed to choose from a variety of aerobic activities, including walking, jogging, cycling, rowing, swimming, *etc.*

2.4. Laboratory Testing Procedures

All testing (see below) was administered pre-intervention (week 0) and post intervention (week 17) between 0600 and 0900, following a 12-h fast and 48-h abstinence from caffeine and alcohol intake, and 48–72 h after the last exercise session to eliminate the acute effects of the last bout of exercise.

2.5. Body Weight and Composition

Body weight was obtained during each visit with a standard digital scale (Befour Inc., Cedarburg, WI, USA). Height was measured without shoes using a stadiometer. Waist circumferences were obtained in centimeters with a standard tape measure. Waist measurement was taken at the area with the smallest circumference between the rib cage and the iliac crest and obtained by the same investigator (PJA). Body Composition was assessed by Dual Energy X-ray Absorptiometry (iDXA; Lunar iDXA; GE Healthcare, Madison, WI, USA; analyzed using Encore software version 13.6; GE Healthcare). Total body adiposity, % body fat, lean body mass, appendicular composition, visceral adipose tissue (VAT), and regional abdominal adiposity were all analyzed from DXA scans as previously described [13].

2.6. Dietary Intake and Feelings of Hunger and Satiety

Throughout the intervention, subjects maintained a daily food log that included all food and beverages consumed each day, including meal timing. To further verify compliance, food intake was analyzed from a representative three-day period of two week days and one weekend day at weeks 0 and 16 using Food Processor SQL Edition (version 10.12.0, 2012; ESHA Research, Salem, OR, USA) as previously described [13,23]. All dietary analyses were performed by the same technician. Visual analog scales (VAS) were administered at baseline and week 16 to evaluate the effects of the lifestyle interventions on hunger, satiation, and desire-to-eat [13].

2.7. Physical Performance Assessments

Measures of one repetition strength of the upper and lower body were assessed via the bench and leg press, respectively, following National Strength and Conditioning Association (NSCA) guidelines, as previously described [20]. Upper body muscular endurance of the chest and abdominals were assessed with push-ups and sit ups completed in one minute, respectively.

For the push-ups, men started in a plank position with arms extended and hands placed under the shoulders and balancing on the toes. A successful push-up was defined as lowering the body so elbows reached 90° followed by a return to the starting plank position. Women started in the plank position balancing on the hands and knees and followed identical procedures as the men. Participants were asked to perform as many push-ups as possible within 60 s in a continuous pattern with no more than two seconds between repetitions.

Sit-ups required participants to start in the supine position with knees bent to 90° and feet flat on the ground and supported by a research team member and arms folded across the chest. A successful sit-up required participants to curl up to a 90° position (vertical) to the floor and then return to the starting position. The sit-up action was continuous, with a single rest of no more than 2 s allowed between repetitions and performed to achieve the maximum number of sit-ups in 60 s.

Postural static standing balance was assessed with the stork balance test. Participants were instructed to balance on the dominant leg with the heel lifted off the ground while the non-dominant leg was bent at the knee to allow the foot to be placed gently against the inside of the dominant knee. Hands were placed on top of the iliac crests. The trial ended when the heel of the dominant leg touched the floor, the hands came off of the hips, or the non-dominant foot was removed from the dominant standing leg. Participants were provided three attempts and the best time was recorded for analysis.

Lower back and hamstring flexibility was assessed with the sit and reach test. This was administered using a standard preassembled metal 30.48 cm by 53.34 cm box (Lafayette Instrument

Company, Lafayette, IN, USA). Participants sat on the floor with legs extended and shoulder width apart with feet flat against the front side of the box and arms fully extended with one hand over the over on the top edge of the box beginning at the zero point. When prompted, they flexed forward from their waist with legs straight and slowly slid their hands along a ruler positioned on top of the box. Following three attempts, the maximal distance traveled with their hands was recorded.

Hand grip strength using a dynamometer (Lafayette Instruments, Model 78011) was performed in the standing position with 90 degrees of elbow flexion. Participants were allowed three trials using the dominant arm only and the highest value was recorded.

2.8. Cardiometabolic Biomarkers

A 12-h fasted venous blood sample was obtained in an ethylenediamine tetraacetic acid (EDTA)-coated vacutainer tube and centrifuged for 15 min at 4 °C. Plasma leptin, adiponectin, and insulin concentrations were determined using commercially available ELISA kits (Millipore, Billerica, MA, USA and Diagnostic Systems Laboratories, Webster, TX, USA). Total cholesterol (TC), high-density lipoprotein cholesterol (HDL-C), low-density lipoprotein cholesterol (LDL-C), triglycerides (TRG), and blood glucose (GLU) were assessed using the Cholestech LDX blood analysis system (Cholestech, Hayward, CA, USA). Insulin sensitivity was estimated with homeostasis model assessment-estimated (HOMA-IR) as previously described [10].

2.9. Resting Energy Expenditure (REE), Heart Rate, and Blood Pressure

On laboratory testing days (week 0 and 17), resting energy expenditure (REE) was measured via indirect calorimetry using the ventilated hood technique (ParvoMedics; analyzed via True One software) as previously described [4]. Participants arrived at the Human Performance Laboratory immediately upon waking (between 0600 and 0730). Following 20 min of quiet lying, REE was measured for 30 min while subjects lay supine in a darkened, temperature controlled room. Only the last 25 min were used for calculation of the REE. Resting heart rate was recorded with telemetry (Polar Electro) and blood pressure was obtained with a standard mercury sphygmomanometer and stethoscope in the supine position following a minimum of 10 min of quiet resting; all measurements were obtained by the same investigator (PJA).

2.10. Internet-Based Healthy Lifestyle

Participants in both groups were provided a unique login and password to a website containing detailed content on relevant exercise and nutrition lifestyle strategies on a weekly basis. Specifically, each week emphasized a different component of the exercise routines and nutritional intervention they were to follow over the course of the 16 weeks study. This internet-based program served as a complement to the content delivery of the interventions by the investigators. However, all exercise routines were closely monitored and administered by at least two members of the research team. Weekly healthy lifestyle strategies provided through the web-based program included: stress reduction techniques; monitoring exercise intensity; protein-pacing; portion control; nutrient density and quality; meal/menu planning; breathing techniques; nutrient timing; non-exercise activity thermogenesis; healthy carbohydrates; phytonutrients; juicing; healthy fats, sleep quality; and supplementation.

2.11. Statistical Analysis

Statistical analyses were performed using SPSS software (version 21; IBM-SPSS, Armonk, NY, USA). A 2 by 2 factor repeated measures ANOVA (group; WP *vs.* FP X time; pre *vs.* post) was used to determine differences between groups and time points. Post-hoc comparisons were analyzed using Tukey's test. Statistical significance was set at $p < 0.05$ for all analyses; and all values are reported as means $\pm$ SE.

3. Results

3.1. Participants and Compliance

A total of 30 individuals (n = 15 women; n = 15 men) were randomized into the interventions. A total of nine participants were removed from statistical analysis due to either non-compliance (<80% compliance) with whey protein supplementation (WP, n = 3), adverse cardiometabolic event unrelated to the study (FP, n = 3) and/or pre-existing injury (FP, n = 3). As such, twenty one participants (Table 1) completed the 16 week intervention (whey protein, WP, n = 9; food protein, FP, n = 12) and results are shown for all outcome measures.

Table 1. Participant Characteristics.

Variable	WP	FP
Sex (M/F)	4/5	7/5
Age (year)	48 ± 4	52 ± 1
Height (cm)	173 ± 3	172 ± 3
Weight (kg)	96 ± 3	97 ± 5
Body mass index	32 ± 2	33 ± 1

WP: whey protein; FP: food protein. All values are means ± SE.

3.2. Physical Performance Assessments

All physical performance measures improved significantly (p < 0.01) for each group following the RISE exercise protocol. In particular, upper and lower body maximal strength were significantly improved (p < 0.01, Figure 2A,B), with no group differences reported. Likewise, core and upper body muscular endurance were improved (p < 0.01, Figure 2C,D) following the RISE exercise protocol. Balance, flexibility and grip strength were also improved (p < 0.01, Figure 2E–G) with no differences between groups observed.

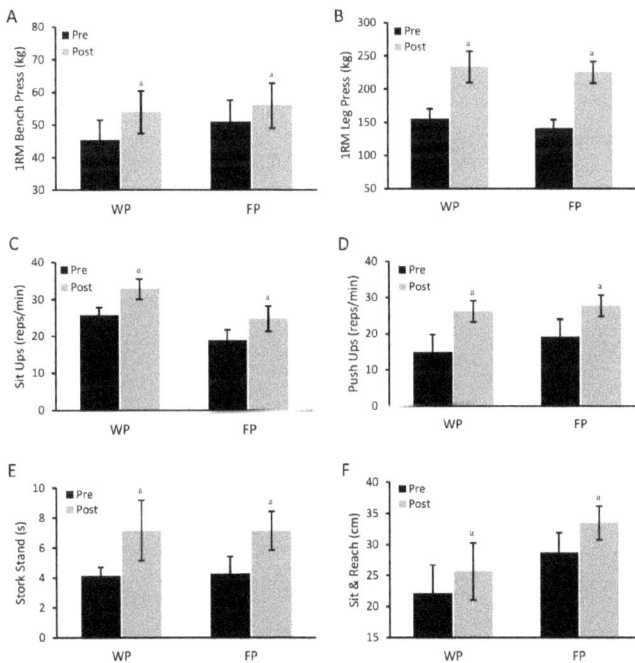

Figure 2. *Cont.*

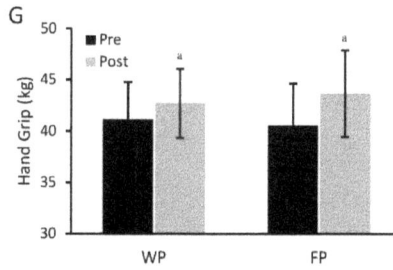

Figure 2. Comparisons of physical performance assessments between the food protein (FP) and the whey protein (WP) groups following the protein-pacing, resistance, interval, stretching, endurance training (PRISE): upper (**A**) and lower body maximal strength (**B**); core (**C**) and upper body muscular endurance (**D**); balance (**E**); flexibility (**F**) and grip strength (**G**). [a] Significantly different from baseline in each group ($p < 0.01$).

3.3. Body Weight and Composition and Resting Energy Expenditure

Significant improvements were observed across all measures of body composition after the 16 week intervention, though no differences were reported between groups (Table 2).

Table 2. Body composition measures at baseline and post-intervention.

Variable	WP			FP		
	Pre	Post	Δ %	Pre	Post	Δ %
Body Mass (kg)	95.8 ± 6.1	90.9 ± 5.5 [a]	−4.8 ± 1.2	96.9 ± 4.8	92.2 ± 4.4 [a]	−4.8 ± 0.9
Waist (cm)	105.2 ± 3.7	94.3 ± 3.0 [a]	−10.1 ± 1.9	104.7 ± 3.1	96.3 ± 3.2 [a]	−7.9 ± 1.3
Fat Mass (kg)	35.8 ± 2.9	31.7 ± 2.6 [a]	−10.9 ± 2.3	38.4 ± 2.8	34.1 ± 2.8 [a]	−11.9 ± 1.8
% Fat Mass	38.8 ± 1.9	36.2 ± 1.8 [a]	−6.8 ± 1.6	41.4 ± 2.4	38.5 ± 2.6 [a]	−7.5 ± 1.2
AbFat Mass (kg)	5.1 ± 0.4	4.2 ± 0.3 [a]	−15.3 ± 4.7	5.5 ± 0.4	4.7 ± 0.4 [a]	−15.9 ± 2.8
VAT (g)	1232.6 ± 219.9	884. 9 ± 173.3 [a]	−29.9 ± 5.6	1816.8 ± 262.2	1498.2 ± 221.9 [a]	−18.1 ± 4.8

Data presented as means ± SE. Pre, baseline; AbFat, abdominal fat; VAT, visceral adipose tissue. [a] Significantly different from baseline ($p < 0.05$).

Of particular interest was the significant improvement ($p < 0.01$) observed in percent lean body mass following the RISE exercise protocol in both groups (WP, 2.7%; FP, 2.9%; Figure 3). Resting energy expenditure (kcal/kg BW) showed a tendency ($p = 0.10$) to decline in both groups (WP; pre 18.9 ± 0.5 *vs.* post 18.1 ± 0.3: FP; pre 18.5 ± 0.7 *vs.* post 17.8 ± 1.0).

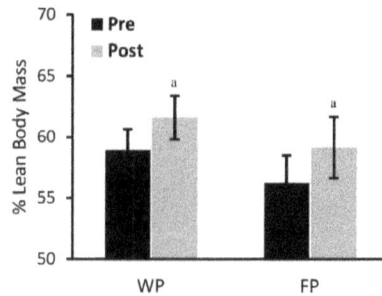

Figure 3. Comparison of percent lean body mass percent (%) lean body mass between the food protein (FP) and the whey protein (WP) groups following the PRISE training. [a] Significantly different from baseline in each group ($p < 0.01$).

3.4. Cardiometabolic Markers

A significant improvement ($p < 0.01$) was seen in systolic blood pressure for each group, while resting heart rate and diastolic blood pressure did not change following the training intervention for either group (Table 3).

Table 3. Cardiometabolic markers at baseline and post-intervention.

Variable	WP		FP	
	Pre	Post	Pre	Post
HR (beats/min)	63.3 ± 4.0	61.1 ± 2.1	64.8 ± 2.8	61.0 ± 2.3
SBP (mmHg)	130.4 ± 5.0	116.0 ± 4.1 [a]	124.3 ± 3.3	119.2 ± 2.9 [a]
DBP (mmHg)	83.6 ± 2.7	80.3 ± 2.3	84.8 ± 2.4	84.0 ± 2.1
TGL (mg/dL)	171.8 ± 29.8	123.2 ± 27.0 [a]	94.2 ± 8.5 [*]	104.4 ± 12.8 [#]
Cholesterol (mg/dL)	192.2 ± 20.0	151.3 ± 10.9 [a]	197.8 ± 8.3	166.3 ± 5.0 [a]
HDL (mg/dL)	42. 6 ± 4.0	46.1 ± 4.6	52.8 ± 4.6 [*]	50.0 ± 4.7 [#]
LDL (mg/dL)	115. 2 ± 20.1	92.0 ± 9.6 [a]	126.2 ±7.8	98.9 ± 5.1 [a]
GLU (mg/dL)	97. 0 ± 4.6	93.6 ± 4.2 [a]	104.0 ± 3.0	94.1 ± 2.0 [a]
Insulin (µg/dL)	21.7 ± 10.5	7.5 ± 2.0 [a]	9.6 ± 2.3 [*]	7.7 ± 2.0 [a]
HOMA-IR (units)	1.0 ± 0.3	1.0 ± 0.3	0.9 ± 0.2	1.2 ± 0.3
LEP (ng/dL)	26.0 ± 4.2	18.7 ± 1.9 [a]	42.4 ± 10.5 [*]	29.8 ± 9.3 [a]
ADI (µg/dL)	18.5 ± 1.5	21.1 ± 1.5 [a]	19.2 ± 1.6	23.5 ± 2.4 [a]

Data presented as means ± SE. Pre, baseline; HR, heart rate; SBP, systolic blood pressure; DBP, diastolic blood pressure; TGL, plasma triglycerides; GLU, fasting plasma glucose; Insulin, fasting plasma insulin; HOMA-IR, homeostasis model assessment-estimated insulin resistance; LEP, leptin; ADI, adiponectin. [a] Significantly different from baseline ($p < 0.05$); [*] significantly different from WP at baseline (<0.05); [#] significantly different from WP post-intervention (<0.05).

A significant improvement was observed in cholesterol, low-density lipoprotein, glucose, insulin, leptin, and adiponectin ($p < 0.01$, Table 3) following the RISE protocol, with no group effect reported. A significant improvement ($p < 0.01$, Table 3) was also reported for triglycerides, and to a significantly greater extent in the WP group (interaction, $p < 0.05$, Table 3). However, the group interaction observed was likely a result of the WP group having significantly higher triglycerides at baseline. The exercise training protocol did not significantly influence high-density lipoprotein or HOMA-IR in either group (Table 3).

3.5. Dietary Intake and Self-Reported Feelings of Hunger, Desire to Eat, and Satiety

All participants met recommended daily intakes at baseline, with no difference between groups (Table 4).

By design, each group significantly increased ($p < 0.01$) protein consumption in absolute (WP, 92 *vs.* 150; FP, 94 *vs.* 140 g/day) and relative amounts (WP, 17% *vs.* 33%; FP, 20% *vs.* 30%: WP, 1.0 *vs.* 1.7; FP, 0.9 *vs.* 1.6 g/kg BW/day). In contrast, carbohydrate intake significantly reduced ($p < 0.05$) in absolute (WP, 253 *vs.* 178; FP, 214 *vs.* 158 g/day) and relative (WP, 48% *vs.* 38%: FP, 43% *vs.* 34%) amounts in both groups. There was no significant change in the intake of fat, fiber, and omega 3 for either group (Table 4). Self-reported feelings of hunger decreased significantly in each group ($p < 0.05$), while feelings of satiety significantly increased ($p < 0.05$, Table 4). Subjective ratings for the desire to eat remained unchanged following the intervention.

Table 4. Dietary intake and hunger ratings at baseline and post-intervention.

Variable	WP		FP	
	Pre	Post	Pre	Post
Kcal	2146 ± 175	1889 ± 148 [a]	2094 ± 194	1833 ± 158 [a]
Protein (g)	92 ± 10	150 ± 14 [a]	94 ± 7	140 ± 8 [a]
Protein (%)	17 ± 2	33 ± 2 [a]	20 ± 1	30 ± 2 [a]
Protein (g/kg)	1.0 ± 0.12	1.7 ± 0.17 [a]	0.9 ± 0.1	1.6 ± 0.2 [a]
Carbohydrates (g)	253 ± 20	178 ± 19 [a]	214 ± 17	158 ± 16 [a]
Carbohydrates (%)	48 ± 2	38 ± 2 [a]	43 ± 2	34 ± 2 [a]
Fat (g)	77 ± 9	62 ± 4	75 ± 9	76 ± 12
Fat (%)	33 ± 2	30 ± 1	33 ± 2	36 ± 3
Fiber (g)	14 ± 1	26 ± 3	22 ± 3	23 ± 4
Omega 3	2 ± 0.5	2 ± 1	1 ± 0.1	2 ± 0.5
Hunger	36 ± 8	31 ± 7 [a]	46 ± 6	30 ± 8 [a]
Satiety	23 ± 7	44 ± 5 [a]	37 ± 6	44 ± 11 [a]
Desire to eat	39 ± 10	38 ± 7	48 ± 6	31 ± 6 [a]

Data presented as means ± SE. Pre, baseline; Post, post-intervention. [a] Significantly different from baseline ($p < 0.05$).

4. Discussion

The primary purpose of the current study was to compare the effects of a protein-pacing diet consisting of either whey protein supplementation (WP; consumed as three of the six daily meals) or food protein from protein-rich food sources (FP; consumed for all six daily meals) combined with RISE training on fitness-related performance outcomes, as well as cardiometabolic and body composition measures. The main findings of this study were that increased dietary protein from either WP or FP combined with RISE exercise training for 16 weeks improved: (1) physical performance outcomes (upper and lower body maximal strength and endurance, flexibility, balance, and handgrip strength) and; (2) body composition (weight, waist circumference, body fat percentage, abdominal fat, visceral fat, and lean mass) and cardiometabolic markers (systolic blood pressure, blood glucose, LDL, total cholesterol, adiponectin) in both groups. Collectively, these results demonstrate, for the first time, increased dietary protein (>30% of total calories; >1.6 g/kg BW/day) from either WP or FP combined with the multimodal RISE protocol improves physical performance outcomes necessary for engaging in an active lifestyle, as well as enhanced cardiometabolic health in obese/overweight adults. Additionally, sources of dietary protein (whey *vs.* whole food) do not appear to be important factors determining such improvements.

4.1. Physical Performance

Diminished physical performance is a common consequence of aging, which may interfere with the ability to perform daily life activities [24]. Such diminution can, however, be reversed with exercise training in combination with increased protein consumption [1]. Despite such knowledge, little is known regarding the effects of lifestyle interventions combined with increased protein consumption on physical performance outcomes. Interestingly, we have recently demonstrated that the combination of the RISE training and whey protein supplementation is more effective in improving body composition and health outcomes than traditional resistance training, although how such improvement may influence physical performance still remains unclear [13].

In the present study, we extended our previous findings by demonstrating that the RISE protocol (16 weeks) combined with varying sources of protein consumption (>1.6 g/kg BW protein/day as five to six meals/day and >0.4 g/kg BW/meal) was effective in improving aspects of physical performance (upper and lower body maximal strength and endurance, flexibility, balance, and handgrip strength) in middle-aged overweight/obese adults (Figure 1). These findings are consistent with current recommendations [22] and previous studies investigating protein consumption and physical performance in healthy adults [20,23,25,26]. Interestingly, we have shown in the present study that whole food protein sources appear to be as effective in improving physical performance as whey protein supplementation, suggesting that increased protein consumption, irrespective of dietary sources, may improve physical performance when combined with exercise training. Our findings suggest that lean whole food protein sources (both animal and plant) are equally effective as whey protein to support body composition and physical performance outcomes in overweight/obese adults engaged with a multi-mode exercise program. Research has consistently shown whey protein's ability to induce rapid absorption kinetics and the ability to stimulate muscle protein synthesis [27–29]. Thus, our finding of similar benefit from consuming lean, whole food protein sources is noteworthy, given the relatively high cost of protein supplementation.

The mechanisms underlying the improved physical performance are likely due to enhanced muscle protein synthesis and reduced protein breakdown [30]. A high plasma concentration of essential amino acids following protein consumption has been shown to work synergistically with the anabolic effect of exercise training (*i.e.*, resistance exercise) to enhance muscle protein synthesis and reduce protein breakdown [30]. In the present study, we utilized the RISE training protocol instead of traditional resistance exercise training based on our previous finding demonstrating its superiority in improving cardiometabolic health compared to traditional resistance training [13]. Collectively, our data suggest that a combination of a high protein diet consumed as five to six meals per day of >0.4 g/kg BW per meal (~32% of total kcals from protein), as either whey protein or lean whole food sources, and the RISE training protocol, are equally effective at improving physical performance outcomes in overweight/obese adults.

4.2. Body Composition

We found similar improvements in body composition, including reductions in weight, waist circumference, body fat percentage, abdominal fat, visceral fat, as well as an increase in percent lean mass (Table 2). It is noteworthy that such improvements occurred regardless of sources of dietary protein, suggesting similar effectiveness of increased protein consumption and exercise training in enhancing body composition. The mechanisms for the increased lean body mass are likely attributable to increased muscle protein synthesis and reduced protein breakdown [30]. In addition, the reduction in total and abdominal fat mass may be induced by enhanced subcutaneous and whole-body lipolysis, resulting in an increase in fat oxidation [31], as well as by enhanced energy expenditure [4].

Our findings are consistent with our previous study [13] that showed reductions in total and abdominal fat mass and an increased lean mass in overweight adults following the RISE training with whey protein supplementation (an addition of 60 g of protein to their daily diet). Most studies document a favorable increase in lean body mass following increased dietary protein (>1.5 g/kg BW/day) combined with exercise training [23], although this is not a universal finding [32]. Such discrepancies may be related to the amount and timing of protein intake. The strength of our study design was the matching of total protein intake in both groups (WP *vs.* FP) and an identical RISE exercise program performed by both groups throughout the 16 week intervention. This allowed us to systematically compare the source of increased dietary protein during exercise training on all outcome measures. Collectively, our findings support protein-pacing (five to six meals of 0.4 g/kg BW of protein) of both whey and food sources combined with multi-mode exercise training (RISE) to improve body composition in middle-aged overweight adults.

4.3. Cardiometabolic Biomarkers

The relationships between obesity, high blood pressure, and dyslipidemia have been well documented [33,34]. Increased adiposity is associated with the release of pro-inflammatory cytokines, leading to vascular wall injuries, arterial stiffening, blood pressure increases, atherosclerosis [35,36], and impaired glucose and fat metabolism [37,38]. Other important factors released from adipocytes are leptin and adiponectin, which play a role in the regulation of insulin sensitivity and body composition [39].

While these factors may be affected by increased levels of adiposity, previous studies have demonstrated that protein supplementation and exercise training may favorably combat obesity-related cardiovascular and metabolic risks [13,19,40]. In the current study, there were similar reductions in systolic blood pressure, total cholesterol, low-density lipoprotein cholesterol, leptin, insulin, and blood glucose concentrations, as well as an increase in adiponectin concentrations in both groups (Table 3). It is important to note that baseline leptin levels were different between groups due to two outliers (100 ng/dL; $>\pm2$ SD of the FP group mean, ±12.4 ng/dL) in the FP group. In fact, omitting these two outliers resulted in similar baseline leptin levels (FP, 23.1 $\pm$ 4.1 *vs.* WP, 26.0 $\pm$ 4.2, ng/dL). The reductions in systolic blood pressure have been attributed to consumption of whey protein and/or isoleucine-tryptophan [41]. The favorable lipid and adipokine changes are likely related to the increased lipolysis following protein supplementation and increased levels of physical activity [28,31].

Although the whey protein group also exhibited a reduction in triglyceride concentration, this was due to the high baseline value compared with the food protein group, whose concentration (mean of 94.2 mg/dL at baseline and 104.4 mg/dL at post-training) was in a healthy range throughout the intervention.

4.4. Satiation and Hunger Ratings, and Dietary Intake

In the present study, both groups exhibited similar improvements in satiation and hunger ratings (Table 4), which corroborates earlier work from our laboratory [42] and others [43] showing increased satiety and reduced hunger with increased protein consumption. It is important to highlight the current study was not caloric-restricted but instead was *ad libitum*. The fact that study participants reported a significant reduction in total calorie intake despite self-reported feelings of increased satiety and decreased hunger at the end of the 16 week intervention provides compelling support to encourage protein-pacing as a public health initiative to combat obesity-related diseases and enhance cardiometabolic and body composition health.

There are several limitations to the current study that are noteworthy and warrant further explanation. First, because previous work documented that the RISE training combined with whey protein supplementation was more effective in improving body composition and cardiometabolic health than whey protein alone or combined with traditional resistance exercise training [13], we did not include a non-protein supplemented RISE group. However, by design, this was intentionally omitted due to the well-known increased protein requirements during exercise training, particularly with obese, sedentary adults embarking on an exercise intervention. Thus, the current design afforded us the greatest degree of scientific rigor and rationale, as well as statistical control. Finally, our results should be interpreted and extrapolated to other ethnicities with caution as our cohort was predominantly white.

5. Conclusions

The current study demonstrates that a high protein diet from WP or from FP (>30% total calories from dietary protein; five to six meals per day (>1.6 g/kg BW/day or 0.4 g/kg BW protein/meal) combined with RISE training are equally effective in improving physical performance outcomes (upper and lower body maximal strength and endurance, flexibility, balance, and handgrip strength), body composition (total and abdominal fat), and cardiometabolic health (systolic blood pressure, blood glucose, LDL, total cholesterol, adiponectin) in middle-aged overweight adults.

Supplementary Materials: The following are available online at http://www.mdpi.com/2072-6643/8/5/288/s1, Table S1: Sample Menus from the FP and WP nutritional intervention diet plans during the 16 week PRISE intervention. Menus were similar in macronutrient distribution, Table S2: RISE exercise training protocol.

Acknowledgments: We are grateful for the assistance of Patricia Bosen NP, Kathy Sikora RN, and Michelle Lapo RN. We are especially thankful for the dedication and hard work of all of our study participants.

Author Contributions: P.J.A. (PI and corresponding author) conceived and designed the study, recruited subjects, performed exercise training, data collection and analysis, and manuscript preparation; R.C.E. assisted in manuscript preparation and data analysis; K.B. assisted with manuscript preparation, study coordination, subject recruitment, exercise training, data collection, and analysis; C.L.G. and M.J.O. assisted in manuscript preparation and data analysis, and C.K., C.D., M.R., Q.Z., J.Z., and J.P. assisted with study coordination, subject recruitment, exercise training, data collection, and analysis.

Conflicts of Interest: Funding was provided by the Skidmore College Student Opportunity Fund Grants to K.B., C.K., C.D., M.R., Q.Z., J.Z. and J.P. All authors have no financial or competing interests regarding the outcomes of this investigation.

Abbreviations

PRISE	protein-pacing, resistance, interval, stretching, endurance training
WP	whey protein
FP	food protein
VAT	visceral adipose tissue
TC	total cholesterol
HDL-C	high density lipoprotein cholesterol
LDL-C	low density lipoprotein cholesterol
TRG	triglycerides
GLU	glucose
REE	resting energy expenditure

References

1. Goisser, S.; Kemmler, W.; Porzel, S.; Volkert, D.; Sieber, C.C.; Bollheimer, L.C.; Freiberger, E. Sarcopenic obesity and complex interventions with nutrition and exercise in community-dwelling older persons—A narrative review. *Clin. Interv. Aging* **2015**, *10*, 1267–1282. [PubMed]

2. Devries, M.C.; Phillips, S.M. Supplemental protein in support of muscle mass and health: Advantage whey. *J. Food Sci.* **2015**, *80* (Suppl. S1), A8–A15. [CrossRef] [PubMed]

3. Martens, E.A.; Westerterp-Plantenga, M.S. Protein diets, body weight loss and weight maintenance. *Curr. Opin. Clin. Nutr. Metab. Care* **2014**, *17*, 75–79. [CrossRef] [PubMed]

4. Arciero, P.J.; Ormsbee, M.J.; Gentile, C.L.; Nindl, B.C.; Brestoff, J.R.; Ruby, M. Increased protein intake and meal frequency reduces abdominal fat during energy balance and energy deficit. *Obesity* **2013**, *21*, 1357–1366. [CrossRef] [PubMed]

5. Ramadas, A.; Quek, K.F.; Chan, C.K.; Oldenburg, B. Web-based interventions for the management of type 2 diabetes mellitus: A systematic review of recent evidence. *Int. J. Med. Inform.* **2011**, *80*, 389–405. [CrossRef] [PubMed]

6. Baker, M.K.; Atlantis, E.; Singh, M.A.F. Multi-modal exercise programs for older adults. *Age Ageing* **2007**, *36*, 375–381. [CrossRef] [PubMed]

7. Marzolini, S.; Oh, P.I.; Brooks, D. Effect of combined aerobic and resistance training *versus* aerobic training alone in individuals with coronary artery disease: A meta-analysis. *Eur. J. Prev. Cardiol.* **2012**, *19*, 81–94. [CrossRef] [PubMed]

8. Lee, J.S.; Kim, C.G.; Seo, T.B.; Kim, H.G.; Yoon, S.J. Effects of 8-week combined training on body composition, isokinetic strength, and cardiovascular disease risk factors in older women. *Aging Clin. Exp. Res.* **2015**, *27*, 179–186. [CrossRef] [PubMed]

9. Sillanpaa, E.; Hakkinen, A.; Nyman, K.; Mattila, M.; Cheng, S.; Karavirta, L.; Laaksonen, D.E.; Huuhka, N.; Kraemer, W.J.; Hakkinen, K. Body composition and fitness during strength and/or endurance training in older men. *Med. Sci. Sports Exerc.* **2008**, *40*, 950–958. [CrossRef] [PubMed]

10. Boutcher, S.H. High-intensity intermittent exercise and fat loss. *J. Obes.* **2011**, *2011*. [CrossRef] [PubMed]

11. Aladro-Gonzalvo, A.R.; Machado-Diaz, M.; Moncada-Jimenez, J.; Hernandez-Elizondo, J.; Araya-Vargas, G. The effect of Pilates exercises on body composition: A systematic review. *J. Bodyw. Mov. Ther.* **2012**, *16*, 109–114. [CrossRef] [PubMed]

12. Telles, S.; Naveen, V.K.; Balkrishna, A.; Kumar, S. Short term health impact of a yoga and diet change program on obesity. *Med. Sci. Monit.* **2010**, *16*, CR35–CR40. [PubMed]

13. Arciero, P.J.; Baur, D.; Connelly, S.; Ormsbee, M.J. Timed-daily ingestion of whey protein and exercise training reduces visceral adipose tissue mass and improves insulin resistance: The PRISE study. *J. Appl. Physiol.* **2014**, *117*, 1–10. [CrossRef] [PubMed]

14. Cermak, N.M.; Res, P.T.; de Groot, L.C.; Saris, W.H.; van Loon, L.J. Protein supplementation augments the adaptive response of skeletal muscle to resistance-type exercise training: A meta-analysis. *Am. J. Clin. Nutr.* **2012**, *96*, 1454–1464. [CrossRef] [PubMed]

15. Pal, S.; Radavelli-Bagatini, S.; Hagger, M.; Ellis, V. Comparative effects of whey and casein proteins on satiety in overweight and obese individuals: A randomized controlled trial. *Eur. J. Clin. Nutr.* **2014**, *68*, 980–986. [CrossRef] [PubMed]

16. Baer, D.J.; Stote, K.S.; Paul, D.R.; Harris, G.K.; Rumpler, W.V.; Clevidence, B.A. Whey protein but not soy protein supplementation alters body weight and composition in free-living overweight and obese adults. *J. Nutr.* **2011**, *141*, 1489–1494. [CrossRef] [PubMed]

17. Joy, J.M.; Lowery, R.P.; Wilson, J.M.; Purpura, M.; de Souza, E.O.; Wilson, S.M.; Kalman, D.S.; Dudeck, J.E.; Jager, R. The effects of 8 weeks of whey or rice protein supplementation on body composition and exercise performance. *Nutr. J.* **2013**, *12*, 86. [CrossRef] [PubMed]

18. Antonio, J.; Peacock, C.A.; Ellerbroek, A.; Fromhoff, B.; Silver, T. The effects of consuming a high protein diet (4.4 g/kg/day) on body composition in resistance-trained individuals. *J. Int. Soc. Sports Nutr.* **2014**, *11*, 19. [CrossRef] [PubMed]

19. Arciero, P.J.; Gentile, C.L.; Pressman, R.; Everett, M.; Ormsbee, M.J.; Martin, J.; Santamore, J.; Gorman, L.; Fehling, P.C.; Vukovich, M.D.; *et al.* Moderate protein intake improves total and regional body composition and insulin sensitivity in overweight adults. *Metabolism* **2008**, *57*, 757–765. [CrossRef] [PubMed]

20. Arciero, P.J.; Gentile, C.L.; Martin-Pressman, R.; Ormsbee, M.J.; Everett, M.; Zwicky, L.; Steele, C.A. Increased dietary protein and combined high intensity aerobic and resistance exercise improves body fat distribution and cardiovascular risk factors. *Int. J. Sport Nutr. Exerc. Metab.* **2006**, *16*, 373–392. [PubMed]

21. Pasiakos, S.M.; Austin, K.G.; Lieberman, H.R.; Askew, E.W. Efficacy and safety of protein supplements for U.S. Armed Forces personnel: Consensus statement. *J. Nutr.* **2013**, *143*, 1811S–1814S. [CrossRef] [PubMed]

22. Phillips, S.M.; Chevalier, S.; Leidy, H.J. Protein "requirements" beyond the RDA: Implications for optimizing health. *Appl. Physiol. Nutr. Metab.* **2016**, *41*, 1–8. [CrossRef] [PubMed]

23. Cribb, P.J.; Williams, A.D.; Carey, M.F.; Hayes, A. The effect of whey isolate and resistance training on strength, body composition, and plasma glutamine. *Int. J. Sport Nutr. Exerc. Metab.* **2006**, *16*, 494–509. [CrossRef] [PubMed]

24. Rolland, Y.; Lauwers-Cances, V.; Cristini, C.; van Kan, G.A.; Janssen, I.; Morley, J.E.; Vellas, B. Difficulties with physical function associated with obesity, sarcopenia, and sarcopenic-obesity in community-dwelling elderly women: The EPIDOS (EPIDemiologie de l'OSteoporose) Study. *Am. J. Clin. Nutr.* **2009**, *89*, 1895–1900. [CrossRef] [PubMed]

25. Hansen, M.; Bangsbo, J.; Jensen, J.; Bibby, B.M.; Madsen, K. Effect of whey protein hydrolysate on performance and recovery of top-class orienteering runners. *Int. J. Sport Nutr. Exerc. Metab.* **2015**, *25*, 97–109. [CrossRef] [PubMed]

26. Phillips, S.M.; Hartman, J.W.; Wilkinson, S.B. Dietary protein to support anabolism with resistance exercise in young men. *J. Am. Coll. Nutr.* **2005**, *24*, 134S–139S. [CrossRef] [PubMed]

27. Mitchell, C.J.; McGregor, R.A.; D'Souza, R.F.; Thorstensen, E.B.; Markworth, J.F.; Fanning, A.C.; Poppitt, S.D.; Cameron-Smith, D. Consumption of milk protein or whey protein results in a similar increase in muscle protein synthesis in middle aged men. *Nutrients* **2015**, *7*, 8685–8699. [CrossRef] [PubMed]

28. Mobley, C.B.; Fox, C.D.; Ferguson, B.S.; Pascoe, C.A.; Healy, J.C.; McAdam, J.S.; Lockwood, C.M.; Roberts, M.D. Effects of protein type and composition on postprandial markers of skeletal muscle anabolism, adipose tissue lipolysis, and hypothalamic gene expression. *J. Int. Soc. Sports Nutr.* **2015**, *12*, 14. [CrossRef] [PubMed]

29. Boirie, Y.; Dangin, M.; Gachon, P.; Vasson, M.P.; Maubois, J.L.; Beaufrere, B. Slow and fast dietary proteins differently modulate postprandial protein accretion. *Proc. Natl. Acad. Sci. USA* **1997**, *94*, 14930–14935. [CrossRef] [PubMed]

30. Morton, R.W.; McGlory, C.; Phillips, S.M. Nutritional interventions to augment resistance training-induced skeletal muscle hypertrophy. *Front. Physiol.* **2015**, *6*, 245. [CrossRef] [PubMed]

31. Ormsbee, M.J.; Choi, M.D.; Medlin, J.K.; Geyer, G.H.; Trantham, L.H.; Dubis, G.S.; Hickner, R.C. Regulation of fat metabolism during resistance exercise in sedentary lean and obese men. *J. Appl. Physiol.* **2009**, *106*, 1529–1537. [CrossRef] [PubMed]
32. Weinheimer, E.M.; Conley, T.B.; Kobza, V.M.; Sands, L.P.; Lim, E.; Janle, E.M.; Campbell, W.W. Whey protein supplementation does not affect exercise training-induced changes in body composition and indices of metabolic syndrome in middle-aged overweight and obese adults. *J. Nutr.* **2012**, *142*, 1532–1539. [CrossRef] [PubMed]
33. Hall, J.E.; do Carmo, J.M.; da Silva, A.A.; Wang, Z.; Hall, M.E. Obesity-induced hypertension: Interaction of neurohumoral and renal mechanisms. *Circ. Res.* **2015**, *116*, 991–1006. [CrossRef] [PubMed]
34. Lavie, C.J.; Milani, R.V.; Ventura, H.O. Obesity and cardiovascular disease: Risk factor, paradox, and impact of weight loss. *J. Am. Coll. Cardiol.* **2009**, *53*, 1925–1932. [CrossRef] [PubMed]
35. Chatterjee, T.K.; Stoll, L.L.; Denning, G.M.; Harrelson, A.; Blomkalns, A.L.; Idelman, G.; Rothenberg, F.G.; Neltner, B.; Romig-Martin, S.A.; Dickson, E.W.; *et al.* Proinflammatory phenotype of perivascular adipocytes: Influence of high-fat feeding. *Circ. Res.* **2009**, *104*, 541–549. [CrossRef] [PubMed]
36. Omar, A.; Chatterjee, T.K.; Tang, Y.; Hui, D.Y.; Weintraub, N.L. Proinflammatory phenotype of perivascular adipocytes. *Arterioscler. Thromb. Vasc. Biol.* **2014**, *34*, 1631–1636. [CrossRef] [PubMed]
37. Abranches, M.V.; Oliveira, F.C.; Conceicao, L.L.; Peluzio, M.D. Obesity and diabetes: The link between adipose tissue dysfunction and glucose homeostasis. *Nutr. Res. Rev.* **2015**, *28*, 121–132. [CrossRef] [PubMed]
38. Berg, A.H.; Combs, T.P.; Du, X.; Brownlee, M.; Scherer, P.E. The adipocyte-secreted protein Acrp30 enhances hepatic insulin action. *Nat. Med.* **2001**, *7*, 947–953. [CrossRef] [PubMed]
39. Upadhyaya, S.; Kadamkode, V.; Mahammed, R.; Doraiswami, C.; Banerjee, G. Adiponectin and IL-6: Mediators of inflammation in progression of healthy to type 2 diabetes in Indian population. *Adipocyte* **2014**, *3*, 39–45. [CrossRef] [PubMed]
40. Ormsbee, M.J.; Rawal, S.R.; Baur, D.A.; Kinsey, A.W.; Elam, M.L.; Spicer, M.T.; Fischer, N.T.; Madzima, T.A.; Thomas, D.D. The effects of a multi-ingredient dietary supplement on body composition, adipokines, blood lipids, and metabolic health in overweight and obese men and women: A randomized controlled trial. *J. Int. Soc. Sports Nutr.* **2014**, *11*, 37. [CrossRef] [PubMed]
41. Martin, M.; Kopaliani, I.; Jannasch, A.; Mund, C.; Todorov, V.; Henle, T.; Deussen, A. Antihypertensive and cardioprotective effects of the dipeptide isoleucine-tryptophan and whey protein hydrolysate. *Acta Physiol.* **2015**, *215*, 167–176. [CrossRef] [PubMed]
42. Gentile, C.L.; Ward, E.; Holst, J.J.; Astrup, A.; Ormsbee, M.J.; Connelly, S.; Arciero, P.J. Resistant starch and protein intake enhances fat oxidation and feelings of fullness in lean and overweight/obese women. *Nutr. J.* **2015**, *14*, 113. [CrossRef] [PubMed]
43. MacKenzie-Shalders, K.L.; Byrne, N.M.; Slater, G.J.; King, N.A. The effect of a whey protein supplement dose on satiety and food intake in resistance training athletes. *Appetite* **2015**, *92*, 178–184. [CrossRef] [PubMed]

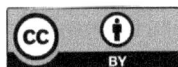

nutrients

MDPI

Article

Protein-Pacing and Multi-Component Exercise Training Improves Physical Performance Outcomes in Exercise-Trained Women: The PRISE 3 Study [†]

Paul J. Arciero [1,*], Stephen J. Ives [1], Chelsea Norton [1], Daniela Escudero [1], Olivia Minicucci [1], Gabe O'Brien [1], Maia Paul [1], Michael J. Ormsbee [2], Vincent Miller [1], Caitlin Sheridan [1] and Feng He [1,3]

[1] Human Nutrition and Metabolism Laboratory, Department of Health and Exercise Sciences, Skidmore College, Saratoga Springs, NY 12866, USA; sives@skidmore.edu (S.J.I.); chelseanorton1@gmail.com (C.N.); descuder@skidmore.edu (D.E.); ominicucci1@gmail.com (O.M.); gobrien@skidmore.edu (G.O.); maiapaul@yahoo.com (M.P.); vin.miller@gmail.com (V.M.); csherida@skidmore.edu (C.S.); fhe@csuchico.edu (F.H.)
[2] Institute of Sports Sciences & Medicine, Department of Nutrition, Food and Exercise Sciences, Florida State University, Tallahassee, FL 32306, USA; mormsbee@fsu.edu
[3] Department of Kinesiology, California State University, Chico, CA 95929, USA
* Correspondence: parciero@skidmore.edu; Tel.: +1-518-580-5366
† This study was registered with ClinicalTrials.gov Identifier: NCT02593656.

Received: 26 April 2016; Accepted: 27 May 2016; Published: 1 June 2016

Abstract: The beneficial cardiometabolic and body composition effects of combined protein-pacing (P; 5–6 meals/day at 2.0 g/kg BW/day) and multi-mode exercise (resistance, interval, stretching, endurance; RISE) training (PRISE) in obese adults has previously been established. The current study examines PRISE on physical performance (endurance, strength and power) outcomes in healthy, physically active women. Thirty exercise-trained women (>4 days exercise/week) were randomized to either PRISE ($n = 15$) or a control (CON, 5–6 meals/day at 1.0 g/kg BW/day; $n = 15$) for 12 weeks. Muscular strength (1-RM bench press, 1-RM BP) endurance (sit-ups, SUs; push-ups, PUs), power (bench throws, BTs), blood pressure (BP), augmentation index, (AIx), and abdominal fat mass were assessed at Weeks 0 (pre) and 13 (post). At baseline, no differences existed between groups. Following the 12-week intervention, PRISE had greater gains ($p < 0.05$) in SUs, PUs (6 ± 7 *vs.* 10 ± 7, 40%; 8 ± 13 *vs.* 14 ± 12, 43% Δreps, respectively), BTs (11 ± 35 *vs.* 44 ± 34, 75% Δwatts), AIx (1 ± 9 *vs.* -5 ± 11, 120%), and DBP (-5 ± 9 *vs.* -11 ± 11, 55% ΔmmHg). These findings suggest that combined protein-pacing (P; 5–6 meals/day at 2.0 g/kg BW/day) diet and multi-component exercise (RISE) training (PRISE) enhances muscular endurance, strength, power, and cardiovascular health in exercise-trained, active women.

Keywords: protein-pacing; exercise-trained women; PRISE; muscular fitness; augmentation index

1. Introduction

There continues to be a heightened interest in healthy lifestyles among women. However, limited data is available on combined nutrition and exercise training interventions that quantify changes in fitness-related outcomes such as muscular strength, power and endurance, aerobic fitness, flexibility, and balance in this population. Recently, we demonstrated that a protein-pacing diet alone (P; 5–6 meals/day at >1.4 g/kg BW protein/day; 20–25 g protein/meal) [1] combined with a multi-mode (RISE; resistance, interval, stretching, endurance) exercise training intervention (PRISE) results in greater reductions in total and regional (abdominal/visceral) fat mass, greater gains in lean mass, and enhanced cardiometabolic health compared to a combined protein-pacing (P) and traditional resistance training intervention in obese/overweight women [2]. Thus, it is of interest to examine the efficacy of the PRISE lifestyle (nutrition/exercise) program in improving physical performance and body composition outcomes in lean, fit women.

Given the paucity of scientific investigations examining fitness/performance outcomes in response to nutrition and exercise interventions in physically active women, the primary aim of the present study was to compare PRISE (5–6 meals/day at 2.0 g/kg BW/day) to normal protein intake and RISE training (CON) on fitness-related performance (strength, power, aerobic fitness, flexibility, balance), body composition, and cardiometabolic outcomes in healthy, exercise-trained women. We hypothesized, given our previous findings in obese adults [2], that PRISE would result in improved fitness-related performance, body composition, and cardiometabolic health outcomes when compared to CON.

2. Materials and Methods

2.1. Participants

A total of 140 women from the Saratoga Springs, NY area, responded to emails, flyers, and local newspapers to advertisements regarding the study. A total of 59 subjects were initially screened, of which 30 were eligible for participation (Figure 1).

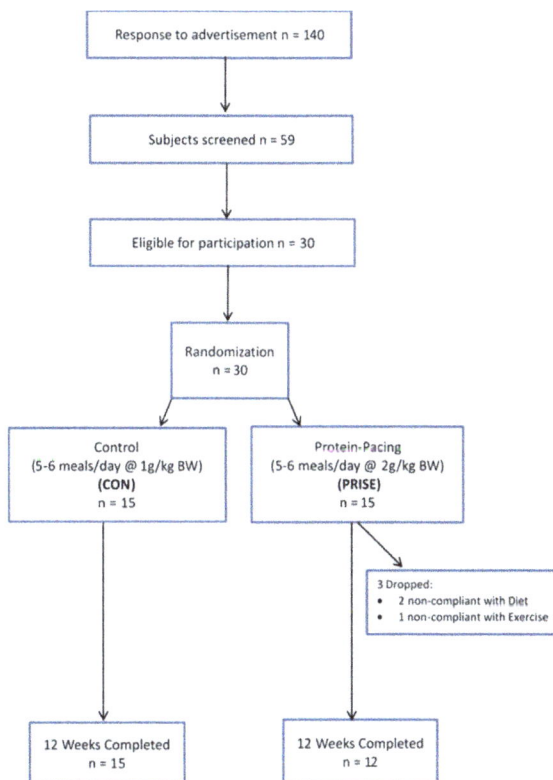

Figure 1. CONSORT flow chart of participants during the intervention.

Participants were nonsmoking, healthy, exercise-trained women with no known cardiovascular, renal, or metabolic diseases as assessed by a medical history and a comprehensive medical examination.

All participants were highly active (minimum of >30 min, 4 day/week of structured physical activity), lean (BMI < 25 kg/m^2; % body fat <30%), middle-aged (25–55 years), and weight stable (± 2 kg) for at least 6 months prior to the beginning of the study assessed through questionnaire. All participants provided informed written consent prior to participation, and the study was approved by the Human Subjects Institutional Review Board of Skidmore College (IRB #: 1401-382). All experimental procedures were performed in accordance with the Federal Wide Assurance and related New York State regulations, which are consistent with the National Commission for the Protection of Human Subjects of Biomedical and Behavioral Research and in agreement with the Helsinki Declaration as revised in 1983. This study was registered with ClinicalTrials.gov Identifier: NCT02593656.

2.2. Experimental Design

Study Timeline

Participants were randomly assigned to one of two groups: (1) protein pacing and multi-mode exercise training (PRISE; *n* = 15; 5–6 meals/day at 2.0 g/kg BW/day) or (2) normal protein and multi-mode exercise training (CON; *n* = 15; 5–6 meals/day at 1.0 g/kg BW/day). This level of protein intake was used ($\leqslant$2.0 g/kg BW per day) because it is regarded as safe and is not associated with any adverse effects on renal function (such as blood urea nitrogen, creatinine, glomerular filtration rate, and creatinine clearance). All participants performed the identical RISE exercise training program consisting of 4 days/week of closely supervised and monitored progressive exercise training for 12 weeks (Table S1). All testing procedures (see below) were administered pre-intervention (Week 0) and post-intervention (Week 13) unless otherwise noted. Upon arrival at the laboratory, anthropometric and body composition measurements and blood sampling for subsequent analysis were performed.

2.3. Nutrition Intervention

Meal plans were identically matched in terms of total kcals, meal frequency and timing, and dietary support. By design, the only difference between the two groups was the amount of protein (1.0 *vs.* 2.0 g/kg BW per day). Additional supplementation (daily multi-vitamin/minerals, and caffeine and electrolytes on workout days) was also provided to participants and differed only by the type of product manufacturer. Participants in both groups were provided detailed meal plans designed by a registered dietitian and instructed to follow the meal plans throughout the 12-week intervention (Table S2). The registered dietitian met with participants weekly for the first two weeks and thereafter on an "as needed" basis. In addition, investigators met with participants a minimum of four days per week to answer questions and reinforce meal plans. To facilitate adherence to the meal plans, food was provided to both groups.

PRISE meal plans included protein-pacing (P; 5–6 meals/day at 2.0 g/kg BW/day) on all days, three of which were whey protein-supplemented (IsaPro®: 150 kcals, 27 g protein, 3 g carbohydrate, 1.5 g fat; IsaLean Pro®: 280 kcals, 36 g protein, 21 g carbohydrate, 6 g fat; and IsaLean Bars®: 210 kcals, 18 g protein, 28 g carbohydrate, 5 g fat—Isagenix LLC, Chandler, AZ, USA). On exercise days, they were supplemented with a caffeine (e+®: 85 mg caffeine, 8 g carbohydrate) and electrolyte beverage (Replenish®: 35 kcals, 9 g carbohydrates, 110 mg sodium, 95 mg potassium—Isagenix LLC, Chandler, AZ, USA), and a multi-vitamin/mineral (Ageless Essentials®—Isagenix LLC, Chandler, AZ, USA) was taken every morning. It is important to note that the protein dosing was equivalent to >0.25 g/kg BW per meal, which has been shown to be the optimal intake for muscle protein synthesis [3]. Recently, it has been shown that women supplementing with whey protein and exercise training have increased lean mass compared to placebo supplements [4,5].

CON participants followed a similar healthy meal plan as PRISE but included a normal protein intake (5–6 meals/day at 1.0 g/kg BW/day on all days), three of which were supplemented (Nature Valley Protein Chewy Bars®: 190 kcals, 10 g protein, 14 g carbohydrate, 12 g fat; Nature Valley Sweet and Salty Nut Granola Bars®: 170, 4 g protein, 20 g carbohydrate, 8 g fat—General Mills, Inc., Minneapolis, MN, USA—and Horizon Organic Milk®: 150 kcals, 8 g protein, 22 g carbohydrate, 2.5 g fat—WhiteWave Foods Company, Inc. Broomfield, CO, USA). On exercise days, they also consumed a caffeine (tea or coffee with sweetener: ~85 mg caffeine, 8 g carbohydrate) and electrolyte beverage (Gatorade G2®: 45 kcals, 12 g carbohydrates, 250 mg sodium, 75 mg potassium—PepsiCo, Purchase, NY, USA) along with a multi-vitamin/mineral (One-A-Day Multivitamins®—Bayer, Whippany, NJ, USA) taken every morning. CON participants were also asked to return empty food packets to monitor compliance. It is important to note, by study design, the only macronutrient that was intentionally different between groups was the protein per kg BW. Participants in both groups were given a 1-week supply of the supplements and asked to return empty packets before they received the next week's supply as a means of assessing their compliance. Both groups were provided equivalent nutritional support and similar caloric intakes throughout the 12-week intervention.

The timing of meals was an important component of the current study, and both groups consumed meals using an identical meal pattern schedule. On resistance (R) and interval (I) exercise days (See below), participants consumed a small snack (~250 kcals) prior and, on stretching (S) and endurance (E) days, arrived fasted but well hydrated and were allowed to consume the electrolyte beverage as needed on all exercise days. Breakfast was consumed after the exercise, and remaining meals were consumed at 3-h intervals throughout the remainder of the day. On non-exercise days, participants consumed breakfast within an hour of waking in the morning and remaining meals at 3-h intervals thereafter (Table S2).

2.4. RISE Exercise Training Protocol

Subjects in both groups underwent the same closely supervised/monitored progressive multiple exercise training regimen as described previously [2]. Briefly, the training program consisted of four specific types of exercise training: (1) resistance exercise; (2) interval sprints; (3) stretching/yoga/Pilates; and (4) endurance exercise (RISE training) (Table S1). Subjects underwent four exercise sessions per week, and the sessions rotated through the four types of exercise such that each of the four exercises was performed 1 day per week. To familiarize participants with the individual exercises and to ensure compliance, all training sessions were performed in the Skidmore College Sports Center under the close supervision of the research team. Intensity level was monitored at every exercise session with heart rate monitors (Polar H7, Polar Electro, Lake Success, NY, USA) to ensure subject safety and proper compliance with the exercise program.

Specific details of the four types of exercises that comprise the RISE training have been previously published [2,6] and are shown in Table S1. Briefly, the resistance (R) training sessions were completed within 60 min and consisted of a dynamic warm-up, footwork and agility, lower and upper body resistance, and core exercises, all performed at a resistance to induce muscular fatigue in 10–15 repetitions and for 2–3 sets. A 30-s recovery was provided between sets, and a 60-s recovery was allowed between different exercises. The sprint interval (I) training sessions were completed within 35 min and consisted of either 7 sets of 30 s "all-out" with a 4-min recovery or 10 sets of 60 s "almost all-out" with 2 min of rest after each interval. Participants were allowed to perform the sprints using any mode of exercise. The stretching (S) routine incorporated traditional yoga poses with additional stretches and Pilates movements, providing a total body stretching, flexibility, and strengthening workout. All sessions were completed within 60 min and were led by a certified yoga instructor. Finally, endurance (E) exercise training was performed for 60 min at a moderate pace (60% of maximal effort). Participants were allowed to choose from a variety of aerobic activities, including running, cycling, rowing, swimming, *etc.*

2.5. Laboratory Testing Procedures

All testing was performed between 0600 and 0900, following a 12-h fast and 48-h abstinence from caffeine and alcohol intake, and 48–72 h after the last exercise session to eliminate the acute effects of the last bout of exercise. These tests were performed at Weeks 0 and 13 and performed by the same investigators for the pre- and post-intervention testing.

2.6. Cardiometabolic Biomarkers

Blood lipids and C-reactive protein: A 12-h fasted venous blood sample (~20 mL) was obtained (Week 0 and Week 13). Blood was collected into EDTA-coated vacutainer tubes and centrifuged (Hettich Rotina 46R5) for 15 min at 2500 rpm at 4 °C. Upon separation, plasma was stored at −70 °C in aliquots until analyzed. Plasma C-reactive protein and insulin concentrations were determined using commercially available ELISA kits (Millipore, Billerica, MA, USA). Total cholesterol (TC), high-density lipoprotein cholesterol (HDL-C), and triglycerides (TRGs) were assessed using the Cholestech LDX blood analysis system (Hayward, CA, USA). The test–retest intraclass correlation (r) and coefficient of variation (CV) in our laboratory with $n = 15$ are as follows: TC and HDL-C (mg/dL); $r = 0.95$, $CV = 3.2\%$; $r = 0.97$, $CV = 5.3\%$, respectively.

Heart rate and blood pressure: Resting heart rate and systolic and diastolic blood pressure (BP) were obtained in the supine position as previously described [2]. Heart rate and BP were obtained following a minimum of 10 min of quiet resting.

Arterial function: Vascular health was assessed using pulse contour analysis (augmentation index) and pulse wave velocity (Arteriograph, version 1.10.0.1, TensioMed Kft., Budapest, Hungary). Augmentation index was determined by the following formula:

$$Aix \ (100\%) = (P_2 - P_1)/PP \times 100$$

where P_1 is the early (direct) wave's amplitude; P_2 is the late (reflected) systolic wave's amplitude; and PP equals the pulse pressure.

The aortic pulse wave velocity (PWVao) was determined by the wave reflection generated from the early direct pulse wave as it is reflected back from the aortic bifurcation. Return time (RT) is determined by measuring the time interval between peaks from the early direct (P_1) and reflected late (P_2) systolic waves. The PWVao calculations were measured using the distance from the upper edge of the pubic bone to the sternal notch (Jugulum-Symphisis $\frac{1}{4}$), as this provides the closest approximation of the actual aortic length. PWVao was calculated with the following formula:

$$PWVao \ (m/s) \ = [Jug - Sy \ (m)]/[(RT/2) \ (s)]$$

where RT is return time; and Jug–Sy is the aortic distance (Jugulum–Symphisis). The test–retest intraclass correlation (r) coefficient of variation (CV) in our laboratory with $n = 10$ are as follows: PWV and RT; $r = 0.94$, $CV = 11.2\%$; $r = 0.90$, $CV = 12.0\%$, respectively.

2.7. Resting Energy Expenditure (REE)

Resting metabolic rate (RMR) was measured (Weeks 0 and 13) using the ventilated hood technique (ParvoMedic; analyzed via True One 2400 software). Specifically, participants arrived at the Human Nutrition and Metabolism Laboratory between 0600 and 0800 with minimal physical movement and fasted for 10–12 h. Following 20 min of relaxed supine lying, REE was measured for 30 min in a darkened, temperature controlled room. The test–retest intraclass correlation (r) and coefficient of variation (CV) in $n = 14$ are as follows: RMR (Kcal/min); $r = 0.92$, 4.2%, respectively.

2.8. Total and Regional Body Composition

Anthropometric and body composition measurements were obtained at Weeks 0 and 13. At each visit, body weight was measured with a standard digital scale (Befour Inc. Cedarburg, WI, USA), height was measured using a stadiometer, and waist circumferences were measured with a standard tape measure placed at the area with the smallest circumference between the rib cage and the iliac crest. As described previously, body composition was assessed by dual energy X-ray absorptiometry (iDXA; Lunar iDXA; GE Healthcare, Madison, WI, USA; analyzed using encore software version 13.6) for total body adiposity, % body fat, lean body mass, visceral adipose tissue (VAT), and regional abdominal adiposity [2]. The test–retest intraclass correlation (r) and coefficient of variation (CV) for body composition analysis using iDXA in our laboratory with $n = 12$ are as follows: LBM and FM; $r = 0.99$, CV = 0.64%; $r = 0.98$, CV = 2.2%, respectively. For regional abdominal body composition analysis, they are as follows: %FAT: $r = 0.99$, CV = 2.4%.

2.9. Dietary Intake and Feelings of Hunger and Satiety

Throughout the intervention, subjects maintained a daily food log that included all food and beverages consumed each day, including meal timing. To further verify compliance, food intake was analyzed from a representative 3-day period at Weeks 0 and 12 using Food Processor SQL Edition (version 10.12.0, 2012; ESHA Research, Salem, OR, USA) [2]. All dietary analyses were performed by the same technician. Visual analog scales (VAS's) were administered at baseline and Week 13 to evaluate the effects of the lifestyle interventions on hunger, satiation, and a desire to eat [2].

2.10. Physical Performance Assessments

Following a familiarization session for all testing procedures, physical performance outcomes were assessed at Weeks 0 and 13 at the same time of day and completed over a 2-day period. For example, aerobic power (5-km TT), muscular endurance (sit-ups/push-ups), flexibility (sit and reach), and balance (standing stork balance) were completed on Day 1, whereas upper and lower body strength (bench press/leg press) and power tests (squat jumps/bench throws) and vertical jumps were completed on Day 2 (See below).

Upper Body Muscular Endurance. Upper body muscular endurance was assessed with timed push-ups in 1 min. Women started in the plank position balancing on the knees with arms extended and hands placed under the shoulders. A successful push-up was defined as lowering the body so that elbows reached 90° followed by a return to the starting plank position. Participants were asked to perform as many push-ups as possible within 60 s in a continuous pattern with no more than two seconds of rest between repetitions.

Core Muscular Endurance. Timed sit-ups were performed in the supine position with arms folded across the chest, knees bent at 90°, and feet flat on the ground and supported by a research team member. A successful sit-up required participants to curl up to a 90° position (vertical) to the floor and then return to the starting position. The sit-up action was continuous, with a rest duration of no more than 2 s allowed between repetitions. Participants were instructed to perform as many sit-ups as possible in 60 s.

Standing Balance. Postural balance was assessed with the stork balance test. While in the standing position, participants were instructed to balance on the dominant leg with the heel lifted off the ground and the non-dominant knee flexed to 90°, with the foot placed gently against the inside of the dominant knee. Hands were placed on the hips at the level of the iliac crests. The trial ended when the heel of the dominant leg touched the floor, the hands came off of the hips, or the non-dominant foot was removed from the dominant standing leg. Participants were provided three attempts and the best time was recorded for analysis.

Flexibility. Lower back and hamstring flexibility were assessed with the sit-and-reach test. This was administered using a standard sit-and-reach box (Lafayette Instrument Company, Lafayette, IN, USA), following a standard technique. The maximal distance reached of 3 trials was recorded.

5-km Cycle Ergometer Time Trial. Subjects arrived to the laboratory for performance testing sessions having consumed a standardized meal (PRISE, IsaLean bar; CON, granola bar) 1 h prior. Before the time trial began, seat and handle bar lengths, height, and tilt were adjusted according to each subject's preferences. Each adjustment was recorded and used for the post-test (Week 13). Following a 5–7 min warm-up at 60% of heart rate reserve (HRR) on the Velotron Dynafit Pro cycle ergometer (Racermate,

CompuTrainer 3D Software, Version 1, Seattle, WA, USA), participants completed a 5-km time trial (5-km TT) as fast as possible. Pedaling cadence and gear ratio were selected freely by the participant during each ride (Weeks 0 and 13). Subjects were permitted to drink water, if needed (*ad libitum*). Total time to complete the time trial and mean and max watts were all recorded. HR and blood pressure were recorded every five minutes during the time trial immediately upon finishing and 5 and 10 min after completion.

Upper and Lower Body Maximal Strength. Measures of one repetition maximal strength (1 RM) of the upper and lower body were assessed via the bench (barbell) and leg press, respectively, as previously described [7]. The test–retest intraclass correlation (r) and coefficient of variation (CV) in $n = 15$ are as follows: chest 1-RM and leg 1-RM; $r = 0.99$, CV = 1.6%; $r = 0.99$, CV = 2.7%, respectively.

Upper and Lower Body Maximal Force and Power. Following 1 RM's of the bench and leg press, dynamic maximal force and power of the upper and lower body were assessed with bench throws (BTs) and jump squats (JS's), respectively, using the Ballistic Measurement System (Innervations Inc., Muncie, IN, USA) interfaced with a commercial smith rack. Prior to performing the tests participants were provided instructions on how to perform the tests safely and with proper techniques. During the familiarization process, subjects performed 3–5 un-weighted practice trials for the BTs and JS's. For the JS's, participants performed three consecutive repetitions with the barbell loaded to 30% of their predetermined IRM for the leg press. Participants began the JS's in the standing position with feet slightly wider than hip width apart and the loaded barbell across the upper trapezius muscles. When instructed, they lowered into the squat position until 90° of knee flexion was achieved, then jumped as high as possible, and landed with bent knees. Immediately upon landing, without pause, participants repeated the same upward jumping movement for a total of three maximal JS's in succession.

For the bench throws (BTs), participants followed identical familiarization procedures as the JS's by performing 3–5 un-weighted practice trials lying supine on a bench with hands positioned on the barbell slightly wider than shoulder width apart and arms fully extended. The bar was then loaded with 20% of the 1 RM of the bench press. To initiate the BTs, subjects lowered the barbell to the chest just above the distal end of the sternum and were instructed to explosively push and then release the barbell with the intent to project the barbell as high as possible. Participants caught the bar on its descent and immediately, without pause, initiated another maximal BT until 3 successive repetitions were completed. Throughout both the JS and BT tests, spotters were present on both sides of the barbell to provide verbal encouragement and ensure safety of the participants. The physical performance variables measured and used for analysis were mean and peak power (watts) taken as an average of the three repetitions.

2.11. Statistical Analysis

Statistical analysis was performed using SPSS software (Ver. 23; IBM). A 2×2 repeated measures ANOVA was performed to assess differences between groups (PRISE *vs.* CON) and time (pre *vs.* post) to determine main effects and interactions. *Post hoc* comparisons (Bonferroni) were performed to determine whether there was an interaction with the addition of between-group independent samples *t*-tests at the pre- and post-time points. One-tailed tests were utilized for this study based on our previous investigation showing improved body composition metrics following PRISE training [2], and the significance was set at $p < 0.05$. All values are reported as means $\pm$ standard deviation unless stated otherwise. Before the start of the study, sample size was determined through power analysis (80%) based on the major outcome variables (muscular strength, body composition, and arterial function). This analysis determined that $n = 12$ was required to detect significant differences between groups. Absolute changes in muscular strength (kg), body weight (kg), and arterial function change were calculated.

3. Results

3.1. Participant Characteristics and Compliance

The participant characteristics are presented in Table 1. Prior to the intervention, all variables in each outcome domain (physical performance, cardiovascular health, body composition, diet, and metabolic profile) were not different between groups. Three participants in the PRISE group were excluded from analysis due to non-compliance to the diet and/or exercise routine, resulting in an 80% adherence rate for both the nutrition and exercise interventions.

Table 1. Baseline subject characteristics ($N = 27$).

	CON ($n = 15$)	PRISE ($n = 12$)
Age (year)	42 ± 7	42 ± 9
Height (cm)	166 ± 6	165 ± 7
Weight (kg)	65 ± 9	65 ± 7
Body Mass Index (kg/m^2)	24 ± 3	24 ± 2
Systolic Blood Pressure (mmHg)	126 ± 11	127 ± 18
Diastolic Blood Pressure (mmHg)	78 ± 8	82 ± 12
Pulse Pressure (mmHg)	48 ± 6	44 ± 6
Heart Rate (beats/min)	59 ± 11	61 ± 7
Total Cholesterol (mg/dL)	184 ± 22	185 ± 37
HDL Cholesterol (mg/dL)	68 ± 17	67 ± 11
LDL Cholesterol (mg/dL)	97 ± 21	107 ± 25
Triglycerides (mg/dL)	88 ± 44	88 ± 43
Glucose (mg/dL)	81 ± 7	81 ± 6

CON: normal protein (5–6 meals/day at 1.0 g/kg BW/day); PRISE: protein-pacing (5–6 meals/day at 2.0 g/kg·BW/day); HDL: High Density Lipoprotein; LDL: Low density lipoprotein. Data are means ± standard deviation.

3.2. Muscular Fitness and Exercise Performance

By design, each of the fitness and performance outcomes was improved following the interventions. Specifically, core (abdominal sit-ups) and upper body muscular endurance (push-ups) were improved (training effect, $p < 0.01$, Figure 2A,D) and to a significantly greater extent in the PRISE group (interaction, $p < 0.01$). Upper and lower body maximal strength, assessed via 1-RM bench press and leg press, respectively, significantly improved ($p < 0.01$, Figure 2B,E), and no group differences were found. Likewise, upper (bench throws) and lower (squat jumps) body muscle power significantly improved as a result of the training ($p < 0.05$, Figure 2C,F), and upper body power increased to a greater extent in the PRISE group (interaction, $p < 0.05$, Figure 2C).

Flexibility, as assessed by the sit-and-reach test, significantly ($p < 0.05$) improved following the intervention (CON: 37 ± 2 *vs.* 40 ± 2; PRISE: 34 ± 2 *vs.* 37 ± 2 cm, pre- *vs.* post-intervention, respectively), though no differences were found between groups. Balance, assessed with the stork stand test, significantly ($p < 0.05$) improved following the intervention, but no differences were found between groups (CON: 6.4 ± 0.8 *vs.* 9.8 ± 2.9 s; PRISE: 3.2 ± 1.0 *vs.* 10.7 ± 3.2 s, pre- *vs.* post-intervention, respectively). Lastly, aerobic power, as assessed by time to complete a 5-km cycling time trial, significantly ($p < 0.05$) improved following the training (CON: 621 ± 11 *vs.* 586 ± 9 s; PRISE: 613 ± 12 *vs.* 592 ± 10 s, pre- *vs.* post-intervention, respectively); however, no differences were found between groups.

3.3. Cardiovascular Health

Both systolic and diastolic blood pressures significantly improved following the exercise intervention ($p < 0.05$, Figure 3A,B), though diastolic blood pressure fell to a greater degree in the PRISE group (interaction, $p < 0.05$). Resting heart rate was unaffected by the exercise intervention or by the protein supplementation ($p > 0.05$, Figure 3C). Augmentation index of both the brachial artery and aorta improved following the training intervention ($p < 0.05$), an effect that was more pronounced in the PRISE group (interaction, $p < 0.01$, Figure 3D,E). Aortic pulse wave velocity and return time were not significantly impacted by the intervention in either group ($p > 0.05$, Figure 3F). The assessment of circulating C-reactive protein was unaffected by the training in either group (CON: 0.47 ± 0.85 *vs.* 0.42 ± 0.57 µg/mL; PRISE: 0.50 ± 1.2 *vs.* 0.72 ± 1.9 µg/mL, pre- *vs.* post-intervention, respectively).

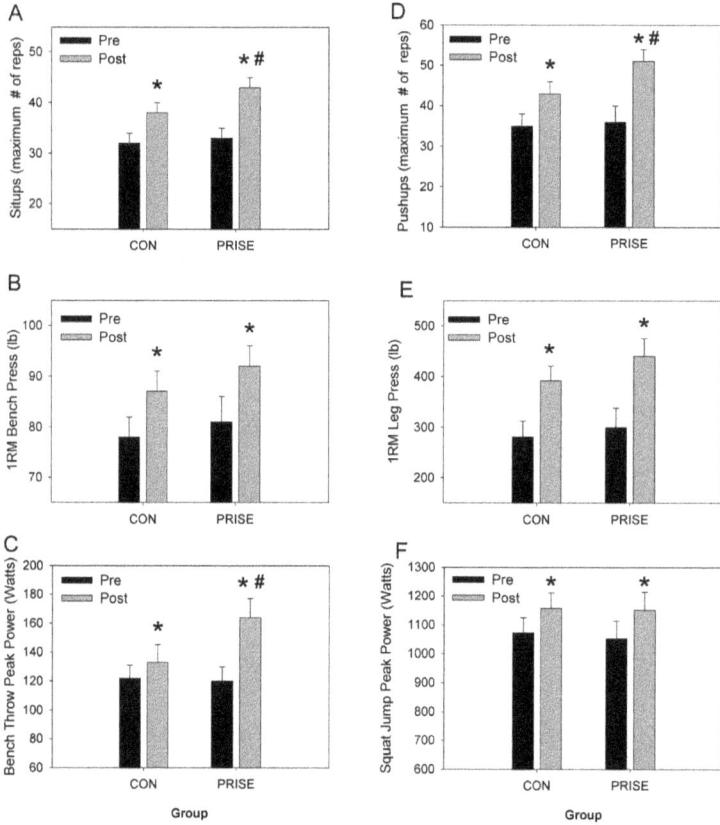

Figure 2. Muscle function parameters at baseline (pre) and after 12 weeks (post) between PRISE and CON. * $p < 0.05$ pre *vs.* post training, # $p < 0.05$ group difference in training response. CON, normal protein; PRISE, protein-pacing. Mean $\pm$ SD.

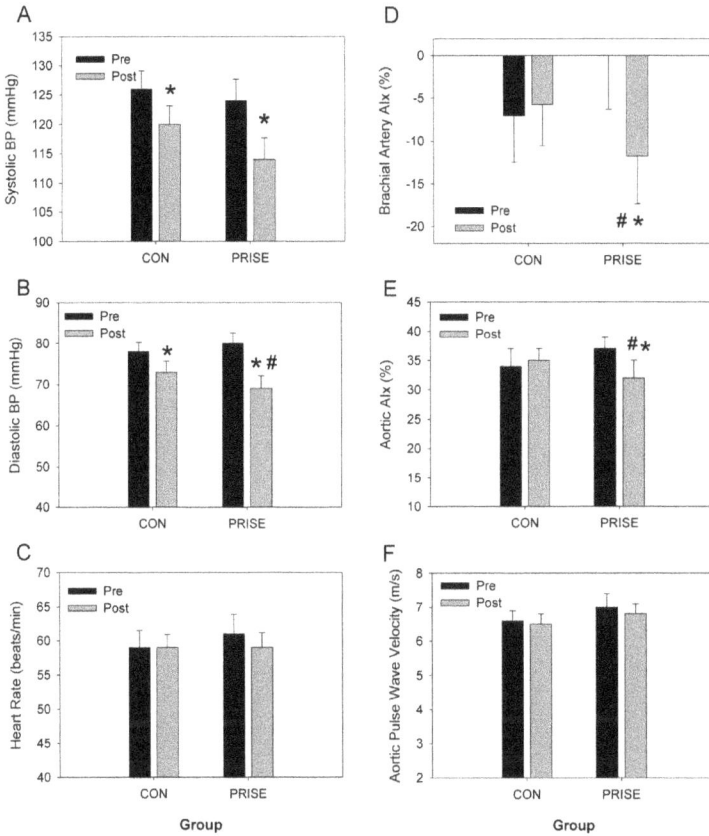

Figure 3. Cardiovascular responses to 12 weeks of PRISE and CON. * $p < 0.05$ pre *vs.* post training, # $p < 0.05$ group difference in training response. CON, normal protein; PRISE, protein-pacing. Mean ± SD.

3.4. Body Composition

Body composition significantly improved in both groups following the training protocol, though no interactions were observed between groups. Independent of changes in body weight, significant improvements were observed in body composition. Of particular note was the significant increase in percent lean body mass and decrease in abdominal and hip fat following the intervention in both groups (Table 2).

Table 2. Changes in body composition pre- and post-intervention.

		Pre	Post
Body Weight (kg)	CON	65.4 ± 9.4	64.8 ± 9.5
	PRISE	64.8 ± 7.3	64.6 ± 7.3
Body Fat (%) *	CON	31.9 ± 6.6	30.9 ± 6.2
	PRISE	30.8 ± 6.1	29.5 ± 7.0
Fat Mass (kg) *	CON	20.3 ± 6.3	19.6 ± 6.1
	PRISE	19.3 ± 5.4	18.6 ± 5.9
Fat Free Mass (kg) *	CON	44.8 ± 5.2	45.2 ± 5.1
	PRISE	45.0 ± 4.1	45.9 ± 4.3
Lean Body Mass (kg) *	CON	42.3 ± 5.0	42.7 ± 4.8
	PRISE	42.6 ± 4.0	43.5 ± 4.2
% Lean Body Mass (%) *	CON	65.2 ± 6.7	66.5 ± 5.9
	PRISE	66.1 ± 5.6	67.7 ± 6.2
Abdominal Fat (%) *	CON	30.8 ± 10.6	29.0 ± 10.0
	PRISE	28.5 ± 9.5	26.7 ± 11.5
Hip Fat (%) *	CON	35.9 ± 5.6	34.7 ± 5.1
	PRISE	35.9 ± 6.4	33.7 ± 7.2

CON: normal protein (5–6 meals/day at 1.0 g/kg BW/day); PRISE: protein-pacing (5–6 meals/day at 2.0 g/kg BW/day). Data are means ± standard deviation. *: denotes significant effect of intervention (pre *vs.* post).

3.5. Diet, Satiety, and Hunger

At baseline, all participants met recommended daily intakes and were not different between groups (Table 3). By design, the PRISE group consumed significantly more protein in absolute (grams) and relative (grams/kg body weight) terms (interaction, $p < 0.05$). The PRISE women experienced a reduction, whereas CON women showed an increase in self-reported VAS question "How much food do you feel like you could eat right now?" (interaction, $p < 0.05$). All other dietary factors remained constant across the intervention and similar between groups (Table 3).

Table 3. Diet, satiety, and hunger ratings pre- and post-intervention.

		Pre	Post
Caloric Intake (kcal/day)	CON	1631 ± 285	1608 ± 282
	PRISE	1662 ± 149	1756 ± 171
Fat Intake (g/day)	CON	58 ± 15	56 ± 20
	PRISE	58 ± 17	53 ± 19
Carbohydrate Intake (g/day)	CON	188 ± 55	193 ± 53
	PRISE	172 ± 63	177 ± 42
Protein Intake (g/day) #	CON	77 ± 12	69 ± 10
	PRISE	75 ± 23	131 ± 16
Protein Intake (g/kg BW/day) #	CON	1.2 ± 0.2	1.1 ± 0.1
	PRISE	1.2 ± 0.4	2.0 ± 0.1
Cholesterol Intake (mg/day) #	CON	212 ± 115	169 ± 99
	PRISE	170 ± 139	286 ± 125
Sodium Intake (mg/day)	CON	1856 ± 920	1993 ± 639
	PRISE	1816 ± 594	1822 ± 620
Fiber Intake (g/day)	CON	21 ± 7	27 ± 11
	PRISE	19 ± 7	23 ± 8
How hungry are you feeling? (0–100)	CON	40 ± 17	45 ± 17
	PRISE	42 ± 22	44 ± 23
How full do you feel? (0–100)	CON	28 ± 18	35 ± 15
	PRISE	24 ± 21	34 ± 23
How much food could you eat? (0–100) #	CON	44 ± 11	54 ± 10
	PRISE	49 ± 20	43 ± 19
What is your desire to eat? (0–100)	CON	42 ± 14	47 ± 17
	PRISE	41 ± 33	43 ± 27

CON: normal protein (5–6 meals/day at 1.0 g/kg BW/day); PRISE: protein-pacing (5–6 meals/day at 2.0 g/kg BW/day). Data are means ± standard deviation. #: denotes significant interaction of group (CON; 1 g/kg of body weight) *vs.* (PRISE; 2 g/kg of body weight).

3.6. Metabolic Profile

The exercise training protocol reduced resting metabolic rate ($p < 0.05$) by ~5%, with no group effect (Table 4). Although fasting blood glucose increased following the intervention in both groups, it remained within normal, healthy levels. Total plasma cholesterol levels declined in both groups ($p = 0.04$), and insulin remained unchanged from baseline (Table 4).

Table 4. Metabolic profile pre- and post-intervention.

		Pre	Post
Resting Metabolic Rate (kcal/day) *	CON	1385 ± 195	1322 ± 147
	PRISE	1453 ± 147	1367 ± 98
Respiratory Exchange Ratio	CON	0.80 ± 0.04	0.80 ± 0.05
	PRISE	0.80 ± 0.05	0.79 ± 0.04
CHOox (%)	CON	34 ± 20	33 ± 17
	PRISE	32 ± 16	30 ± 14
FATox (%)	CON	66 ± 20	67 ± 17
	PRISE	68 ± 16	70 ± 14
Fasting Blood Glucose (mg/dL) *	CON	81 ± 7	83 ± 5
	PRISE	81 ± 6	84 ± 6
Insulin (uU/mL)	CON	2.7 ± 1.2	2.5 ± 0.5
	PRISE	2.5 ± 0.4	2.5 ± 0.4
Total Cholesterol (mg/dL) *	CON	185 ± 22	182 ± 21
	PRISE	185 ± 37	175 ± 27
HDL Cholesterol (mg/dL)	CON	68 ± 17	69 ± 13
	PRISE	67 ± 11	67 ± 12
LDL Cholesterol (mg/dL)	CON	93 ± 21	94 ± 25
	PRISE	107 ± 25	96 ± 27
Total Cholesterol/HDL	CON	2.9 ± 0.9	2.7 ± 0.6
	PRISE	2.6 ± 0.4	2.6 ± 0.3
Triglycerides (mg/dL)	CON	92 ± 40	87 ± 31
	PRISE	88 ± 43	89 ± 28

CON: normal protein (5–6 meals/day at 1.0 g/kg BW/day); PRISE: protein-pacing (5–6 meals/day at 2.0 g/kg BW/day). CHOox: relative contribution of carbohydrate to energy expenditure; FATox: relative contribution of fat to energy expenditure; HDL: High Density Lipoprotein; LDL: Low density lipoprotein. Data are means ± standard deviation. * denotes significant effect of intervention (pre *vs.* post).

4. Discussion

The aim of this study was to determine the effect of a 12-week protein-pacing (P) diet (PRISE, 5–6 meals/day at 2.0 g/kg·BW/day) compared to a normal protein intake (CON, 5–6 meals/day at 1.0 g/kg·BW/day), both of which included a multimodal RISE training program (Resistance, Interval, Stretch and Endurance) on physical performance (muscular fitness; strength, power, flexibility; and aerobic fitness), cardiovascular measures, and body composition in exercise-trained, healthy women. The main findings of the current study are as follows: (1) The RISE protocol elicited significant improvements in performance (5-km TT, upper and lower body maximal strength and power, flexibility, and balance), and some of these improvements were enhanced in the PRISE group (2.0 g/kg/day), specifically abdominal and upper body strength and power; (2) in terms of the effects of RISE training on cardiovascular outcomes (systolic and diastolic blood pressure as well as augmentation index, AIx) and body composition (% fat, fat free mass, fat mass, abdominal fat, and hip fat), all improved with training, and the PRISE group exhibited greater reductions in DBP and Aix; and (3), following the intervention, the PRISE group exhibited an enhanced satiety compared to the CON group (1.0 g/kg· BW/day).

Collectively, these results demonstrate, for the first time, that the multimodal RISE protocol improves all aspects of performance (muscle strength, power, flexibility, balance, and endurance) in active healthy females. In addition, adding a protein-pacing dietary intake pattern (5–6 meals/day at 2.0 g/kg·BW/day) confers additional benefit from training, enhancing the increases in upper body muscle strength and power, abdominal strength, as well as eliciting greater reductions in diastolic blood pressure and augmentation index in active women.

4.1. Fitness and Performance Outcomes

Previously, the multimodal RISE training protocol was used in overweight/obese men and women, targeting improvements in body composition and cardiometabolic risk reductions [2]. Thus, it remained unanswered whether RISE may enhance physical performance outcomes. Research on concurrent strength and endurance training has revealed that either endurance capacity [8] or muscle strength [9] may be compromised due to conflicting physiological mechanisms or perhaps the reallocation of training volume or overtraining. In the current study, there was no apparent blunting of improvements in endurance performance (5-km TT), muscle strength (1 RM), muscle power (jump squat or bench throw), flexibility (sit and reach), balance (stork stand), or muscle endurance (maximum # of push-ups and sit-ups). Thus, we contend that a multimodal training paradigm is not detrimental to fitness-specific performance gains and may actually be complementary for facilitating improvements, possibly promoting the avoidance of injury and symptoms of over training (*i.e.*, burn out).

Ingestion of whey protein or protein supplements is highly prevalent in both the athletic and recreational populations, ranging from 13% to 75% [10–12]. In recreational athletes, Cantarow *et al.* [10] reported that 75% of males consumed protein supplements. While lower than males, 50% of females reported the use of a protein supplement. Thus, understanding the effects of high dietary protein on performance is warranted. Some studies have demonstrated that increasing protein intake above RDA levels can positively influence body composition and/or athletic performance measures. Our data are in agreement with these studies. Despite this, the majority of studies suggest an acute benefit to muscle protein synthesis [13–17] and/or recovery [18,19]. In support of this, our findings are in agreement with those of others showing a training-induced improvement in performance outcomes [4,5,20], and we extend these findings to demonstrate this in recreationally active healthy women. A recent review on the topic reported that protein ingestion of 0.4 g/kg/meal optimally stimulates muscle protein synthesis [3]. Interestingly, our protein intake per meal in the current study was 0.41 g/kg/meal, which may have partly accounted for the significant improvement in physical performance outcomes in PRISE compared to CON. The lack of differences in body composition between groups despite the maximally stimulating dose of protein ingestion per meal in the PRISE group suggests that body composition changes may be delayed compared to muscular performance adaptations to the higher protein per meal ingestion in women. As such, a longer intervention may be required to detect changes in body composition. Work in mice has suggested that ingestion of high dietary protein (whey) increased muscle strength and endurance [21]. Indeed, in humans, supplemental protein ingestion has improved running endurance performance by 4 km over a one-week intensive training camp [20] and may prevent decline during such training [22]. On the contrary, another study found that acute protein ingestion [23] did not improve aerobic performance. However, participants with the lowest level of fitness/performance were found to benefit from the protein ingestion.

In the current study, we found, as expected, that the RISE training improved every aspect of performance (muscle strength, power, balance, flexibility, endurance performance); additionally, protein-pacing resulted in a synergistic effect, further improving upper body and abdominal muscle strength and endurance (maximum # of push-ups and sit-ups, respectively) and upper body muscle power (bench throw) (Figure 2) in previously active women. Most previous studies investigating the potential performance benefits of protein ingestion have almost exclusively focused on men [17,20,22–24]. Thus, the current study is in agreement with previous investigations documenting an increased protein intake and enhanced performance outcomes [5,20]. It remains to be seen if such protein supplementation might extend to other populations, such as highly-trained athletes, and whether greater amounts of dietary protein (2.0–4.0 g/kg· BW/day) are warranted.

4.2. Cardiovascular Health

Previous investigations of training on vascular health have revealed positive responses to either resistance, interval [25], flexibility (e.g., yoga) [26], or endurance exercise training [25], and very few have combined these training modalities [27,28]. Acute ingestion of milk and/or whey proteins alone has been demonstrated to improve vascular health or factors contributing to CVD risk [29–31]. In the current study, we demonstrate that 12 weeks of a mixed modality training program targeting multiple aspects of fitness (muscular endurance, strength and power, flexibility, aerobic power, and balance) resulted in significant reductions in both systolic and diastolic blood pressure. Specifically, on average, the groups reduced both systolic and diastolic blood pressure by ~8 mmHg (Figure 3). Such changes are known to significantly reduce risk of coronary heart disease events and stroke, by approximately 25% and 36%, respectively [32]. It is also important to note that the PRISE group experienced a tendency for a greater reduction in systolic (Δ10 *vs.* Δ6 mmHg, PRISE *vs.* CON) and a significantly greater reduction in diastolic blood pressure (Δ11 *vs.* Δ5 mmHg, PRISE *vs.* CON), which, again, might translate into a meaningful reduction in risk for CV related events. Augmentation index (AIx), but not pulse wave velocity, corroborates the blood pressure findings, indicating a significant reduction with training, which was enhanced in the PRISE group (Figure 3) and likely translates into a reduction in CV risk [33]. Taken together, these findings suggest that the multimodal RISE training improves vascular health, which can be further enhanced with protein-pacing intake.

As exercise paradigms shift and new guidelines are developed, it is important to understand how each fitness component may influence vascular health and the importance of performing more than one type of exercise training (RISE protocol). In light of previous investigations that suggest resistance training elevates vascular stiffness [34], the current study highlights that, using a multimodal training protocol, central pulse wave velocity was not altered, and, in fact, augmentation index was reduced. In combination with the reductions in diastolic blood pressure, this reduction in AIx is suggestive of a training-induced reduction in peripheral resistance, which was enhanced with protein-pacing (PRISE).

4.3. Body Composition

Our previous work in overweight and obese men and women [2] demonstrated that the PRISE protocol elicited a significantly greater improvement in lean body mass, reductions in fat mass, and visceral adipose tissue over a protein-pacing diet with and without a concomitant resistance training program. Here, we demonstrate that the RISE protocol enhances body composition (increases lean body mass, decreases total and abdominal fat mass) in healthy, normal-weight women. The prior investigation compared protein-pacing alone with protein-pacing with resistance training, or with the RISE protocol (PRISE) [2], and showed that, in overweight/obese individuals, PRISE was more efficacious in improving body composition than protein-pacing combined with resistance training, or protein-pacing alone [2]. In the current study, RISE training significantly improved body composition (total and abdominal fat mass, hip fat, and lean body mass) in normal-weight women, regardless of protein intake (Table 2).

While increased protein [35] and/or increased meal frequency [1] alone, or when combined with exercise [3,36], have been shown to improve body composition in normal- and overweight adults, we did not see additional benefit of protein-pacing on body composition in active normal-weight women performing RISE training. However, recent work by Antonio *et al.* [37] indicated that high protein intake in combination with heavy resistance training did elicit additional improvement in body composition, namely, a greater reduction in fat mass and % body fat. However, it is important to note that the definition of high protein in that study [37] was 3.4 g/kg· body weight/day *versus* the 2.0 g/kg· BW/day used in the current study. While the recommended dietary intake for protein is 0.8 g/kg· BW/day, Antonio *et al.* assigned participants to 3.4 g/kg· BW/day and observed no adverse effects on metabolic profile, including markers of kidney function with intakes as high as 4.4 g/kg·BW/day [38]. Thus, it is possible that additional protein intake beyond 2.0 g/kg·BW/day may provide additional body composition benefit over the RISE training alone and warrants further investigation.

4.4. Hunger Ratings and Dietary Intake

In the current study we find that feelings of satiation ("*How much food do you feel you could eat right now?*") were significantly enhanced in the PRISE group but not the CON group following the intervention (Table 3). While the other indicators of satiety or hunger were not significantly different between groups, this finding of improved satiety is supported by previous work from our lab and by others that also suggest increased satiety with increased protein intake [39,40]. By design, macronutrient intake, specifically protein intake, was different between groups and on target for the protein goals of both the control (CON, 1 g/kg·BW/day) and the PRISE (2 g/kg·BW/day) groups (Table 3). All other dietary factors were not different between groups (with the exception of dietary cholesterol intake). Thus, any differences observed between the groups were likely attributed to the PRISE and warrants further investigation.

4.5. Metabolic Profile

Prior investigations of high dietary protein intake suggest that elevated protein intake has the potential to either acutely [30] or chronically improve cardiometabolic profile [31]. Though, it is important to note that the magnitude of protein ingestion (g/kg·BW) as well as the population studied (healthy *vs.* disease) likely play a role in whether PRISE alters metabolic profile and the degree to which it is improved. The current study demonstrated a slightly improved metabolic efficiency (~5% reduction in RMR), which corroborates previous investigations [41]. Additionally, the reduction in total cholesterol supports previous work demonstrating an improved cardiovascular risk profile in response to exercise training [42].

5. Conclusions

The multimodal RISE training protocol improves multiple aspects of performance (core and upper body maximal strength and power, aerobic power, balance, and flexibility), cardiovascular health, and body composition. Furthermore, inclusion of protein-pacing (P, 2.0 g/kg·BW/day) confers additional benefit in core and upper body strength and power, as well as cardiovascular health (DBP and AIx) in active normal-weight women. The results from this study provide compelling evidence that increasing dietary protein intake to more than twice the current RDA may further augment the training-induced adaptations to multimodal exercise training programs with additional cardiovascular benefits.

Supplementary Materials: The following are available online at http://www.mdpi.com/2072-6643/8/6/332/s1.

Acknowledgments: We are grateful for the assistance from Jake Robinson, Kathryn Curran, Kayla Rose, Nathaniel Robinson, J. Matthew McCrary, and Gail Picillo, and TJ Docherty for their excellent training of the participants and Kindy Peaslee RD for her nutritional consulting expertise. We would like to acknowledge the participation of our research volunteers.

Author Contributions: S.J.I. assisted in manuscript preparation and data collection and analysis; C.N. assisted with study coordination, subject recruitment, exercise training, and data collection and analysis; D.E., O.M., G.O., M.P., and C.S. assisted with exercise training and data collection and analysis; F.H. and V.M. assisted in data collection and analysis; P.J.A. (senior corresponding author) assisted in the design of the study, subject recruitment, exercise training, data collection and analysis, manuscript preparation, obtained the grant, and served as the study PI. All authors read and approved the final manuscript.

Conflicts of Interest: This study was funded by Isagenix International, LLC through an unrestricted research grant to Skidmore College and P.J.A. P.J.A. received honoraria for travel to present preliminary data from Isagenix International LLC. All authors have no financial interests regarding the outcomes of this investigation. All other authors declare no conflict of interests.

Abbreviations

The following abbreviations are used in this manuscript:

PRISE	protein-pacing, resistance, interval, stretching, endurance training
CON	control
AIx,	augmentation index
PWV	pulse wave velocity
SUs	sit-ups
PUs,	push-ups
5-km TT	five kilometer time-trial
BT's	bench throws
JS's	jump squats
DBP	diastolic blood pressure
SBP	systolic blood pressure
TC	total cholesterol
HDL-C	high density lipoprotein cholesterol;
LDL-C	low density lipoprotein cholesterol
TRGs	triglycerides
GLU	glucose
REE	resting energy expenditure

References

1. Arciero, P.J.; Ormsbee, M.J.; Gentile, C.L.; Nindl, B.C.; Brestoff, J.R.; Ruby, M. Increased protein intake and meal frequency reduces abdominal fat during energy balance and energy deficit. *Obesity* **2013**, *21*, 1357–1366. [CrossRef] [PubMed]
2. Arciero, P.J.; Baur, D.; Connelly, S.; Ormsbee, M.J. Timed-daily ingestion of whey protein and exercise training reduces visceral adipose tissue mass and improves insulin resistance: The prise study. *J. Appl. Physiol.* **2014**, *117*, 1–10. [CrossRef] [PubMed]
3. Morton, R.W.; McGlory, C.; Phillips, S.M. Nutritional interventions to augment resistance training-induced skeletal muscle hypertrophy. *Front. Physiol.* **2015**, *6*, 245. [CrossRef] [PubMed]
4. Volek, J.S.; Volk, B.M.; Gomez, A.L.; Kunces, L.J.; Kupchak, B.R.; Freidenreich, D.J.; Aristizabal, J.C.; Saenz, C.; Dunn-Lewis, C.; Ballard, K.D.; et al. Whey protein supplementation during resistance training augments lean body mass. *J. Am. Coll. Nutr.* **2013**, *32*, 122–135. [CrossRef] [PubMed]
5. Wilborn, C.D.; Taylor, L.W.; Outlaw, J.; Williams, L.; Campbell, B.; Foster, C.A.; Smith-Ryan, A.; Urbina, S.; Hayward, S. The effects of pre- and post-exercise whey vs. Casein protein consumption on body composition and performance measures in collegiate female athletes. *J. Sports Sci. Med.* **2013**, *12*, 74–79. [CrossRef] [PubMed]
6. Arciero, P.J.; Miller, V.J.; Ward, E. Performance enhancing diets and the prise protocol to optimize athletic performance. *J. Nutr. Metab.* **2015**, *2015*, 715859. [CrossRef] [PubMed]
7. Arciero, P.J.; Gentile, C.L.; Martin-Pressman, R.; Ormsbee, M.J.; Everett, M.; Zwicky, L.; Steele, C.A. Increased dietary protein and combined high intensity aerobic and resistance exercise improves body fat distribution and cardiovascular risk factors. *Int. J. Sport Nutr. Exerc. Metab.* **2006**, *16*, 373–392. [PubMed]
8. Glowacki, S.P.; Martin, S.F.; Maurer, A.; Baek, W.; Green, J.S.; Crouse, S.F. Effects of resistance, endurance, and concurrent exercise on training outcomes in men. *Med. Sci. Sports Exerc.* **2004**, *36*, 2119–2127. [CrossRef] [PubMed]
9. Bell, G.J.; Syrotuik, D.; Martin, T.P.; Burnham, R.; Quinney, H.A. Effect of concurrent strength and endurance training on skeletal muscle properties and hormone concentrations in humans. *Eur. J. Appl. Physiol.* **2000**, *81*, 418–427. [CrossRef] [PubMed]
10. Cantarow, M.E.; Livermore, A.A.; McEntee, K.B.; Brown, L.S. Differences in the use of protein supplements and protein-rich food as seen among us recreational athletes. *Top. Clin. Nutr.* **2015**, *30*, 167–173. [CrossRef]
11. Lieberman, H.R.; Marriott, B.P.; Williams, C.; Judelson, D.A.; Glickman, E.L.; Geiselman, P.J.; Dotson, L.; Mahoney, C.R. Patterns of dietary supplement use among college students. *Clin. Nutr.* **2015**, *34*, 976–985. [CrossRef] [PubMed]

12. Heikkinen, A.; Alaranta, A.; Helenius, I.; Vasankari, T. Dietary supplementation habits and perceptions of supplement use among elite finnish athletes. *Int. J. Sport Nutr. Exerc. Metab.* **2011**, *21*, 271–279. [PubMed]
13. Moore, D.R.; Soeters, P.B. The biological value of protein. *Nestle Nutr. Inst. Workshop Ser.* **2015**, *82*, 39–51. [PubMed]
14. Arentson-Lantz, E.; Clairmont, S.; Paddon-Jones, D.; Tremblay, A.; Elango, R. Protein: A nutrient in focus. *Appl. Physiol. Nutr. Metab.* **2015**, *40*, 755–761. [CrossRef] [PubMed]
15. Churchward-Venne, T.A.; Murphy, C.H.; Longland, T.M.; Phillips, S.M. Role of protein and amino acids in promoting lean mass accretion with resistance exercise and attenuating lean mass loss during energy deficit in humans. *Amino Acids* **2013**, *45*, 231–240. [CrossRef] [PubMed]
16. Phillips, S.M. A brief review of critical processes in exercise-induced muscular hypertrophy. *Sports Med.* **2014**, *44* (Suppl. 1), S71–S77. [CrossRef] [PubMed]
17. Phillips, S.M.; Hartman, J.W.; Wilkinson, S.B. Dietary protein to support anabolism with resistance exercise in young men. *J. Am. Coll. Nutr.* **2005**, *24*, 134s–139s. [CrossRef] [PubMed]
18. Buckley, J.D.; Thomson, R.L.; Coates, A.M.; Howe, P.R.; DeNichilo, M.O.; Rowney, M.K. Supplementation with a whey protein hydrolysate enhances recovery of muscle force-generating capacity following eccentric exercise. *J. Sci. Med. Sport* **2010**, *13*, 178–181. [CrossRef] [PubMed]
19. Cooke, M.B.; Rybalka, E.; Stathis, C.G.; Cribb, P.J.; Hayes, A. Whey protein isolate attenuates strength decline after eccentrically-induced muscle damage in healthy individuals. *J. Int. Soc. Sports Nutr.* **2010**, *7*, 30. [CrossRef] [PubMed]
20. Hansen, M.; Bangsbo, J.; Jensen, J.; Bibby, B.M.; Madsen, K. Effect of whey protein hydrolysate on performance and recovery of top-class orienteering runners. *Int. J. Sport Nutr. Exerc. Metab.* **2015**, *25*, 97–109. [CrossRef] [PubMed]
21. Chen, W.C.; Huang, W.C.; Chiu, C.C.; Chang, Y.K.; Huang, C.C. Whey protein improves exercise performance and biochemical profiles in trained mice. *Med. Sci. Sports Exerc.* **2014**, *46*, 1517–1524. [CrossRef] [PubMed]
22. Witard, O.C.; Jackman, S.R.; Kies, A.K.; Jeukendrup, A.E.; Tipton, K.D. Effect of increased dietary protein on tolerance to intensified training. *Med. Sci. Sports Exerc.* **2011**, *43*, 598–607. [CrossRef] [PubMed]
23. Vegge, G.; Ronnestad, B.R.; Ellefsen, S. Improved cycling performance with ingestion of hydrolyzed marine protein depends on performance level. *J. Int. Soc. Sports Nutr.* **2012**, *9*, 14. [CrossRef] [PubMed]
24. Phillips, S.M. A brief review of higher dietary protein diets in weight loss: A focus on athletes. *Sports Med.* **2014**, *44*, 149–153. [CrossRef] [PubMed]
25. Rakobowchuk, M.; Tanguay, S.; Burgomaster, K.A.; Howarth, K.R.; Gibala, M.J.; MacDonald, M.J. Sprint interval and traditional endurance training induce similar improvements in peripheral arterial stiffness and flow-mediated dilation in healthy humans. *Am. J. Physiol.* **2008**, *295*, R236–R242. [CrossRef] [PubMed]
26. Sivasankaran, S.; Pollard-Quintner, S.; Sachdeva, R.; Pugeda, J.; Hoq, S.M.; Zarich, S.W. The effect of a six-week program of yoga and meditation on brachial artery reactivity: Do psychosocial interventions affect vascular tone? *Clin. Cardiol.* **2006**, *29*, 393–398. [CrossRef] [PubMed]
27. Okamoto, T.; Masuhara, M.; Ikuta, K. Combined aerobic and resistance training and vascular function: Effect of aerobic exercise before and after resistance training. *J. Appl. Physiol.* **2007**, *103*, 1655–1661. [CrossRef] [PubMed]
28. Figueroa, A.; Park, S.Y.; Seo, D.Y.; Sanchez-Gonzalez, M.A.; Baek, Y.H. Combined resistance and endurance exercise training improves arterial stiffness, blood pressure, and muscle strength in postmenopausal women. *Menopause* **2011**, *18*, 980–984. [CrossRef] [PubMed]
29. Fekete, A.A.; Givens, D.I.; Lovegrove, J.A. The impact of milk proteins and peptides on blood pressure and vascular function: A review of evidence from human intervention studies. *Nutr. Res. Rev.* **2013**, *26*, 177–190. [CrossRef] [PubMed]
30. Ballard, K.D.; Kupchak, B.R.; Volk, B.M.; Mah, E.; Shkreta, A.; Liptak, C.; Ptolemy, A.S.; Kellogg, M.S.; Bruno, R.S.; Seip, R.L.; *et al.* Acute effects of ingestion of a novel whey-derived extract on vascular endothelial function in overweight, middle-aged men and women. *Br. J. Nutr.* **2013**, *109*, 882–893. [CrossRef] [PubMed]
31. Clifton, P.M.; Bastiaans, K.; Keogh, J.B. High protein diets decrease total and abdominal fat and improve cvd risk profile in overweight and obese men and women with elevated triacylglycerol. *Nutr. Metab. Cardiovasc. Dis. NMCD* **2009**, *19*, 548–554. [CrossRef] [PubMed]

32. Law, M.R.; Morris, J.K.; Wald, N.J. Use of blood pressure lowering drugs in the prevention of cardiovascular disease: Meta-analysis of 147 randomised trials in the context of expectations from prospective epidemiological studies. *BMJ* **2009**, *338*, b1665. [CrossRef] [PubMed]

33. Weber, T.; Auer, J.; O'Rourke, M.F.; Kvas, E.; Lassnig, E.; Berent, R.; Eber, B. Arterial stiffness, wave reflections, and the risk of coronary artery disease. *Circulation* **2004**, *109*, 184–189. [CrossRef] [PubMed]

34. Miyachi, M. Effects of resistance training on arterial stiffness: A meta-analysis. *Br. J. Sports Med.* **2013**, *47*, 393–396. [CrossRef] [PubMed]

35. Arciero, P.J.; Gentile, C.L.; Pressman, R.; Everett, M.; Ormsbee, M.J.; Martin, J.; Santamore, J.; Gorman, L.; Fehling, P.C.; Vukovich, M.D.; *et al.* Moderate protein intake improves total and regional body composition and insulin sensitivity in overweight adults. *Metabolism* **2008**, *57*, 757–765. [CrossRef] [PubMed]

36. Campbell, W.W.; Kim, J.E.; Amankwaah, A.F.; Gordon, S.L.; Weinheimer-Haus, E.M. Higher total protein intake and change in total protein intake affect body composition but not metabolic syndrome indexes in middle-aged overweight and obese adults who perform resistance and aerobic exercise for 36 weeks. *J. Nutr.* **2015**, *145*, 2076–2083. [CrossRef] [PubMed]

37. Antonio, J.; Ellerbroek, A.; Silver, T.; Orris, S.; Scheiner, M.; Gonzalez, A.; Peacock, C.A. A high protein diet (3.4 g/kg/day) combined with a heavy resistance training program improves body composition in healthy trained men and women—A follow-up investigation. *J. Int. Soc. Sports Nutr.* **2015**, *12*, 39. [CrossRef] [PubMed]

38. Antonio, J.; Peacock, C.A.; Ellerbroek, A.; Fromhoff, B.; Silver, T. The effects of consuming a high protein diet (4.4 g/kg/day) on body composition in resistance-trained individuals. *J. Int. Soc. Sports Nutr.* **2014**, *11*, 19. [CrossRef] [PubMed]

39. MacKenzie-Shalders, K.L.; Byrne, N.M.; Slater, G.J.; King, N.A. The effect of a whey protein supplement dose on satiety and food intake in resistance training athletes. *Appetite* **2015**, *92*, 178–184. [CrossRef] [PubMed]

40. Gentile, C.L.; Ward, E.; Holst, J.J.; Astrup, A.; Ormsbee, M.J.; Connelly, S.; Arciero, P.J. Resistant starch and protein intake enhances fat oxidation and feelings of fullness in lean and overweight/obese women. *Nutr. J.* **2015**, *14*, 1–10. [CrossRef] [PubMed]

41. Henderson, G.C. Sexual dimorphism in the effects of exercise on metabolism of lipids to support resting metabolism. *Front. Endocrinol.* **2014**, *5*, 162.

42. Rossi, F.E.; Fortaleza, A.C.; Neves, L.M.; Buonani, C.; Picolo, M.R.; Diniz, T.A.; Kalva-Filho, C.A.; Papoti, M.; Lira, F.S.; Freitas Junior, I.F. Combined training (aerobic plus strength) potentiates a reduction in body fat but demonstrates no difference on the lipid profile in postmenopausal women when compared to aerobic training with a similar training load. *J. Strength Cond. Res.* **2015**. [CrossRef] [PubMed]

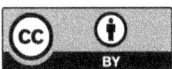

nutrients

MDPI

Brief Report

Effects of Beer, Non-Alcoholic Beer and Water Consumption before Exercise on Fluid and Electrolyte Homeostasis in Athletes

Mauricio Castro-Sepulveda [1,*]**, Neil Johannsen** [2,3]**, Sebastián Astudillo** [4]**, Carlos Jorquera** [5]**, Cristian Álvarez** [6]**, Hermann Zbinden-Foncea** [1] **and Rodrigo Ramírez-Campillo** [7]

[1] Exercise Science Laboratory, Faculty of Medicine, Universidad Finis Terrae, Av. Pedro de Valdivia 1509, Providencia, Santiago 7500000, Chile; hzbinden@uft.cl
[2] Department of Preventive Medicine, Pennington Biomedical Research Center, Baton Rouge, LA 70808, USA; neil.johannsen@pbrc.edu
[3] School of Kinesiology, Louisiana State University, Baton Rouge, LA 70803, USA
[4] Family Health Center, El Peral s/n Sector La Pirca, Panquehue 2210000, Chile; bote_seba15@hotmail.com
[5] Nutrition and Exercise Laboratory, Faculty of Medicine, Universidad Mayor, Santiago 8320000, Chile; cjorquera6@hotmail.com
[6] Family Health Center, Los Lagos 5170000, Chile; profecristian.alvarez@gmail.com
[7] Department of Physical Activity Sciences, Universidad de Los Lagos, Osorno 5290000, Chile; r.ramirez@ulagos.cl
* Correspondence: m.castro.med@gmail.com; Tel.: +56-2-2420-7100

Received: 11 April 2016; Accepted: 31 May 2016; Published: 7 June 2016

Abstract: Fluid and electrolyte status have a significant impact on physical performance and health. Pre-exercise recommendations cite the possibility of consuming beverages with high amounts of sodium. In this sense, non-alcoholic beer can be considered an effective pre-exercise hydration beverage. This double-blind, randomized study aimed to compare the effect of beer, non-alcoholic beer and water consumption before exercise on fluid and electrolyte homeostasis. Seven male soccer players performed 45 min of treadmill running at 65% of the maximal heart rate, 45 min after ingesting 0.7 L of water (W), beer (AB) or non-alcoholic beer (NAB). Body mass, plasma Na^+ and K^+ concentrations and urine specific gravity (USG) were assessed before fluid consumption and after exercise. After exercise, body mass decreased ($p < 0.05$) in W (-1.1%), AB (-1.0%) and NAB (-1.0%). In the last minutes of exercise, plasma Na^+ was reduced ($p < 0.05$) in W (-3.9%) and AB (-3.7%), plasma K^+ was increased ($p < 0.05$) in AB (8.5%), and USG was reduced in W (-0.9%) and NAB (-1.0%). Collectively, these results suggest that non-alcoholic beer before exercise could help maintain electrolyte homeostasis during exercise. Alcoholic beer intake reduced plasma Na^+ and increased plasma K^+ during exercise, which may negatively affect health and physical performance, and finally, the consumption of water before exercise could induce decreases of Na^+ in plasma during exercise.

Keywords: hydration before-exercise; fluid balance during-exercise; blood electrolytes

---

1. Introduction

Fluid and electrolyte status have a significant impact on physiological homeostasis and may impact physical performance [1,2], cognitive performance [3] and overall health [4,5]. Physical performance decrements have been observed with less than 2% loss of body mass. Fluid loss during exercise or sport competitions can be as high as 5 L per hour [6], with heterogeneous sodium (Na^+) and potassium (K^+) losses in sweat that can affect plasma osmolality, health and performance [7].

In spite of current recommendations for improving fluid and electrolyte status in sports, hydration strategies of athletes are far from optimal [8,9] with hypohydration and dehydration being common.

Recent research has demonstrated a high proportion of soccer players become hypohydrated during practice and competition [10–12], where hydration status is particularly important. Small changes in hydration status in these athletes have been shown to increase the perception of fatigue [13], reduce performance in sport-specific tasks and alter cognitive performance [14]. In addition, soccer matches may last up to 120 min, under conditions of high temperature and humidity in certain geographical regions [15] increasing the probabilities of reaching a dehydration state. Although hydration strategies during and after exercise are fundamental, hydration before the onset of exercise or sport could be an equally important strategy for maintaining optimal performance and physiologic function during exercise and competition [16]. Specifically, pre-exercise recommendations cite the possibility of consuming foods and beverages with high amounts of sodium to reduce the amount of fluid loss and improve fluid balance [6,17]. In this sense, sport drinks are a common option due to their considerable sodium content (e.g., 300–400 mg/L). However, another beverage that has considerable sodium content (80–100 mg/L), though less than sports drinks, but with higher preference among athletes [18] and relatively reduced economic cost, is beer. Previously, light beer (2.3% alcohol) was shown to improve hydration status after exercise [19]. Nowadays, there is a commercial explosion in non-alcoholic beers, which claim to have a similar nutrient composition without the negative effects of alcohol consumption. These negative effects are associated with a delay of muscle recovery, given the diuretic effect that leads to a known and well-recognized electrolyte imbalance making non-alcoholic beer a potentially attractive rehydration drink [20].

The aim of this study was to compare the acute effects of consuming 0.7 L of beer (4.6% alcohol), non-alcoholic beer (0% alcohol) or water, 45 min prior to exercise at 65% of the maximal heart rate (HRmax) on urine volume, sweat rate, evaporative water loss, plasma electrolytes (Na^+ and K^+), and USG in young athletes. We hypothesized that, compared to alcoholic beer or water, non-alcoholic beer would be more effective at maintaining fluid homeostasis.

2. Materials and Methods

2.1. Participants

Seven soccer players (19.1 ± 0.4 years) were recruited from two different professional soccer teams with similar training and competitive schedules (four training sessions and one competitive game per week). Subject descriptive characteristics are provided in Table 1. All subjects were over 18 years of age (*i.e.*, above the legal age for drinking in Chile, where the study was conducted). Subjects fulfilled the following inclusion criteria: (1) a background of more than six years of consecutive soccer training and competition experience; (2) continuous soccer training in the last two years; (3) low daily consumption of beer (*i.e.*, <1 L per week). All subjects were carefully informed about the experimental procedures and the possible risks and benefits associated with participation in the study and signed an informed consent document before any of the tests were performed. The study was conducted in accordance with the Declaration of Helsinki and was approved by the ethics committee of the responsible department in Chile. The sample size was computed according to the changes observed (*i.e.*, previous study) in peak urine specific gravity (d = 0.01 g/mL; SD = 0.005) in a group of soccer players submitted to the same exercise and non-alcoholic beer protocol applied in this study. A statistical power analysis revealed that a total of four participants per group would yield a power of 90% and α = 0.01.

Table 1. Baseline descriptive characteristics of athletes.

Characteristics	$n = 7$
Age (years)	19.1 ± 0.4
Height (cm)	173 ± 11.4
Body mass index (kg/m^2)	22.7 ± 1.3
Soccer experience (years)	7.0 ± 1.3
VO$_{2max}$ (mL/kg/min)	62.5 ± 2.1

All the data is presented as means $\pm$ SD.

2.2. Experimental Protocol

Athletes participated in three trials completed in a randomized order and separated by at least one week. Training and competition was kept relatively constant during this period. Three-day diet (food) and physical activity diaries were kept and replicated before each trial. Considering that under "real" training and competition settings, soccer players might be under a non-optimal hydration status [11,12], to achieve better ecological validity, no hydration recommendations were made before trials. Trials consisted of ingesting 0.7 L (about 1% of body mass) of commercially available bottled water (W—Vital®, Chanqueahue, Chile), beer (AB; 4.6% of alcohol—Cristal®, Santiago, Chile) or non-alcoholic beer (NAB; 0% of alcohol—Cristal®, Santiago, Chile) 45 min before exercise (see drinks characteristic in Table 2).

Table 2. Nutritional characteristics of drinks *.

Characteristics	Water	Beer	Non-Alcoholic Beer
Energy (Kcal)	0	153	110
Carbohydrates (g)	0	12.64	26
Fat (g)	0	0	0.3
Protein (g)	0	1.64	0.89
Na (mg)	0.06	14	32
K (mg)	0.03	96	104
Alcohol (%)	0	4.6	0
Osmolality (mOsmol/kg)	0	997	323

* Values expressed per 350 mL.

During AB, subjects consumed 0.48 ± 0.06 g of alcohol per kilogram of body weight. All beverages were provided at ~10 °C. AB and NAB were delivered in a double-blind manner. The beverages were coded; thus, neither the investigators nor the participants were aware of the contents until completion of the analyses. The beverages were provided by a staff member of our research laboratory who did not have any participation in the data acquisition, analyses, and interpretation. Regarding the efficacy of blinding, at the end of the study participants were questioned about the beverage ingested and the percentage of correct answers was compared between three drinks, with similar results between groups. Upon arrival to the laboratory, each subject's body mass and height were measured using a mechanical scale with stadiometer (SECA, model M20812, Hamburg, Germany). Urine was analyzed for USG using a portable refractometer (Robinair, model Spx, Michigan, USA). USG was classified by previously described values [16] as an indicator of hydration status. A Teflon indwelling catheter was placed into an antecubital vein and blood samples (4 mL) were taken before (in the standing position) and during the last minute of exercise (*i.e.*, 45-min). Blood samples were placed in lithium heparin collection tubes and centrifuged at 300 g for 10 min (Gelec, model G-20 digital, Buenos Aires, Argentina). The resultant plasma samples were analyzed for sodium and potassium using ion-selective probes (IC, Wiener lab, Rosario, Argentina). The normal ranges of plasma sodium and potassium are 140–148 and 3.60–5.20 mmol/L, respectively [21]. Body mass, USG, and plasma Na$^+$ and K$^+$ were measured before fluid consumption. Na$^+$ and K$^+$ measurements were repeated in the last minute of exercise (*i.e.*, 45-min), whereas body mass and USG were repeated within 5 min after cessation of exercise. Subjects urinated in a glass graduated cylinder to quantify the urine volume produced during exercise and to determine total urinary fluid losses. Urine was collected at two time points, immediately before the 0.7 L drinks and within 5 min after exercise.

Evaporative water loss and sweat rate were calculated according to the following formulas (for practical purposes, 1 mg was considered equivalent to 1 mL):

$$\text{Evaporative water loss (mL)} = \text{body mass change between pre-post 45 min of aerobic running at 65\% of maximal heart rate (mg)} - \text{volume of collected after running (mL)} \tag{1}$$

$$\text{Sweat rate (L/h)} = \text{evaporative water loss (L)} - \text{experimental trial duration (\textit{i.e.}, 1.5 h)} \tag{2}$$

2.3. Exercise

Steady-state exercise was performed at 65% of HRmax (134 ± 7 bpm) on a motorized treadmill (Oxford SIX BE6546, Santiago, Chile), for a period of 45 min. Room conditions were 26 °C and relative humidity of 36%. Heart rate was checked every 5 min using a heart rate monitor (Polar, RS 800, Kempele, Finland). No fluids were provided during the exercise protocol. To facilitate the blood withdrawl in the last minute of exercise, subjects placed their hands on the handles of the treadmill.

2.4. Statistical Analyses

All values are reported as mean $\pm$ standard deviation (SD). Relative changes (%) for dependent variables and effect size (ES—changes as a fraction or multiple of baseline SD) are expressed with 90% confidence limits (CL). Normality and homoscedasticity assumptions for all data were checked with Shapiro-Wilk and Levene tests, respectively. A two-way repeated measures analysis of variance (ANOVA) with repeated measurements (three treatments $\times$ two time points) was applied. In addition, a one-way repeated measures ANOVA was used to compare relative changes between trial conditions and for urine volumes, sweat rate and evaporative water loss. When a significant F value was achieved across time or between experimental conditions, Tukey's *post hoc* procedures were performed to locate the pairwise differences between the means. The α level was set at $p < 0.05$ for statistical significance. All statistical calculations were performed using STATISTICA statistical package (Version 8.0; StatSoft Inc., Tulsa, OK, USA). In addition to this null hypothesis testing, data were also assessed using an approach based on the magnitudes of ES. Threshold values for assessing magnitudes of ES were 0.20, 0.60, 1.2, and 2.0 for small, moderate, large, and very large, respectively [22]. We obtained high intra-class correlation coefficients for the performance measurements, varying between 0.86 and 0.98.

3. Results

Baseline body mass (mean of all trials) was 68.8 ± 6.2 kg, without significant differences between trials ($p = 0.97$ to 0.99). After exercise, all trials showed a significant ($p < 0.01$) body mass reduction, although no significant differences were observed between trials regarding relative changes (%) or after-exercise absolute values (Table 3).

Table 3. Effects (with 90% confidence limits) of water (W), alcoholic beer (AB) or non-alcoholic beer (NAB) intake on body mass and hydroelectrolitic status after 45 min of running at 65% of maximal heart rate.

Variables/group	Baseline	Change (%)	Effect Size
Body mass (kg) [a]			
W	68.4 (5.4)	−1.1 (−1.6, −0.6) [†]	−0.08 (−0.09, −0.01)
AB	68.8 (6.8)	−1.0 (−1.2, −0.8) [†]	−0.08 (−0.10, −0.06)
NAB	68.9 (7.5)	−1.0 (−1.7, −0.3) [†]	−0.07 (−0.13, −0.02)
Plasma Na⁺ (mmol/L)			
W	145 (3.0)	−3.9 (−5.0, −2.8) [†]	−1.91 (−2.46, −1.37) ***
AB	144 (2.0)	−3.7 (−4.9, −2.5) [†]	−2.23 (−2.97, −1.49) ****
NAB	142 (3.3)	−1.2 (−2.9, 0.6)	−0.48 (−1.24, 0.27) *
Plasma K⁺ (mmol/L)			
W	4.1 (0.4)	7.8 (4.2, 11.4)	0.74 (0.41, 1.07) **
AB	4.5 (0.5)	8.5 (3.1, 14.1) [‡]	0.64 (0.24, 1.04) **
NAB	4.4 (0.6)	7.3 (1.0, 14.1)	0.57 (0.08, 1.07) *
Urine specific gravity (g/mL)			
W	1.024 (0.006)	−0.9 (−1.4, −0.4) [‡]	−1.50 (−2.28, −0.72) ***
AB	1.023 (0.007)	−0.6 (−1.2, 0.1)	−0.69 (−1.49, 0.12) **
NAB	1.023 (0.005)	−1.0 (−1.5, −0.4) [‡]	−1.38 (−2.17, −0.59) ***

[a] Denotes that baseline body mass represents values before fluid intake and the change is in relation with values after exercise; *, **, ***, **** denote small, moderate, large and very large effect size, respectively; [‡] denotes significant difference from before to after exercise ($p < 0.05$); [†] denotes significant difference from before to after exercise ($p < 0.01$). Baseline data is presented as means (±SD).

Baseline USG (mean of all trials) was 1.025 ± 6.1 g/mL, without significant differences between trials ($p = 0.21$ to 0.95). During trials only two participants showed a basal USG <1.020 g/mL. A significant ($p < 0.05$) time effect was noted for USG, with W and NAB showing a reduction after exercise, although no time group × time interaction was observed. No significant differences were observed between trials regarding relative changes (%) or after-exercise absolute values (Table 3). Baseline plasma Na⁺ and K⁺ (mean of all trials) were 143 ± 2.9 mmol/L and 4.3 ± 0.5 mmol/L, respectively, without significant (Na⁺, $p = 0.3$ to 0.93; K⁺, $p = 0.5$ to 0.97) differences between trials. W and AB trials showed a significant decrease in plasma Na⁺ ($p < 0.01$) in the last minute (*i.e.*, 45-min) of exercise (Table 3), although no group × time interaction was noted. Plasma K⁺ showed a significant ($p < 0.05$) increase in the last minute of exercise only with the AB trial, with no group × time interaction (Table 3). In the last minute of exercise, no significant differences were observed between trials for plasma Na⁺ or K⁺ regarding relative changes (%) or absolute values (Table 3).

No significant differences were observed between trials regarding the excretion of urine ($p = 0.35$), sweat rate ($p = 0.2$), or total evaporative water loss ($p = 0.36$) (Table 4).

Table 4. Effects of water (W), alcoholic (AB) or non-alcoholic beer (NAB) intake on excretion of urine, sweat rate, and evaporative water loss.

Variables	W	AB	NAB
Excretion of urine (mL)	117 ± 146	285 ± 252	239 ± 196
Sweat rate (L/h)	0.63 ± 0.13	0.68 ± 0.07	0.64 ± 0.20
Evaporative water loss (mL)	903 ± 105	1080 ± 72	1094 ± 129

4. Discussion

Results showed no significant change of plasma Na⁺ with NAB or of plasma K⁺ with NAB and W. Regarding USG, a significant reduction was observed after NAB and W. Although previous studies suggested the favorable effect of post-exercise non-alcoholic and low-alcoholic beer on hydration status [19,23], to our knowledge, this is the first study to compare the effect of beer, non-alcoholic beer, and water consumption before exercise on fluid homeostasis.

Body mass significantly decreased after exercise in all trials, and urine losses, sweat rates and evaporative water losses were not significantly different among trials. However, USG was significantly reduced after exercise in the W and NAB trials. These results suggest that kidney function is altered with non-alcoholic beer, similarly to water consumption, and that consumption of non-alcoholic beer before exercise might aid in hydration status regulation during exercise in the same way as water, although the former might be preferred due to its flavor. More studies with better and more reliable hydration markers are needed to confirm the previous statement.

Plasma Na^+ regulation is essential for athletic performance and the health of the athletes [24]. Our results showed that plasma Na^+ decreased significantly in the W and AB trials, and remained unchanged in the NAB trial (Table 3). However, plasma Na^+ values remained within normal physiological limits, reflecting eunatremic status after all trials. In our study, fluid intake was not allowed during exercise since the main objective was to evaluate the effects of three beverages as a pre-exercise hydration strategy. Future research could focus on the effect of non-alcoholic beer ingestion before exercise on fluid ingested during and after exercise, through its effects on thirst [25].

Plasma K^+ increases during exercise [26], which may be associated with muscle fatigue [27] and reduced muscular strength [28]. Our results showed that plasma K^+ was higher in the last minutes of exercise ($p < 0.05$) in the alcoholic beer trial only, while no significant alterations in plasma K^+ were observed after the non-alcoholic beer and water trials. Therefore, water and non-alcoholic beer consumed before exercise helped to maintain plasma K^+ homeostasis. Future studies should focus on the effects of non-alcoholic beer consumed before exercise on muscle performance during prolonged exercise.

One of the limitations of this study is that continuous steady-state exercise was used as a model to assess the effects of pre-exercise hydration beverages; however, the evaluated athletes usually perform intermittent, high-intensity bouts of activity. Future studies may incorporate exercise models with better ecological validity (e.g., Loughborough Intermittent Shuttle Test). In the same line, future studies may incorporate exercise models with a longer duration (e.g., >60 min) and greater environmental thermal stress (e.g., >27 °C and >80% of relative humidity), as soccer matches may last up to 120 min under conditions of high temperature and humidity in certain geographical regions where this sport is very popular (e.g., Brazil), although strict ethical and safety considerations should be taken. Another potential limitation of this study is the low number of participants. Although not a main objective of study, our results suggested that athletes (*i.e.*, soccer players) showed a relatively high prevalence of hypohydration before exercise trials (*i.e.*, mean USG = 1.024 g/mL), which appears to be common among soccer players. For instance, among elite Brazilian young male soccer players, a mean USG value of 1.021 g/mL was found before competitive games [11]. Most recently a mean USG value of 1.026 g/mL was reported in Chilean soccer players before training practice [12]. Within these considerations, it is our hope that the study's findings provide the impetus for further investigation regarding the use of non-alcoholic beer in intermittent sports athletes and that these findings now need to be replicated in larger clinical trials, considering the limitations previously raised.

Similarly, replication studies might consider hydration assessment recommendations with more consensus [29] and the comparison of NAB with well established hydration beverages (e.g., sports drinks). Also, although subjects reported no gastrointestinal-related symptoms after NAB (or AB) consumption, further investigations should consider the possible effects of gas contained in beer on stomach disturbances and fluid emptying [30].

5. Conclusions

The consumption of 0.7 L of non-alcoholic beer before exercise could help maintain blood electrolyte homeostasis during exercise. The consumption of 0.7 L of alcoholic beer before exercise increased plasma K^+ and decreased plasma Na^+ during exercise, which could negatively affect sport performance and health. Water ingestion before exercise also resulted in a decrease in plasma Na^+

during exercise. Non-alcoholic beer, but not alcoholic beer or water, may be an effective sports drinks before exercise.

Acknowledgments: Author and co-authors did not receive any funding.

Author Contributions: The study was designed by M.C.-S., N.J. and S.A.; data were collected and analyzed by M.C.-S., S.A. and R.R.-C.; data interpretation and manuscript preparation were undertaken by M.C.-S., N.J., S.A., C.J., C.A., H.Z.-F. and R.R.-C. All authors approved the final version of the paper.

Conflicts of Interest: The authors declare no conflict of interest.

Abbreviations

The following abbreviations are used in this manuscript:

W	Water
AB	Beer
NAB	Non-alcoholic beer
USG	Urine specific gravity

References

1. Stearns, R.L.; Casa, D.J.; Lopez, R.M.; McDermott, B.P.; Ganio, M.S.; Decher, N.R.; Scruggs, I.C.; West, A.E.; Armstrong, L.E.; Maresh, C.M. Influence of hydration status on pacing during trail running in the heat. *J. Strength Cond. Res.* **2009**, *23*, 2533–2541. [CrossRef] [PubMed]
2. Barr, S.I. Effects of dehydration on exercise performance. *Can. J. Appl. Physiol.* **1999**, *24*, 164–172. [CrossRef] [PubMed]
3. Tomporowski, P.D.; Beasman, K.; Ganio, M.S.; Cureton, K. Effects of dehydration and fluid ingestion on cognition. *Int. J. Sports Med.* **2007**, *28*, 891–896. [CrossRef] [PubMed]
4. Greenland, K. Exercise-associated hyponatraemia or hypo-osmolarity? *Emerg. Med. Australas.* **2004**, *16*, 482–484. [CrossRef] [PubMed]
5. Cheuvront, S.N.; Haymes, E.M. Thermoregulation and marathon running: Biological and environmental influences. *Sports Med.* **2001**, *31*, 743–762. [CrossRef] [PubMed]
6. Sawka, M.N.; Burke, L.M.; Eichner, E.R.; Maughan, R.J.; Montain, S.J.; Stachenfeld, N.S. American College of Sports Medicine position stand. Exercise and fluid replacement. *Med. Sci. Sports Exerc.* **2007**, *39*, 377–390. [PubMed]
7. Shirreffs, S.M.; Maughan, R.J. Whole body sweat collection in humans: An improved method with preliminary data on electrolyte content. *J. Appl. Physiol.* **1997**, *82*, 336–341. [PubMed]
8. Castro-Sepúlveda, M.; Ramirez-Campillo, R.; Astudillo, S.; Burgos, C.; Henríquez-Olguín, C. Prevalence of dehydration and fluid intake practices rally Dakar drivers. *Sci. Sports* **2014**, *29*, 327–330. [CrossRef]
9. Palmer, M.S.; Spriet, L.L. Sweat rate, salt loss, and fluid intake during an intense on-ice practice in elite Canadian male junior hockey players. *Appl. Physiol. Nutr. Metab.* **2008**, *33*, 263–271. [CrossRef] [PubMed]
10. Aragón-Vargas, L.F.; Moncada-Jiménez, J.; Hernández-Elizondo, J.; Barrenechea, A.; Monge-Alvarado, M. Evaluation of pre-game hydration status, heat stress, and fluid balance during professional soccer competition in the heat. *Eur. J. Sport Sci.* **2009**, *9*, 269–276. [CrossRef]
11. Da Silva, R.P.; Mundel, T.; Natali, A.J.; Filho, M.G.; Alfenas, R.C.; Lima, J.R.; Belfort, F.G.; Lopes, P.R.; Marins, J.C. Pre-game hydration status, sweat loss, and fluid intake in elite Brazilian young male soccer players during competition. *J. Sports Sci.* **2012**, *30*, 37–42. [CrossRef] [PubMed]
12. Castro-Sepúlveda, M.; Astudillo, S.; Álvarez, C.; Zapata-Lamana, R.; Zbinden-Foncea, H.; Ramírez-Campillo, R.; Jorquera, C. Prevalence of dehydration before training in professional Chilean soccer players. *Nutr. Hosp.* **2015**, *32*, 308–311. [PubMed]
13. Mohr, M.; Krustrup, P.; Bangsbo, J. Fatigue in soccer: A brief review. *J. Sports Sci.* **2005**, *23*, 593–599. [CrossRef] [PubMed]

14. Edwards, A.M.; Mann, M.E.; Marfell-Jones, M.J.; Rankin, D.M.; Noakes, T.D.; Shillington, D.P. Influence of moderate dehydration on soccer performance: Physiological responses to 45 min of outdoor match-play and the immediate subsequent performance of sport-specific and mental concentration tests. *Br. J. Sports Med.* **2007**, *41*, 385–391. [CrossRef] [PubMed]

15. Shirreffs, S.M.; Sawka, M.N. Fluid and electrolyte needs for training, competition, and recovery. *J. Sports Sci.* **2011**, *29*, S39–S46. [CrossRef] [PubMed]

16. Casa, D.J.; Armstrong, L.E.; Hillman, S.K.; Montain, S.J.; Reiff, R.V.; Rich, B.S.; Roberts, W.O.; Stone, J.A. National athletic trainers' association position statement: Fluid replacement for athletes. *J. Athl. Train.* **2000**, *35*, 212–224. [PubMed]

17. Savoie, F.A.; Dion, T.; Asselin, A.; Goulet, E.D. Sodium-induced hyperhydration decreases urine output and improves fluid balance compared with glycerol- and water-induced hyperhydration. *Appl. Physiol. Nutr. Metab.* **2015**, *40*, 51–58. [CrossRef] [PubMed]

18. Maughan, R.J. Alcohol and football. *J. Sports Sci.* **2006**, *24*, 741–748. [CrossRef] [PubMed]

19. Desbrow, B.; Murray, D.; Leveritt, M. Beer as a sports drink? Manipulating beer's ingredients to replace lost fluid. *Int. J. Sport Nutr. Exerc. Metab.* **2013**, *23*, 593–600. [PubMed]

20. Barnes, M.J. Alcohol: Impact on sports performance and recovery in male athletes. *Sports Med.* **2014**, *44*, 909–919. [CrossRef] [PubMed]

21. Langhof, E.; Stelness, I. Potentiometric analysis for sodium and potassium in biological fluids. *Clin. Chem.* **1982**, *28*, 170–172.

22. Hopkins, W.G.; Marshall, S.W.; Batterham, A.M.; Hanin, J. Progressive statistics for studies in sports medicine and exercise science. *Med. Sci. Sports Exerc.* **2009**, *41*, 3–13. [CrossRef] [PubMed]

23. Jiménez-Pavón, D.; Cervantes-Borunda, M.S.; Díaz, L.E.; Marcos, A.; Castill, M.J. Effects of a moderate intake of beer on markers of hydration after exercise in the heat: A crossover study. *Int. Soc. Sports Nutr.* **2015**, *12*, 26. [CrossRef] [PubMed]

24. Baker, L.B.; Jeukendrup, A.E. Optimal composition of fluid-replacement beverages. *Compr. Physiol.* **2014**, *4*, 575–620. [PubMed]

25. Johannsen, N.M.; Sullivan, Z.M.; Warnke, N.R.; Smiley-Oyen, A.L.; King, D.S.; Sharp, R.L. Effect of preexercise soup ingestion on water intake and fluid balance during exercise in the heat. *Int. J. Sport Nutr. Exerc. Metab.* **2013**, *23*, 287–296. [PubMed]

26. Medbo, J.I.; Seiersted, O.M. Plasma potassium changes with high intensity exercise. *J. Physiol.* **1990**, *421*, 105–122. [CrossRef] [PubMed]

27. Clausen, T. Regulation of active Na^+-K^+ transport in skeletal muscle. *Physiol. Rev.* **1986**, *66*, 542–580. [PubMed]

28. Atanasovska, T.; Petersen, A.C.; Rouffet, D.M.; Billaut, F.; Nq, I.; McKenna, M.J. Plasma K^+ dynamics and implications during and following intense rowing exercise. *J. Appl. Physiol.* **2014**, *117*, 60–68. [CrossRef] [PubMed]

29. Cheuvront, S.N.; Kenefick, R.W.; Zambraski, E.J. Spot urine concentrations should not be used for hydration assessment: A methodology review. *Int. J. Sport Nutr. Exerc. Metab.* **2015**, *25*, 293–297. [CrossRef] [PubMed]

30. Ploutz-Snyder, L.; Foley, J.; Ploutz-Snyder, R.; Kanaley, J.; Sagendorf, K.; Meyer, R. Gastric gas and fluid emptying assessed by magnetic resonance imaging. *Eur. J. Appl. Physiol. Occup. Physiol.* **1999**, *79*, 212–220. [CrossRef] [PubMed]

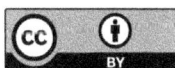

nutrients

MDPI

Article

25(OH)D Status of Elite Athletes with Spinal Cord Injury Relative to Lifestyle Factors

Kelly Pritchett [1,*], Robert Pritchett [1], Dana Ogan [1], Phil Bishop [2], Elizabeth Broad [3] and Melissa LaCroix [4]

[1] Department of Nutrition, Exercise, and Health Sciences, Central Washington University,
   400 E. University Way, Ellensburg, WA 98926, USA; pritchettr@cwu.edu (R.P.); ogand@cwu.edu (D.O.)
[2] Department of Kinesiology, the University of Alabama, P.O. Box 870312, Tuscaloosa, AL 35487, USA;
   pbishop@bamaed.ua.edu
[3] US Olympic Committee, 2800 Olympic Parkway, Chula Vista, CA 91915, USA; elizabeth.broad@usoc.org
[4] Canadian Sport Institute Pacific, 6111 River Rd, Richmond, BC V7C 0A2, Canada; mlacroix@csipacific.ca
* Correspondence: pritchettk@cwu.edu; Tel.: +1-509-963-2786; Fax: +1-509-963-1848

Received: 18 April 2016; Accepted: 9 June 2016; Published: 17 June 2016

Abstract: Background: Due to the potential negative impact of low Vitamin D status on performance-related factors and the higher risk of low Vitamin D status in Spinal Cord Injury (SCI) population, research is warranted to determine whether elite athletes with SCI have sufficient 25(OH)D levels. The purposes of this study were to examine: (1) the seasonal proportion of vitamin D insufficiency among elite athletes with SCI; and (2) to determine whether lifestyle factors, SCI lesion level, and muscle performance/function are related to vitamin D status in athletes with SCI. **Methods:** Thirty-nine members of the Canadian Wheelchair Sports Association, and the US Olympic Committee Paralympic program from outdoor and indoor sports were recruited for this study. Dietary and lifestyle factors, and serum 25(OH)D concentrations were assessed during the autumn (October) and winter (February/March). An independent t-test was used to assess differences in 25(OH)D status among seasons, and indoor and outdoor sports in the autumn and winter, respectively. **Results:** Mean $\pm$ SD serum 25(OH)D concentration was 69.6 $\pm$ 19.7 nmol/L (range from 30 to 107.3 nmol/L) and 67.4 $\pm$ 25.5 nmol/L (range from 20 to 117.3 nmol/L)in the autumn and winter, respectively. In the autumn, 15.4% of participants were considered vitamin D deficient (25(OH)D < 50 nmol/L) whereas 51.3% had 25(OH)D concentrations that would be considered insufficient (<80 nmol/L). In the winter, 15.4% were deficient while 41% of all participants were considered vitamin D insufficient. **Conclusion:** A substantial proportion of elite athletes with SCI have insufficient (41%–51%) and deficient (15.4%) 25(OH)D status in the autumn and winter. Furthermore, a seasonal decline in vitamin D status was not observed in the current study.

Keywords: 25(OH)D; sun exposure; spinal cord injuries; athletes

1. Introduction

The Third National Health and Nutrition Examination Survey (NHANES III) determined that over 77% of Americans are considered vitamin D insufficient [1]. Vitamin D is well known for its role in bone health [2], but recent research has linked vitamin D to other important processes in the body including: hormone synthesis, signaling gene response, immunity, protein synthesis, and cell turnover [3–7]. These rates of insufficiency (25(OH)D < 80 nmol/L), together with the essential metabolic properties of vitamin D, have led researchers to examine the influence of vitamin D not only on bone health, but also on physical performance and injury in athletes.

Vitamin D receptors have recently been identified in skeletal muscle, which has led to further examination of the influence of vitamin D on athletic performance [7]. Therefore, the risk of vitamin D insufficiency among athletes has received growing interest. In the last decade, researchers have examined 25(OH)D (criterion measure for vitamin D concentration levels) among various groups of athletes including: gymnasts [8], runners [4,9,10], rugby players [10], and jockeys [11] and have suggested that athletes are at a high risk for vitamin D insufficiencies [7]. Blood 25(OH)D concentrations are largely dependent on geographical location (latitude) and type of sport (indoor *vs.* outdoor) [3,7].

Individuals with spinal cord injury (SCI) may be at increased risk for vitamin D insufficiency due to inadequate diet [12], anticonvulsant medications, and reduced sunlight exposure [13]. The ability of individuals with spinal cord injury to go outdoors and synthesize vitamin D from sunlight may be limited due to decreased functional mobility, impaired thermoregulation, amount of skin exposed, season of the year, and latitude. Oleson *et al.* (2006) found that 65% of patients with acute SCI, and 81% of patients with chronic SCI had insufficient 25(OH)D levels in the summer, despite living in Birmingham, AL (33°N) [13]. These rates increased to 84% and 96% in the winter months [13]. Hummel *et al.* (2012) found that 39% of individuals ($n = 62$) with chronic SCI had insufficient 25(OH)D regardless of supplementation use [14]. Furthermore, Hummel *et al.* (2012) suggested that optimal serum 25(OH)D levels for SCI may be higher than in an able bodied population due to an increased 25(OH)D needed to suppress parathyroid hormone (PTH) release and absorb calcium [14]. Considering individuals with SCI are already at high risk for osteoporosis [13,15,16], a low serum 25(OH)D puts them at an even greater risk for bone injuries and fractures given that the onset of bone loss occurs quickly post injury [13,14,17]. Although performance trials are limited in an athletic population, a number of studies support vitamin D's indirect role in enhancing exercise performance [18–22], however recent studies do not support the benefits of vitamin D supplementation [23,24]. A recent meta-analysis suggested that vitamin D supplementation has a small, but positive, impact on muscle strength in healthy individuals [22]. Favorable 25(OH)D levels may reduce the risk of debilitating stress fracture among athletes, indirectly influencing performance through prevention of injury [25,26]. Finally, because vitamin D is used in numerous metabolic pathways, it has been suggested that the athlete may need a higher vitamin D status to ensure acceptable energy availability and storage [27].

Knowledge regarding the vitamin D status of athletes with SCI is lacking. Due to the potential negative impact of low vitamin D status on performance-related factors and the potentially higher risk of vitamin D insufficiency in SCI population, research is warranted to determine whether elite athletes with SCI have sufficient 25(OH)D levels. The purposes of this study were to examine (1) the seasonal proportion of vitamin D insufficiency among elite athletes with SCI; and (2) to determine whether lifestyle factors, SCI lesion level, and muscle performance/function are related to vitamin D status in athletes with SCI. Based on previous studies conducted in athletes [9,10], we hypothesized that a seasonal decline in 25(OH)D status will be observed from autumn to winter. In addition, rates of vitamin D insufficiency will be higher among elite athletes with SCI participating in indoor sports compared to those participating in an outdoor sport, which may be related to increased time spent indoors [13], decreased mobility, and vitamin/mineral deficiencies that are commonly a problem in individuals with SCI [12].

2. Methods

2.1. Subjects

Male and female athletes, ⩾18 years old, were recruited via the sport medicine staff from The Canadian Wheelchair Sports Association, and the US Olympic Committee Paralympic programs. Athletes were screened for eligibility and then recruited via members of the sports medicine team. Only athletes eligible for participation were approached. Participating athletes with SCI were required to have an impairment of their spinal cord (e.g., spinal cord injury, spina bifida) and were selected from tennis, athletics, basketball and rugby. Exclusion criteria included athletes with a diagnosis of fat malabsorption, thyroid, kidney, or bone disease. Based on data from previous studies [13] using a mean of 37.4 ± 24.9 nmol/L, a power of 0.8 and alpha = 0.05, an a priori power analysis (G Power version 3.1) indicated the need for 40 participants. This study was approved by the Central Washington University (CWU) Human Subjects Review Committee (HSRC) (Project # H14114). Subjects provided written consent prior to participating in the study.

2.2. Study Design

A longitudinal, observational trial examined seasonal changes (summer, winter) in 25(OH)D status. Participants reported to the testing facility on two separate data collection sessions (involving 2 days), initially at the beginning of autumn (October 2014, for maximal cumulative sun exposure) and for a follow up in the winter (February/March 2015, for minimal cumulative sun exposure).

Descriptive characteristics including height, weight, injury level, and history of injury were recorded. Prior to testing, participants were asked to sustain normal hydration levels, and consume their usual breakfast for both testing sessions (autumn, winter), which was recorded and analyzed for macronutrient (carbohydrate, protein, and fat) content. In addition, participants were asked to complete a Diet and Lifestyle Questionnaire. Participants' supplement routine was recorded for each trial to account for any changes.

The following measurements were collected:

2.3. 25(OH)D Assay

The 25(OH)D levels were assessed during each data collection session. Blood samples consisted of 5–10 drops of blood obtained from the fingertips using a lancet and sterile procedures. Drops of whole blood were pipetted onto blood spot cards. Blood spots were air dried for at least 30 min and sent in batches to a certified laboratory (ZRT Laboratory, Beaverton, OR, USA) for 25(OH)D assay. Blood spot assay has shown excellent correlation ($r = 0.97$; with a lower limit of detection of 1.9 ng/mL) with liquid chromatography/tandem mass spectrometry assay and has been suggested to provide a convenient alternative [28]. Results were compared to reference values (Table 1), and various other published 25(OH)D concentrations from studies conducted in healthy adults [9,29–31].

Table 1. Reference 25(OH)D Values.

Category	25(OH) D Level (nmol/L)
Deficient	<50
Insufficient	<80
Sufficient	80–250
Optimal	100–200
High	>250

Reference values from other published studies reporting 25(OH)D concentrations [9,27,29–31].

2.4. Diet and Lifestyle Questionnaire

Participants completed a self-administered questionnaire at each data collection session that focused on factors that could potentially influence vitamin D status including dietary intake, supplement use (vitamin D, multivitamin, and calcium), UVB exposure, sunscreen use, injuries and illness. Instructions were provided prior to administration of the questionnaire. The questionnaire was replicated, with permission, from Halliday *et al.* (2010) [9]. This frequency questionnaire addressed dietary intake, supplement use, UVB exposure, sunscreen use, injuries and illness. Participants rated how often they consumed vitamin D-containing foods and supplements (never or <1 per month, 1–3 per month, 1 per week, 2–4 per week, 5–6 per week, 1 per day, 2–3 per day, 4–5 per day, or 6 or more per day). In addition, the frequency of time spent outdoors (never or <10 min per week, 1–3 h per month, 1 h per week, 2–4 h per week, 5–6 h per week, 0.5–1 h per day or >2 h per day), time of day when sun exposure occurred (6–10 a.m., 10 a.m. to 2 p.m., 2–6 p.m.), tanning bed use (never or <10 min per week, 10–20 min per week, 20–30 min per week, 30–40 min per week, 40–50 min per week, 50–60 min per week or >60 min per week), sunscreen use (on 100 mm scale with left anchor of

NEVER, and right anchor of ALWAYS), Sun protection factor (SPF) of sunscreen used, type clothing worn, and frequency of illness was self-reported [9]. Participants reported their responses based on their location during the previous three months.

The average vitamin D content of food listed in the questionnaire was calculated from the United States Department of Agriculture (USDA) national nutrient database for standard reference [32], and food labels as derived from Halliday *et al.* (2010). Daily average intakes, expressed in international units (IU), were calculated by "multiplying the frequency midpoint by the average" vitamin D content in each food or supplement [9].

2.5. Performance Tests

The 20 m SPRINT A self-regulated, warm up was matched with autumn, and winter trials. 20 m sprint tests were completed using 4 sets of timing lights (Brower Timing Systems, Draper, UT, USA) to measure 5 m, 10 m, and 20 m to splits. Where timing gates were not accessible, a hand held stopwatch was used to record time for the 20 m sprint. A 20 M sprint test is commonly used to assess anaerobic performance in athletes with SCI.

Handgrip strength was assessed using a handgrip dynamometer (model 68812 County Technology INC, Gays Mills, WI, USA) using the dominant hand first. The grip width was adjusted until the second joint of the participant's forefinger was bent at 90 degrees during the grasp. The indicator was set to zero before each trial. In a seated position and relaxed, with their elbows at 90 degrees participants gripped the dynamometer with their dominant hand to exert full force without letting their arms touch their body or rest on any part of their wheelchair. These procedures were repeated twice on both the left and right hands, and the highest score was recorded for a sum of the two hands.

2.6. Data Analysis

Data were analyzed using IBM SPSS for Windows version 18.0 software (SPSS Inc, Chicago, IL, USA). Basic descriptive statistics (mean $\pm$ SD) were computed to describe the sample population, and to quantify 25(OH)D status in this population. Data were examined for normalcy using the Komogorov-Smirnov test for skewness and kurtosis. The results indicated a normal distribution, therefore means $\pm$ SD, and parametric tests were used to describe and examine the sample. Given there were no differences in 25(OH)D status and geographical location, USA and CAN athletes were analyzed as one group. Pearson *r* correlations were used to examine the relationship between 25(OH)D levels and vitamin D intake. Spearman rank correlations were used to assess the relationship between serum 25(OH)D concentrations and non-continuous variables, including frequency of intake of vitamin D–containing foods and supplements, leisure time spent outdoors, tanning bed use, and frequency of illness. A one-way repeated measures analysis of variance (ANOVA) was used to examine differences in 25(OH)D status based on level of lesion. A Tukey *post hoc* test was applied in the case of significant ($p \leqslant 0.05$). A paired *t*-test was used to assess difference in 25(OH)D status among seasons, and indoor and outdoor sports in the autumn, and winter. A Pearson correlation was used to analyze associations between 25(OH)D and muscle function measures. Cohen's d effect size was calculated for mean difference between indoor and outdoor sports in the autumn and winter, respectively. The alpha level was set at 0.05.

3. Results

Volunteers (height: 131.5 + 13.6 cm; weight: 59.5 + 13.5 kg; age: 27.7 + 6.5 years) (*n* = 39: 19 male, and 20 female; 1 African American, 1 White Hispanic, 3 Asian, and 30 Caucasian) from outdoor: tennis (*n* = 1) and athletics (track and field) (*n* = 14), and indoor sports: rugby (*n* = 12), and basketball (*n* = 12). All athletes with SCI were analysed in a single group, due to the small sample size which is typical for research examining athletes with SCI. Seven participants did not complete the winter testing session due to not being selected for the next team camp or travel. Therefore, only 32 athletes completed the final testing session in the winter. Baseline characteristics were not significantly different between dropouts and those who finished the study. Descriptive characteristics and seasonal 25(OH)D status organized by sport are displayed in Table 2.

Table 2. Descriptive characteristics and seasonal 25(OH)D status organized by indoor and outdoor sport.

	Outdoor		Indoor		
	Athletics	Tennis	Basketball	Rugby	*p*-Value
Autumn 25(OH)D (nmol/L) (*n* = 39)	76.4 ± 5.2 (*n* = 14)	47.4 (*n* = 1)	70.4 ± 5.7 (*n* = 12)	62.9 ± 5.7 (*n* = 12)	*p* = 0.19
Winter 25(OH)D (nmol/L) (*n* = 32)	70.4 ± 21.7 (*n* = 13)	49.9 (*n* = 1)	60.2 ± 29.5 (*n* = 10)	74.6 ± 27.5 (*n* = 7)	*p* = 0.75

Data are means ± SD. Note: No differences were found in 25(OH)D between indoor (basketball and rugby) and outdoor sports (athletics and tennis) in the autumn or winter, respectively, using an independent samples *t*-test.

3.1. The 25(OH)D Status

In the autumn, mean 25(OH)D concentrations averaged 69.6 ± 19.7 nmol/L (range 30 to 107.3 nmol/L). 15.4% (*n* = 6) of participants were considered vitamin D deficient (25(OH)D < 50 nmol/L) whereas 51.3% (*n* = 20) had 25(OH)D concentrations that would be considered insufficient (50–79.9 nmol/L). 6% of outdoor athletes were classified as deficient and 60% as insufficient for 25(OH)D status compared to 21% of indoor athletes classified as deficient and 46% insufficient. 33% of participants in both groups were classified as sufficient for 25(OH)D status. There was no significant difference (*p* = 0.19) in 25(OH)D among indoor and outdoor sports, respectively (indoor 66.3 ± 21.5 nmol/L; outdoor 74.8 ± 16.2 nmol/L; ES = 0.45).

In the winter, mean 25(OH)D concentrations averaged 67.4 ± 25.5 nmol/L (ranging from 20 to 117.3 nmol/L). There was no significant difference (*p* = 0.68) in Vitamin D status between autumn and winter (autumn: 69.6 ± 19.7 nmol/L, winter 67.4 ± 25.5) for the total group. 41% of all participants were considered vitamin D insufficient, while 15.4% were deficient. Furthermore, 6% of outdoor athletes were classified as deficient and 56% as insufficient for 25(OH)D status compared to 21% of indoor athletes classified as deficient and 30% insufficient. 23% of all participants in the winter were classified as sufficient. In addition, there was no significant difference (*p* = 0.75) in 25(OH)D among indoor and outdoor sports, respectively (indoor 66.1 ± 28.5 nmol/L; outdoor 69.8 ± 21.5 nmol/L; ES = 0.16).

For all participants, 25(OH)D concentration in the autumn was correlated with 25(OH)D concentrations in the winter (*r* = 0.59, *n* = 32, *p* < 0.001). Plasma 25(OH)D was not significantly different between sports team during autumn or winter (Table 2) or between gender in the autumn (*p* = 0.29) (females 73.1 ± 18.5; males 66.1 ± 21.2) or winter (*p* = 0.59) (females 65.2 ± 23.2; males 70.1 ± 28). Furthermore, the mean differences observed between 25(OH)D concentrations and level of lesion were not statistically different in the autumn (*p* = 0.15) and winter (*p* = 0.59), respectively (Table 3).

Table 3. 25(OH)D status relative to level of Spinal Cord Injury (SCI) lesion.

	C Level	T1–T6	T7–T12	Lumbar	*p*-Value
Autumn 25(OH)D (nmol/L) (*n* = 39)	58.4 ± 23.7 (*n* = 11)	75.1 ± 18 (*n* = 10)	74.9 ± 16.5 (*n* = 11)	74.4 ± 20.5 (*n* = 5)	*p* = 0.15
Winter 25(OH)D (nmol/L) (*n* = 32)	73.9 ± 30.2 (*n* = 8)	71.9 ± 28.7 (*n* = 7)	64.9 ± 2.3 (*n* = 11)	62.9 ± 25.5 (*n* = 6)	*p* = 0.59

Data are means ± SD. Note: No differences were found in 25(OH)D between level of SCI lesion in the autumn or winters, respectively, using one-way ANOVA.

3.2. *Dietary Intake of Vitamin D and Vitamin D Status*

Frequency of consumption of vitamin D containing foods is displayed in Table 4. The average dietary intake of vitamin D from food sources was 121.1 ± 9.8 IU/day in the autumn, and 115 ± 12.25 IU/day in the winter. Milk consumption in the autumn and winter averaged 2 to 4 servings per week. In the autumn and winter, the estimated average frequency for multivitamin (MVI) intake was "never". Vitamin D status was correlated with milk consumption in the autumn ($r = 0.27$, $p \leqslant 0.05$), and in the winter ($r = 0.58$, $p \leqslant 0.05$). However, no other correlations were found between 25(OH)D status and supplements, or vitamin D containing foods. In the winter, vitamin D status was correlated with calcium supplementation ($r = 0.33$, $p = 0.04$).

Table 4. Reported Frequency of Consumption of Dietary Vitamin D by Season.

Food/Vitamin D Content (IU)	Autumn (n = 39)	Winter (n = 32)
Milk (8 oz), 100 IU		
never, <1/month	9	5
1–2/month	2	5
2–4/week	1	10
5–6/week	6	2
1/day	9	7
2–3/day	4	3
Cereal (6–8 oz), 40 IU		
never, <1/month	11	7
1–3/month	7	12
1/week	1	4
2–4/week	2	6
5–6/week	1	2
1/day	1	1
Fortified Orange Juice (8 oz), 100 IU		
never, <1/month	13	12
1–2/month	7	11
1/week	5	2
2–4/week	7	3
5–6/week	3	3
1/day	2	1
2–3/day	1	0
Egg (1 whole), 18 IU		
never, <1/month	4	5
1–3/month	3	2
1/week	3	3
2–4/week	15	11
5–6/week	6	3
1/day	3	5
2–3/day	3	3
6+/day	1	0
Salmon (3.5 oz), 815 IU		
never, <1/month	10	8
1–3/month	12	13
1/week	5	6
2–4/week	11	5
MVI, 400 IU		
never, <1/month	28	26
1–3/month	1	2
2–4/week	2	0
1/week	0	1
1/day	5	2
2–3/day	1	1

Note: Derived from Halliday *et al.*, 2011 [4].

3.3. UVB Exposure and Vitamin D Status

Reported leisure time spent outdoors was significantly different across seasons ($p \leqslant 0.001$) and averaged 5.5 ± 1.6 h/week^{-1} in the autumn, and 2 ± 1.5 h/week^{-1} winter, respectively. Leisure time spent outdoors was significantly ($r = 0.41$, $p \leqslant 0.05$) correlated with vitamin D status in the autumn, but not in the winter ($r = -0.02$, $p = 0.46$). However, the time of day spent outdoors (daylight hours independent of hours spent outdoors), geographical location, sunscreen use, or SPF (sun protection factor) was not correlated with 25(OH)D status for either season.

3.4. Muscle Function and Vitamin D Status

Pearson correlations for 20 M sprint time and 25(OH)D were not significant during the autumn ($r = -0.16$, $p = 0.17$) or winter ($r = -0.03$, $p = 0.45$), or for handgrip strength and 25(OH)D during the autumn ($r = 0.2$, $p = 0.14$) or winter ($r = 0.08$, $p = 0.35$), respectively.

4. Discussion

Our findings suggest that a substantial proportion (41%–51%) of elite athletes with SCI have insufficient vitamin D status in the winter, and autumn. Although a seasonal decline in vitamin D status was not observed in the current study, a higher proportion of athletes were considered sufficient in the autumn compared to the winter (33% *vs.* 23%, respectively). Furthermore, there was no significant difference in 25(OH)D among indoor and outdoor sports. The proportion of vitamin D insufficiency observed in these athletes with SCI was lower than vitamin D insufficiency rates reported in a group of sedentary individuals with SCI (81%), and the general U.S. population (77%) from 2001 to 2004 [1,13]. These findings support other literature suggesting that high-risk athletes, such as indoor athletes and those who avoid peak daylight hours, should have 25(OH)D levels assessed annually [7,9]. Because vitamin D status may play a role in the development of osteoporosis [13–15], injury risk [13,14,17] and exercise performance [18–24], further research is warranted to appropriately identify serum 25(OH)D goal levels in athletes with SCI and to determine the magnitude of effect from vitamin D status on muscle strength and performance.

Similar to studies conducted in able-bodied athletes [9,10], 15% of our participants were considered vitamin D deficient while 51% had 25(OH)D concentrations that would be considered insufficient in the autumn. Furthermore, 6% of outdoor athletes with SCI were deficient compared to 21% of indoor athletes with SCI in the autumn. In contrast, a study conducted in Laramie, WY (41.3°N), found lower vitamin D insufficiency rates (12%) athletes ($n = 41$) after the summer months compared to the autumn [4]. Another study suggested that 73% of indoor athletes (gymnasts and dancers) were vitamin D insufficient despite living at favorable latitude for UVB exposure (Israel 31.8°N) [33].

Recent findings by Flueck *et al.* (2016) suggested that 73.2% of Paralympic athletes have insufficient/deficient 25(OH)D status [34]. Furthermore, 25(OH)D levels were significantly lower during the winter months [31], however it should be noted that the study was cross sectional in nature and did not examine the within subject change from autumn to winter. The authors concluded that athletes need to be tested for 25(OH)D status in the autumn, and again in the winter/early spring months as performed in the current study. Contrary to findings in able-bodied athletes [9,10], and in a group of sedentary individuals with SCI [13], a seasonal decline in vitamin D status was not observed in the current study. In the winter, comparable rates of vitamin D insufficiency (41%) and deficiency (15%) were observed in athletes with SCI.

In the current study, sunlight was the primary source of vitamin D during the summer months leading into autumn. Sun exposure significantly ($p \leqslant 0.001$) decreased from autumn to winter (5.5 ± 1.6 h/week^{-1} in autumn, and 2 ± 1.5 h/week^{-1} in winter). Furthermore, time spent outdoors was associated with vitamin D status in the autumn, but not in the winter. Oleson *et al.* (2006) found that patients with chronic SCI had sub therapeutic 25(OH)D levels in the summer despite living in Birmingham, AL (33°N) and these rates increased to 84% and 96% in the winter months [13]. It should be noted that heat and humidity may create a barrier for individuals with SCI to go outdoors during the summer months due to difficulties with thermoregulation. Similar to previous research, geographical location (latitude) and gender did not appear to be the major risk factors for vitamin D insufficiency in athletes with SCI [9,10]. As seen in able-bodied indoor athletes, lack of sun exposure may increase the risk for vitamin D insufficiency [7].

The average vitamin D intake observed in the current study did not meet the minimum Dietary Recommended Intake (DRI; 600 IU/day for adults 18–70 years of age) to prevent a clinical vitamin D deficiency [21]. According to National Health and Nutrition Examination Survey (NHANES) data, only 9.4% of individuals with a disability (n = 11,811) meet the recommendations for vitamin D intake from food alone [35]. Krempien *et al.* (2011) suggested that vitamin D intake from food alone was inadequate in a group of elite Canadian athletes with SCI (Males 87 ± 66 IU/day, Females 166 ± 130 IU/day) [12]. In addition, the estimated prevalence of inadequate intake was the highest for vitamin D when compared to other vitamins or minerals [12]. However, it should be noted that vitamin D intake from foods was the major source of vitamin D in the winter months.

Finally, it has been suggested that vitamin D supplementation may be necessary to maintain adequate levels during the winter even in athletes who spend ample time outdoors [7,36], however this has yet to be examined in athletes with SCI. Furthermore, Storlie *et al.* (2011) suggested that supplementation with 1000 IU/day of vitamin D was not enough to prevent seasonal decline of vitamin D status in male athletes [10]. Hummel *et al.* (2012) found that 39% of individuals (n = 62) with chronic SCI had suboptimal 25(OH)D levels, although a large majority of subjects were taking vitamin D supplements [14]. Therefore, vitamin D supplementation protocols for athletes with SCI needs to be established.

Athletes with SCI exemplify a fascinating group to examine due to the diversity of physical impairment resulting in a variety of physiological abilities [37]. In the current study, measures of muscle function/performance (handgrip strength and sprint time) were not associated with 25(OH)D status during the autumn or winter. Muscle wasting below the level of the lesion (which reflects both level and completeness of injury) may hinder the demonstration of any possible relationship between 25(OH)D levels and muscle strength tests in individuals with SCI. We can only speculate that the ability to detect a change in performance measures may be limited given that the subjects in the current study are highly trained, elite athletes with SCI. In a study by Barbonetti *et al.* (2016), lower 25(OH)D levels showed a significant independent association with poorer physical function outcomes, after adjusting for several confounders in individuals with chronic SCI [38]. Other studies have suggested that 25(OH)D status may have an effect on muscle performance and injury prevention, therefore possibly influencing athletic performance [7,39,40]. Foo *et al.* (2009) suggested that poor vitamin D status (<50 nmol/L) was associated with reduced forearm strength (using a handgrip dynamometer) when compared to individuals with vitamin D levels > 50 nmol/L in a group of Chinese adolescent females (n = 301) [33]. Although controversial, a recent meta-analysis suggested that vitamin D supplementation had a small, but positive, impact on muscle strength [19]. Researchers have suggested that it may be necessary to increase 25(OH)D levels above 100 nmol/L before a performance benefit can be observed [11,20]. Therefore, further research is warranted to determine the magnitude of effect of vitamin D supplementation on muscle strength and performance in athletes with SCI.

This study is not without limitations, despite the strengths of this well controlled study conducted in elite Paralympic athletes. One limitation of this study is the small sample size when compared to research with an able bodied population. Although our findings may not be generalizable due to the lower power, it should be noted that a sample size of this magnitude in the current study is uncommon for a population of athletes with SCI, but is comparable to the sample sizes used in studies examining able-bodied athletes [9,10]. The ability to detect to detect a small difference in 25(OH)D among indoor and outdoor sports, which is further supported by the low effect sizes, may have been due to the small sample size. As seen in most studies examining athletes with SCI the variation in level of lesion among athletes resulted in differences in physiological capabilities. Furthermore, although there was no correlation observed among geographical location and 25(OH)D, athletes resided in multiple locations throughout the US and Canada. Given there were no differences in 25(OH)D status and geographical location, USA and CAN athletes were analyzed as one group. Although we reported a high proportion of insufficiency and deficiency in our population, since this study did not examine age matched to able-bodied athletes or sedentary subjects with SCI, it is difficult to make comparisons to previously published data in able bodied athletes or sedentary individuals with SCI.

5. Conclusions

In conclusion, the findings suggest that a substantial proportion of elite athletes with SCI have low vitamin D status even after the summer months. Contrary to our hypothesis, a seasonal decline in 25(OH)D status was not observed in the current study, regardless of the decrease in sun exposure from autumn to winter. However, it should be noted that a higher proportion of athletes were considered sufficient in autumn compared to winter. In addition, a higher percentage of indoor athletes compared to outdoor athletes were classified as deficient during both the autumn and winter months. Finally, research is warranted to appropriately identify serum 25(OH)D goal levels in athletes with SCI and routine screening and supplementation protocols need to be instituted to prevent vitamin D insufficiencies [7,13].

Acknowledgments: The authors and co-authors did not receive any funding to conduct this study.

Author Contributions: The study was designed by K.P., E.B., M.L., R.P., P.B.; data were collected and analyzed by K.P., E.B., M.L., R.P.; data interpretation and manuscript preparation were undertaken by K.P., E.B., M.L., R.P., P.B., and D.O. All authors approved the final version of the paper.

Conflicts of Interest: The authors declare no conflict of interest.

References

1. Ginde, A.A.; Liu, M.C.; Camargo, C.A. Demographic differences and trends of vitamin D insufficiency in the US population, 1988–2004. *Arch. Intern. Med.* **2009**, *169*, 626–632. [CrossRef] [PubMed]
2. Tsugawa, N. Bone and nutrition. Vitamin D intake and bone. *Clin. Calcium* **2015**, *25*, 973–981. [PubMed]
3. Larsen-Meyer, D.E.; Willis, K.S. Vitamin D and athletes. *Curr. Sports Med. Rep.* **2010**, *9*, 220–226. [CrossRef] [PubMed]
4. Willis, K.S.; Smith, D.T.; Broughton, K.S.; Larson-Meyer, D.E. Vitamin D status and biomarkers of inflammation in runners. *Open Access J. Sports Med.* **2012**, *3*, 35–42. [PubMed]
5. Campbell, P.M.F.; Allain, T.J. Muscle strength and vitamin D in older people. *Gerontology* **2006**, *52*, 335–338. [CrossRef] [PubMed]
6. Ceglia, L. Vitamin D and skeletal muscle tissue and function. *Mol. Aspects Med.* **2008**, *29*, 407–414. [CrossRef] [PubMed]
7. Ogan, D.; Pritchett, K. Vitamin D and the athlete: Risks, recommendations, and benefits. *Nutrients* **2013**, *5*, 1856–1868. [CrossRef] [PubMed]
8. Lovell, G. Vitamin D status of females in an elite gymnastics program. *Clin. J. Sport Med.* **2008**, *18*, 159–161. [CrossRef] [PubMed]
9. Halliday, T.M.; Peterson, N.J.; Thomas, J.J.; Kleppinger, K.; Hollis, B.W.; Larson-Meyer, D.E. Vitamin D status relative to diet, lifestyle, injury, and illness in college athletes. *Med. Sci. Sports Exerc.* **2011**, *43*, 335–343. [CrossRef] [PubMed]
10. Storlie, D.M.; Pritchett, K.; Pritchett, R.; Cashman, L. 12-week vitamin D supplementation trial does not significantly influence seasonal 25(OH)D status in male collegiate athletes. *Int. J. Health Nutr.* **2011**, *2*, 8–13.
11. Close, G.L.; Leckey, J.; Patterson, M.; Bradley, W.; Owens, D.J.; Fraser, W.D.; Morton, J.P. The effects of vitamin D(3) supplementation on serum total 25[OH]D concentration and physical performance: A randomised dose-response study. *Br. J. Sports Med.* **2013**, *47*, 692–696. [CrossRef] [PubMed]
12. Krempien, J.L.; Barr, S.I. Risk of nutrient inadequacies in elite Canadian athletes with spinal cord injury. *Int. J. Sport Nutr. Exerc. Metab.* **2011**, *21*, 417–425. [PubMed]

13. Oleson, C.V.; Chen, D.; Wuermser, L.A. Vitamin D deficiency in traumatic spinal cord injury. In *Conference Proceedings of Contemporary Diagnosis and Treatment of Vitamin D-Related Disroders*, Proceedings of the American Society of Bone and Mineral Research, Arlington, VA, USA, 4–6 December 2006; p. 41.

14. Hummel, K.; Craven, B.C.; Giangregorio, L. Serum 25(OH)D, PTH and correlates of suboptimal 25(OH)D levels in persons with chronic spinal cord injury. *Spinal Cord* **2012**, *50*, 812–816. [CrossRef] [PubMed]

15. Bauman, W.A.; Zhong, Y.-G.; Schwartz, E. Vitamin D deficiency in veterans with chronic spinal cord injury. *Metabolism* **1995**, *44*, 1612–1616. [CrossRef]

16. Vaziri, N.D.; Pandian, M.R.; Segal, J.L.; Winer, R.L.; Eltorai, I.; Brunnemann, S. Vitamin D, parathormone, and calcitonin profiles in persons with long-standing spinal cord injury. *Arch. Phys. Med. Rehabil.* **1994**, *75*, 766–769. [PubMed]

17. Nemunaitis, G.A.; Mejia, M.; Nagy, J.A.; Johnson, T.; Chae, J.; Roach, M.J. A descriptive study on vitamin D levels in individuals with spinal cord injury in an acute inpatient rehabilitation setting. *PM R* **2010**, *2*, 202–208. [CrossRef] [PubMed]

18. Wyon, M.A.; Wolman, R.; Nevill, A.M.; Cloak, R.; Metsios, G.S.; Gould, D.; Ingham, A.; Koutedakis, Y. Acute effects of vitamin D$_3$ supplementation on muscle strength in judoka athletes: A randomized placebo-controlled, double-blind trial. *Clin. J. Sport Med.* **2015**. [CrossRef] [PubMed]

19. Ceglia, L.; Harris, S.S. Vitamin D and its role in skeletal muscle. *Calcif. Tissue Int.* **2013**, *92*, 151–162. [CrossRef] [PubMed]

20. Close, G.L.; Russell, J.; Cobley, J.N.; Owens, D.J.; Wilson, G.; Gregson, W.; Fraser, W.D.; Morton, J.P. Assessment of vitamin D concentration in non-supplemented professional athletes and healthy adults during the winter months in the UK: Implications for skeletal muscle function. *J. Sports Sci.* **2013**, *31*, 344–353. [CrossRef] [PubMed]

21. Girgis, C.M.; Clifton-Bligh, R.J.; Hamrick, M.W.; Holick, M.F.; Gunton, J.E. The roles of vitamin D in skeletal muscle: Form, function, and metabolism. *Endocr. Rev.* **2013**, *34*, 33–83. [CrossRef] [PubMed]

22. Beaudart, C.; Buckinx, F.; Rabenda, V.; Gillain, S.; Cavalier, E.; Slomian, J.; Petermans, J.; Reginster, J.Y.; Bruyère, O. The effects of vitamin D on skeletal muscle strength, muscle mass, and muscle power: A systematic review and meta-analysis of randomized controlled trials. *J. Clin. Endocrinol. Metab.* **2014**, *99*, 4336–4345. [CrossRef] [PubMed]

23. Owens, D.J.; Fraser, W.D.; Close, G.L. Vitamin D and the athlete: Emerging insights. *Eur. J. Sport Sci.* **2015**, *15*, 73–84. [CrossRef] [PubMed]

24. Owens, D.; Webber, D.; Impey, S.G.; Tang, J.; Donovan, T.F.; Fraser, W.D.; Morton, J.P.; Close, G.L. Vitamin D supplementation does not improve human skeletal muscle contractile properties in insufficient young males. *Eur. J. Appl. Physiol.* **2014**, *114*, 1309–1320. [CrossRef] [PubMed]

25. Välimäki, V.V.; Alfthan, H.; Lehmuskallio, E.; Löyttyniemi, E.; Sahi, T.; Stenman, U.H.; Suominen, H.; Välimäki, M.J. Vitamin D status as a determinant of peak bone mass in young Finnish men. *J. Clin. Endocrinol. Metab.* **2004**, *89*, 76–80. [CrossRef] [PubMed]

26. Lappe, J.; Cullen, D.; Haynatzki, G.; Recker, R.; Ahlf, R.; Thompson, K. Calcium and vitamin D supplementation decreases incidence of stress fractures in female navy recruits. *J. Bone Miner. Res.* **2008**, *23*, 741–749. [CrossRef] [PubMed]

27. Willis, K.S.; Peterson, N.J.; Larson-Meyer, D.E. Should we be concerned about the vitamin D status of athletes? *Int. J. Sport Nutr. Exerc. Metab.* **2008**, *18*, 204–224. [PubMed]

28. Newman, M.S.; Brandon, T.R.; Groves, M.N.; Gregory, W.L.; Kapur, S.; Zava, D.T. A Liquid chromatography/tandem mass spectrometry method for determination of 25-hydroxy vitamin D$_2$ and 25-hydroxy vitamin D$_3$ in dried blood spots: A potential adjunct to diabetes and cardiometabolic risk screening. *J. Diabetes Sci. Technol.* **2009**, *3*, 156–162. [CrossRef] [PubMed]

29. Heaney, R.P. Vitamin D in health and disease. *Clin. J. Am. Soc. Nephrol.* **2008**, *3*, 1535–1541. [CrossRef] [PubMed]

30. Holick, M.F. Vitamin D: A D-Lightful health perspective. *Nutr. Rev.* **2008**, *66*, S182–S194. [CrossRef] [PubMed]

31. Holick, M.F. The vitamin D epidemic and its health consequences. *J. Nutr.* **2005**, *135*, 2739S–2748S. [PubMed]

32. United States Department of Agriculture (USDA). National Nutrient Database for Standard Reference. Available online: http://www.ars.usda.gov/nutrientdata (accessed on 16 January 2016).

33. Constantini, N.W.; Arieli, R.; Chodick, G.; Dubnov-Raz, G. High prevalence of vitamin D insufficiency in athletes and dancers. *Clin. J. Sport Med.* **2010**, *20*, 368–371. [CrossRef] [PubMed]

34. Flueck, J.L.; Hartmann, K.; Strupler, M.; Perret, C. Vitamin D deficiency in Swiss elite wheelchair athletes. *Spinal Cord* **2016**. [CrossRef] [PubMed]

35. An, R.; Chiu, C.Y.; Zhang, Z.; Burd, N.A. Nutrient intake among US adults with disabilities. *J. Hum. Nutr. Diet.* **2015**, *28*, 465–475. [CrossRef] [PubMed]

36. Hamilton, B. Vitamin D and athletic performance: The potential role of muscle. *Asian J. Sports Med.* **2011**, *2*, 211–219. [CrossRef] [PubMed]

37. Goosey-Tolfrey, V.L.; Leicht, C.A. Field-based physiological testing of wheelchair athletes. *Sports Med.* **2013**, *43*, 77–91. [CrossRef] [PubMed]

38. Barbonetti, A.; Sperandio, A.; Micillo, A.; D'Andrea, S.; Pacca, F.; Felzani, G.; Francavilla, S.; Francavilla, F. Independent association of vitamin D with physical function in people with chronic spinal cord injury. *Arch. Phys. Med. Rehabil.* **2016**. [CrossRef] [PubMed]

39. Foo, L.H.; Zhang, Q.; Zhu, K.; Ma, G.; Hu, X.; Greenfield, H.; Fraser, D.R. Low vitamin D status has an adverse influence on bone mass, bone turnover, and muscle strength in Chinese adolescent girls. *J. Nutr.* **2009**, *139*, 1002–1007. [CrossRef] [PubMed]

40. Ward, K.A.; Das, G.; Berry, J.L.; Roberts, S.A.; Rawer, R.; Adams, J.E.; Mughal, Z. Vitamin D status and muscle function in post-menarchal adolescent girls. *J. Clin. Endocrinol. Metab.* **2009**, *94*, 559–563. [CrossRef] [PubMed]

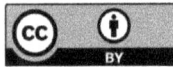

nutrients

Review

Dietary Recommendations for Cyclists during Altitude Training

Małgorzata Michalczyk [1], Miłosz Czuba [2,*], Grzegorz Zydek [1], Adam Zając [2] and Józef Langfort [1]

[1] Department of Nutrition & Supplementation, the Jerzy Kukuczka Academy of Physical Education in Katowice, Faculty of Physical Education, Mikołowska 72A, Katowice 40-065, Poland; m.michalczyk@awf.katowice.pl (M.M.); g.zydek@awf.katowice.pl (G.Z.); j.langfort@awf.katowice.pl (J.L.)

[2] Department of Sports Training, the Jerzy Kukuczka Academy of Physical Education in Katowice, Faculty of Physical Education, Mikołowska 72A, Katowice 40-065, Poland; a.zajac@awf.katowice.pl

* Correspondence: m.czuba@awf.katowice.pl; Tel.: +48-32-207-51-63

Received: 4 May 2016; Accepted: 12 June 2016; Published: 18 June 2016

Abstract: The concept of altitude or hypoxic training is a common practice in cycling. However, several strategies for training regimens have been proposed, like "live high, train high" (LH-TH), "live high, train low" (LH-TL) or "intermittent hypoxic training" (IHT). Each of them combines the effect of acclimatization and different training protocols that require specific nutrition. An appropriate nutrition strategy and adequate hydration can help athletes achieve their fitness and performance goals in this unfriendly environment. In this review, the physiological stress of altitude exposure and training will be discussed, with specific nutrition recommendations for athletes training under such conditions. However, there is little research about the nutrition demands of athletes who train at moderate altitude. Our review considers energetic demands and body mass or body composition changes due to altitude training, including respiratory and urinary water loss under these conditions. Carbohydrate intake recommendations and hydration status are discussed in detail, while iron storage and metabolism is also considered. Last, but not least the risk of increased oxidative stress under hypoxic conditions and antioxidant supplementation suggestions are presented.

Keywords: altitude training; hypoxia; nutrition; cycling

1. Altitude and Hypoxic Training

Cycling is an endurance sport discipline in which the athlete encounters significant training and competition loads and is often exposed to extreme environmental conditions. Therefore, in cycling numerous performance-enhancing nutritional and physiological aids are used to improve the efficiency of the cardio-respiratory system. One of the legal and natural performance enhancing methods used in cycling includes altitude training, which significantly improves the cardio-respiratory potential.

The concept of altitude or hypoxic training is a common practice in cycling not only for improving sport performance at sea level but also at moderate altitude [1–3]. Cyclists often compete in races (e.g., Tour de France, Giro d 'Italia and Vuelta a España) at moderate altitudes (from 1000 to 3000 m a.s.l); what requires a specific adaptation to a hypoxia environment. At these conditions increasing altitude and the consequent reduction of air density is beneficial from the aerodynamic perspective [4], but on the other hand acute hypoxia deteriorates exercise performance [5,6]. In particular, the maximal aerobic workload that can be sustained during exercise involving large muscle groups (e.g., cycling) is considerably lower in hypoxia compared with normoxia. The origin of human performance limitation in hypoxia is attributed to a decrease in VO_{2max}. Dempsey and Wagner [7] observed that each 1% decrement in SaO_2% below the 95% level approximates to a 1%–2% decrement in maximal oxygen uptake (VO_{2max}). Diminished VO_{2max} in hypoxia is accompanied by a lowered O_2 partial pressure in arterial blood (PaO$_2$), which reduces O$_2$ delivery to tissues and negatively affects muscle metabolism and contraction [8,9], leading to so-called peripheral fatigue.

After 40 years of altitude training, several strategies of such training regimens have been proposed, like "live high, train high" (LH-TH), "live high, train low" (LH-TL) or "intermittent hypoxic training" (IHT). Each of them combines the effect of acclimatization and different training protocols, which requires specific nutrition [3,10,11]. These nutrition concepts are due to different time of exposure to hypoxia at rest and different combinations of training under hypoxia and exposure to these conditions. In the LH-TH and LH-TL methods the acclimatization depends primarily on the iron status of the body, as well as on the maintenance of acid-base and energy equilibrium, what can significantly influence erythropoiesis. In the IHT method the dietary recommendations for athletes are less strict, and concentrate on pre-, mid- and post training unit nutrition. The specific demands of IHT relate to greater delivery of carbohydrates and better hydration.

According to the first mentioned method, athletes live and train in a natural hypobaric hypoxic environment at moderate altitude for a few weeks. Chronic exposure to moderate altitudes (2000–3000 m) improves oxygen transport capacity by enhancing erythropoietin secretion and the consequential increase in total hemoglobin mass [12,13]. This adaptive change improves maximal oxygen uptake (VO$_{2max}$) and enhances physical performance [14]. Chronic exposure to hypoxia may also reduce the energy cost of exercise at sea level by more efficient cellular metabolism [13]. The mechanism responsible for the decreased energy cost of exercise at sea level after altitude training is related to the increase of ATP production per molecule of O$_2$ utilized [15], and/or a decreased ATP breakdown during muscular contractions [16]. These adaptive changes can be seen already after 3 to 4 weeks of exposure to moderate altitudes, but the main factor limiting the effectiveness of the LH-TH concept is that many athletes cannot maintain the required training intensity while staying at an altitude for a longer period of time, and consequently decrease their level of endurance and technical abilities [11]. In response to this weak point of LH-TH method, the LH-TL method was proposed by Levine and Stray-Gundersen [10]. The LH-TL protocol allows athletes to "live high (2000–3000 m)" for altitude acclimatization while "training low" (below 1000 m) for the purpose of replicating low-altitude training intensity and oxygen flux, thereby inducing beneficial metabolic and neuromuscular adaptations [11]. In this method athletes can live in a natural hypobaric environment, or use special technology based on nitrogen dilution or oxygen filtration, to simulate physiological adaptive changes by creating a normobaric hypoxia environment [17,18]. However, the current results of research on the efficacy of the LH-TL method are controversial. There are some studies which support the performance enhancing effects of LH-TL training on endurance performance and aerobic capacity [1,17,18], and those that do not confirm such effects [19,20].

Recently, significant attention in sport sciences, as well as in competitive cycling has been given to IHT, which theoretically, may cause more pronounced adaptive changes in muscle tissues in comparison to traditional training under normoxic conditions [21]. In this method, athletes live under normoxic conditions and train in a natural hypobaric or simulated normobaric hypoxic environment. The improvement in sea-level performance and an increase in VO$_{2max}$ after IHT cannot be explained by changes in blood variables alone, but is also associated with non-hematological adaptive mechanisms [3]. The results of our previous studies [3,13] and other well-controlled studies [22,23] indicate that the improvements in aerobic capacity and endurance performance are caused by muscular and systemic adaptations, which are either absent or less developed after training under normoxia. These changes include increased skeletal muscle mitochondrial density, elevated capillary-to-fiber ratio, and increased fiber cross-sectional area [24,25].

Acute and chronic exposure to hypoxia induces serval metabolic consequences in the body and combined with physical exercise under hypoxic conditions presents an enormous challenge for athletes [26–29]. A significantly lower oxygen concentration in the blood, forces the body to produce the energy primarily from other substrates than in normoxia [30]. The athlete's body needs 2–3 weeks to adapt to the low level of oxygen, or else they feel fatigue, headaches and a decrease in appetite [31].

An appropriate nutrition strategy can help athletes achieve their fitness and performance goals in this unfriendly environment.

In this review the physiological stress of altitude exposure and training will be discussed, with specific nutrition recommendations for athletes training under such conditions [32]. However, there is little research about the nutrition demands of athletes who train at moderate altitude (2000–3000 m) [33,34]. Only in a few studies the authors assessed the nutritional habits of athletes training under hypoxia [31,32]. The data and nutrition recommendations in this review relate primarily to cycling, but they can be applied to other aerobic endurance sport disciplines such as the triathlon, Nordic skiing or the biathlon.

2. Body Composition during Altitude Training

There are some evidences that body composition of athletes exposed to altitude may be significantly changed after training. First of all, during acute exposure there may be a slight reduction in total body mass due to increased respiratory and urinary water loss. However, chronic oxygen deprivation observed initiates many physiological changes, with the most prominent changes being loss of body mass and protein stores especially at high altitudes (above 5000 m) [35], as well as fat content [36,37]. However, chronic exposure to moderate altitudes has also been reported to be an important factor in skeletal muscle atrophy [3,38]. Changes in fat and muscle mass in athletes may be a consequence of increased basal metabolic rate [39], as well as increased training loads [40] in combination with decreased caloric intake. However, Kayser [40] stated that people can prevent body composition changes by maintaining an adequate caloric intake, when they stay below 5000 m. This fact is very meaningful to athletes because altitude training camps are typically located at elevations from 2000 to 3000 m. Therefore proper nutrition strategy is a key factor determining the effectiveness of altitude training (LH-TH). For example Svedenhag *et al.* [41] and Gore *et al.* [42] reported insignificant differences in body composition in endurance athletes (runners and cyclists) after few weeks of altitude training conducted at moderate altitude (2000 and 2700 m). According to the authors, these athletes experienced this effect despite proper nutrition and adequate hydration.

On the other hand, Etheridge *et al.* [43] indicated that breathing normobaric hypoxic air (FiO_2 = 12%) in a post-absorptive state did not modify muscle protein synthesis at rest, but rather blunted the increase in protein synthesis induced by exercise. Acute hypoxia (intermittent hypoxic training) was also shown to inhibit muscle protein synthesis [44] primarily by inhibiting mechanistic target of rapamycin complex 1 (mTORC1) via activation of the AMP-activated protein kinase (AMPK) [45].

3. Hydration during Altitude Training

The maintenance of proper fluid balance during cycling training and competition is a key factor determining sport performance. However, creating a successful nutrition strategy, especially in a hot and humid environment is a great challenge. Proper hydration seems even more important for athletes training at altitude. Within the first few days at altitude, there is a tendency toward dehydration due to increased respiratory water loss by enhanced ventilation [26], and increased urinary water loss secondary to downregulation of the renin-angiotensin-aldosterone hormone mechanism [46]. Therefore, at moderate altitudes up to 4000 m respiratory water loss may be increased to 1900 mL per day in men [39] and 850 mL per day in women [47]. Besides, urinary water loss may increase up to 500 mL per day [48]. Cyclists during altitude training need to maintain fluid balance through regular hydration, in conjunction with daily workouts as well as during the restitution period of the day. Fluid intake in the form of water, isotonic carbo-electrolyte drinks, and juices should be increased even up to 7 L per day to insure adequate hydration [38,49]. Saris [38] reported that during the Tour de France mountain stages of the race, several cyclists drank more than 10 L of fluid per day. On the other hand cyclists must be cautious not to overhydrate their bodies, as this may hinder the adaptive processes and decrease performance. According to the authors of this review regular monitoring of body mass and urine osmolality during altitude training is absolutely necessary. This relates to the range altitude used for training purposes (2000–3500 m) and training loads. Athletes and coaches must take into consideration the fact that diuretic drinks like coffee and tea, as well as energy drinks with caffeine, can increase the diuretic effect but on the other hand can help increase the intensity of exercise and reduce the perception of fatigue.

The natural high altitude environment in addition to low oxygen concentration is often accompanied by low air temperature. To cope with these unfavourable conditions, and to maintain optimal body temperature, athletes must increase their basic metabolic rate to prevent hypothermia [31,39,40]. The acclimatization to hypoxia may induce different molecular adaptive responses. Decreased oxygen concentration under hypoxic conditions causes the muscle cells to accumulate large amounts of multi gene transcription protein like HIF-1 (Hypoxia Inducible Factor), which is known to regulate the synthesis of EPO (Erythropoietin) and VEGF (Vascular Endothelial Growth Factor), proteins required for erythropoiesis and angiogenesis. HIF-1 also regulates transcription oxidative pathway enzymes like pyruvate dehydrogenase (PHD), increases activity of lactate dehydrogenase (LDH), inhibits mitochondrial biogenesis, and activates the transcription of genes encoding glucose (GLUT1) and lactate MCT4 transporters as well as glycolytic enzymes. Because of lower oxygen tension, energy synthesis, both at rest and during exercise is mainly supplied by the glycolysis pathway. In short acute hypoxia exposure, lactate (La) concentration for submaximal exercise is higher than in normoxia, without peak La value changes. Gore *et al.* [50] showed an almost 10% improvement of efficiency during submaximal exercise after altitude acclimatization. Hoppler [51] indicated that training in hypoxia results in an increase of phosphofructokinase (PFK) mRNA, an enzyme which is involved in the glycolytic pathway, HIF-1mRNA, myoglobin mRNA and VEGF mRNA as well as mitochondria density [51,52] which may lead to increased oxidative metabolism. However, Lundby *et al.* [53] did not confirm that 8 weeks of exposure to hypoxia increases muscular VEGF m RNA expression and capillary density.

Energy expenditure in athletes who train and live at high altitude could be 2.5–3 times higher than at sea level [31,39,54]. However, during the Tour de France, elite cyclists recorded a 3.6–5.3 higher energy expenditure than the resting metabolic rate [34]. Duc found that energy cost during ski mountaineering racing at high altitude increases by approximately 15% [55]. Lack of critical macronutrients like carbohydrates, fats and proteins can enhance hypothermia, decrease metabolic rate, disturb optimal performance and decrease body mass [30,56]. It is believed that food intake may limit exercise performance in cycling events at altitude like the Tour de France, and the main factors limiting this performance include the ability to maintain energy balance and muscle mass [34].

Carbohydrates and protein must be delivered during high altitude physical activity to maintain body weight, replenish glycogen stores, and provide adequate protein to build and repair tissue [32,39]. Fat intake should also be sufficient to provide essential fatty acids and fat-soluble vitamins, and to contribute energy for weight maintenance. During an expedition to Mt. Everest Reynolds *et al.* [31] observed a significant decrease in energy consumption in climbers at increasing altitude but no changes in total carbohydrate, fat and protein consumption. Between climbers it is commonly assumed that there is a natural tendency to increase the consumption of carbohydrate intake at higher altitudes [57]. Carbohydrate consumption before exercise in hypoxia alleviates some of the negative symptoms of high altitude, like decreased appetite, less oxygen saturation and less ventilation [58]. Golja *et al.* [58] showed that carbohydrate consumption 40 min prior to acute hypoxia exposure increases ventilation and oxygen saturation, thereby oxygen delivery to the tissues.

Vitamin and mineral supplements are not needed for athletes at high altitude if adequate energy to maintain body weight is consumed from a variety of foods [59–61]. On the other hand, athletes who restrict energy intake due to lack of appetite, eliminating one or more food groups from their diet because of intolerance, or consuming unbalanced diets with low micronutrient density may require additional supplements.

4. Dietary Carbohydrate Intake Recommendations

Athletes training or competing at high altitude dramatically increase the rate of energy expenditure compared to normoxia [54]. It is critical to obtain sufficient energy intake to support total energy requirements including those for muscle activity but also for tissue maintenance and repair. Athletes training and competing under such conditions should make a conscious effort to eat at frequent intervals. It is important that athletes and their coaches understand how appropriate energy intake and energy substrate utilization enhance mental and muscle function. It is well known that the higher the exercise intensity, the greater the amount of carbohydrates used as fuel for working muscles. For athletes like road cyclists who train with extremely high loads for several hours a day, the most important source of energy for working muscles includes carbohydrates [62–65]. These substrates need less oxygen than fats and protein to be metabolized for ATP resynthesis. Consumption of adequate amounts of carbohydrates is especially important where cold stress and shivering occurs [66].

Athletes should provide the right amount of carbohydrates before, during and after exercise at high altitude [49]. It is absolutely clear that low pre-exercise muscle glycogen stores result in reduced exercise intensity [67]. A cyclist's diet during altitude training and competition should contain more than 60% CHO with one-third coming from liquid CHO due to reduced hunger at altitude [33]. Brouns [49] reported that during exhausting training sessions at altitude CHO intake increased up to 80% of consumed calories per day. It is suggested that cyclists consume 12–13 g of CHO per kg of body mass per day [33], what was confirmed by Rehrer's research [34], which presented values of 12.9 g CHO/kg of body mass per day in the Tour de France race. It is suggested that in endurance athletes like cyclists, inadequate carbohydrate consumption before and during training or competitions at high altitude may result in a reduction of exercise capacity. Adequate carbohydrate consumption before exercise increases glycogen stores in the muscle and liver. Eventually, insufficient intake of carbohydrates at high altitude may also cause low blood glucose levels, which leads to central fatigue [68]. Sufficient carbohydrate consumption after training or competition provides quick glycogen resynthesis, reduced muscle soreness and enhanced muscle recovery [63].

Athletes who train in hypoxia must consume carbohydrates to provide quickly and easily assimilated sources of energy for muscle and brain, between meals and during exercise, to optimize glycogen stores before and after exercise, and to enhance muscle recovery after physical activity. Additionally the carbohydrates must provide the energy to maintain blood glucose level between the main meal and during exercise. According to the International Society of Sports Nutrition, carbohydrates should provide 55%–65% of total caloric intake [69]. These authors indicate that while determining the optimal amount of carbohydrate intake the conversion to body weight should be applied. The carbohydrate intake recommendation for endurance trained athletes range from 7 to 10 g/kg of body mass per day [62]. Road cyclists after very intensive high altitude competition, which lasts from 4 to 6 h, should consume up to 12 g of carbohydrate per kilogram of body mass per day [62]. Some authors suggest that the average amount of carbohydrate which enhances cyclists performance is 300–400 g for meals consumed 3–4 h before exercise [70,71].

It is very difficult to deliver that quantity of carbohydrates in the form of traditional meals. Taking this into consideration, athletes consume a large part of their carbohydrates in the form of supplements, usually liquid form. In addition during high altitude training or competitions athletes suffer from appetite suppression and other gastrointestinal problems, which may contribute to inadequate energy intake [64]. They often suffer from weight loss, especially muscle mass, which negatively affects endurance and strength capacity [72]. The amount of consumed carbohydrates is not the only important factor determining the delivered energy during exercise. Attention should be paid to other factors like meal temperature, osmolality and exercise intensity, as these factors determine gastric empting and intestines absorption [64,73]. However, in order to calculate the individual carbohydrate recommendations for high altitude, other factors like gender, body weight and training status should also be considered [64].

Between regular meals or training sessions conducted at altitude, athletes should consume high-carbohydrate, nutrient-rich snacks, which are a good alternative energy supply [54]. All these recommendations should be adjusted to individual requirements of athletes. It is also important to choose recovery meals that contain various components besides carbohydrates. Several authors suggest that carbohydrates consumed with proteins after exercise aid glycogen resynthesis [74].

Road and off-road cyclists often modify their diets 1–2 days before competition, using the carbohydrate loading procedure to enhance muscle glycogen [63]. This procedure assumes that to achieve muscle glycogen super compensation, ingestion of 10 g of carbohydrate per kilogram of body mass per day is recommended [54]. It is critical for athletes to consume different kinds of carbohydrates. During and immediately after exercise, carbohydrate products with a high glycaemic index should be preferred. They can include glucose or disaccharides derived from liquid, semiliquid and solid foods, like sport drinks and fruit bars [64]. On the other hand, during main meals, athletes should consume rather complex low glycaemic carbohydrates, derived from solid foods like cereals and grains, breads, vegetables, fruits and legumes [64]. To optimize muscle glycogen resynthesis after training or competition, it is recommended that cyclists consume 1.37–1.72 g $CHO \cdot kg^{-1} \cdot h^{-1}$ [33] or 1.5 g/$kg^{-1} \cdot h^{-1}$ carbohydrates, for the first 4 h after exercise [62]. Post training and post competition meals should contain carbohydrate rich foods and fluids with a high and medium glycaemic index [62]. When less than 1 g of carbohydrates per kilogram per hour is ingested, the meal should also contain proteins to provide a higher rate of glycogen synthesis [74].

In addition to suitable calories and carbohydrate consumption, athletes who train under conditions of inadequate oxygen concentration should provide adequate amounts of B vitamins like folic acid, vitamin B_{12} and iron [60,75]. A healthy individually balanced diet should supply most of the needed macronutrients, which are necessary to produce haemoglobin, but otherwise some vitamin and mineral supplementation should be considered [69].

5. Antioxidants

Performing endurance training at high altitude requires an increased demand not only for energy but also for vitamins and minerals [76]. In the past decade or so, we have observed increased antioxidant supplementation in competitive athletes, especially in endurance sport disciplines, such as road cycling, long distance running and Nordic skiing [77–79]. However numerous controversies have risen about the benefits of antioxidant supplementation in athletes. Some authors argue that antioxidants can protect muscle cells against oxidative damage [77,80], while others argue the contrary [78,81–83]. Many authors suggest that vitamin and mineral supplementation should be considered by athletes before exposure to high altitude, because under those conditions muscle cells release a lot of free radicals which are highly reactive [28]. During typical cycling training at high altitudes, were hypoxia occurs, muscle cells release large amounts of reactive oxygen/nitrogen species (RONS), which can damage cell lipids, proteins and DNA structure causing cell dysfunction and, eventually, apoptosis [84–86]. Oxidative damage of polyunsaturated lipid membranes seems especially harmful, as it results in a decrease of membrane fluidity, compromised integrity, and inactivation of membrane bound protein receptors and enzymes [79,84].

If muscle cells produce large amounts of RONS, they can provide significant oxidative stress [85,87]. In essence oxidative stress presents an imbalance between production and degradation of free RONS [88,89]. Such conditions may lead to a physiological imbalance in cells and tissues and cause inflammation, overloading or even overtraining. However it is still unclear whether oxidative stress is harmful to athletes [82,86]. RONS play an important role in the regulation of the body's immune system, counteract tissue insulin resistance and cell signalling [90]. Researches generally confirm that in athletes oxidative stress can promote mitochondria biogenesis, cellular growth, proliferations and increased antioxidant enzymes gene expression [82,83]. During typical endurance training or competitions the primary source of RONS includes the mitochondrial respiratory chain, where almost 2% of all oxygen consumption is converted to damaging superoxide radicals [91]. A different source of

RONS includes xanthine oxidase reactions during ischemia/reperfusion—transient tissue hypoxia conditions, catecholamine auto oxidation and lactic acid reactions [79,92]. Scientists also discovered that especially haem proteins like haemoglobin or myoglobin in the Fenton reaction can generate highly reactive hydroxyl radicals, while during auto oxidation of those proteins superoxide radicals can be produced [90]. These states are very frequent during road cycling training in normoxia conditions, as a response to muscle damage [80,93]. These processes are even intensified in athletes training under hypoxia [85,87]. To protect against oxidative damage muscle cells contain complex endogenous cellular defence mechanisms [92]. There are several enzymes and small scavengers which are involved in converting or removal of RONS. Antioxidant enzymes like superoxide dismutase (SOD), glutathione peroxidase (GPX), catalase (CAT) or glutathione reductase (GR) form the first line of defence against free radicals [79,92]. The second line of defence includes small scavengers like vitamin E and vitamin A, located in the cell membrane [84] as well as glutathione and vitamin C located inside the cells [92].

Recently numerous research projects regarding antioxidant supplementation in athletes have been conducted [94,95]. Most authors used typical supplements like vitamin C, A and E [94,96] or their combinations [80,95,97]. Some authors confirm positive effects of antioxidants/vitamin C supplementation [98,99]. Maxwell and Aschton suggest that pre exercise vitamin C supplementation attenuates the level of exercise induced free radicals and reduces exercise induced muscle damage [98]. Bryant confirms that supplementation with 400 IU of vitamin E per kg of body mass is more effective than 1 g per day vitamin C supplementation or a combination of 1 g vitamin C per day plus 200 IU vitamin E per kg, to reduce lipid peroxidation level in trained cyclists at sea level [99]. However Purkayastha [100] suggests that in men 400 mg/day vitamin E supplementation prevented stress at moderate altitude (3700 m). On the other hand supplementation of 400 IU vitamin E per day, did not significantly affect markers of oxidative stress associated with increased energy expenditure at high altitude [101]. In recent years, growing evidence indicates that exercise-induced production of reactive oxygen species serves as a signal to promote the expression of numerous skeletal muscle proteins, including antioxidant enzymes, mitochondrial proteins, and heat shock proteins [102,103]. Furthermore, two recent reports indicate that antioxidant supplementation with high levels of vitamins E and C (*i.e.*, 16 times higher than the recommended dietary allowance for adults) can blunt the training adaptation to exercise under normoxia [79,83].

In another study, Bentley showed that acute supplementation of trained cyclists 4 h prior to an exercise trial with antioxidant pine bark extract increased maximal oxygen uptake and extended time to exhaustion [104]. Nieman used quercetin supplementation as a form of an antioxidant, and showed improved exercise performance and increased muscle mitochondrial biogenesis [105]. Most well-controlled studies report no attenuating or even negative effect of antioxidant supplementation on oxidative stress markers [79–83]. Some authors suggest that antioxidant supplementation may promote muscle damage and cause longer recovery [81,106].

Numerous recent research projects have concentrated on the beneficial biological effects of antioxidants contained in vegetables and fruits that can currently be identified and measured [107–109]. In contrast to antioxidant supplements, plant foods contain many different kinds of antioxidants, like vitamin E and C, carotenoids and other phytochemicals that can act as synergists [110,111].

Most researches have confirmed that cyclists who undertake very high training loads, either living and/or training at moderate to high altitudes, or who participate in ultra-endurance competitions have an antioxidant imbalance [85,87,112]. There are reports indicating that cyclists who train under intermittent hypoxia conditions show lower plasma antioxidant levels [85]. It seems that under such circumstances the athletes can benefit from natural antioxidant supplementation. Considering the present state of knowledge, it seems that the best natural source of antioxidants comes from a diet full of fresh vegetables, fruits and flavours [107,113]. A well balanced diet full of natural antioxidants can minimize the level of oxidative stress produced during high volume and high intensity training [114]. While training at altitude, athletes, should consume high amounts of different kinds of micellar lyophilized fruit like blueberry, acai berry, goy berry, red grapes, raspberry, orange, papaya, blackcurrant, cherry, kiwi, strawberry, red grapes, mango, melon, grapefruit and lemon [115,116]. Those fruits are rich in naturally occurring vitamin C, carotenes, polyphenols and many others phytochemicals [108,110,113]. A cyclist's diet should also contain large amounts of vegetables, especially lyophyilizate products, like tomato, carrot, spinach, beetroot, broccoli, parsley, avocado, which are naturally full of antioxidants, such as vitamin A, vitamin C, carotenes, glutathione, resveratrol and quercetin [105,108,109]. In additions to vegetables and fruit, it is suggested that endurance athletes also consume flavouring, especially cloves, cinnamon, oregano, curcumin seed, cumin seed, basil, curry powder, pepper, with many bioactive compounds like flavonoids and anthocyanins which may directly or through their metabolism affect the total antioxidant capacity of plasma and tissue [87,113,117].

6. Iron Storage

Apart from antioxidant vitamins and phytochemicals, minerals like copper, zinc, manganese, selenium and iron, which act as cofactors of antioxidant enzymes, are very important in an athlete's diet [92,114]. Iron status in particular should be at a high level before attempting altitude training. In addition to the previously mentioned role of iron in the production of red blood cells, it plays an important role in the antioxidant defence not only as an antioxidant microelement but also because appropriate supply of oxygen to the working muscles depends indirectly on the level of iron [60].

As a result of acclimatization to altitude due to an increase in erythropoiesis, a decline in iron storage in the blood is observed [118]. In studies conducted by Roberts and Smith [119] and Pauls *et al.* [118], a significant reduction in the concentration of ferritin in the blood at altitudes above 2000 m was observed. Low levels of ferritin and iron in the blood can impair the increase in haemoglobin concentration in athletes exposed to hypoxia. It should also be noted, that in early research with altitude training [120–123] scientists did not control the concentration of iron and ferritin in the blood. The lack of this data makes it difficult to explain the improvement of aerobic capacity of the blood after altitude training. This interpretation is supported by data obtained by Stray-Gundersen *et al.*, [27], which show an improvement in erythropoiesis at altitude in case of low concentration of ferritin in the blood. These authors also reported, a lack of changes in haematological variables during altitude training when serum ferritin was less than 30 ng·mL^{-1} in men and 20 ng·mL^{-1} in women. The results of these studies have provided evidence that the level of ferritin must be monitored regularly, before and during altitude training. Additionally, in many studies athletes were supplemented with iron (even up to 100 mg daily) during altitude training to prevent potential anaemia from occurring.

Due to the slow replenishment, iron deficit should be completed several months before high altitude training [28]. The best source of iron is red meat like beef, offal and seafood. Vegetarian cyclists to provide appropriate amounts of iron should consume higher amounts of soya beans, beans, and green vegetables like parsley, broccoli and sprout. Unfortunately, the iron of those products due to significant contents of fibre is poorly absorbable. Grains, seeds and nuts are a very good source of other minerals mentioned above.

7. Vitamin D

The identification of the vitamin D receptor in the heart and blood vessels raised a possibility of potential cardiovascular effects of vitamin D [124,125], and thereby most likely on aerobic exercise, which is known to induce cardiovascular changes associated with marked increases of aerobic power and endurance performance [126]. There is evidence that vitamin D causes vascular relaxation by suppressing the renin-angiotensin-aldosterone system [127,128] and improves cardiomyocyte contractility [129] that may create physiological conditions for more efficient skeletal muscle oxygenation. Moreover, some data indicate that vitamin D is necessary for maintenance of skeletal muscle structural integrity and function [130]. This study raises a question if vitamin D supplementation may take part in protection of skeletal muscle against atrophic changes seen under hypobaric hypoxia conditions [39,131]. Findings confirming the high prevalence of vitamin D deficiency in the general population, as well as in athletes [132], and a significant decrease of serum vitamin D level in alpinists after their return from mountaineering expeditions (14 days, 3200–3616 m above sea level) [133] suggests that vitamin D supplementation should be considered in athletes who stay at high altitude. Such an assumption is further supported by the fact that the conversion of 25(OH)D into1,25(OH)2D$_3$ within the kidney by the enzyme 1alfa-hydroxylase is O$_2$-dependent and hypoxic conditions induce enzyme inhibition [134].

At altitude the intensity of UV radiation increases, creating favorable conditions for vitamin D synthesis, but to take full advantage of these environmental conditions the athlete's body has to be exposed to sunlight. It seems logical that during the summer months, when light clothing is worn during training, vitamin D synthesis should be increased, as opposed to colder parts of the year, when the body is usually fully covered. Unfortunately there are no data regarding this topic.

8. Alkalizing Agents

Considering the course of adaptive changes to altitude training supplementation with alkalizing agents (beta-alanine and bicarbonate) seems unjustified. One of the main adaptive changes induced by hypoxia training includes the increased buffering of the blood and muscle tissues. One of the acute as well as chronic adaptive changes to hypoxia is hyperventilation, with the objective of maintaining vacuole PO$_2$ at a steady level. Do to altitude hyperventilation, an increased diffusion of vacuole CO$_2$ occurs what causes the so called respiratory alkalosis. This response may improve the buffering capacity of tissues through a decrease in pH and an increased excretion of bicarbonates through the kidneys. An increased buffering capacity can significantly improve high intensity exercise potential. This has been confirmed by research of Mizuno *et al.*, [135], in which the authors observed a 6% increase of buffering capacity in the gastrocnemius muscle, as well as a 17% increase in the time to exhaustion performed on a treadmill in elite Nordic skiers living at an altitude of 2100 m and training at 2700 m for 2 weeks. According to these training concepts, cyclists exposed to hypoxia improved their muscle buffering capacity by 18%, and afterwards improved their results significantly during a specific cycling test performed under normoxic conditions [1]. The mechanism responsible for increased buffering capacity of muscle tissues under conditions of hypoxia is not fully examined, yet most likely it may occur do to the buffering properties of phosphocreatine and the concentration of muscle proteins [135]. On the other hand the improvement of blood buffering capacity is related to the higher concentration of hemoglobin and bicarbonates [136].

9. Conclusions and Recommendations

Considering the above reviewed data, it is not easy to create specific nutrition recommendations for cyclists and other endurance athletes training at altitude. This stems from a lack of well-controlled research under these conditions in competitive athletes. Precise dietary recommendations are difficult because of the great range of altitude at which exercise and exposure take place, which varies from 2000 to 3500 m. Additionally, athletes use different volume and intensity of exercise, depending on their sports level and part of the season. The most important aspects of nutrition strategy for altitude training for competitive athletes include proper hydration and optimal energy balance. According to the authors, it is difficult to recommend a strictly defined intake of fluids, as it is dependent on several variables such as range of altitude, air temperature, humidity, and most of all, the entire training load. Thus fluid intake should be monitored on a daily basis through body mass measurement and urine osmolality. Several reports are available that indicate an intake of close to 10 L daily for cyclists undertaking heavy training loads at moderate altitude. Monitoring of fluid intake is also of great significance because of the threat of over hydration which has shown effects of decreased adaptation to hypoxia. Another important aspect of nutrition during altitude training includes increased energy intake through the consumption of greater amounts of CHO. One must also consider the fact that exposure to altitude suppresses hunger and appetite, what can lead to a negative energy balance.

A high carbohydrate diet is recommended for athletes exercising intensively at altitude with the upper daily range of CHO consumption close to 12 g/kg. A well-balanced diet with an increased caloric intake should provide a sufficient amount of all antioxidants, so we do not recommend additional supplements which could hinder the adaptive processes related to aerobic endurance. Antioxidant supplementation should be considered only when natural food sources such as fruits and vegetables are not available at altitude. One of the more significant elements of altitude nutrition relates to the monitoring of iron, for which intake needs to amount to at least 100 mg/day. A deficit of iron may disturb erythropoiesis. Despite the increased UVB radiation from sunlight, it is recommended to supplement athletes training at altitude with up to 4000 IU/day of vitamin D, especially in the winter months of the year.

The presented data clearly shows great deficits in research related to nutrition and dietary recommendations for competitive athletes training at altitude. General guidelines for altitude nutrition can be proposed, but specific recommendations require further, well controlled research.

Acknowledgments: The presented manuscript was supported by grants from Ministry of Science and Higher Education of Poland (N RSA3 04153) and National Science Centre, Poland (UMO-2013/09/B/NZ7/00726).

Conflicts of Interest: The authors declare no conflict of interest.

References

1. Gore, C.J.; Hahn, A.G.; Aughey, R.J.; Martin, D.T.; Ashenden, M.J.; Clark, S.A.; Garnham, A.P.; Roberts, A.D.; Slater, G.J.; McKenna, M.J. Live high: train low increases muscle buffer capacity and submaximal cycling efficiency. *Acta Physiol. Scand.* **2001**, *173*, 275–286. [CrossRef] [PubMed]
2. Green, H.J.; Roy, B.; Grant, S. Increases in submaximal cycling efficiency mediated by altitude acclimatization. *J. Appl. Physiol.* **2000**, *89*, 1189–1197. [PubMed]
3. Czuba, M.; Waskiewicz, Z.; Zajac, A.; Poprzecki, S.; Cholewa, J.; Roczniok, R. The effects of intermittent hypoxic training on aerobic capacity and endurance performance in cyclists. *J. Sports Sci. Med.* **2011**, *10*, 175–183. [PubMed]
4. Péronnet, F.; Thibault, G.; Cousineau, D.L. A theoretical analysis of the effect of altitude on running performance. *J. Appl. Physiol.* **1991**, *70*, 399–404. [PubMed]
5. Amann, M.; Eldridge, M.W.; Lovering, A.T.; Stickland, M.K.; Pegelow, D.F.; Dempsey, J.A. Arterial oxygenation influences central motor output and exercise performance via effects on peripheral locomotor muscle fatigue in humans. *J. Physiol.* **2006**, *575*, 937–952. [CrossRef] [PubMed]
6. Peltonen, J.E.; Rusko, H.K.; Rantamaki, J.; Sweins, K.; Nittymaki, S.; Vitasalo, J.T. Effects of oxygen fraction in inspired air on force production and electromyogram activity during ergometer rowing. *Eur. J. Appl. Physiol.* **1997**, *76*, 495–503. [CrossRef] [PubMed]
7. Dempsey, J.A.; Wagner, P.D. Exercise-induced arterial hypoxemia. *J. Appl. Physiol.* **1999**, *87*, 1997–2006. [PubMed]
8. Adams, R.P.; Welch, H.G. Oxygen uptake, acid-base status, and performance with varied inspired oxygen fractions. *J. Appl. Physiol.* **1980**, *49*, 863–868. [PubMed]
9. Hogan, M.C.; Richardson, R.S.; Haseler, L.J. Human muscle performance and PCr hydrolysis with varied inspired oxygen fraction: A ^{31}P-MRS study. *J. Appl. Physiol.* **1999**, *86*, 1367–1373. [PubMed]
10. Levine, B.D.; Stray-Gundersen, J. "Living high-training low": Effect of moderate-altitude acclimatization with low-altitude training on performance. *J. Appl. Physiol.* **1997**, *83*, 102–112. [PubMed]
11. Wilber, R.L.; Stray-Gundersen, J.; Levine, B.D. Effect of hypoxic "dose" on physiological responses and sea-level performance. *Med. Sci. Sports Exerc.* **2007**, *39*, 1590–1599. [CrossRef] [PubMed]
12. Bunn, H.F.; Poyton, R.O. Oxygen sensing and molecular adaptation to hypoxia. *Physiol. Rev.* **1996**, *76*, 839–885. [PubMed]
13. Czuba, M.; Maszczyk, A.; Gerasimuk, D.; Roczniok, R.; Fidos-Czuba, O.; Zając, A.; Gołaś, A.; Mostowik, A.; Langfort, J. The effects of hypobaric hypoxia on erythropoiesis, maximal oxygen uptake and energy cost of exercise in normoxia in elite biathletes. *J. Sports Sci. Med.* **2014**, *13*, 912–920. [PubMed]

14. Ferretti, G.; Kayser, B.; Schena, F.; Turner, D.L.; Hoppeler, H. Regulation of perfusive O_2 transport during exercise in humans: Effects of changes in haemoglobin concentration. *J. Physiol.* **1992**, *455*, 679–688. [CrossRef] [PubMed]

15. Hochachka, P.W.; Stanley, C.; Matheson, G.O.; McKenzie, D.C.; Allen, P.S.; Parkhouse, W.S. Metabolic and work efficiencies during exercise in Andean natives. *J. Appl. Physiol.* **1991**, *70*, 1720–1730. [PubMed]

16. Ponsot, E.; Dufour, S.P.; Zoll, J.; Doutrelau, S.; N'Guessan, B.; Geny, B.; Hoppeler, H.; Lampert, E.; Mettauer, B.; Ventura-Clapier, R.; *et al.* Exercise training in normobaric hypoxia in endurance runners. II. Improvement of mitochondrial properties in skeletal muscle. *J. Appl. Physiol.* **2006**, *100*, 1249–1257. [CrossRef] [PubMed]

17. Mattila, V.; Rusko, H. Effect of living high and training low on sea level performance in cyclists. *Med. Sci. Sports Exerc.* **1996**, *28*, 157. [CrossRef]

18. Roberts, A.D.; Clark, S.A.; Townsend, N.E.; Anderson, M.E.; Gore, C.; Hahn, A.G. Changes in performance, maximal oxygen uptake and maximal accumulated oxygen deficit after 5, 10 and 15 days of live high: train low altitude exposure. *Eur. J. Appl. Physiol.* **2003**, *88*, 390–395. [CrossRef] [PubMed]

19. Ashenden, M.J.; Gore, C.J.; Dobson, G.P.; Hahn, A.G. Simulated moderate altitude elevates serum erythropoietin but does not increase reticulocyte production in well-trained runners. *Eur. J. Appl. Physiol.* **2000**, *81*, 428–435. [CrossRef] [PubMed]

20. Hinckson, E.A.; Hopkins, W.G. Changes in running endurance performance following intermittent altitude exposure simulated with tents. *Eur. J Sport Sci.* **2005**, *5*, 15–24. [CrossRef]

21. Czuba, M.; Zając, A.; Maszczyk, A.; Roczniok, R.; Poprzęcki, S.; Garbaciak, W.; Zając, T. The effects of high intensity interval training in normobaric hypoxia on aerobic capacity in basketball players. *J. Hum. Kinet.* **2012**, *39*, 103–114. [CrossRef] [PubMed]

22. Dufour, S.P.; Ponsot, E.; Zoll, J.; Doutreleau, S.; Lonsdorfer-Wolf, E.; Geny, B.; Lampert, E.; Flück, M.; Hoppeler, H.; Billat, V.; *et al.* Exercise training in normobaric hypoxia in endurance runners. I. Improvements in aerobic performance capacity. *J. Appl. Physiol.* **2006**, *100*, 1238–1248. [CrossRef] [PubMed]

23. Zoll, J.; Ponsot, E.; Dufour, S.; Doutreleau, S.; Ventura-Clapier, R.; Vogt, M.; Hoppeler, H.; Richard, R.; Flück, M. Exercise training in normobaric hypoxia in endurance runners. III. Muscular adjustments of selected gene transcripts. *J. Appl. Physiol.* **2006**, *100*, 1258–1266. [CrossRef] [PubMed]

24. Desplanches, D.; Hoppeler, H. Effects of training in normoxia and normobaric hypoxia on human muscle ultrastructure. *Pflügers Arch. Eur. J. Physiol.* **1993**, *425*, 263–267. [CrossRef]

25. Vogt, M.; Puntschart, A.; Geiser, J.; Zuleger, C.; Billeter, R.; Hoppeler, H. Molecular adaptations in human skeletal muscle to endurance training under simulated hypoxic conditions. *J. Appl. Physiol.* **2001**, *91*, 173–182. [PubMed]

26. Kayser, B. Nutrition and energetics of exercise at altitude. Theory and possible practical implications. *Sports Med.* **1994**, *17*, 309–323. [CrossRef] [PubMed]

27. Stray-Gundersen, J.; Alexander, C.; Hochstein, A.; deLomos, D.; Levine, B.D. Failure of red cell volume to increase to altitude exposure in iron deficient runners. *Med. Sci. Sports Exerc.* **1992**, *24*, 90–98. [CrossRef]

28. Askew, E.W. Environmental and physical stress and nutrient requirements. *Am. J. Clin. Nutr.* **1995**, *61*, 631–637.

29. Clark, S.A.; Aughey, R.J.; Gore, C.J.; Hahn, A.G.; Townsend, N.E.; Kinsman, T.A. Effects of live high, train low hypoxic exposure on lactate metabolism in trained humans. *J. Appl. Physiol.* **2004**, *96*, 517–525. [CrossRef] [PubMed]

30. Zamboni, M.; Armellini, F.; Turcato, E.; Robbi, R.; Micciolo, R.; Todesco, T.; Mandragona, R.; Angelini, G.; Bosello, O. Effect of altitude on body composition during mountaineering expeditions: Interrelationships with changes in dietary habits. *Ann. Nutr. Metab.* **1996**, *40*, 315–324. [CrossRef] [PubMed]

31. Reynolds, R.D.; Lickteig, J.A.; Howard, M.P.; Deuster, P.A. Intakes of high fat and high carbohydrate foods by humans increased with exposure to increasing altitude during an expedition to Mt. Everest. *J. Nutr.* **1998**, *128*, 50–55. [PubMed]

32. Praz, C.; Granges, M.; Burtin, C.; Kayser, B. Nutritional behaviour and beliefs of ski-mountaineers: A semi-quantitative and qualitative study. *J. Int. Soc. Sports Nutr.* **2015**, *9*, 12–46. [CrossRef] [PubMed]

33. Saris, W.H.; van Erp-Baart, M.A.; Brouns, F.; Westerterp, K.R.; Ten Hoor, F. Study on food intake and energy expenditure during extreme sustained exercise: The tour de France. *Int. J. Sports Med.* **1989**, *10* (Suppl. 1), 26–31. [CrossRef] [PubMed]

34. Rehrer, N.J.; Hellemans, I.J.; Rolleston, A.K.; Rush, E.; Miller, B.F. Energy intake and expenditure during a 6-day cycling stage race. *Scand. J. Med. Sci. Sports* **2010**, *20*, 609–618. [CrossRef] [PubMed]

35. Macdonald, J.H.; Oliver, S.J.; Hillyer, K.; Sanders, S.; Smith, Z.; Williams, C.; Yates, D.; Ginnever, H.; Scanlon, E.; Roberts, E.; *et al.* Body composition at high altitude: A randomized placebo-controlled trial of dietary carbohydrate supplementation. *Am. J. Clin. Nutr.* **2009**, *90*, 1193–1202. [CrossRef] [PubMed]

36. Hoppeler, H.; Kleinert, E.; Schlegel, C.; Claassen, H.; Howald, H.; Kayar, S.R.; Cerretelli, P. Morphological adaptations of human skeletal muscle to chronic hypoxia. *Int. J. Sports Med.* **1990**, *11*, 3–9. [CrossRef] [PubMed]

37. MacDougall, J.D.; Green, H.J.; Sutton, J.R.; Coates, G.; Cymerman, A.; Young, P.; Houston, C.S. Operation Everest II: Structural adaptations in skeletal muscle in response to extreme simulated altitude. *Acta Physiol. Scand.* **1991**, *142*, 421–427. [CrossRef] [PubMed]

38. Bharadwaj, H.; Prasad, J.; Pramanik, S.N.; Krishnani, S.; Zachariah, T.; Chaudhary, K.L.; Sridharan, K.; Srivastava, K.K. Effect of prolonged exposure to high altitude on skeletal muscle of Indian soldiers. *Def. Sci. J.* **2000**, *50*, 167–176. [CrossRef]

39. Butterfield, G.E.; Gates, J.; Fleming, S.; Brooks, G.A.; Sutton, J.R.; Reeves, J.T. Increased energy intake minimizes weight loss in men at high altitude. *J. Appl. Physiol.* **1992**, *72*, 1741–1748. [PubMed]

40. Kayser, B. Nutrition and high altitude exposure. *Int. J. Sports Med.* **1992**, *13*, 129–132. [CrossRef] [PubMed]

41. Svedenhag, J.; Saltin, B.; Johansson, C.; Kaijser, L. Aerobic and anaerobic exercise capacities of elite middle-distance runners after two weeks of training at moderate altitude. *Scand. J. Med. Sci. Sports* **1991**, *1*, 205–214. [CrossRef]

42. Gore, C.J.; Hahn, A.; Rice, A.; Bourdon, P.; Lawrence, S.; Walsh, C.; Stanef, T.; Barnes, P.; Parisotto, R.; Martin, D.; *et al.* Altitude training at 2690 m does not increase total Haemoglobin mass or sea level $\dot{V}O_{2max}$ in world champion track cyclists. *J. Sci. Med. Sport* **1998**, *1*, 156–170. [CrossRef]

43. Etheridge, T.; Atherton, P.J.; Wilkinson, D.; Selby, A.; Rankin, D.; Webborn, N.; Smith, K.; Watt, P.W. Effects of hypoxia on muscle protein synthesis and anabolic signaling at rest and in response to acute resistance exercise. *Am. J. Physiol. Endocrinol. Metab.* **2011**, *301*, 697–702. [CrossRef] [PubMed]

44. Koumenis, C.; Wouters, B.G. "Translating" tumor hypoxia: Unfolded protein response (UPR)-dependent and UPR-independent pathways. *Mol. Cancer Res.* **2006**, *4*, 423–436. [CrossRef] [PubMed]

45. Liu, L.; Cash, T.P.; Jones, R.G.; Keith, B.; Thompson, C.B.; Simon, M.C. Hypoxia-induced energy stress regulates mRNA translation and cell growth. *Mol. Cell* **2006**, *21*, 521–531. [CrossRef] [PubMed]

46. Hogan, R.P.; Kotchen, T.A.; Boyd, A.E.; Hartley, L.H. Effect of altitude on renin-aldosterone system and metabolism of water and electrolytes. *J. Appl. Physiol.* **1973**, *35*, 385–390. [PubMed]

47. Mawson, J.T.; Braun, B.; Rock, P.; Moore, L.G.; Mazzeo, R.S.; Butterfield, G.E. Women at altitude: Energy requirement at 4300 m. *J. Appl. Physiol.* **2000**, *88*, 272–281. [PubMed]

48. Butterfield, G.E. Maintenance of body weight at altitude: In search of 500 kcal/day. In *Nutritional Needs in Cold and High-Altitude Environments: Applications for Personnel in Field Operations*; Marriott, B.M., Carlson, S.J., Eds.; National Academy Press: Washington, DC, USA, 1996; pp. 357–378.

49. Brouns, F.; Saris, W.H.; Stroecken, J.; Beckers, E.; Thijssen, R.; Rehrer, N.J.; ten Hoor, F. Eating, drinking, and cycling. A controlled Tour de France simulation study, Part I. *Int. J. Sports Med.* **1989**, *10* (Suppl. 1), 32–40. [CrossRef] [PubMed]

50. Gore, C.J.; Clark, S.A.; Saunders, P.U. Nonhematological mechanisms of improved sea-level performance after hypoxic exposure. *Med. Sci. Sports Exerc.* **2007**, *39*, 1600–1609. [CrossRef] [PubMed]

51. Hoppeler, H.; Vogt, M. Muscle tissue adaptations to hypoxia. *J. Exp. Biol.* **2001**, *204*, 3133–3139. [PubMed]

52. Hoppeler, H.; Vogt, M.; Weibel, E.R.; Flück, M. Response of skeletal muscle mitochondria to hypoxia. *Exp. Physiol.* **2003**, *88*, 109–119. [CrossRef] [PubMed]

53. Lundby, C.; Pilegaard, H.; Andersen, J.L.; van Hall, G.; Sander, M.; Calbet, J.A. Acclimatization to 4100 m does not change capillary density or mRNA expression of potential angiogenesis regulatory factors in human skeletal muscle. *J. Exp. Biol.* **2004**, *207*, 3865–3671. [CrossRef] [PubMed]

54. Praz, C.; Léger, B.; Kayser, B. Energy expenditure of extreme competitive mountaineering skiing. *Eur. J. Appl. Physiol.* **2014**, *114*, 2201–2211. [CrossRef] [PubMed]

55. Duc, S.; Cassirame, J.; Durand, F. Physiology of ski mountaineering racing. *Int. J. Sports Med.* **2011**, *32*, 856–863. [CrossRef] [PubMed]

56. Worme, J.D.; Lickteig, J.A.; Reynolds, R.D.; Deuster, P.A. Consumption of a dehydrated ration for 31 days at moderate altitudes: Energy intakes and physical performance. *J. Am. Diet. Assoc.* **1991**, *91*, 1543–1549. [PubMed]

57. Fulco, C.S.; Cymerman, A.; Pimental, N.A.; Young, A.J.; Maher, J.T. Anthropometric changes at high altitude. *Aviat. Space Environ. Med.* **1985**, *56*, 220–224. [PubMed]

58. Golja, P.; Flander, P.; Klemenc, M.; Maver, J.; Princi, T. Carbohydrate ingestion improves oxygen delivery in acute hypoxia. *High Alt. Med. Biol.* **2008**, *9*, 53–62. [CrossRef] [PubMed]

59. Singh, A.; Moses, F.M.; Deuster, P.A. Chronic multivitamin-mineral supplementation does not enhance physical performance. *Med. Sci. Sports Exerc.* **1992**, *24*, 726–732. [CrossRef] [PubMed]

60. Lukaski, H.C. Vitamin and mineral status: Effects on physical performance. *Nutrition* **2004**, *20*, 632–644. [CrossRef] [PubMed]

61. Fry, A.C.; Bloomer, R.J.; Falvo, M.J.; Moore, C.A.; Schilling, B.K.; Weiss, L.W. Effect of a liquid multivitamin/mineral supplement on anaerobic exercise performance. *Res. Sports Med.* **2006**, *14*, 53–64. [CrossRef] [PubMed]

62. Burke, L.M.; Hawley, J.A.; Wong, S.H.; Jeukendrup, A.E. Carbohydrates for training and competition. *J. Sports Sci.* **2011**, *29*, 17–27. [CrossRef] [PubMed]

63. Jeukendrup, A.E.; McLaughlin, J. Carbohydrate ingestion during exercise: Effects on performance, training adaptations and trainability of the gut. In *Sports Nutrition: More Than Just Calories—Triggers for Adaptation*; Maughan, R.J., Burke, L.M., Eds.; Karger AG: Basel, Switzerland, 2011; Volume 69, pp. 1–17.

64. Jeukendrup, A. A step towards personalized sports nutrition: Carbohydrate intake during exercise. *Sports Med.* **2014**, *44*, 25–33. [CrossRef] [PubMed]

65. Stellingwerff, T.; Cox, G.R. Systematic review: Carbohydrate supplementation on exercise performance or capacity of varying durations. *Appl. Physiol. Nutr. Metab.* **2014**, *39*, 998–1011. [CrossRef] [PubMed]

66. Febbraio, M.A. *Exercise at Climatic Extremes, in Nutrition in Sport*; Blackwell Science Ltd.: Oxford, UK, 2000.

67. Stellingwerff, T.; Maughan, R.J.; Burke, L.M. Nutrition for power sports: Middle-distance running, track cycling, rowing, canoeing/kayaking, and swimming. *J. Sports Sci.* **2011**, *29*, 79–89. [CrossRef] [PubMed]

68. Jeukendrup, A.E.; Jentjens, R.L.; Moseley, L. Nutritional considerations in triathlon. *Sports Med.* **2005**, *35*, 163–181. [CrossRef] [PubMed]

69. Kreider, R.B.; Wilborn, C.D.; Taylor, L.; Campbell, B.; Almada, A.L.; Collins, R.; Cooke, M.; Earnest, C.P.; Greenwood, M.; Kalman, D.S.; *et al.* ISSN exercise & sport nutrition review: Research & recommendations. *J. Int. Soc. Sports Nutr.* **2010**, *7*, 1–43.

70. Sherman, W.M.; Doyle, J.A.; Lamb, D.R.; Strauss, R.H. Dietary carbohydrate, muscle glycogen, and exercise performance during 7 day of training. *Am. J. Clin. Nutr.* **1993**, *57*, 27–31. [PubMed]

71. Wright, D.A.; Sherman, W.M.; Dernbach, A.R. Carbohydrate feedings before, during, or in combination improve cycling endurance performance. *J. Appl. Physiol.* **1991**, *71*, 1082–1088. [PubMed]

72. Hill, N.E.; Stacey, M.J.; Woods, D.R. Energy at high altitude. *J. R. Army Med. Corps* **2011**, *157*, 43–48. [CrossRef] [PubMed]

73. Brouns, F.; Beckers, E. Is the gut an athletic organ? Digestion, absorption and exercise. *Sports Med.* **1993**, *15*, 242–257. [CrossRef] [PubMed]

74. Beelen, M.; Burke, L.M.; Gibala, M.J.; van Loon, L.J.C. Nutritional strategies to promote postexercise recovery. *Int. J. Sport Nutr. Exerc. Metab.* **2010**, *20*, 515–532. [PubMed]

75. Peeling, P.; Blee, T.; Goodman, C.; Dawson, B.; Claydon, G.; Beilby, J.; Prins, A. Effect of iron injections on aerobic-exercise performance of iron-depleted female athletes. *Int. J. Sport Nutr. Exerc. Metab.* **2007**, *17*, 221–231. [PubMed]

76. Sridharan, K.; Ranganathan, S.; Mukherjee, A.K.; Kumria, M.L.; Vats, P. Vitamin status of high altitude (3660 m) acclimatized human subjects during consumption of tinned rations. *Wilderness Environ. Med.* **2004**, *15*, 95–101. [CrossRef]

77. Tauler, P.; Aguiló, A.; Gimeno, I.; Fuentespina, E.; Tur, J.A.; Pons, A. Response of blood cell antioxidant enzyme defences to antioxidant diet supplementation and to intense exercise. *Eur. J. Nutr.* **2006**, *45*, 187–195. [CrossRef] [PubMed]

78. Gomez-Cabrera, M.C.; Domenech, E.; Romagnoli, M.; Arduini, A.; Borras, C.; Pallardo, F.V.; Sastre, J.; Viña, J. Oral administration of vitamin C decreases muscle mitochondrial biogenesis and hampers training-induced adaptations in endurance performance. *Am. J. Clin. Nutr.* **2008**, *87*, 142–149. [PubMed]

79. Fisher-Wellman, K.; Bloomer, R.J. Acute exercise and oxidative stress: A 30 years history. *Dyn. Med.* **2009**, *13*, 1–25. [CrossRef] [PubMed]

80. Goldfarb, A.H.; McKenzie, M.J.; Bloomer, R.J. Gender comparisons of exercise-induced oxidative stress: Influence of antioxidant supplementation. *Appl. Physiol. Nutr. Metab.* **2007**, *32*, 1124–1131. [CrossRef] [PubMed]

81. Teixeira, V.H.; Valente, H.F.; Casal, S.I.; Marques, A.F.; Moreira, P.A. Antioxidants do not prevent postexercise peroxidation and may delay muscle recovery. *Med. Sci. Sports Exerc.* **2009**, *41*, 1752–1760. [CrossRef] [PubMed]

82. Peternelj, T.T.; Coombes, J.S. Antioxidant supplementation during exercise training: Beneficial or detrimental? *Sports Med.* **2011**, *41*, 1043–1069. [CrossRef] [PubMed]

83. Ristow, M.; Zarse, K.; Oberbach, A.; Klöting, N.; Birringer, M.; Kiehntopf, M.; Stumvoll, M.; Kahn, C.R.; Blüher, M. Antioxidants prevent health-promoting effects of physical exercise in humans. *Proc. Natl. Acad. Sci. USA* **2009**, *106*, 8665–8670. [CrossRef] [PubMed]

84. Clarkson, P.M.; Thompson, H.S. Antioxidants: What role do they play in physical activity and health? *Am. J. Clin. Nutr.* **2000**, *72*, 637–646.

85. Pialoux, V.; Mounier, R.; Rock, E.; Mazur, A.; Schmitt, L.; Richalet, J.P.; Robach, P.; Brugniaux, J.; Coudert, J.; Fellmann, N. Effects of the 'live high-train low' method on prooxidant/antioxidant balance on elite athletes. *Eur. J. Clin. Nutr.* **2009**, *63*, 756–762. [CrossRef] [PubMed]

86. Pialoux, V.; Brugniaux, J.V.; Rock, E.; Mazur, A.; Schmitt, L.; Richalet, J.P.; Robach, P.; Clottes, E.; Coudert, J.; Fellmann, N.; *et al.* Antioxidant status of elite athletes remains impaired 2 weeks after a simulated altitude training camp. *Eur. J. Nutr.* **2010**, *49*, 285–292. [CrossRef] [PubMed]

87. García-Flores, L.A.; Medina, S.; Cejuela, R.; Martínez-Sanz, J.M.; Oger, C.; Galano, J.M.; Durand, T.; Casas-Pina, T.; Martínez-Hernández, P.; Ferreres, F.; *et al.* Assessment oxidative stress biomarkers—Neuroprostanes and dihomo-isoprostanes—In elite triathletes urine after two weeks of moderate altitude training. *Free Radic. Res.* **2015**, *27*, 1–24. [CrossRef] [PubMed]

88. Pingitore, A.; Lima, G.P.; Mastorci, F.; Quinones, A.; Iervasi, G.; Vassalle, C. Exercise and oxidative stress: Potential effects of antioxidant dietary strategies in sports. *Nutrition* **2015**, *31*, 916–922. [CrossRef] [PubMed]

89. Valko, M.; Leibfritz, D.; Moncol, J.; Cronin, M.T.; Mazur, M.; Telser, J. Free radicals and antioxidants in normal physiological functions and human disease. *Int. J. Biochem. Cell Biol.* **2007**, *39*, 44–84. [CrossRef] [PubMed]

90. Vollaard, N.B.; Shearman, J.P.; Cooper, C.E. Exercise-induced oxidative stress: Myths, realities and physiological relevance. *Sports Med.* **2005**, *35*, 1045–1062. [CrossRef] [PubMed]

91. Boveris, A.; Oshino, N.; Chance, B. The cellular production of hydrogen peroxide. *Biochem. J.* **1972**, *128*, 617–630. [CrossRef] [PubMed]

92. Powers, S.K.; DeRuisseau, K.C.; Quindry, J.; Hamilton, K.L. Dietary antioxidants and exercise. *J. Sports Sci.* **2004**, *22*, 81–94. [CrossRef] [PubMed]

93. Michalczyk, M.; Poprzęcki, S.; Czuba, M.; Zydek, G.; Jagsz, S.; Sadowska-Krępa, E.; Zając, A. Blood antioxidant status in road cyclists during progressive (VO_{2max}) and constant cyclist intensity test (MLSS). *J. Sports Med. Phys. Fit.* **2015**, *55*, 855–864.

94. Sacheck, J.M.; Milbury, P.E.; Cannon, J.G.; Roubenoff, R.; Blumberg, J.B. Effect of vitamin E and eccentric exercise on selected biomarkers of oxidative stress in young and elderly men. *Free Radic. Biol. Med.* **2003**, *34*, 1575–1588. [CrossRef]

95. Bloomer, R.J.; Goldfarb, A.H.; McKenzie, M.J. Oxidative stress response to aerobic exercise: Comparison of antioxidant supplements. *Med. Sci. Sports Exerc.* **2006**, *38*, 1098–1105. [CrossRef] [PubMed]

96. Nakhostin-Roohi, B.; Babaei, P.; Rahmani-Nia, F.; Bohlooli, S. Effect of vitamin C supplementation on lipid peroxidation, muscle damage and inflammation after 30-min exercise at 75% VO_2max. *J. Sports Med. Phys. Fit.* **2008**, *48*, 217–224.

97. Rokitzki, L.; Logemann, E.; Sagredos, A.N.; Murphy, M.; Wetzel-Roth, W.; Keul, J. Lipid peroxidation and antioxidative vitamins under extreme endurance stress. *Acta Physiol. Scand.* **1994**, *151*, 149–158. [CrossRef] [PubMed]

98. Maxwell, S.R.; Jakeman, P.; Thomason, H.; Leguen, C.; Thorpe, G.H. Changes in plasma antioxidant status during eccentric exercise and the effect of vitamin supplementation. *Free Radic. Res. Commun.* **1993**, *19*, 191–202. [CrossRef] [PubMed]
99. Bryant, R.J.; Ryder, J.; Martino, P.; Kim, J.; Craig, B.W. Effects of vitamin E and C supplementation either alone or in combination on exercise-induced lipid peroxidation in trained cyclists. *J. Strength Cond. Res.* **2003**, *17*, 792–800. [CrossRef] [PubMed]
100. Purkayastha, S.S.; Sharma, R.P.; Ilavazhagan, G.; Sridharan, K.; Ranganathan, S.; Selvamurthy, W. Effect of vitamin C and E in modulating peripheral vascular response to local cold stimulus in man at high altitude. *Jpn. J. Physiol.* **1999**, *49*, 159–167. [CrossRef] [PubMed]
101. Subudhi, A.W.; Jacobs, K.A.; Hagobian, T.A.; Fattor, J.A.; Fulco, C.S.; Muza, S.R.; Rock, P.B.; Hoffman, A.R.; Cymerman, A.; Friedlander, A.L. Antioxidant supplementation does not attenuate oxidative stress at high altitude. *Aviat. Space Environ. Med.* **2004**, *75*, 881–888. [PubMed]
102. Powers, S.K.; Jackson, M.J. Exercise-induced oxidative stress: Cellular mechanisms and impact on muscle force production. *Physiol. Rev.* **2008**, *88*, 1243–1276. [CrossRef] [PubMed]
103. Sen, C.K. Antioxidants in exercise nutrition. *Sports Med.* **2001**, *31*, 891–908. [CrossRef] [PubMed]
104. Bentley, D.J.; Dank, S.; Coupland, R.; Midgley, A.; Spence, I. Acute antioxidant supplementation improves endurance performance in trained athletes. *Res. Sports Med.* **2012**, *20*, 1–12. [PubMed]
105. Nieman, D.C.; Williams, A.S.; Shanely, R.A.; Jin, F.; McAnulty, S.R.; Triplett, N.T.; Austin, M.D.; Henson, D.A. Quercetin's influence on exercise performance and muscle mitochondrial biogenesis. *Med. Sci. Sports Exerc.* **2010**, *42*, 338–345. [CrossRef] [PubMed]
106. Dawson, B.; Henry, G.J.; Goodman, C.; Gillam, I.; Beilby, J.R.; Ching, S.; Fabian, V.; Dasig, D.; Morling, P.; Kakulus, B.A. Effect of vitamin C and E supplementation on biochemical and ultrastructural indices of muscle damage after a 21 km run. *Int. J. Sports Med.* **2002**, *23*, 10–15. [CrossRef] [PubMed]
107. Chun, O.K.; Kim, D.O.; Smith, N.L.; Schroeder, D.; Han, J.T.; Lee, C.Y. Daily consumption of phenolics and total antioxidant capacity from fruit and vegetables in the American diet. *J. Sci. Food Agric.* **2005**, *85*, 1715–1724. [CrossRef]
108. Mangels, A.; Holden, J.; Beecher, G.; Forman, M.; Lanza, E. Carotenoid content of fruits and vegetables: An evaluation of analytic data. *J. Am. Diet. Assoc.* **1993**, *93*, 284–296. [CrossRef]
109. Gahler, S.; Otto, K.; Böhm, V. Alterations of vitamin C, total phenolics, and antioxidant capacity as affected by processing tomatoes to different products. *J. Agric. Food Chem.* **2003**, *51*, 7962–7968. [CrossRef] [PubMed]
110. Baur, J.A.; Sinclair, D.A. Therapeutic potential of resveratrol: The *in vivo* evidence. *Nat. Rev. Drug Discov.* **2006**, *5*, 493–506. [CrossRef] [PubMed]
111. George, T.W.; Waroonphan, S.; Niwat, C.; Gordon, M.H.; Lovegrove, J.A. Effects of acute consumption of a fruit and vegetable purée-based drink on vasodilation and oxidative status. *Br. J. Nutr.* **2013**, *109*, 1442–1452. [CrossRef] [PubMed]
112. Pialoux, V.; Mounier, R.; Ponsot, E.; Rock, E.; Mazur, A.; Dufour, S.; Richard, R.; Richalet, J.P.; Coudert, J.; Fellmann, N. Effects of exercise and training in hypoxia on antioxidant/pro-oxidant balance. *Eur. J. Clin. Nutr.* **2006**, *60*, 1345–1354. [CrossRef] [PubMed]
113. United States Department of Agriculture. *Agricultural Research Service. Database for the Flavonoid Content of Selected Foods*; USDA: Washington, DC, USA, 2003.
114. Palazzetti, S.; Rousseau, A.S.; Richard, M.J.; Favier, A.; Margaritis, I. Antioxidant supplementation preserves antioxidant response in physical training and low antioxidant intake. *Br. J. Nutr.* **2004**, *91*, 91–100. [CrossRef] [PubMed]
115. McAnulty, L.S.; Nieman, D.C.; Dumke, C.L.; Shooter, L.A.; Henson, D.A.; Utter, A.C.; Milne, G.; McAnulty, S.R. Effect of blueberry ingestion on natural killer cell counts, oxidative stress, and inflammation prior to and after 2.5 h of running. *Appl. Physiol. Nutr. Metab.* **2011**, *36*, 976–984. [CrossRef] [PubMed]
116. Bowtell, J.L.; Sumners, D.P.; Dyer, A.; Fox, P.; Mileva, K.N. Montgomery cherry juice reduces muscle damage caused by intensive strength exercise. *Med. Sci. Sports Exerc.* **2010**, *43*, 1544–1551. [CrossRef] [PubMed]
117. Lotito, S.B.; Frei, B. Consumption of flavonoid-rich foods and increased plasma antioxidant capacity in humans: Cause, consequence, or epiphenomenon? *Free Radic. Biol. Med.* **2006**, *41*, 1727–1746. [CrossRef] [PubMed]
118. Pauls, D.W.; van Duijnhoven, H.; Stray-Gundersen, J. Iron insufficient erythropoiesis at altitude-speed skating. *Med. Sci. Sports Exerc.* **2002**, *34*, 252S. [CrossRef]

119. Roberts, D.; Smith, D.J. Training at moderate altitude: Iron status of elite male swimmers. *J. Lab. Clin. Med.* **1992**, *120*, 387–391. [PubMed]
120. Daniels, J.; Oldridge, N. The effects of alternate exposure to altitude and sea level on world-class middle distance runners. *Med. Sci. Sports* **1970**, *2*, 107–112. [CrossRef] [PubMed]
121. Adams, W.C.; Bernauer, E.M.; Dill, D.B.; Bomar, J.B. Effects of equivalent sea level and altitude training on VO_{2max} and running performance. *J. Appl. Physiol.* **1975**, *39*, 262–266. [PubMed]
122. Dill, D.B.; Adams, W. Maximal oxygen uptake at sea level and at 3090-m altitude in high school champion runners. *J. Appl. Physiol.* **1971**, *3*, 854–859.
123. Terrados, N.; Melichna, J.; Sylvén, C.; Jansson, E.; Kaijser, L. Effects of training at simulated altitude on performance and muscle metabolic capacity in competitive road cyclists. *Eur. J. Appl. Physiol.* **1988**, *57*, 203–209. [CrossRef]
124. Walters, M.R.; Wicker, D.C; Riggle, P.C. 1,25-Dihydroxyvitamin D3 receptors identified in the rat heart. *J. Mol. Cell Cardiol.* **1986**, *18*, 67–72. [CrossRef]
125. Merke, J.; Hofmann, W.; Goldschmidt, D.; Ritz, E. Demonstration of 1,25(OH)2 vitamin D3 receptors and actions in vascular smooth muscle cells *in vitro. Calcif. Tissue Int.* **1987**, *41*, 112–114. [CrossRef] [PubMed]
126. Hellsten, Y.; Nyberg, M. Cardiovascular adaptations to exercise training. *Compr. Physiol.* **2015**, *6*, 1–32. [PubMed]
127. Wacker, M.; Holick, M.F. Vitamin D—Effect on skeletal and extra skeletal health and the need for supplementation. *Nutrients* **2013**, *5*, 111–148. [CrossRef] [PubMed]
128. Li, Y.C.; Qiao, G.; Uskokovic, M.; Xiang, W.; Zheng, W.; Kong, J. Vitamin D: A negative endocrine regulation of the renin-angiotensis system and blood pressure. *J. Steroid Biochem. Mol. Biol.* **2004**, *89–90*, 387–392. [CrossRef] [PubMed]
129. Reid, I.R.; Bolland, M.J. Role of vitamin D deficiency in cardiovascular disease. *Heart* **2012**, *98*, 609–614. [CrossRef] [PubMed]
130. Polly, P.; Tan, T.C. The role of vitamin D in skeletal and cardiac muscle function. *Front. Physiol.* **2014**, *16*, 145. [CrossRef] [PubMed]
131. Magalhaes, J.; Ascensao, A.; Soares, J.M.; Ferreira, R.; Neuparth, M.J.; Marques, F.; Duarte, J.A. Acute and severe hypobaric hypoxia increases oxidative stress and impairs mitochondrial function in mouse skeletal muscle. *J. Appl. Physiol.* **2005**, *99*, 1247–1253. [CrossRef] [PubMed]
132. Williams, S.; Heuberger, R. Outcoms of vitamin D supplementation in adults who are deficient on critically Ill: A review of the literature. *Am. J. Ther.* **2015**. [CrossRef] [PubMed]
133. Kasprzak, Z.; Śliwocka, E.; Henning, K.; Pilaczyńska-Szczesniak, Ł.; Huta-Osiecka, A.; Nowak, A. Vitamin D, Iron metabolism, and diet in alpinists during a 2-week high-altitude climb. *High Alt. Med. Biol.* **2015**, *16*, 230–235. [CrossRef] [PubMed]
134. Kawashima, H.; Kurokawa, K. Metabolism and sites of action of vitamin D in the kidney. *Kidney Int.* **1986**, *29*, 98–107. [CrossRef] [PubMed]
135. Mizuno, M.; Juel, C.; Bro-Rasmussen, T.; Mygind, E.; Schibye, B.; Rasmussen, B.; Saltin, B. Limb skeletal muscle adaptation in athletes after training at altitude. *J. Appl. Physiol.* **1990**, *68*, 496–502. [PubMed]
136. Nummela, A.; Rusko, H. Acclimatization to altitude and normoxic training improve 400-m running performance at sea level. *J. Sports Sci.* **2000**, *18*, 411–419. [CrossRef] [PubMed]

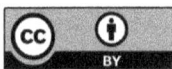

nutrients

MDPI

Article

Substrate Utilization and Cycling Performance Following Palatinose™ Ingestion: A Randomized, Double-Blind, Controlled Trial

Daniel König [1,*], Denise Zdzieblik [1], Anja Holz [2], Stephan Theis [2] and Albert Gollhofer [1]

[1] Section for Nutrition and Sports, Department of Sports and Sports Science, University of Freiburg, Schwarzwaldstrasse 175, Freiburg 79117, Germany; Denise.Zdzieblik@sport.uni-freiburg.de (D.Z.); AG@sport.uni-freiburg.de (A.G.)

[2] BENEO-Institute, Wormserstrasse 11, Obrigheim 67283, Germany; Anja.Holz@beneo.com (A.H.); Stephan.Theis@beneo.com (S.T.)

* Correspondence: Daniel.Koenig@sport.uni-freiburg.de; Tel.: +49-761-203-4542

Received: 1 May 2016; Accepted: 16 June 2016; Published: 23 June 2016

Abstract: (1) Objective: To compare the effects of isomaltulose (Palatinose™, PSE) vs. maltodextrin (MDX) ingestion on substrate utilization during endurance exercise and subsequent time trial performance; (2) Methods: 20 male athletes performed two experimental trials with ingestion of either 75 g PSE or MDX 45 min before the start of exercise. The exercise protocol consisted of 90 min cycling (60% VO_2max) followed by a time trial; (3) Results: Time trial finishing time (-2.7%, 90% CI: $\pm3.0\%$, 89% likely beneficial; $p = 0.147$) and power output during the final 5 min ($+4.6\%$, 90% CI: $\pm4.0\%$, 93% likely beneficial; $p = 0.053$) were improved with PSE compared with MDX. The blood glucose profile differed between trials ($p = 0.013$) with PSE resulting in lower glycemia during rest (95%–99% likelihood) and higher blood glucose concentrations during exercise (63%–86% likelihood). In comparison to MDX, fat oxidation was higher (88%–99% likelihood; $p = 0.005$) and carbohydrate oxidation was lower following PSE intake (85%–96% likelihood; $p = 0.002$). (4) Conclusion: PSE maintained a more stable blood glucose profile and higher fat oxidation during exercise which resulted in improved cycling performance compared with MDX. These results could be explained by the slower availability and the low-glycemic properties of Palatinose™ allowing a greater reliance on fat oxidation and sparing of glycogen during the initial endurance exercise.

Keywords: isomaltulose; athletic performance; fat oxidation; glycemic index; endurance

1. Introduction

Carbohydrates and fats are the most important energy sources during exercise [1–4]. It is well established that both a high carbohydrate diet before exercise as well as carbohydrate (CHO) ingestion during prolonged endurance exercise significantly improve endurance performance. However, for endurance athletes, there are several situations in training and competition in which high carbohydrate oxidation rates may not be desirable. These situations comprise phases of basic training in which fat metabolism should be improved or segments in endurance competitions (e.g., road cycling) in which the intensity is in the aerobic range and carbohydrate stores could be spared.

The human body has a distinct metabolic flexibility to switch between fat and carbohydrate utilization [3,5]. A major regulatory factor for substrate utilization is the presence or relative preponderance of one macronutrient over the other. Another important possibility of modulating substrate utilization consists in the modulation of the glycemic index (GI) of foods in the diet.

In recent years, the role of CHO in sports nutrition has been studied with respect to the GI. The GI provides a method of classifying foods based on their postprandial blood glucose response compared to a reference (i.e., white bread or glucose). At a given quantity, foods with a low GI result in lower postprandial blood glucose and generally also in a lower insulin response compared with high GI foods [6]. Insulin is the strongest hormone in suppressing fat oxidation. It has been shown that the GI of a meal has a significant effect on the postprandial fuel metabolism, both under resting conditions and during exercise [7,8]. Most investigations have found that the consumption of a low glycemic meal prior to physical exercise increased fat oxidation during endurance exercise compared with a higher glycemic meal [9–13]. Therefore, there is a rationale to consider the GI in the athlete's diet as well as in consumed CHO before and during exercise since increased fat oxidation could promote endurance stamina and glycogen sparing in liver and skeletal muscles [14,15].

Commercial sports drinks most often contain high GI carbohydrates like for instance maltodextrin where the glucose monomers are linked by rapidly digestible α-1,4-glycosidic bonds. Isomaltulose (Palatinose™) is a disaccharide with glucose and fructose linked by an α-1,6-glycosidic bond. The low GI of Palatinose™ of 32 [16] results from the slow hydrolysis of the α-1,6-glycosidic bond by the sucrose-isomaltase complex situated on the brush border membrane of the small intestinal cells [17]. Therefore, the rate of absorption of Palatinose™ is rather slow. Nevertheless, after hydrolysis, glucose and fructose are efficiently taken up in the small intestine, and it has been shown that Palatinose™ is a fully digestible carbohydrate [18].

The aim of the present investigation was to analyze the influence of isomaltulose (Palatinose™) vs. maltodextrin ingestion on substrate utilization during endurance exercise and subsequent time trial performance in trained cyclists. The hypothesis was that isomaltulose ingestion before exercise would favor fat oxidation during the initial endurance exercise leading to glycogen sparing in the muscle and liver. The spared glycogen would then be available for improved performance during the time trial.

2. Materials and Methods

2.1. Subjects

Twenty male athletes participated in this study (age 29 ± 3 years; weight 75.6 ± 1.1 kg; height 183 ± 1.1 cm; VO_2max 61.3 ± 1 mL/kg/min). Subjects were eligible if they were healthy experienced endurance cyclists (VO_2max > 55 mL/kg/min) having participated in previous tests on cycling ergometers with time trial events. All subjects completed a comprehensive medical examination and routine blood testing. Written informed consent was given by all subjects and the study protocol was approved by the ethical committee of the University of Freiburg. The exercise tests was performed at the Cycling Lab (Radlabor) Freiburg.

2.2. Design

The study employed a randomized, double-blind, controlled cross-over design. Each subject attended the laboratory on 4 occasions (2 preliminary sessions followed by 2 experimental trials). During the first preliminary session, the individual VO_2max was determined using a ramp test (cycling 3 min at 100 W and 3 min at 150 W, then increasing 10 W/10 s until exhaustion). During the second preliminary session, subjects performed a pre-test with a commercial sports beverage for better familiarization with the exercise protocol (conditions were identical to that used in the experimental trials described later). The implementation of such a familiarization has been shown to increase the reliability of subsequent tests [19].

During the remaining two test sessions, subjects performed the exercise protocol following ingestion of 750 mL of a beverage containing either 75 g isomaltulose (Palatinose™, PSE) or maltodextrin (MDX) (10% *w*/*v*). Both drinks were of comparable sweetness and identical in terms of taste and appearance. After an overnight fast, the different carbohydrate drinks were ingested in randomized order 45 min prior to the start of the exercise protocol. Randomization as well as the preparation of the different carbohydrate drinks was carried out by a person not actively involved in the conduct of the study. The exercise protocol commenced with 90 min of endurance exercise (cycling at the individual 60% VO_2max as determined during the first preliminary session). After the endurance exercise, a time trial test followed immediately; the test was finished when a workload of 6.5 kJ/kg bodyweight was achieved. Subjects were instructed to finish the test as fast as possible. All exercise protocols were performed on the same day of the week (i.e., at least 1 week apart) and at the same time of the day in order to minimize effects of circadian variation. All testing was done using the same cycle ergometer.

In the evenings before the tests, subjects ingested a standardized supper at 7 pm consisting of a commercially available pasta meal (670 kcal, 21.5 g protein, 61.5 g carbohydrate, 38.5 g fat). Afterwards, they were only allowed to consume water or unsweetened tea until the beginning of the test sessions. During their participation in the study, subjects maintained a constant duration and intensity of training.

2.3. Parameters

The primary outcome parameter in this study was the time needed to finish the time trial. Secondary outcome parameters comprised the power output during the final 5 min of the time trial as well as the profiles of several physiological parameters including blood glucose and lactate concentrations, changes in substrate oxidation, and heart rate.

Capillary blood samples were drawn at −45 min (i.e., before ingestion of the drinks), −30, −15 and 0 min (i.e., immediately before the start of exercise) as well as after 15, 30, 45, 60, 75, and 90 min of endurance exercise and upon completion of the time trial. Blood glucose and lactate concentrations were determined enzymatically with ESAT 6660 (Medingen, Germany). Mean oxygen uptake (VO_2) and carbon dioxide production (VCO_2) were determined over 3-min intervals at −45, −30, −15, 0, 15, 30, 45, 60, 75, and 90 min using ZAN 600 CPET (nSpire Health Care, Oberthulba, Germany). The ratio of carbon dioxide production to oxygen consumption (respiratory quotient, RQ) was calculated and energy expenditure, carbohydrate and fat oxidation were determined according the equation of Weir [20]. Heart rate was recorded throughout the protocol (Polar Electro GmbH, Buettelborn, Germany).

2.4. Statistical Methods

Data were analyzed using the probabilistic magnitude-based inference approach as recommended for studies in sports medicine and exercise sciences. A published spreadsheet [21], designed to examine post-only crossover trials, was used to determine the mechanistic and clinical significance between conditions based on guidelines by Hopkins [22]. Analysis was done using Microsoft Excel version 2010 (Microsoft, Redmond, WA, USA).

Physiological outcomes were described by mechanistic inferences. The magnitude of the effect was tested for substantiveness against the standardized (Cohen) change of 0.2 times the between-athlete standard deviation for the reference condition (i.e., the maltodextrin trial). Interpretation of the magnitude of the effect was based on Cohen's effect size (ES) scores of standardized differences and classified according to the following modified system: trivial (0–0.2), small (0.2–0.6), moderate (0.6–1.2), large (1.2–2.0), and very large (>2.0) [22].

Performance data were described by clinical inferences. The threshold for a substantial change was given by 0.3 times the typical within-athlete variability (coefficient of variation) to test for a small effect; moderate and large performance effects were described by 0.9 and 1.6 of the typical within-athlete variation [22]. The coefficients of variation for finishing time and power output following familiarization in a simulated cycling time trial of a comparable distance as in the current study have been determined previously and were reported as 1.5% and 3.6%, respectively [19].

An effect was unclear if the confidence interval (CI) overlapped both the upper and lower thresholds for substantiveness. Otherwise, the likelihood of a substantial increase or decrease was classified as follows: almost certainly not (<0.5%), very unlikely (1%–5%), unlikely (5%–25%), possibly (25%–75%), likely (75%–95%), very likely (95%–99.5%), and almost certainly (>99.5%). For mechanistic inferences, the threshold chances for substantial magnitudes were set at 5%. For clinical inferences, the threshold chances for harmful ("non-beneficial") and beneficial effects were set at 0.5% and 25%, whereas an effect was declared beneficial if the odds ratio of beneficial/non-beneficial was >66 [22].

Unless otherwise stated, data are reported as raw means ± SD. Mean differences between trials are presented as the percentage change with the associated 90% CI. All metabolic and performance data were log-transformed prior to analysis to reduce non-uniformity of error and to express outcomes as percent [22].

Besides the probabilistic magnitude-based inferential analysis, statistical p-values for the comparisons between the MDX and PSE trial for all physiological and performance related parameters are also reported. A repeated measures analysis of variance (ANOVA) was used to identify significant effects attributable to time, trial, or both. Mauchly's test was consulted and, if the assumption of sphericity was violated, the Greenhouse-Geisser correction was applied. If a significant time × trial interaction existed, simple main effects of trial were examined. A p-value of < 0.05 was considered statistically significant. Statistical analysis was done using SPSS Statistics Version 21 (SPSS Inc., Chicago, IL, USA).

3. Results

All twenty subjects completed the study and were included in the final analysis. Due to missing spirometric data from three subjects, results for fat and CHO oxidation were evaluated for $n = 17$.

The time to complete the time trial was 31.08 ± 6.27 min for the MDX and 30.05 ± 4.70 min for the PSE trial (mean change: −2.7%, 90% CI: ±3.0%; $p = 0.147$), corresponding to a likely small (89% likelihood) to moderate (77% likelihood) benefit of Palatinose™ (Figure 1).

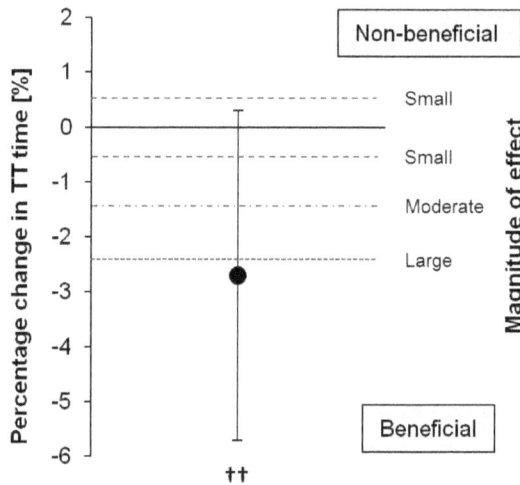

Figure 1. Percentage change and 90% confidence interval (CI) of cycling time trial finishing time between the Palatinose™ (PSE) and maltodextrin (MDX) trial ($N = 20$). Thresholds for small, moderate, and large effects are indicated by dashed lines. †† denotes a likely small to moderate benefit, i.e., faster time trial performance with PSE compared with MDX.

The power output was consistently higher with PSE vs. MDX (Figure 2), yet a clinically relevant benefit was detected only during the final 5 min of the time trial (290.61 ± 45.85 W vs. 279.42 ± 55.91 W). The higher power output with PSE corresponds to a mean change of +0.8% (90% CI: ±2.8%, $p = 0.608$)

and +2.0% (90% CI: ±3.5%, $p = 0.327$) during the first 5 min and until the final 5 min of the time trial, respectively. When the final 5 min of the time trial were analyzed, power output with PSE, compared with MDX, was higher by +4.6% (90% CI: ±4.0%; $p = 0.053$), which corresponds to a likely small benefit of Palatinose™ (93% likelihood).

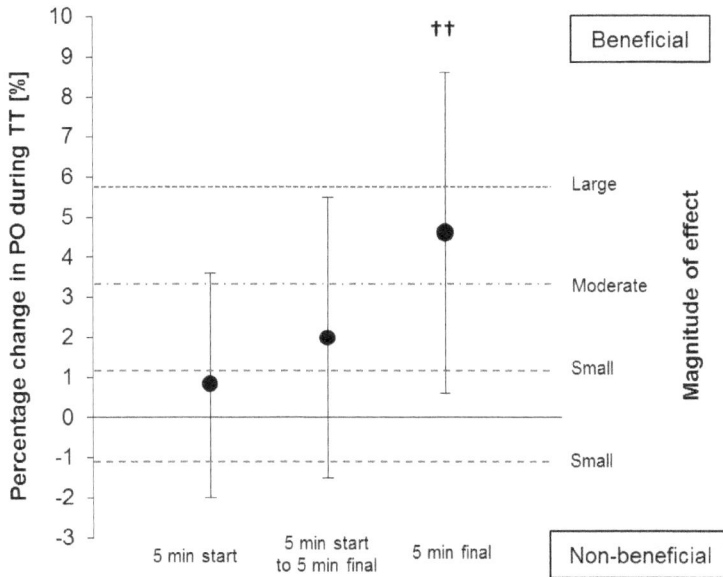

Figure 2. Percentage change and 90% CI of power output between the PSE and MDX trials during the first 5 min, the final 5 min, and the intermediate period of the time trial ($N = 20$). Thresholds for small, moderate, and large effects are indicated by dashed lines. ⁺⁺ denotes a likely small benefit, i.e., higher power output with PSE compared with MDX.

Heart rate was similar between trials (time × trial interaction: $p = 0.961$), and no differences between the PSE and MDX trials, neither during rest nor during the endurance exercise, were detected (Table 1).

Table 1. Average heart rate at rest and during endurance exercise for the PSE and MDX trials, presented as mean ± SD ($N = 20$).

	Palatinose™	Maltodextrin
Heart rate at rest (beats/min)	65.7 ± 8.8	65.6 ± 9.2
Heart rate during endurance exercise (beats/min)	159.2 ± 13.9	158.7 ± 13.6

Figure 3 shows that the blood glucose profile differed between trials (time × trial interaction: $p = 0.013$). At rest, i.e., 30 min, 15 min, and 0 min prior to the start of exercise, consumption of PSE resulted in lower blood glucose concentrations compared with the ingestion of MDX (95% to 99% likelihood, ES = −0.61 to −0.87, moderate effect; $p < 0.05$ for all time points). After 30 min, 45 min, 60 min, and 75 min of endurance exercise, blood glucose concentrations were higher with PSE compared with MDX (63% to 86% likelihood, ES = 0.29 to 0.52, small effect; $p > 0.05$ for all time points). The reduction in glycemia following the onset of exercise was attenuated with PSE vs. MDX (93% likelihood, ES = 0.64, moderate effect; $p = 0.034$).

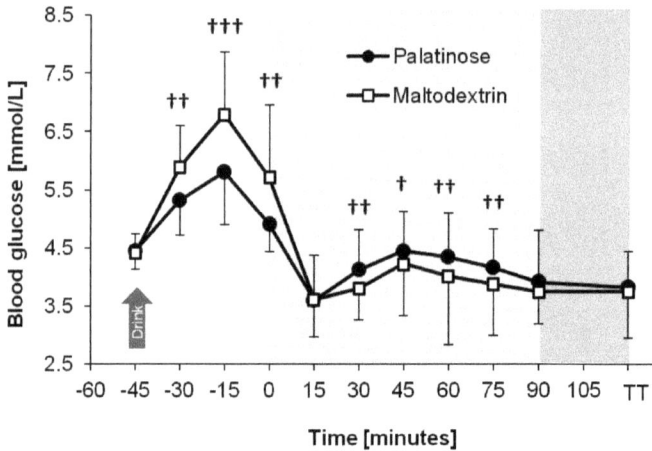

Figure 3. Plasma glucose profiles during the PSE and MDX trials, presented as mean ± SD (*N* = 20). The symbols [†], [††], and [†††] denote a possible, likely, and very likely difference between the PSE and MDX trials at the corresponding time point, respectively. From 0 min to 90 min: endurance exercise. TT = blood sample drawn upon completion of the time trial.

Figure 4 demonstrates that plasma lactate concentrations were similar between trials (time × trial interaction: $p = 0.562$), and no differences could be detected.

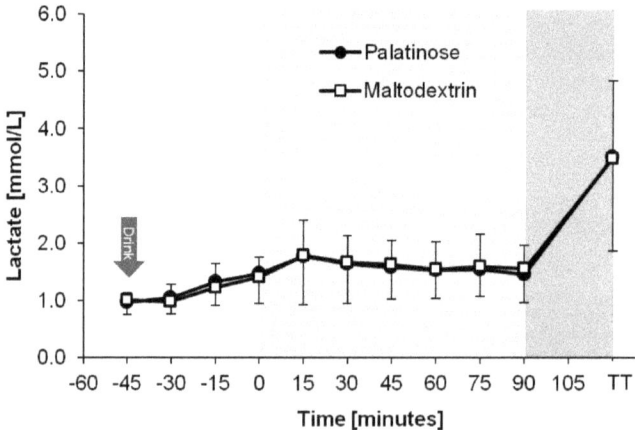

Figure 4. Plasma lactate profiles during the PSE and MDX trials, presented as mean ± SD (*N* = 20). From 0 min to 90 min: endurance exercise. TT = blood sample drawn upon completion of the time trial.

Figure 5 shows that the exercise-induced increase in fat and carbohydrate oxidation differed between the MDX and PSE trial (time × trial interactions: $p = 0.005$ and $p = 0.002$). During the endurance exercise, PSE resulted in higher fat oxidation (88% to 99% likelihood, ES = 0.65 to 1.60, moderate to large effect; $p < 0.05$ for all time points from 30 to 90 min) and lower carbohydrate oxidation compared with MDX (85% to 96% likelihood, ES = −0.44 to −0.63, small to moderate effect; $p < 0.05$ for all time points from 0 to 75 min and $p = 0.069$ at 90 min). Total energy expenditure was similar between trials (1306 kcal vs. 1316 kcal for the PSE and MDX trials until 90 min, respectively; $p = 0.579$).

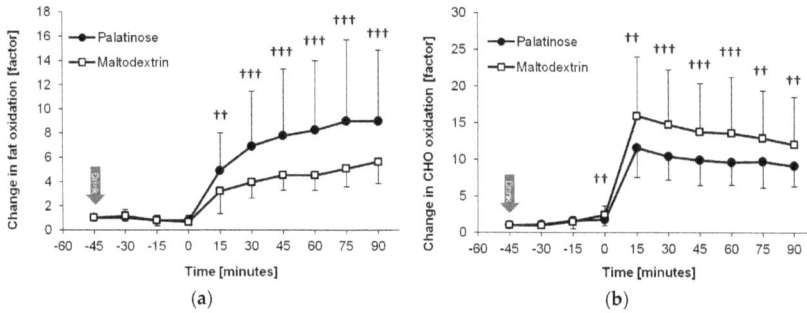

Figure 5. Changes in (**a**) fat oxidation and (**b**) carbohydrate (CHO) oxidation during the PSE and MDX trials, presented as mean ± SD (*N* = 17). The symbols ⁺⁺ and ⁺⁺⁺ denote a likely and very likely difference between the PSE and MDX trials at the corresponding time point, respectively. From 0 min to 90 min: endurance exercise.

During the entire examination period, no adverse or unintended effects were observed. None of the subjects complained about bad palatability or gastrointestinal discomfort following ingestion of either test beverage.

4. Discussion

The most important finding in the present study was that cycling time trial finishing time was 30.05 ± 4.70 min following pre-exercise ingestion of low glycemic Palatinose™ and 31.08 ± 6.27 min when an isocaloric high glycemic maltodextrin beverage was consumed. The effect size of 1 min is impressive, even though under this study design the difference achieved did not reach the level of statistical significance. Using the probabilistic magnitude-based inference approach as recommended for studies in sports medicine and exercise sciences, this effect corresponds to a likely benefit of Palatinose™. This was also accompanied by a likely benefit of Palatinose™ for power output during the final 5 min of the time trial. Furthermore, pre-exercise ingestion of a low glycemic Palatinose™ beverage increased fat oxidation while reducing carbohydrate oxidation during the endurance exercise, as compared with the high glycemic maltodextrin drink. Palatinose™ ingestion also resulted in a more stable blood glucose profile with lower blood glucose increases shortly after consumption and a sustained blood glucose response during the subsequent endurance exercise protocol at 60% VO$_2$max.

Official guidelines recommend that, in endurance-type sports, CHO should be the predominant source of energy within the athlete's diet [22]. According to current guidelines, athletes should aim at increasing the amount of CHO within their diet to 6–10 g CHO/kg bodyweight/day in accordance with training duration or intensity of competition [23]; the GI of CHO is not sufficiently addressed in current guidelines.

However, the GI of ingested CHO has a distinct influence on important metabolic processes under both resting or pre-exercise conditions and during exercise. It has been previously demonstrated that the course of blood glucose and insulin levels following ingestion of low GI CHO favored a higher level of free fatty acids during exercise and was associated with enhanced fat oxidation and improved blood glucose homeostasis [6,7,24–27]. During submaximal endurance exercise, the maintenance of higher fat oxidation leads to a sparing of glycogen in muscles and particularly in the liver. It has been speculated that this glycogen sparing could lead to enhanced endurance capacity. This is the most likely theory that explains the better performance in the time trial following Palatinose™ ingestion.

An improved performance following low GI CHO ingestion could be found in some [8,10,13,26,28] but not all studies [27,29,30]. This may be due to differences in the quantity and timing of CHO ingested as well as the type, duration, and intensity of the exercise protocol. It is evident that the glycogen sparing effect of low GI CHO will not be relevant during short or high intensity exercise.

Our data show that pre-exercise ingestion of Palatinose™ was associated with higher blood glucose concentrations during the 90 min endurance exercise. The drop in glycemia following the onset of exercise, i.e., the "exercise-induced rebound glycemic response", was substantially attenuated with PSE compared with MDX. This could be explained by the lower pre-exercise glucose and insulin response following Palatinose™ ingestion, the slow release kinetic of the monosaccharides glucose and fructose contributing to a more constant energy supply, and, of course, the higher amount of fat oxidized during the PSE trial [6,24,25].

Apart from the energy provision by CHO during exercise, there is also evidence that higher glucose concentrations improve mental performance. It has been shown that ingestion of slowly available, low GI Palatinose™ improves mental performance compared with higher GI CHO [31]. In addition, it has been demonstrated that also relatively short and highly intense exercise may be improved by pre-exercise CHO ingestion [32,33]. Therefore, it could be speculated that the higher glucose levels during the 90-min endurance exercise improved cognitive performance and reduced mental fatigue, thereby further improving stamina during the time trial [32].

Nevertheless, the study has several limitations: The number of subjects is relatively small, and some variables such as ratings of perceived exertion, muscle glycogen content, and the rate of appearance and disappearance of glucose or hormones such as cortisol have not been measured. In addition, while parameters such as blood glucose, fat, and carbohydrate oxidation were beneficial in both the magnitude-based inference approach and the conventional ANOVA, the improvement of time trial performance and power output by Palatinose™ was only beneficial in the magnitude-based inference approach and did not reach significance in the conventional statistical analysis ($p = 0.147$ and $p = 0.053$, respectively). However, we feel that the magnitude-based inference approach is well suited to determine whether a performance-enhancing effect is truly beneficial for athletes or simply an effect that is statistically significant but without any practical value in training or competition.

5. Conclusions

The results of the present study have shown that cycling performance was improved following pre-exercise ingestion of a low GI Palatinose™ beverage (750 mL, 10% w/v) compared with an isocaloric high GI maltodextrin drink. In the preceding 90 min endurance exercise at 60% VO$_2$max, Palatinose™ resulted in a sustained blood glucose response while maintaining a higher rate of fat oxidation compared with maltodextrin, thereby reducing the reliance on CHO oxidation. These differences may have contributed to the better performance indices in the time trial test.

Acknowledgments: This study was funded by BENEO GmbH, Mannheim, Germany, a member of the Südzucker Group. The study results and data contained in the publication have been developed by and/or for BENEO. BENEO reserves the exclusive right to use the results and data for possible Health Claim requests. The planning, organization, monitoring and analysis of the study were performed independently by the University of Freiburg. The exercise testing was performed by the Cycling Lab (Radlabor) Freiburg.

Author Contributions: D.K., D.Z., A.H., S.T., and A.G. were involved in the design and realization of the study or manuscript preparation. All authors read and approved the final manuscript.

Conflicts of Interest: A.H. and S.T. are employees of BENEO/Südzucker Group.

Abbreviations

The following abbreviations are used in this manuscript:

ANOVA	analysis of variance
CHO	carbohydrate
ES	effect size
CI	confidence interval
GI	glycemic index
MDX	maltodextrin
PSE	Palatinose™
SD	standard deviation

References

1. Hargreaves, M.; Hawley, J.A.; Jeukendrup, A. Pre-exercise carbohydrate and fat ingestion: Effects on metabolism and performance. *J. Sports Sci.* **2004**, *22*, 31–38. [CrossRef] [PubMed]
2. Jeukendrup, A.E. Modulation of carbohydrate and fat utilization by diet, exercise and environment. *Biochem. Soc. Trans.* **2003**, *31*, 1270–1273. [CrossRef] [PubMed]
3. Kelley, D.E. Skeletal muscle fat oxidation: Timing and flexibility are everything. *J. Clin. Investig.* **2005**, *115*, 1699–1702. [CrossRef] [PubMed]
4. Rodriguez, N.R.; di Marco, N.M.; Langley, S. American College of Sports Medicine position stand: Nutrition and athletic performance. *Med. Sci. Sports Exerc.* **2009**, *41*, 709–731. [PubMed]
5. Shah, M.; Garg, A. High-fat and high-carbohydrate diets and energy balance. *Diabetes Care* **1996**, *19*, 1142–1152. [CrossRef] [PubMed]
6. Van Can, J.G.; van Loon, L.J.; Brouns, F.; Blaak, E.E. Reduced glycaemic and insulinaemic responses following trehalose and isomaltulose ingestion: Implications for postprandial substrate use in impaired glucose-tolerant subjects. *Br. J. Nutr.* **2012**, *108*, 1210–1217. [CrossRef] [PubMed]
7. Siu, P.M.; Wong, S.H. Use of the glycemic index: Effects on feeding patterns and exercise performance. *J. Physiol. Anthropol. Appl. Hum. Sci.* **2004**, *23*, 1–6. [CrossRef]
8. DeMarco, H.M.; Sucher, K.P.; Cisar, C.J.; Butterfield, G.E. Pre-exercise carbohydrate meals: Application of glycemic index. *Med. Sci. Sports Exerc.* **1999**, *31*, 164–170. [CrossRef] [PubMed]
9. Stevenson, E.; Williams, C.; McComb, G.; Oram, C. Improved recovery from prolonged exercise following the consumption of low glycemic index carbohydrate meals. *Int. J. Sport Nutr. Exerc. Metab.* **2005**, *15*, 333–349. [PubMed]
10. Thomas, D.E.; Brotherhood, J.R.; Brand, J.C. Carbohydrate feeding before exercise: Effect of glycemic index. *Int. J. Sports Med.* **1991**, *12*, 180–186. [CrossRef] [PubMed]
11. Stevenson, E.J.; Williams, C.; Mash, L.E.; Phillips, B.; Nute, M.L. Influence of high-carbohydrate mixed meals with different glycemic indexes on substrate utilization during subsequent exercise in women. *Am. J. Clin. Nutr.* **2006**, *84*, 354–360. [PubMed]
12. Brand-Miller, J.C.; Holt, S.H.; Pawlak, D.B.; McMillan, J. Glycemic index and obesity. *Am. J. Clin. Nutr.* **2002**, *76*, 281S–285S. [PubMed]
13. Wu, C.L.; Williams, C. A low glycemic index meal before exercise improves endurance running capacity in men. *Int. J. Sport Nutr. Exerc. Metab.* **2006**, *16*, 510–527. [PubMed]
14. Kirwan, J.P.; O'Gorman, D.J.; Cyr-Campbell, D.; Campbell, W.W.; Yarasheski, K.E.; Evans, W.J. Effects of a moderate glycemic meal on exercise duration and substrate utilization. *Med. Sci. Sports Exerc.* **2001**, *33*, 1517–1523. [CrossRef] [PubMed]
15. Wee, S.L.; Williams, C.; Tsintzas, K.; Boobis, L. Ingestion of a high glycemic index meal increases muscle glycogen storage at rest but augments its utilisation during subsequent exercise. *J. Appl. Physiol.* **2005**, *99*, 707–714. [CrossRef] [PubMed]
16. Atkinson, F.S.; Foster-Powell, K.; Brand-Miller, J.C. International tables of glycemic index and glycemic load values: 2008. *Diabetes Care* **2008**, *31*, 2281–2283. [CrossRef] [PubMed]
17. Lina, B.A.; Jonker, D.; Kozianowski, G. Isomaltulose (Palatinose): A review of biological and toxicological studies. *Food Chem. Toxicol.* **2002**, *40*, 1375–1381. [CrossRef]
18. Holub, I.; Gostner, A.; Theis, S.; Nosek, L.; Kudlich, T.; Melcher, R.; Scheppach, W. Novel findings on the metabolic effects of the low glycaemic carbohydrate isomaltulose (Palatinose™). *Br. J. Nutr.* **2010**, *103*, 1730–1737. [CrossRef] [PubMed]
19. Zavorsky, G.S.; Murias, J.M.; Gow, J.; Kim, D.J.; Poulin-Harnois, C.; Kubow, S.; Lands, L. Laboratory 20-km cycle time trial reproducibility. *Int. J. Sports Med.* **2007**, *28*, 743–748. [CrossRef] [PubMed]
20. Weir, J. New methods for calculating metabolic rate with special reference to protein metabolism. *J. Physiol.* **1949**, *109*, 1–9. [CrossRef] [PubMed]
21. Hopkins, W. Sportscience. Available online: newstats.org/xPostOnlyCrossover.xls (accessed on 7 July 2015).
22. Hopkins, W.G.; Marshall, S.W.; Batterham, A.M.; Hanin, J. Progressive statistics for studies in sports medicine and exercise science. *Med. Sci. Sports Exerc.* **2009**, *41*, 3–13. [CrossRef] [PubMed]

23. Rodriguez, N.R.; DiMarco, N.M.; Langley, S. Position of the American Dietetic Association, Dietitians of Canada, and the American College of Sports Medicine: Nutrition and athletic performance. *J. Am. Diet. Assoc.* **2000**, *100*, 1543–1556.

24. Konig, D.; Theis, S.; Kozianowski, G.; Berg, A. Postprandial substrate use in overweight subjects with the metabolic syndrome after isomaltulose (Palatinose) ingestion. *Nutrition* **2012**, *28*, 651–656. [CrossRef] [PubMed]

25. Oosthuyse, T.; Carstens, M.; Millen, A.M. Ingesting isomaltulose versus fructose-maltodextrin during prolonged moderate-heavy exercise increases fat oxidation but impairs gastrointestinal comfort and cycling performance. *Int. J. Sport Nutr. Exerc. Metab.* **2015**, *25*, 427–438. [CrossRef] [PubMed]

26. Wu, C.L.; Nicholas, C.; Williams, C.; Took, A.; Hardy, L. The influence of high-carbohydrate meals with different glycaemic indices on substrate utilisation during subsequent exercise. *Br. J. Nutr.* **2003**, *90*, 1049–1056. [CrossRef] [PubMed]

27. Febbraio, M.A.; Keenan, J.; Angus, D.J.; Campbell, S.E.; Garnham, A.P. Pre exercise carbohydrate ingestion, glucose kinetics, and muscle glycogen use: Effect of the glycemic index. *J. Appl. Physiol.* **2000**, *89*, 1845–1851. [PubMed]

28. Kirwan, J.P.; O'Gorman, D.; Evans, W.J. A moderate glycemic meal before endurance exercise can enhance performance. *J. Appl. Physiol.* **1998**, *84*, 53–59. [PubMed]

29. Thomas, D.E.; Brotherhood, J.R.; Miller, J.B. Plasma glucose levels after prolonged strenuous exercise correlate inversely with glycemic response to food consumed before exercise. *Int. J. Sport Nutr.* **1994**, *4*, 361–373. [PubMed]

30. Wee, S.L.; Williams, C.; Gray, S.; Horabin, J. Influence of high and low glycemic index meals on endurance running capacity. *Med. Sci. Sports Exerc.* **1999**, *31*, 393–399. [CrossRef] [PubMed]

31. Young, H.; Benton, D. The effect of using isomaltulose (Palatinose) to modulate the glycaemic properties of breakfast on the cognitive performance of children. *Eur. J. Nutr.* **2015**, *54*, 1013–1020. [CrossRef] [PubMed]

32. Meeusen, R. Exercise, nutrition and the brain. *Sports Med.* **2014**, *44*, S47–S56. [CrossRef] [PubMed]

33. Lee, C.L.; Cheng, C.F.; Astorino, T.A.; Lee, C.J.; Huang, H.W.; Chang, W.D. Effects of carbohydrate combined with caffeine on repeated sprint cycling and agility performance in female athletes. *J. Int. Soc. Sports Nutr.* **2014**, *11*, 17. [CrossRef] [PubMed]

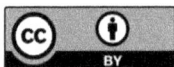

nutrients

Article

Slow-Absorbing Modified Starch before and during Prolonged Cycling Increases Fat Oxidation and Gastrointestinal Distress without Changing Performance

Daniel A. Baur [1], Fernanda de C. S. Vargas [1], Christopher W. Bach [1], Jordan A. Garvey [1] and Michael J. Ormsbee [1,2,*]

[1] Institute of Sport Sciences and Medicine, Department of Nutrition, Food, and Exercise Sciences, Florida State University, Tallahassee, FL 32306, USA; dab13b@my.fsu.edu (D.A.B.); fd14c@my.fsu.edu (F.d.C.S.V.); cwb12b@my.fsu.edu (C.W.B.); jag12h@my.fsu.edu (J.A.G.)
[2] Department of Biokinetics, Exercise and Leisure Sciences, University of KwaZulu-Natal, Durban 4000, South Africa
*   Correspondence: mormsbee@fsu.edu; Tel.: +1-850-644-4793

Received: 20 May 2016; Accepted: 22 June 2016; Published: 25 June 2016

Abstract: While prior research reported altered fuel utilization stemming from pre-exercise modified starch ingestion, the practical value of this starch for endurance athletes who consume carbohydrates both before and during exercise is yet to be examined. The purpose of this study was to determine the effects of ingesting a hydrothermally-modified starch supplement (HMS) before and during cycling on performance, metabolism, and gastrointestinal comfort. In a crossover design, 10 male cyclists underwent three nutritional interventions: (1) a commercially available sucrose/glucose supplement (G) 30 min before (60 g carbohydrate) and every 15 min during exercise (60 g·h^{-1}); (2) HMS consumed at the same time points before and during exercise in isocaloric amounts to G (Iso HMS); and (3) HMS 30 min before (60 g carbohydrate) and every 60 min during exercise (30 g·h^{-1}; Low HMS). The exercise protocol (~3 h) consisted of 1 h at 50% W$_{max}$, 8 × 2-min intervals at 80% W$_{max}$, and 10 maximal sprints. There were no differences in sprint performance with Iso HMS vs. G, while both G and Iso HMS likely resulted in small performance enhancements (5.0%; 90% confidence interval = ±5.3% and 4.4%; ±3.2%, respectively) relative to Low HMS. Iso HMS and Low HMS enhanced fat oxidation (31.6%; ±20.1%; very likely (Iso); 20.9%; ±16.1%; likely (Low), and reduced carbohydrate oxidation (−19.2%; ±7.6%; most likely; −22.1%; ±12.9%; very likely) during exercise relative to G. However, nausea was increased during repeated sprints with ingestion of Iso HMS (17 scale units; ±18; likely) and Low HMS (18; ±14; likely) vs. G. Covariate analysis revealed that gastrointestinal distress was associated with reductions in performance with Low HMS vs. G (likely), but this relationship was unclear with Iso HMS vs. G. In conclusion, pre- and during-exercise ingestion of HMS increases fat oxidation relative to G. However, changes do not translate to performance improvements, possibly owing to HMS-associated increases in gastrointestinal distress, which is not attenuated by reducing the intake rate of HMS during exercise.

Keywords: glycemic index; gastrointestinal distress; blood glucose; ergogenic aids; carbohydrate

1. Introduction

Carbohydrate is a well-documented ergogenic aid for endurance performance, and benefits are dose-responsive within intestinal absorption capacity limits (~90 g·h^{-1}) [1]. As such, current recommendations suggest athletes consume large amounts of carbohydrate before and during prolonged ($\geqslant$120 min) exercise to optimize performance [2]. Notably, studies have found that endurance athletes generally comply with these recommendations [3,4].

Recent research has highlighted the importance of carbohydrate type on metabolic and performance outcomes. For instance, composite solutions containing glucose and fructose (1 to 0.8–1.0 ratio) ingested during exercise seem to enhance performance relative to glucose/maltodextrin-only solutions [5,6]. This effect is likely due to faster carbohydrate absorption and oxidation with glucose/fructose mediated by non-competitive intestinal transport [7]. Interestingly, there is also evidence that reducing the rate of carbohydrate absorption with slow-digesting carbohydrate benefits exercise metabolism and performance. For example, studies have reported enhanced endurance capacity (70% VO_{2max} to exhaustion) or time trial performance (pre-loaded 16-km run) following a pre-exercise meal composed primarily of slow-absorbing and/or low glycemic index carbohydrates [8,9]. This ergogenic effect may be the result of more efficient substrate utilization patterns. Indeed, reported performance improvements are often associated with enhanced exercise fat oxidation, possibly resulting from attenuated blood glucose and insulin responses to feeding [8,9]. Benefits may also be partially explained by a prolonged glucose release from the small intestine maintaining euglycemia during exercise and consequent attenuation of central fatigue [10]. Of interest, this extended energy release into the bloodstream combined with enhanced fat oxidation may permit the intake of fewer overall carbohydrates during exercise. If true, this may be desirable for certain athletes, as carbohydrate intake rates, while associated with performance benefits, are also associated with gastrointestinal distress [3].

Nevertheless, the utility of slow-absorbing carbohydrates for endurance athletes is uncertain. Even if potentially required in lesser amounts, the carbohydrate demands of endurance exercise necessitate ingesting carbohydrate both before and during exercise to maximize performance [11]. Most slow-absorbing carbohydrates are in starch form, a semi-crystalline granular polymer typically found in whole foods like legumes, potatoes, and lentils [12]. Thus, because of the physical form of most starches, athletes are likely limited in their capacity to consume them during exercise due to logistical and palatability concerns. Moreover, any benefits conferred by pre-exercise slow-absorbing carbohydrate are substantially attenuated when traditional fast-absorbing carbohydrates are consumed during exercise [13]. As such, realizing the benefits of a pre-exercise slow-absorbing carbohydrate meal likely requires the continued intake of slow-absorbing carbohydrates during exercise.

Importantly, the macromolecular structure of starch can be modified via various processing techniques to alter its solubility and rate of absorption. Recently, a slow-absorbing and water-soluble waxy maize starch-based exercise supplement was developed through hydrothermal modification. Roberts et al. [14] found that, relative to maltodextrin, ingestion of this modified starch 30 min prior to cycling resulted in very likely increased fat oxidation combined with increased plasma concentrations of free fatty acids (FFA) and glycerol. While endurance capacity in a 100% VO_{2max} time to exhaustion trial following 150 min of cycling (70% VO_{2max}) was unchanged with pre-exercise modified starch, subjects in the study did not consume additional carbohydrate during exercise despite the lengthy nature of the exercise protocol. This may have attenuated any performance benefit stemming from early exercise metabolic alterations. Furthermore, this feeding strategy contrasts with current recommendations and current practice among athletes. As such, the purpose of this study was to investigate the impact of consuming a slow-absorbing modified starch supplement both before and during exercise relative to an isocaloric, fast-absorbing carbohydrate solution in trained male athletes. A secondary purpose was to determine whether the extended glucose release profile and associated metabolic effects of a slow-absorbing modified starch permits the ingestion of less total carbohydrate without impairing performance.

2. Methods

2.1. Subjects

Ten trained male cyclists and triathletes (age = 26 $\pm$ 8 years, mass = 75.2 $\pm$ 9.2 kg, VO_{2max} = 59.4 $\pm$ 3.2 mL·kg^{-1}·min^{-1}, and peak power (W_{max} = 343.3 $\pm$ 37.7 W) participated in the study. All subjects had $\geqslant$2 years cycling experience and had cycled $\geqslant$ 3 day·week^{-1} and $\geqslant$ 7 h·week^{-1} for the preceding two months, while regularly competing in races. Prior to giving their oral and written informed consent, all subjects received information regarding the requirements of the study and potential risks. All procedures were approved by the Florida State University Institutional Review Board.

2.2. Study Design

This was a double-blinded, randomized, counterbalanced, and crossover study. It consisted of baseline testing to determine VO_{2max} and W_{max}, a familiarization trial, and three experimental trials. Each experimental trial was separated by seven days. For the duration of the study, subjects were asked to maintain consistent dietary and training habits. Prior to each experimental trial, exercise and diet were standardized. Specifically, two days prior to each experimental trial, subjects visited the laboratory and completed a standardized training ride (90 min at 50% W_{max}). The day prior to each trial, subjects were asked to refrain from exercise. Additionally, subjects were asked to replicate their diets (2444 $\pm$ 609 kcals; 103 $\pm$ 23 g protein, 299 $\pm$ 123 g carbohydrate, 97 $\pm$ 33 g fat) the day prior to each trial. This was achieved by requiring subjects to complete a 24 h dietary log prior to the first trial. Following this trial, subjects were given a copy of their completed dietary log and asked to replicate it exactly for proceeding trials. Subjects were also asked to abstain from alcohol and caffeine for the 24 h preceding each trial.

2.3. Baseline Testing and Familiarization

During the initial visit to the laboratory, subjects were assessed for VO_{2max} and W_{max}. This consisted of a continuous graded exercise test to exhaustion on a cycle ergometer (Velotron, Racermate, Inc., Seattle, WA, USA). During a self-selected warm-up, a power output corresponding to a "moderately difficult intensity for a 1 h ride" was determined. Commencing at this intensity, power was increased by 25 W every 2 min until volitional exhaustion. VO_{2max} was assessed with a calibrated metabolic cart (TrueOne 2400, Parvo Medics, Inc., Sandy, UT, USA) and was classified as the highest average 20-s oxygen consumption (mL·kg^{-1}·min^{-1}) recorded. W_{max} was the wattage attained in the last completed stage plus the fraction completed of the stage at which exhaustion occurred.

A familiarization trial was completed 2–3 days following baseline testing. The familiarization trial consisted of the entire exercise protocol (see below) without the recording of data.

2.4. Experimental Beverages

The current study evaluated two commercially available sport supplements. Specifically, we investigated the impact of ingesting different amounts of a hydrothermally-modified waxy maize starch (HMS; UCAN®, The UCAN Co., Woodbridge, CT, USA) relative to a sucrose- and glucose-based control solution (G; Gatorade®, PepsiCo, Inc., Purchase, NY, USA). Treatments were as follows: (1) 10% G consumed 30 min before exercise and 7.5% G every ~15 min during exercise; (2) 10% HMS consumed 30 min before exercise and 7.5% HMS every ~15 min during exercise (Iso HMS); and (3) 10% HMS consumed 30 min before exercise and 15% HMS every 60 min (at 60 min and following sprint two of the performance test) during exercise (Low HMS). The dosing strategy for the Low HMS trial was chosen based on recommendations available on the company's website. In order to blind subjects to the dosing strategy, a non-caloric placebo was also ingested in the Low HMS condition during exercise at time points that matched G and Iso HMS beverage ingestion times. All beverages were flavor and texture-matched by the addition of non-caloric additives (e.g., sucralose and guar gum). Pre-exercise beverages contained 600 mL of fluid while during-exercise beverages were 200 mL. As such, carbohydrate delivery rates for G and Iso HMS were 60 g before and 60 g·h^{-1} during exercise. For Low HMS, 60 g carbohydrate was ingested before and 30 g·h^{-1} during exercise. These carbohydrate delivery rates were chosen as they represent the uppermost (60 g·h^{-1}) and lowermost (30 g·h^{-1}) amounts of the currently recommended range for during-exercise ingestion of carbohydrate from a single source [15]. Beverage osmolality was determined via the freezing point depression method (Model 3250 Osmometer, Advanced Instruments, Inc., Norwood, MA, USA). Osmolalities were 363, 278, 51, 37, 53, and 8 mOsm·kg^{-1} for pre-exercise G, during-exercise G, pre-exercise Iso/Low HMS, during-exercise Iso HMS, during-exercise Low HMS, and placebo, respectively.

2.5. Experimental Trials

Subjects reported to the laboratory at 0500–0700 h following an overnight fast (8–10 h). Arrival times were replicated for subsequent trials. Following 5 min of rest in the seated position, resting heart rate (Polar® FTM4, Polar, Inc., Kempele, Finland) was assessed and a fingerprick blood sample was collected for immediate measurement of blood glucose and lactate (YSI 2300 Stat, YSI, Inc., Yellow Springs, OH, USA). Thereafter, a 5-min indirect calorimetry measurement was taken with the final 3 min being used in subsequent analysis. Subjects then received a pre-exercise treatment beverage, which they consumed within 3 min, and remained seated for 30 min. Blood and indirect calorimetry measurements were repeated 15 min and 30 min following ingestion. Next, subjects commenced exercise beginning with a 5-min warm-up at 30% W_{max}. The exercise protocol is presented in Figure 1. It consisted of a 95-min pre-load after which subjects were allowed to stretch and use the restroom (3–5 min). This was followed by a repeated maximal sprint performance assessment, which has been previously described [6]. Specifically, the entire protocol consisted of the following: (1) 60 min at 50% W_{max}; (2) two sets of 4 × 2-min intervals at 80% W_{max} with intervals and sets separated by 2 min and 5 min at 50% W_{max}, respectively; and (3) 10 maximal sprints assessed for mean power. For each sprint and recovery period of the performance test, subjects were required to complete a given amount of work based on their W_{max} (kilocalories = 0.125 × W_{max}). For the sprints, subjects completed the prescribed work as quickly as possible (2–3 min). During recovery periods, the work was completed while subjects cycled at 40% W_{max} (5–6 min). Total exercise time was 183.0 ± 2.9 min.

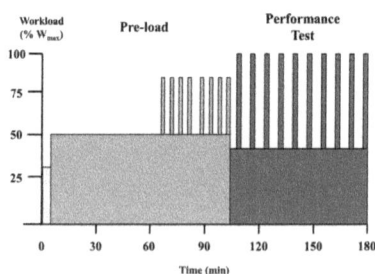

Figure 1. Exercise protocol. W_{max}, peak cycling power.

Treatment beverages were consumed every 15 min during the pre-load portion and at the start and every second sprint during the performance assessment. Physiological measurements were as follows: (1) heart rate was measured every 15 min during the first 60 min of exercise and at the midpoint of each sprint and recovery segment of the performance test; (2) indirect calorimetry measurements were taken every 15 min for 5-min collection periods during the first 60 min of exercise; and (3) blood glucose and lactate were assessed every 15 min during the first 60 min of exercise, and following sprint 5 and sprint 10.

All testing was completed in thermoneutral conditions (22 °C, 45%–50% humidity). Subjects were cooled by a pedestal fan on the medium setting in each trial for uniform cooling. During the performance testing portion of the exercise protocol, subjects received no verbal encouragement and were only permitted to see the amount of work completed.

2.6. Perceptual Response Assessment

Gastrointestinal distress (nausea, abdominal cramp, and fullness) and perceived exertion (effort of cycling, tiredness, and leg strength) were assessed via a 100-mm Likert scale, as previously described [6,16]. Specifically, subjects rated the magnitude of these symptoms by placing a line in relation to specific descriptors including: nothing at all, extremely weak, very weak, weakor mild, moderate, strong, very strong, extremely strong, and absolute maximum. The height (mm) of the line marked by subjects was recorded for subsequent analysis. All measurements of line height were made via ruler by the same researcher. Perceptual responses were assessed every 15 min during the first 60 min of exercise, at the midpoint of the 5-min recovery period between 80% W_{max} intervals, and after the first and every third sprint of the performance test.

2.7. Calculations

Total carbohydrate and fat oxidation at rest and during the first 60 min of exercise were calculated from indirect calorimetry measurements via stoichiochemical equations described elsewhere [17].

2.8. Statistics

Sample size was determined as that which provided sufficient power to detect the smallest worthwhile benefit to cycling performance given the expected typical error (CV) for mean sprint power and anticipated effect size (ES) [18]. Prior studies have reported CV of 1.1%–3.1% for mean sprint power [6,19,20]. To account for inter-laboratory differences, we chose to conservatively estimate a CV of 3.1% with an anticipated moderate 0.9 CV effect size (2.79%). Using 0.5% and 25% as the rates for Type I and Type II clinical errors, respectively, a sample size of 10 was determined.

Probabilistic magnitude-based inferences were utilized to assess physiological and perceptual changes via a published spreadsheet [21]. The spreadsheet derives confidence intervals based on the unequal variances *t* statistic. All physiological data (i.e., performance and metabolic variables) were analyzed following log-transformation to account for any heteroscedasticity of error. Perceptual response raw data were analyzed without transformation. Uncertainty for all variables was expressed as 90% confidence intervals. Changes in performance were evaluated with the clinical version of magnitude-based inferences in which clear effects are classified as having >25% chance of benefit and <0.5% chance of harm. All other variables were assessed non-clinically; differences were deemed unclear if confidence intervals overlapped thresholds for both small positive and negative effects. ES was determined by standardizing all differences to the SD of the control, and small sample bias was accounted for by dividing the control SD by $1 - 3 (4v - 1)$, where v is equal to the degrees of freedom [18]. Threshold values for assessing performance were as follows: 0.3 (0.93%), 0.9 (2.79%), 1.6 (4.96%), 2.5 (7.75%), and 4.0 (12.4%) for small, moderate, large, very large, and extremely large, respectively [18]. Thresholds for small, moderate, large, very large, and extremely large changes in all non-performance variables were 0.2, 0.6, 1.2, 2.0, and 4.0, respectively, multiplied by the SD of the control condition (or the mean SD of the control for a given time period (e.g., the entire performance assessment)). Likelihoods for reaching the substantial change threshold were classified as follows: 5%–25%, unlikely; 25%–75%, possible; 75%–95%, likely; 95%–99%, very likely; and >99%, most likely. Log-transformed data is presented as back-transformed mean (CV). All other data is presented as the mean ± SD (or confidence intervals, where indicated). Differences are described as clear if the probability of a difference is likely or higher and non-trivial in size.

To examine the mechanistic impact of gastrointestinal distress on performance outcomes, correlation coefficient values were calculated using Microsoft Excel by plotting changes in performance against changes in gastrointestinal distress variables. Correlation coefficient confidence intervals were calculated via an additional published spreadsheet [22]. Correlation coefficient strength was qualified as follows: small 0.1, moderate 0.3, large 0.5, very large 0.7, and extremely large 1.0 [18]. Covariate analysis was utilized to assess the impact of changes in gastrointestinal distress on performance. Specifically, a linear model was utilized to assess the impact of individual symptoms of gastrointestinal distress on performance by adding the change in symptom values as a covariate in the primary published spreadsheet [21]. To evaluate the combined effect of multiple gastrointestinal distress symptoms, linear and positional coefficients from a polynomial model were calculated using the LINEST function in Microsoft Excel. An overall gastrointestinal distress covariate was then calculated as the sum of each coefficient multiplied by their respective symptom for each subject. The effect of the covariate was classified as the impact of adjusting performance effects to the mean value of the covariate. The effect, independent of the covariate, was determined by adjusting the impact of the covariate to zero.

3. Results

3.1. Performance

Time course changes in sprint power and pairwise comparisons in mean sprint power are presented in Figure 2. Mean sprint power was 290.9 (10.8), 289.2 (10.7), and 276.0 (11.4) W for G, Iso HMS, and Low HMS, respectively. There were likely small increases in mean sprint power with G vs. Low HMS (ES = 0.46) and Iso HMS vs. Low HMS (ES = 0.40), respectively. Differences in mean sprint power with Iso HMS vs. G were likely trivial (ES = 0.05).

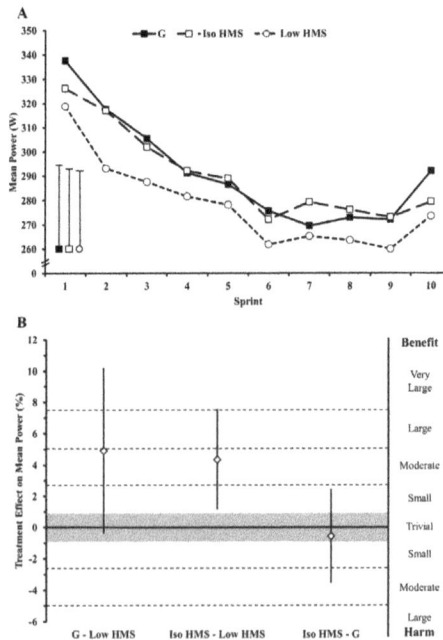

Figure 2. Effect of a hydrothermally-modified starch supplement on cycling performance. (**A**) Mean sprint power for each sprint of the performance test. Bars represent the mean standard deviation for all repeated sprints; and (**B**) mean effects (%) of treatment condition on mean sprint power. Bars represent the 90% confidence interval. G, a sucrose/glucose supplement; Iso HMS, an isocaloric dose (relative to G) of a hydrothermally-modified starch; Low HMS, low dose of a hydrothermally-modified starch.

3.2. Metabolic Parameters

Means and changes in VO_2, total carbohydrate, and fat oxidation during rest and exercise are presented in Table 1. There were no clear differences in resting or exercise VO_2. At rest and during exercise, Iso HMS (ES = 0.76 (rest) and 0.74 (exercise)) and Low HMS (ES = 0.73 and 0.63) enhanced fat oxidation relative to G. Additionally, Iso HMS (ES = 1.33 and 2.35) and Low HMS (ES = 1.77 and 2.20) reduced carbohydrate oxidation relative to G at rest and during exercise. Differences in substrate utilization with Iso HMS vs. Low HMS were unclear.

Table 1. Means and pairwise comparisons for oxygen consumption, total carbohydrate oxidation, and fat oxidation during steady state exercise.

Mean		VO_2 (L·min^{-1})	CHO Oxidation (g·min^{-1})	Fat Oxidation (g·min^{-1})
Rest	G	0.33 (23.5)	0.22 (58.6)	0.07 (82.1)
	Iso HMS	0.33 (7.9)	0.11 (89.6)	0.12 (23.8)
	Low HMS	0.32 (14.7)	0.09 (144.5)	0.12 (49.6)
Exercise	G	2.51 (9.0)	1.95 (8.7)	0.44 (40.6)
	Iso HMS	2.46 (9.3)	1.58 (21.0)	0.58 (34.7)
	Low HMS	2.48 (10.0)	1.60 (23.3)	0.56 (38.4)
Relative Difference (%); ±90% Confidence Interval *				
Rest	Low HMS–G — Mean effect	−2.2; ±11.2	−144.7; ±162.7	38.2; ±17.1
	Low HMS–G — Inference	unclear	very likely large	very likely moderate
	Iso HMS–G — Mean effect	−0.9; ±10.9	−48.9; ±21.4	64.0; ±62.2
	Iso HMS–G — Inference	unclear	very likely moderate	very likely moderate
	Iso HMS–Low HMS — Mean effect	1.3; ±7.6	48.1; ±127.7	1.5; ±27.2
	Iso HMS–Low HMS — Inference	unclear	unclear	unclear
Exercise	Low HMS–G — Mean effect	−1.2; ±3.0	−22.1; ±12.9	20.9; ±16.1
	Low HMS–G — Inference	possibly trivial	very likely very large	likely moderate
	Iso HMS–G — Mean effect	−2.1; ±2.3	−19.2; ±7.6	31.6; ±20.1
	Iso HMS–G — Inference	possibly small	most likely very large	very likely moderate
	Iso HMS–Low HMS — Mean effect	−1.0; ±1.9	−1.4; ±12.8	4.1; ±22.1
	Iso HMS–Low HMS — Inference	likely trivial	unclear	unclear

Note: Data for mean responses is presented as mean (CV). Exercise data was collected during 0–60 min of exercise. G, a glucose and sucrose-based supplement; Low HMS, low dose of hydrothermally-modified starch; Iso HMS, an isocaloric dose (relative to G) of hydrothermally-modified starch; CHO, carbohydrate. * Determination of inferences and effect sizes is described in the methods section.

Time course blood glucose and lactate data are presented in Figure 3. For resting blood glucose, there were clear differences between HMS (Iso and Low) and G at −15 min (ES − 1.49 (Iso); 1.56 (Low)) and 0 min (ES = 1.64; 1.36). During steady-state exercise (0 min–60 min), blood glucose seemed to be higher with HMS vs. G at 15 min (ES = 0.36; 0.44), but was not clearly different at 30 min. Conversely, blood glucose was clearly higher with G vs. Low HMS at 45 min (ES = 0.53), and with G vs. HMS (Iso and Low) at 60 min (ES = 0.62; 1.14). There were no clear differences between HMS and G following sprint 5; however, blood glucose was very likely enhanced following sprint 10 with G vs. HMS (Iso and Low; ES = 0.77; 0.65). For Iso HMS vs. Low HMS, the only clear differences were at 45 min (ES = 0.36) and 60 min (ES = 0.51) where blood glucose was clearly elevated with Iso HMS. For lactate, HMS (Iso and Low) was clearly lower than G at rest (−15 min (ES = 1.13; 1.49), 0 min (ES = 2.56; 2.88)) and during steady state exercise (15 min (ES = 1.23; 1.41), 30 min (ES = 0.77; 0.57), 45 min (ES = 0.85; 0.77), and 60 min (ES = 1.04; 1.00)). The only clear difference during repeated sprints was a reduced blood lactate with Low HMS vs. G following sprint 10 (ES = −0.30). There were no differences in blood lactate levels between Iso HMS and Low HMS at any time point.

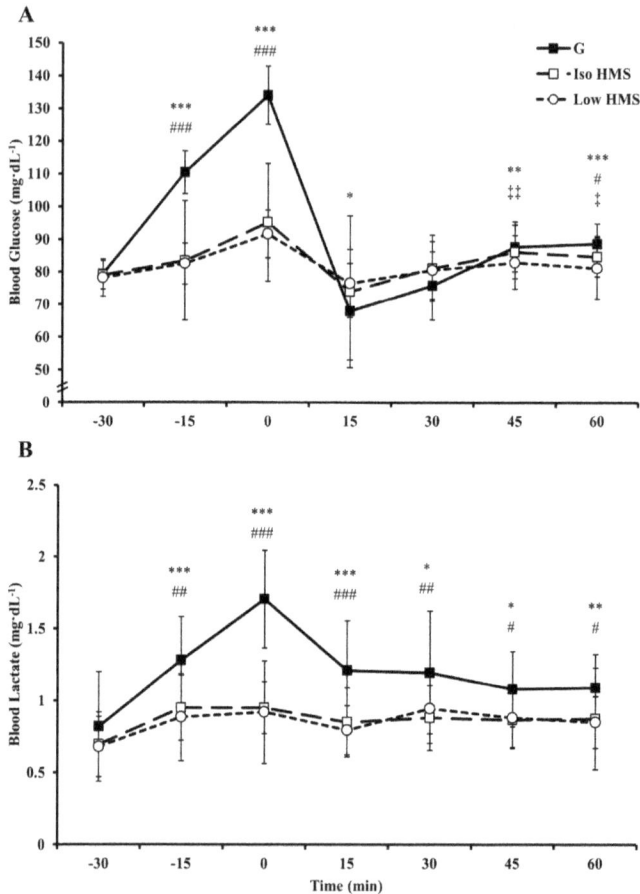

Figure 3. Time course changes in blood glucose and blood lactate. (**A**) Mean blood glucose values; and (**B**) mean blood lactate values. For (**A**,**B**), bars represent standard deviation. G, a sucrose/glucose supplement; Iso HMS, an isocaloric dose (relative to G) of a hydrothermally-modified starch; Low HMS, low dose of a hydrothermally-modified starch; *** denotes most likely different with G vs. Low HMS; ** denotes very likely different with G vs. Low HMS; * denotes likely different with G vs. Low HMS; ### denotes most likely different with G vs. Iso HMS; ## denotes very likely different with G vs. Iso HMS; # denotes likely different with G vs. Iso HMS; † denotes possibly different with G vs. Iso HMS; ‡‡ denotes very likely different with Iso HMS vs. Low HMS; ‡ denotes likely different with Iso HMS vs. Low HMS.

3.3. Heart Rate

There was a likely small and possibly small increase in mean heart rate during steady state exercise with G vs. Iso HMS (136 ± 7 vs. 133 ± 7; ES = 0.49) and G vs. Low HMS (136 ± 7 vs. 134 ± 6; ES = 0.25), respectively. There were no clear differences for mean heart rate during repeated sprints.

3.4. Perceptual Responses

Time course changes in select gastrointestinal symptoms and differences in mean perceptual responses during repeated sprints are presented in Table 2 and Figure 4. There were clear differences for mean ratings of nausea during repeated sprints with HMS (Iso and Low) vs. G (31.2 ± 26.8 (Iso) and 31.9 ± 27.2 (Low) vs. 14.0 ± 18.9; ES = 0.83; 0.86). Additionally, mean ratings of abdominal cramp (14.3 ± 14.9 vs. 9.4 ± 6.9) were increased (ES = 0.65) with Low HMS vs. G during repeated sprints.

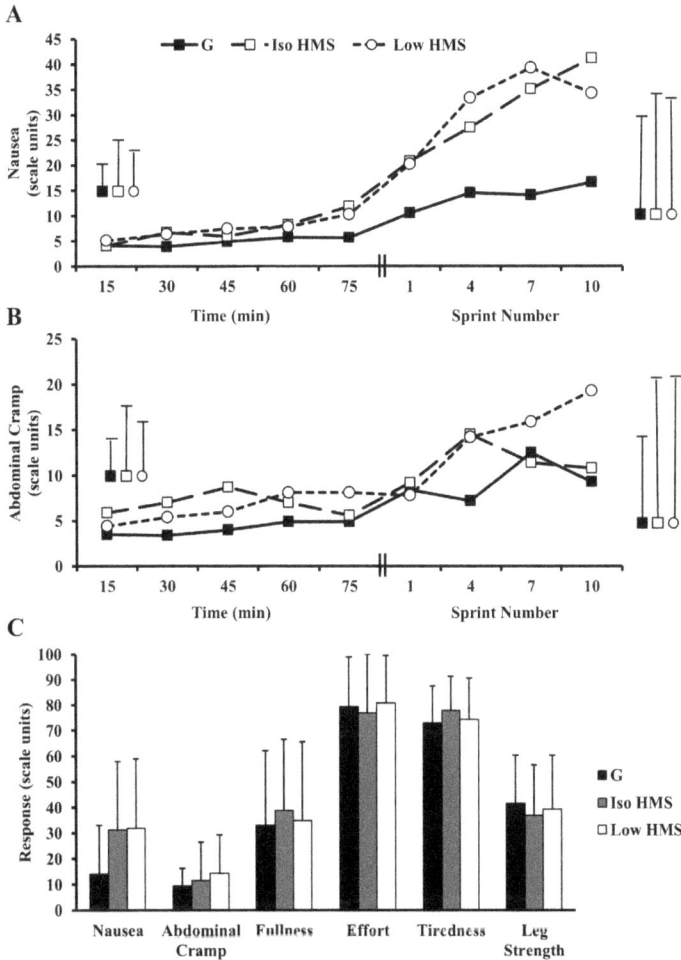

Figure 4. Changes in ratings of gastrointestinal distress and perceived exertion. (**A**) Ratings of nausea during exercise; (**B**) ratings of abdominal cramp during exercise. For (**A**,**B**), bars on the left represent mean standard deviation during the pre-load, and bars on the right represent mean standard deviation during the performance test; (**C**) Mean ratings of gastrointestinal distress and perceived exertion during the performance test. Specific changes are described in text. Mean nausea was likely increased with Iso and Low HMS vs. G during repeated sprints. Mean abdominal cramp was likely elevated with Low HMS vs. G during repeated sprints. Bars represent standard deviation. For effect magnitudes and inferences see text and Table 2. G, a sucrose/glucose supplement; Iso HMS, an isocaloric dose (relative to G) of a hydrothermally-modified starch; Low HMS, low dose of a hydrothermally-modified starch.

Table 2. Pairwise comparisons for perceptual responses during repeated sprints.

Treatment Comparisons		Perceptual Response Difference (Scale Units)					
		Nausea	Abdominal Cramp	Fullness	Effort	Tiredness	Leg Strength
Low HMS–G	Mean effect	17.9; ±14.1	5.0; ±6.1	1.9; ±8.0	1.5; ±3.5	1.4; ±5.6	−2.4; ±7.5
	Inference*	likely moderate	likely moderate	unclear	likely trivial	unclear	unclear
Iso HMS–G	Mean effect	17.2; ±18.2	2.1; ±7.1	5.9; ±11.8	−2.3; ±4.0	4.9; ±5.5	−4.8; ±5.6
	Inference	likely moderate	unclear	unclear	likely trivial	possibly small	possibly small
Iso HMS–Low HMS	Mean effect	−0.7; ±16.9	−2.8; ±4.1	4.0; ±7.8	−3.8; ±6.3	3.6; ±4.5	−2.4; ±6.6
	Inference	unclear	possibly small	possibly trivial	possibly trivial	possibly small	unclear

Note: Data is presented as scale unit differences between treatments ±90% confidence interval. G, a glucose and sucrose-based supplement; Low HMS, low dose of hydrothermally-modified starch; Iso HMS, an isocaloric dose (relative to G) of hydrothermally-modified starch; * determination of inferences and effect sizes is described in the methods section.

3.5. Gastrointestinal Distress-Mediated Effects on Performance

The influence of gastrointestinal distress on mean sprint performance is presented in Table 3. With Iso HMS vs. G, there were likely large correlations between mean sprint nausea ($r = -0.51$; ±0.45 (confidence interval)) and total gastrointestinal distress (nausea and abdominal cramp combined; $r = -0.53$; ±0.44) and performance. With Low HMS vs. G, there were very likely and most likely very large correlations for individual symptoms (nausea ($r = -0.79$; ±0.26) and abdominal cramp ($r = -0.71$; ±0.32)), and total gastrointestinal distress ($r = -0.86$; ±0.19) and changes in mean performance. Finally, there were very likely large correlations between nausea ($r = -0.63$; ±0.38) and total gastrointestinal distress ($r = -0.65$; ±0.37) and performance for Iso HMS vs. Low HMS.

Table 3. Effect of gastrointestinal distress on mean sprint power.

	Relative Difference (%) in Mean Sprint Power		
	Low HMS–G	Iso HMS–G	Iso HMS–Low HMS
Unadjusted mean sprint power	−5.0; ±5.3 likely small	−0.6; ±3.0 likely trivial	4.4; ±3.2 likely small
Effect of gastrointestinal distress	−5.5; ±2.2 very likely small **	−1.4; ±1.4 unclear	−0.3; ±0.2 Unclear **
Effect independent of gastrointestinal distress	0.4; ±3.5 Unclear **	0.8; ±3.1 likely trivial	4.7; ±2.7 likely small
Effect of Individual Symptoms			
Effect of nausea	−5.2; ±2.7 Unclear **	−1.4; ±1.6 likely trivial **	0.1; ±0.1 Unclear **
Effect independent of nausea	0.1; ±4.2 Unclear **	0.9; ±3.2 likely trivial **	4.4; ±2.7 likely small
Effect of abdominal cramp	−2.9; ±2.0 ** unclear	−0.3; ±0.6 most likely trivial **	0.4; ±1.4 Unclear **
Effect independent of abdominal cramp	−2.0; ±4.4 ** possibly trivial	−0.2; ±3.1 Unclear **	4.0; ±3.7 possibly small **

Note: Data is presented as relative differences between treatments ±90% confidence interval. G, a glucose and sucrose-based supplement; Low HMS, low dose of hydrothermally-modified starch; Iso HMS, an isocaloric dose (relative to G) of hydrothermally-modified starch; * gastrointestinal distress refers only to effects of nausea and abdominal cramp because ratings of fullness did not correlate with changes in performance; ** indicates a change in effect magnitude and/or inference mediated by the covariate.

Adding gastrointestinal distress as a covariate revealed that changes in nausea and abdominal cramp mediated changes in performance. The influence of gastrointestinal distress increased the difference between G and HMS (Iso and Low) so that adjusting out the effects of gastrointestinal distress attenuated performance differences. Importantly, adjustment for gastrointestinal distress resulted in clear differences becoming unclear (G vs. Low HMS) or likely trivial impairments in performance becoming likely trivial enhancements (Iso HMS vs. G). The effects of individual symptoms were unclear or trivial; however, adjusting out either nausea or abdominal cramp altered inferences and/or effect magnitudes for performance.

4. Discussion

In prior research examining the effects of ingesting slow-absorbing carbohydrates on endurance performance, interventions have typically been confined to the pre-exercise window, likely as a consequence of carbohydrate physical form and palatability. This timing contradicts current nutritional guidelines and common practice among endurance athletes to ingest carbohydrate both before and during exercise. The present study examined the effects of ingesting a slow-absorbing HMS supplement both before and during exercise on exercise metabolism, gastrointestinal comfort, and high-intensity cycling performance. Primary findings were as follows: (1) fat oxidation was increased and carbohydrate oxidation decreased at rest and during exercise with HMS relative to G; (2) euglycemia was maintained with HMS relative to G; (3) performance was unchanged with ingestion of HMS relative to an isocaloric amount of G; (4) performance was impaired when the during-exercise ingestion rate of HMS was halved relative to G and Iso HMS; (5) incidences of gastrointestinal distress were increased with HMS ingestion; and (6) HMS-mediated increases in gastrointestinal distress seemed to be a major mechanistic determinant of changes in performance.

Fat oxidation was enhanced and carbohydrate oxidation reduced with HMS ingestion relative to G in the current study. This finding is generally supported by studies examining pre-exercise slow-absorbing carbohydrate ingestion [14,23,24]. In the only other study to examine the effect of HMS ingestion on metabolic and performance outcomes, there was a very likely increase in fat oxidation combined with increases in plasma markers of lipolysis (i.e., glycerol and FFA) [14]. While this prior study did not report differences in total carbohydrate oxidation, our finding of reduced total carbohydrate oxidation is in line with a number of other studies examining pre-exercise intake of low glycemic index carbohydrate meals [23,24]. With during-exercise ingestion of slow-absorbing carbohydrates, metabolic findings are mixed. Specifically, increases in fat oxidation have been reported by some [16,25], but not others [26,27]. To our knowledge, this is the first study to examine the impact of a combined pre- and during-exercise slow-absorbing carbohydrate intervention. Importantly, a prior investigation revealed that ingestion of fast-absorbing carbohydrates (i.e., glucose) during exercise attenuates changes in substrate utilization induced by pre-exercise ingestion of a slow-absorbing carbohydrate meal [13]. Our data suggests that any pre-exercise-mediated alterations in substrate utilization induced by HMS are maintained (i.e., not attenuated) by continued during-exercise HMS intake.

Differences in blood glucose responses and/or carbohydrate availability provide potential mechanisms for altered substrate utilization with HMS vs. G. With HMS, pre-exercise elevations in blood glucose were reduced ~20%–23% relative to G. Although not measured in the current study, this likely resulted in an attenuated elevation in insulin [8,9,14,28]. Further evidence comes from the substantially increased levels of blood lactate during exercise with G, which is likely attributable to enhanced blood glucose uptake and glycolysis mediated by insulin binding [29]. Importantly, insulin is potently antilipolytic providing a plausible, albeit speculative, mechanism for alterations in fat utilization [30]. Additionally, carbohydrate oxidation is heavily influenced by exogenous carbohydrate absorption rates [31]. With G, there were presumably substantially faster absorption rates relative to HMS due to non-competitive transport of glucose and fructose (products of sucrose) via separate intestinal transporters [7]. Moreover, digestion of HMS would be slower vs. G due to its increased complexity and/or extensive amylose/amylopectin branching which can impede amylase infiltration [12]. These factors likely enhanced carbohydrate delivery to skeletal muscle with G vs. HMS, thereby increasing carbohydrate oxidation at the expense of fat oxidation.

Despite substantial alterations in metabolism, performance was unchanged with Iso HMS relative to G. This finding is in agreement with Roberts et al. (2011) in which endurance capacity in a 100% VO_{2max} time to exhaustion bout following 150 min of submaximal cycling (70% VO_{2max}) was unchanged with pre-exercise ingestion of HMS or maltodextrin (1 g·kg^{-1}) despite evidence for increased fat utilization with HMS. Additionally, a recent study by Oosthuyse et al. (2015) [16] found that, despite enhanced fat oxidation, cycling performance was impaired in a 16 km time trial following a 2 h pre-load (60% W_{max}) with during-exercise isomaltulose (63 g·h^{-1}) compared to a maltodextrin/fructose composite. It is possible that enhancing fat oxidation with slow-absorbing carbohydrate (which would presumably be beneficial due to possible glycogen sparing [32]), simply does not translate to any meaningful changes in performance. Indeed, a number of studies have reported no change in time trial performance with a low glycemic index pre-exercise meal despite increased exercise fat oxidation [32,33]. Moreover, a recent study found that pharmacological abolishment of lipolysis via nicotinic acid infusion had no impact on half-marathon running performance suggesting that endurance performance may be primarily carbohydrate dependent [34].

It is also possible that any beneficial metabolic effects stemming from slow-absorbing carbohydrate intake are counterbalanced or overridden by non-metabolic mechanisms. For example, gastrointestinal distress was increased in the present study, and mechanistic analysis revealed this to be a negative, albeit unclear, mediator of performance with Iso HMS vs. G. In support, Oosthuyse et al. (2015) reported that during-cycling isomaltulose ingestion resulted in increased gastrointestinal distress coupled with impaired time trial performance. However, differences in performance in the current study with Iso HMS vs. G were trivial even after adjustment for gastrointestinal distress. As such, it is possible that the severity of symptoms was insufficient to alter performance, or that any negative impact of gastrointestinal distress may have been counterbalanced by metabolic benefits (e.g., enhanced fat oxidation). Another possibility is that the impact of gastrointestinal distress may be more apparent in time trial scenarios, which require persistent concentration and pacing, relative to repeated sprint protocols that are more unrestrained in nature [6]. This might help to explain clear performance impairments in the Oosthuyse et al. study, but unclear effects of gastrointestinal distress on performance with Iso HMS vs. G in the current study. However, this notion seems less likely considering the impact of gastrointestinal distress on performance with G vs. Low HMS (discussed below). Regardless, more research is clearly warranted to elucidate the precise impact of gastrointestinal distress on performance and how these effects are altered by metabolic factors.

Perceptual response findings in the current study add further evidence to the notion that malabsorption is the primary pathophysiologic mechanism of carbohydrate-induced gastrointestinal distress during exercise. Indeed, while others have reported associations between beverage osmolality and gastrointestinal distress [35], symptoms of nausea in the present study were elevated despite very low solution osmolalities with Iso HMS and Low HMS vs. G (37–53 vs. 278–363 mOsm·kg^{-1}). Similarly, others have reported clear differences in gastrointestinal comfort with during-exercise ingestion of slow- vs. fast-absorbing carbohydrates despite consuming solutions of the same approximate osmolality (245 vs. 212 mOsm·kg^{-1}) [16]. Taken together, this data suggests that solution osmolality has a minor role in mediating gastrointestinal comfort during exercise. Rather, it seems likely that carbohydrate-induced gastrointestinal distress is primarily mediated by malabsorption, which would presumably be increased with during-exercise ingestion of slow-absorbing carbohydrate. In line with this hypothesis, others have reported increased incidences of gastrointestinal distress when carbohydrate is ingested during exercise at rates exceeding absorption capacity [6,36]. It is worth noting that ratings of nausea were similarly elevated with Iso HMS and Low HMS despite substantial differences in during-exercise intake rates. Assuming that malabsorption was primarily responsible for elevations in feelings of nausea, one might expect that Iso HMS would result in more severe symptoms as a result of a presumably greater degree of malabsorption. It is possible that malabsorption-induced nausea does not respond sensitively to carbohydrate dose. Alternatively, the methods used to assess differences in gastrointestinal distress may have lacked sensitivity to determine subtle differences in symptom severity. More research is clearly warranted to further elucidate the mechanisms governing carbohydrate-induced gastrointestinal distress during exercise.

Our finding that performance was enhanced with Iso HMS and G relative to Low HMS is in line with studies reporting dose-responsive effects of during-exercise carbohydrate ingestion on endurance performance [37,38]. However, prior investigations have only reported a dose-response effect for fast-absorbing carbohydrates (i.e., maltodextrin, glucose, and fructose) with the effect seemingly being mediated by carbohydrate oxidation efficiency. Specifically, performance is optimized when the maximal amount of carbohydrate is ingested than can feasibly be absorbed. Maltodextrin/fructose composites ingested at maximally-absorbable rates (90 g·h^{-1}) maximize performance relative to the same dose of maltodextrin (or lower doses of maltodextrin/fructose) because it can be taken up via separate intestinal transporters permitting absorption of a greater total amount of carbohydrate relative to what is ingested for a given unit of time (e.g., g·min^{-1}) [7]. While oxidation efficiency of HMS has not been measured, it would be expected to be relatively low based on its low glycemic index of 32 and studies reporting that exogenous oxidation rates of similarly slow-absorbing carbohydrates is roughly half that of glucose [27,39]. Thus, this previously-reported dose-response effect may not be a function of oxidation efficiency, but rather is solely a function of carbohydrate quantity. Indeed, while G outperformed Low HMS, Iso HMS and G performance was no different, despite likely different oxidation efficiencies.

Nevertheless, our finding of a slow-absorbing carbohydrate dose-response for performance is uncertain in light of our mechanism analyses. Gastrointestinal distress had a clear negative effect on performance with Low HMS vs. G. In fact, the likely 5% performance impairment with Low HMS vs. G became an unclear 0.4% enhancement when adjustments were made for gastrointestinal distress. This finding would suggest that, independent of gastrointestinal distress, carbohydrate dose had no impact on performance. However, adjusting for gastrointestinal distress had no clear impact on the 4.4% improvement in performance with Iso HMS vs. Low HMS suggesting that higher doses of HMS relative to lower doses improve performance even independent of gastrointestinal distress. For an explanation for these seemingly conflicting findings, it is likely that the similar levels of gastrointestinal distress between Iso and Low HMS trials confounded any adjustment for this covariate. More research is warranted to determine the extent to which performance responds (if at all) to HMS dose and how it is impacted by gastrointestinal distress.

Other interesting findings of the present study include an attenuated heart rate during steady state exercise and attenuated blood glucose concentrations following sprint 10 with HMS vs. G. The elevations in heart rate with G may have been due to the well-documented stimulatory effect of oral glucose on motivation and pleasure centers in the brain augmenting motor output [40]. Indeed, in a recent, (but yet to be published), study examining the impact of mouth rinsing with glucose on fatigued cyclists (following ~2.5 h of cycling), heart rate was elevated during subsequent steady-state exercise (50% W_{max}) following the glucose, but not placebo, rinse (Dr. Nicholas Luden, personal communication [41]). Late-exercise differences in blood glucose were likely the result of a mismatch between muscle uptake of blood glucose, which was likely high late in exercise, and exogenous blood glucose delivery, which would presumably be slower/reduced with HMS relative to G.

5. Conclusions

Findings from the present study suggest that ingesting HMS at currently-recommended rates before and during exercise maintains euglycemia, increases fat oxidation, and reduces carbohydrate oxidation during exercise in trained male cyclists. However, HMS has no impact on high-intensity cycling performance compared to fast-absorbing carbohydrate and is associated with gastrointestinal distress. Reducing the intake rate of HMS during exercise does not attenuate the risk of gastrointestinal distress, and it impairs performance. As such, the value of HMS as a during-exercise supplement seems limited. Future research should examine alternative dosing strategies designed to enhance gastrointestinal tolerance and examine the influence of gut trainability for HMS supplements. Additionally, continued research on potential applications of HMS as a pre-exercise supplement should be explored.

Acknowledgments: We are grateful to The UCAN Co. and Dymatize Nutrition Sport Performance Institute for donating product for this study. We also thank Joseph Schlenoff and Behtash Shakeri for assisting with beverage osmolality testing. Finally, we thank Palmer Johnson for assisting with treatment beverages and David Rowlands of Massey University for his advice and expertise regarding use of the repeated sprint performance protocol. This project was supported by the Florida State University Institute of Sport Sciences and Medicine.

Author Contributions: D.A.B. and M.J.O. conceived and designed the study. D.A.B., M.J.O., F.d.C.S.V., C.W.B., and J.A.G. carried out data collection. D.A.B. analyzed the data. D.A.B. drafted the manuscript. All authors edited and approved the final draft of the manuscript.

Conflicts of Interest: The authors declare no conflict of interest.

Abbreviations

The following abbreviations are used in this manuscript:

CV	coefficient of variation
ES	effect size
FFA	free fatty acids
G	glucose and sucrose-based carbohydrate supplement
HMS	hydrothermally modified starch
VO_2	oxygen consumption
VO_{2max}	maximal oxygen consumption
W_{max}	maximal cycling power

References

1. Stellingwerff, T.; Cox, G.R. Systematic review: Carbohydrate supplementation on exercise performance or capacity of varying durations. *Appl. Physiol. Nutr. Metab.* **2014**, *14*, 1–14. [CrossRef] [PubMed]
2. Thomas, D.T.; Erdman, K.A.; Burke, L.M. Nutrition and Athletic Performance. *Med. Sci. Sports Exerc.* **2016**, *48*, 543–568. [PubMed]
3. Pfeiffer, B.; Stellingwerff, T.; Hodgson, A.B.; Randell, R.; Pottgen, K.; Res, P.; Jeukendrup, A.E. Nutritional Intake and Gastrointestinal Problems during Competitive Endurance Events. *Med. Sci. Sports Exerc.* **2011**, *44*, 344–351. [CrossRef] [PubMed]
4. Havemann, L.; Goedecke, J.H. Nutritional practices of male cyclists before and during an ultraendurance event. *Int. J. Sport Nutr. Exerc. Metab.* **2008**, *18*, 551–566. [PubMed]
5. Currell, K.; Jeukendrup, A.E. Superior endurance performance with ingestion of multiple transportable carbohydrates. *Med. Sci. Sports Exerc.* **2008**, *40*, 275–281. [CrossRef] [PubMed]
6. Rowlands, D.S.; Swift, M.; Ros, M.; Green, J.G. Composite versus single transportable carbohydrate solution enhances race and laboratory cycling performance. *Appl. Physiol. Nutr. Metab.* **2012**, *37*, 425–436. [CrossRef] [PubMed]
7. Shi, X.; Summers, R.W.; Schedl, H.P.; Flanagan, S.W.; Chang, R.; Gisolfi, C.V. Effects of carbohydrate type and concentration and solution osmolality on water absorption. *Med. Sci. Sports Exerc.* **1995**, *27*, 1607–1615. [CrossRef] [PubMed]
8. Wong, S.H.S.; Siu, P.M.; Lok, A.; Chen, Y.J.; Morris, J.; Lam, C.W. Effect of the glycaemic index of pre-exercise carbohydrate meals on running performance. *Eur. J. Sport Sci.* **2008**, *8*, 23–33. [CrossRef]
9. DeMarco, H.M.; Sucher, K.P.; Cisar, C.J.; Butterfield, G.E. Pre-exercise carbohydrate meals: Application of glycemic index. *Med. Sci. Sports Exerc.* **1999**, *31*, 164–170. [CrossRef] [PubMed]
10. Karelis, A.D.; Smith, J.W.; Passe, D.H.; Péronnet, F. Carbohydrate administration and exercise performance: What are the potential mechanisms involved? *Sports Med.* **2010**, *40*, 747–763. [CrossRef] [PubMed]
11. Febbraio, M.A.A.; Chiu, A.; Angus, D.J.J.; Arkinstall, M.J.J.; Hawley, J.A.A. Effects of carbohydrate ingestion before and during exercise on glucose kinetics and performance. *J. Appl. Physiol.* **2000**, *89*, 2220–2226. [PubMed]
12. Miao, M.; Jiang, B.; Cui, S.W.; Zhang, T.; Jin, Z. Slowly Digestible Starch—A Review. *Crit. Rev. Food Sci. Nutr.* **2015**, *55*, 1642–1657. [CrossRef] [PubMed]
13. Burke, L.; Claassen, A. Carbohydrate intake during prolonged cycling minimizes effect of glycemic index of preexercise meal. *J. Appl. Physiol.* **1998**, *85*, 2220–2226. [PubMed]
14. Roberts, M.D.; Lockwood, C.; Dalbo, V.J.; Volek, J.; Kerksick, C.M. Ingestion of a high-molecular-weight hydrothermally modified waxy maize starch alters metabolic responses to prolonged exercise in trained cyclists. *Nutrition* **2011**, *27*, 659–665. [CrossRef] [PubMed]

15. Jeukendrup, A.E. A step towards personalized sports nutrition: Carbohydrate intake during exercise. *Sports Med.* **2014**, *44*, S25–S33. [CrossRef] [PubMed]
16. Oosthuyse, T.; Carstens, M.; Millen, A.M. Ingesting Isomaltulose versus Fructose-Maltodextrin during Prolonged Moderate-Heavy Exercise Increases Fat Oxidation but Impairs Gastrointestinal Comfort and Cycling Performance. *Int. J. Sport Nutr. Exerc. Metab.* **2015**, *25*, 427–438. [CrossRef] [PubMed]
17. Jeukendrup, A.E.; Wallis, G.A. Measurement of Substrate Oxidation during Exercise by Means of Gas Exchange Measurements. *Int. J. Sports Med.* **2005**, *26*, S28–S37. [CrossRef] [PubMed]
18. Hopkins, W.G.; Marshall, S.W.; Batterham, A.M.; Hanin, J. Progressive statistics for studies in sports medicine and exercise science. *Med. Sci. Sports Exerc.* **2009**, *41*, 3–13. [CrossRef] [PubMed]
19. O'Brien, W.J.; Stannard, S.R.; Clarke, J.A.; Rowlands, D.S. Fructose-maltodextrin ratio governs exogenous and other cho oxidation and performance. *Med. Sci. Sports Exerc.* **2013**, *45*, 1814–1824. [CrossRef] [PubMed]
20. Rowlands, D.S.; Thorp, R.M.; Rossler, K.; Graham, D.F.; Rockell, M.J. Effect of protein-rich feeding on recovery after intense exercise. *Int. J. Sport Nutr. Exerc. Metab.* **2007**, *17*, 521–543. [PubMed]
21. Hopkins, W.G. Spreadsheets for analysis of controlled trials, with adjustment for a subject characteristic. *Sports Sci.* **2006**, *10*, 46–50.
22. Hopkins, W.G. A spreadsheet for deriving a confidence interval, mechanistic inference and clinical inference from a p value. *Sports Sci.* **2007**, *11*, 16–20.
23. Stevenson, E.; Astbury, N.M.; Simpson, E.J.; Taylor, M.A.; Macdonald, I.A. Fat oxidation during exercise and satiety during recovery are increased following a low-glycemic index breakfast in sedentary women. *J. Nutr.* **2009**, *139*, 890–897. [CrossRef] [PubMed]
24. Sun, F.-H.; O'Reilly, J.; Li, L.; Wong, S.H.-S. Effect of the glycemic index of pre-exercise snack bars on substrate utilization during subsequent exercise. *Int. J. Food Sci. Nutr.* **2013**, *64*, 1001–1006. [CrossRef] [PubMed]
25. Too, B.W.; Cicai, S.; Hockett, K.R.; Applegate, E.; Davis, B.A.; Casazza, G.A. Natural versus commercial carbohydrate supplementation and endurance running performance. *J. Int. Soc. Sports Nutr.* **2012**, *9*, 27. [CrossRef] [PubMed]
26. Leijssen, D.P.; Saris, W.H.; Jeukendrup, A.E.; Wagenmakers, A.J. Oxidation of exogenous [13C]galactose and [13C]glucose during exercise. *J. Appl. Physiol.* **1995**, *79*, 720–725. [PubMed]
27. Achten, J.; Jentjens, R.L.; Brouns, F.; Jeukendrup, A.E. Exogenous oxidation of isomaltulose is lower than that of sucrose during exercise in men. *J. Nutr.* **2007**, *137*, 1143–1148. [PubMed]
28. Stevenson, E.; Thelwall, P.; Thomas, K.; Smith, F.; Brand-Miller, J.C.; Trenell, M.I. Dietary glycemic index influences lipid oxidation but not muscle or liver glycogen oxidation during exercise. *Am. J. Physiol. Endocrinol. Metab.* **2009**, *296*, E1140–E1147. [CrossRef] [PubMed]
29. Beitner, R.; Kalant, N. Stimulation of glycolysis by insulin. *J. Biol. Chem.* **1971**, *246*, 500–503. [PubMed]
30. Horowitz, J.F.; Mora-Rodriguez, R.; Byerley, L.O.; Coyle, E.F. Lipolytic suppression following carbohydrate ingestion limits fat oxidation during exercise. *Am. J. Physiol.* **1997**, *273*, E768–E775. [CrossRef] [PubMed]
31. Jeukendrup, A.E. Carbohydrate and exercise performance: The role of multiple transportable carbohydrates. *Curr. Opin. Clin. Nutr. Metab. Care* **2010**, *13*, 452–457. [CrossRef] [PubMed]
32. Febbraio, M.; Keenan, J.; Angus, D.; Campbell, S.; Garnham, A. Preexercise carbohydrate ingestion, glucose kinetics, and muscle glycogen use: Effect of the glycemic index. *J. Appl. Physiol.* **2000**, *89*, 1845–1851. [PubMed]
33. Chen, Y.J.; Wong, S.H.; Wong, C.K.; Lam, C.W.; Huang, Y.J.; Siu, P.M. Effect of preexercise meals with different glycemic indices and loads on metabolic responses and endurance running. *Int. J. Sport Nutr. Exerc. Metab.* **2008**, *18*, 281–300. [PubMed]
34. Leckey, J.J.; Burke, L.M.; Morton, J.P.; Hawley, J.A. Altering fatty acid availability does not impair prolonged, continuous running to fatigue: Evidence for carbohydrate dependence. *J. Appl. Physiol.* **2016**, *120*, 107–113. [CrossRef] [PubMed]
35. Rehrer, N.J.; van Kemenade, M.; Meester, W.; Brouns, F.; Saris, W.H. Gastrointestinal complaints in relation to dietary intake in triathletes. *Int. J. Sport Nutr.* **1992**, *2*, 48–59. [PubMed]
36. Triplett, D.; Doyle, J.A.; Rupp, J.C.; Benardot, D. An isocaloric glucose-fructose beverage's effect on simulated 100-km cycling performance compared with a glucose-only beverage. *Int. J. Sport Nutr. Exerc. Metab.* **2010**, *20*, 122–131. [PubMed]

37. Smith, J.; Zachwieja, J.J.; Péronnet, F.; Passe, D.H.; Massicotte, D.; Lavoie, C.; Pascoe, D.D. Fuel selection and cycling endurance performance with ingestion of [13C]glucose: Evidence for a carbohydrate dose response. *J. Appl. Physiol.* **2010**, *108*, 1520–1529. [CrossRef] [PubMed]

38. Smith, J.; Pascoe, D.D.; Passe, D.H.; Ruby, B.C.; Stewart, L.K.; Baker, L.B.; Zachwieja, J.J. Curvilinear Dose-Response Relationship of Carbohydrate (0–120 g· h^{-1}) and Performance. *Med. Sci. Sport Exerc.* **2013**, *45*, 336–341. [CrossRef] [PubMed]

39. Correia, C.E.; Bhattacharya, K.; Lee, P.J.; Shuster, J.J.; Theriaque, D.W.; Shankar, M.N.; Smit, G.P.A.; Weinstein, D.A. Use of modified cornstarch therapy to extend fasting in glycogen storage disease types Ia and Ib. *Am. J. Clin. Nutr.* **2008**, *88*, 1272–1276. [PubMed]

40. Gant, N.; Stinear, C.M.; Byblow, W.D. Carbohydrate in the mouth immediately facilitates motor output. *Brain Res.* **2010**, *1350*, 151–158. [CrossRef] [PubMed]

41. Luden, D.N.; James Madison University, Harrisonburg, VA, USA. Personal communication, 2016.

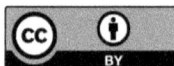

nutrients   MDPI

Article

Improvements in Cycling but Not Handcycling 10 km Time Trial Performance in Habitual Caffeine Users

Terri Graham-Paulson [1], Claudio Perret [2] and Victoria Goosey-Tolfrey [1,*]

[1] School of Sport, Exercise and Health Sciences, Peter Harrison Centre for Disability Sport, Loughborough University, Epinal Way, Loughborough LE113TU, UK; t.s.graham@lboro.ac.uk
[2] Swiss Paraplegic Centre, Institute of Sport Medicine, Guido A. Zäch-Strasse, Nottwil 6207, Switzerland; claudio.perret@paraplegie.ch
*   Correspondence: v.l.tolfrey@lboro.ac.uk; Tel.: +44-0-150-922-6386

Received: 9 May 2016; Accepted: 20 June 2016; Published: 25 June 2016

Abstract: Caffeine supplementation during whole-/lower-body exercise is well-researched, yet evidence of its effect during upper-body exercise is equivocal. The current study explored the effects of caffeine on cycling/handcycling 10 km time trial (TT) performance in habitual caffeine users. Eleven recreationally trained males (mean (SD) age 24 (4) years, body mass 85.1 (14.6) kg, cycling/handcycling peak oxygen uptake ($\dot{V}_{peak}$) 42.9 (7.3)/27.6 (5.1) mL·kg·min^{-1}, 160 (168) mg/day caffeine consumption) completed two maximal incremental tests and two familiarization sessions. During four subsequent visits, participants cycled/handcycled for 30 min at 65% mode-specific $\dot{V}_{peak}$ (preload) followed by a 10 km TT following the ingestion of 4 mg·kg^{-1} caffeine (CAF) or placebo (PLA). Caffeine significantly improved cycling (2.0 (2.0)%; 16:35 vs. 16:56 min; $p = 0.033$) but not handcycling (1.8 (3.0)%; 24:10 vs. 24:36 min; $p = 0.153$) TT performance compared to PLA. The improvement during cycling can be attributed to the increased power output during the first and last 2 km during CAF. Higher blood lactate concentration (Bla) was reported during CAF compared to PLA ($p < 0.007$) and was evident 5 min post-TT during cycling (11.2 $\pm$ 2.6 and 8.8 $\pm$ 3.2 mmol/L; $p = 0.001$) and handcycling (10.6 $\pm$ 2.5 and 9.2 $\pm$ 2.9 mmol/L; $p = 0.006$). Lower overall ratings of perceived exertion (RPE) were seen following CAF during the preload ($p < 0.05$) but not post-TT. Lower peripheral RPE were reported at 20 min during cycling and at 30 min during handcycling, and lower central RPE was seen at 30 min during cycling ($p < 0.05$). Caffeine improved cycling but not handcycling TT performance. The lack of improvement during handcycling may be due to the smaller active muscle mass, elevated (Bla) and/or participants' training status.

Keywords: exercise; ergogenic; upper-body; sport; supplement

---

1. Introduction

Low-moderate doses of caffeine (3–6 mg per kilogram of body weight (mg·kg^{-1})) have been shown to positively influence cycling time-trial (TT) performance [1,2]. During cycling, the leg musculature provides the speed-generating force. However, there are numerous sports and activities such as kayaking, handcycling, double-poling and wheelchair sports during which the arms produce this force. It is apparent that nutritional supplements such as caffeine are commonly used in both able-bodied (AB) [3,4] and disability sports [5], including many that involve upper-body exercise (UBE). The physiological responses to whole- and lower-body exercise (LBE) differ to those of UBE [6], and it is therefore debatable whether the findings from the aforementioned cycling studies are transferable to an UBE sport such as handcycling.

A potential mechanism of caffeine is its influence on the central nervous system (CNS) by which it acts as an adenosine receptor (most likely A$_1$ and A$_{2a}$) antagonist [7,8]. Antagonism reduces the influence of adenosine and produces motor-activating and arousing effects. Caffeine can therefore have a positive influence on subjective feelings such as ratings of perceived exertion (RPE), mood and cognitive performance [9,10]. Lower RPE during submaximal exercise has been reported following caffeine ingestion, and/or similar RPE when a higher workload has been achieved [2,11,12]. Caffeine has also been shown to produce hypoalgesic effects during submaximal cycling in male and female participants [13,14]. It has been suggested that the inhibition of adenosine receptors following caffeine ingestion could also influence motor unit recruitment or have a direct effect on muscle [8,15]. It is likely that a combination of factors contribute to improved endurance performance but with caffeine's influence on the CNS in mind, a similar ergogenic benefit could be expected during UBE as has been reported during LBE. However, the evidence for a positive influence of caffeine during UBE remains equivocal.

An 8 km double-poling TT performance lasting ~34 min was enhanced following the consumption of 6 mg·kg^{-1} caffeine in regular caffeine users [12]. Double-poling is considered primarily to be an UBE; however, the trunk and legs also play a role in the performance of this technique. On the other hand, when LBE and asynchronous UBE were directly compared in very low caffeine users (<40 mg/day) during a preloaded 10 min all-out performance trial (40 min total exercise time), caffeine (5 mg·kg^{-1}) improved LBE but failed to statistically impact UBE in a mixed AB group [16]. The opposing results may be linked to differences in the exercise testing protocols, caffeine dose, training status of the participants', or the participants' level of habitual caffeine consumption. The contrasting responses may also be due to a number of factors related to the physiology of the leg and arm muscles. Firstly, the arms possess a smaller muscle mass and hence a reduced absolute muscle force. Arm muscles may possess a higher percentage of fast-twitch muscle fibers [17,18] and have a lower oxygen extraction capacity compared to the legs [6]. The onset of anaerobic metabolism during UBE therefore occurs at a lower level of oxygen uptake, and lactate concentrations are reported to be higher than during a comparable bout of LBE [6,19]. These factors can be altered with training however [20] and may help explain differences between performance outcomes in recreationally active participants and those that are specifically UBE trained.

It has been previously reported that caffeine increases muscular strength (maximal voluntary contraction) and motor unit recruitment in the knee extensors but not in the elbow flexors [15,16]. These observations may help to explain the lack of performance improvement during short-term UBE in AB participants [21]. The influence of caffeine on longer UBE endurance performance, however, requires further investigation given the protocols of Stadheim et al. [12] and Black et al. [16] both allowed involvement of the trunk to some extent to produce force yet report opposing effects. Black et al. [16] also used a mixed male and female participant pool of very low caffeine users, which makes their findings less applicable to the many competitive athletes who consume caffeine regularly. Therefore, the purpose of the current study was to explore the effects of caffeine on both LBE and UBE endurance performance. The study will employ an ecologically valid LBE and UBE endurance protocol whereby male habitual caffeine users will complete preloaded (30 min at 65% peak oxygen uptake ($\dot{V}_{peak}$) 10 km TTs following the ingestion of caffeine and placebo. Importantly, they will adopt a synchronous handcycling modality for the UBE aspect, which is akin to the sports of handcycling and the cycling discipline of Para-Triathlon.

2. Materials and Methods

2.1. Participants

Eleven recreationally active, healthy males (age 24 (4) year, body mass 85.1 (14.6) kg, lower and upper body $\dot{V}_{peak}$ 42.9 (7.3) and 27.6 (5.1) mL·kg·min^{-1}) participated in the current study. Caffeine users, with average daily caffeine intake 160 (168) mg/day were recruited to represent the usual dietary habits of athletes. All procedures were approved by the Loughborough University Ethics Approvals Sub-committee (R14-P79, 10/04/14) and performed in accordance with the Declaration of

Helsinki. All participants provided written informed consent and none revealed contraindications for participating in the study.

2.2. Experimental Design

The study employed a double-blind, placebo-controlled, repeated measures design. Participants attended the laboratory on eight separate occasions, which consisted of a $\dot{V}_{peak}$ test, a familiarization and two (caffeine and placebo) experimental trials (Figure 1) for both cycling and handcycling. Familiarization sessions aimed to limit a potential learning effect. Familiarization procedures were the same as the experimental procedures described in Figure 1 with the exception of capsule consumption and blood sampling. Experimental trials were separated by $\geqslant 48$ h and were conducted at the same time of day within participants (7:30–09:30 a.m.) to avoid any influence of circadian rhythm [22].

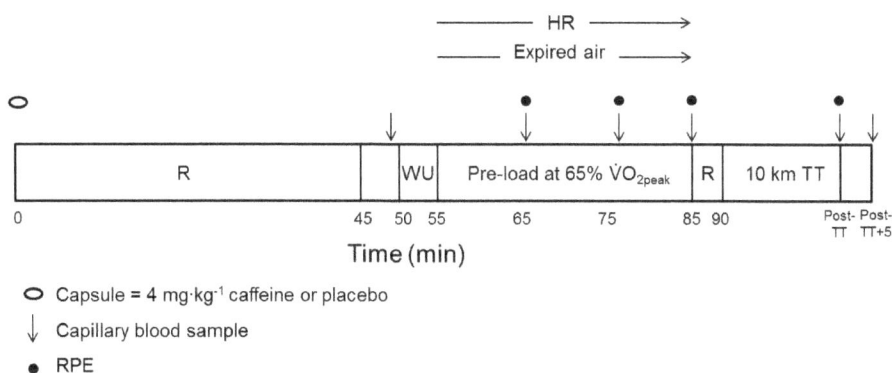

Figure 1. Schematic outline of the preloaded time trial (TT) experimental protocol. HR = heart rate; R = rest; WU = warm-up; and RPE = ratings of perceived exertion.

2.3. Preliminary Trials

The cycling trials were performed on a Viking Jetstream 14 road bike and the handcycling trials were performed on a Draft handbike (operating in synchronous crank mode). Both pieces of equipment were mounted on a Cyclus II ergometer (Avantronic Richter, Leipzig, Germany). Bike settings were individually adjusted and standardized for each participant across trials. The differentiated RPE scale was explained to participants prior to the commencement of preliminary trial testing.

On separate occasions, participants performed incremental cycling and handcycling tests until exhaustion to determine mode-specific $\dot{V}_{peak}$. The ergometer was set in power control mode, which ensured a pre-set power output (PO) was automatically regulated independent of cadence or gear selection by continuous adjustment of the degree of electromagnetic braking. The participants' performed a 5-min warm-up at a self-selected pace. The continuous step tests consisted of 3-min submaximal stages with an initial load of 70 W for the cycling and 20 W for the handcycling test. Increments of 30 W for the cycling and 10 W for the handcycling test were then applied. Participants reported differentiated RPE scores at the end of each stage and upon completion. Blood lactate concentrations (Bla) were determined using a Biosen C-Line (EKF Diagnostic GmbH, Barleben, Germany) at the end of each stage from earlobe capillary blood samples. When the participant's (Bla) increased beyond 4 mmol·L the resistance was increased by 5 W every 15 s until volitional exhaustion (failure to maintain a cadence of $\geqslant 50$ rpm following 2 warnings and an overall RPE = 19–20). Online respiratory gas analysis was carried out via a breath-by-breath system (MetaLyzer 3B, Cortex Biophysik GmbH, Leipzig, Germany). Prior to each test, gases were calibrated according to the manufacturer's recommendations. The highest 30 s rolling average $\dot{V}$ value was used as the participant's $\dot{V}_{peak.}$ Heart rate (HR) was monitored continuously (Polar RS400, Polar, Kempele, Finland).

2.4. Experimental Trials

Participants refrained from exercise, caffeine and alcohol consumption in the 24 h preceding each trial, as previously utilized [23]. They completed 24 h dietary diaries prior to the first experimental trial and were asked to replicate their diet for all subsequent trials. Participants were asked to consume a self-selected standardized meal 1.5 h prior to arriving at the laboratory, which was noted upon arrival (62 (10)% carbohydrate, 18 (9)% protein, 20 (9)% fat) and replicated prior to all subsequent trials.

The experimental trials involved the consumption of either 4 mg·kg^{-1} caffeine anhydrous (CAF) or dextrose placebo (PLA) capsules (Bulk Powders, Colchester, UK) 45 min prior to the warm-up. A 4 mg·kg^{-1} caffeine dose has previously increased plasma caffeine concentrations to 14.6 μM, 50 min post-ingestion [23] and was therefore deemed suitable for the current study. The protocol can be seen in Figure 1 and is based on that used previously to assess the effects of glucose ingestion on UBE performance [24]. Participants were instructed to complete the 10 km TT in the shortest time possible, during which they could change gear at any time. Cycling 10 km TTs have been shown to be reproducible in active and endurance-trained participants with a coefficient of variation of 1.5% for performance time [25]. No motivation was provided during the TT and, to avoid test–retest influence, the only feedback provided was cumulative distance covered. Experimental trial conditions were temperature 19.7 (1.1) °C, pressure 1004 (11) hPa and humidity 52 (12)%.

The 6–20 RPE scale [26] was used as a measure of perceived exertion during exercise at 10, 20 and 30 min during the preload, and post-TT. Participants were asked for three RPE scores: peripheral (muscle and joint exertion) (RPE$_P$), central (ventilatory and circulatory exertion) (RPE$_C$) and overall (integrated) (RPE$_O$).

2.5. Statistical Analyses

Statistical Package for the Social Sciences version 20 software (SPSS Inc., Chicago, IL, USA) was used to analyze the data. Normal distribution was confirmed using the Shapiro–Wilk test and consequently (Bla) performance times, HR, power output (PO), respiratory exchange ratio (RER) and $\dot{V}$ data are reported as mean (standard deviation) (SD). Repeated measures analysis of variance (ANOVA) was used to examine differences in (Bla) and preload HR, RER and PO. Post-hoc paired samples t-tests using the Bonferroni correction were applied following significant findings. Ten km TT performance was also analyzed using a repeated measures two-way ANOVA, with time and treatment as within participant factors and trial order as a covariate. Cohen's d effect sizes (ES) are included to supplement important findings. An ES of 0.2 was considered small, 0.5 moderate and 0.8 large. One-way ANOVAs with habitual caffeine intake (low, moderate, and high users) as a factor were also employed. Nonparametric ordinal RPE data are reported as median (quartiles) and were analyzed using Friedman and Wilcoxon tests. Statistical significance was accepted at $p < 0.05$.

3. Results

3.1. Performance Tests

Caffeine significantly improved 10 km TT performance during cycling by 2.0 (2.0)% compared to PLA (ES = -0.4, $p = 0.033$) (995 (46) s and 1016 (58) s, respectively). Ten (of 11) participants cycled faster during CAF (Figure 2). Participants (7 of 11) also handcycled 1.8 (3.0)% faster during CAF compared to PLA (1450 (86) and 1476 (67) s, respectively) (Figure 2); however, this failed to reach significance (ES = -0.34, $p = 0.153$). There was no significant influence of trial order during cycling ($p = 0.164$) or handcycling ($p = 0.298$). The PO was significantly greater during CAF compared to PLA during cycling only ($p = 0.003$), and this was apparent during the first and last 2 km of the TT ($p < 0.006$). There was no influence of habitual caffeine intake on TT performance ($p > 0.470$). Participants with a handcycling $\dot{V}_{peak}$ greater than the mean value (27.6 ml·kg·min^{-1}) ($n = 7$) improved their handcycling TT performance by 3.2% whereas those with a $\dot{V}_{peak}$ less than the mean ($n = 4$) had a 0.3% reduction in handcycling performance (Figure 2).

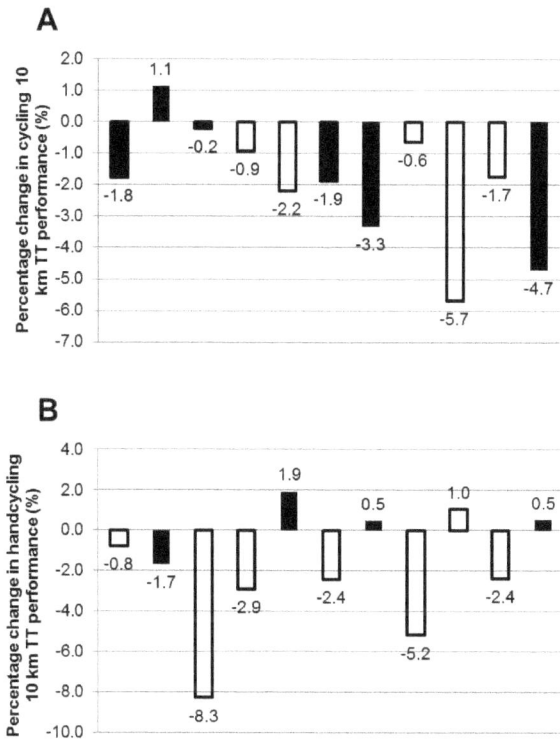

Figure 2. Individual percentage change in 10 km (a) cycling and (b) handcycling time trial (TT) performance. Negative responses indicate a reduction in time to complete the TT during caffeine (CAF) compared to placebo (PLA). Open/filled bars indicate participants with a $\dot{V}_{peak}$ above/below the mode-specific mean. Participant data are ordered the same in A and B.

A significantly lower $\dot{V}_{peak}$ was recorded during handcycling compared to cycling (27.6 (5.1) and 42.9 (7.3) mL·kg·min^{-1}, $p = 0.001$). The target relative exercise intensity of the 65% $\dot{V}_{peak}$ during the preload was matched experimentally with average $\dot{V}$ values of 64.5 (2.5)% during cycling, and 59.7 (4.8)% during handcycling but importantly, did not differ between mode-specific CAF and PLA trials ($p > 0.217$). Average preload HR and RER did not differ between CAF and PLA ($p > 0.180$).

3.2. Blood Lactate Concentration

There was a significant increase in (Bla) over time during all trials ($p = 0.001$). This was evident between 10 and 20 min during cycling following CAF only ($p = 0.006$), and at both 20 and 30 min compared to 10 min during handcycling following both CAF and PLA ($p < 0.005$). The TT resulted in a significant increase in (Bla) post-TT and five min post-TT during all trials ($p < 0.017$). The ingestion of CAF resulted in significantly higher (Bla) compared to PLA during cycling ($p = 0.001$) and handcyling ($p = 0.007$), but differences were only evident post-TT ($p < 0.012$) (Figure 3). The handcycling preload (despite a slightly lower relative workload) produced significantly greater (Bla) than during cycling regardless of trial (p = 0.004 and 0.016 during PLA and CAF, respectively). However, there was no difference in (Bla) pre-exercise or post-TT between modalities (p > 0.134).

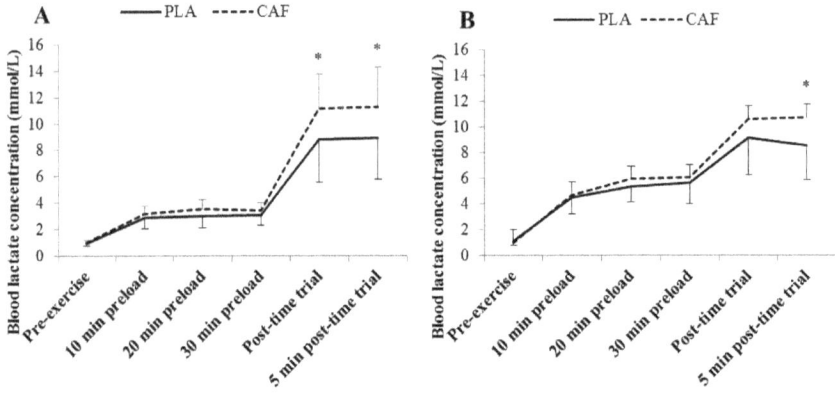

Figure 3. Group mean (SD) blood lactate concentrations (mmol/L) throughout the 30-min preloaded (65% $\dot{V}_{peak}$) 10 km time trial protocol during cycling (**a**) and handcycling (**b**) following the consumption of 4 mg·kg^{-1} caffeine (CAF) or placebo (PLA). * Significantly different from placebo (PLA).

3.3. Subjective Feelings

Participants' RPE responses can be seen in Table 1. Only one participant, a low caffeine user, experienced side effects during CAF, which were reported as feelings of sickness post-preload. Only two participants correctly identified the treatment in all four trials.

Table 1. Overall, central and peripheral ratings of perceived exertion (RPE) at 10, 20 and 30 min during the preload and immediately post-time trial.

		Preload 10 min	Preload 20 min	Preload 30 min	Post-Time Trial
Overall RPE	C PLA	13 (12, 13)	13 (13, 14) [†]	14 (13, 14) [†,‡]	19 (17, 20) [†,‡,#]
	C CAF	12 (11, 13) *	13 (12, 14) [†,*]	13 (12, 14) [†,*]	19 (18, 20) [†,‡,#]
	HC PLA	13 (12, 14)	14 (12, 15) [†]	14 (13, 16) [†,‡]	19 (18, 20) [†,‡,#]
	HC CAF	12 (11, 13) *	13 (12, 14) [†,*]	14 (12, 15) [†]	19 (18, 20) [†,‡,#]
Central RPE	C PLA	12 (11, 13)	12 (11, 13) [†]	13 (11, 14) [†,‡]	18 (17, 20) [†,‡,#]
	C CAF	12 (11, 13)	13 (12, 14) [†]	13 (12, 14)[*,†,‡]	19 (18, 20) [†,‡,#]
	HC PLA	12 (11, 13)	12 (11, 13) [†]	13 (12, 14) [†,‡]	17 (16, 18) [†,‡,#]
	HC CAF	11 (11, 12)	13 (11, 13) [†]	13 (11, 14) [†]	17 (17, 19) [†,‡,#]
Peripheral RPE	C PLA	13 (12, 13)	13 (13, 15) [†]	14 (13, 16) [†,‡]	19 (18, 20) [†,‡,#]
	C CAF	13 (11, 13)	13 (12, 14) [*,†]	14 (13, 15) [†,‡]	19 (17, 20) [†,‡,#]
	HC PLA	14 (13, 15)	15 (13, 16) [†]	15 (13, 16) [†,‡]	19 (19, 20) [†,‡,#]
	HC CAF	13 (11, 14)	14 (12, 15)	15 (12, 16) [*,†]	19 (18, 20) [†,‡,#]

Note: Data are median (quartiles). * Significantly different from placebo (PLA), [†] significantly different from Preload 10 min, [‡] significantly different from Preload 20 min and [#] significantly different from Preload 30 min (p < 0.05).

4. Discussion

This is the first study to assess the effect of caffeine on 10 km TT performance during both cycling and handcycling in habitual caffeine users. The main finding was that the ingestion of caffeine (4 mg·kg^{-1}) significantly improved cycling 10 km TT performance, whereas the same dose did not statistically improve handcycling performance. This study compliments the work of Black et al. [16] by investigating the influence of caffeine on longer-term endurance performance during

LBE (~47 vs. 40 min) and UBE (~54 vs. 40 min) in the same habitual caffeine users. It also supports a large body of evidence on the positive impact of caffeine on endurance cycling performance [1,11,16,27].

4.1. Preload

The ingestion of CAF during the submaximal preload resulted in changes in RPE but not average RER, HR or $\dot{V}$, which agrees with earlier studies [28,29]. While there was a trend for greater (Bla) during the preload following CAF, in contrast to previous steady state exercise data [16] this did not reach significance.

Recent reviews on caffeine and its ergogenic effects propose the antagonism of adenosine receptors as the primary mode of action leading to enhanced performance [30,31]. This mechanism of action has been shown to influence the CNS [7], through which perceived pain, effort and fatigue are reduced. The current results show caffeine to reduce RPE during constant rate LBE and UBE. During cycling, RPE_O was lower at all preload time-points and RPE_P and RPE_C was lower at 20 and 30 min following CAF, respectively. During handcycling, RPE_O was lower at 10 and 20 min and RPE_P was lower at 30 min only following CAF. The reduction in perceived effort during the preload may have influenced the participant's effort during the subsequent cycling TT yet appears not to have impacted the handcycling TT.

4.2. Time Trial Performance

The 10 km TT provided data from which the influence of caffeine on endurance performance could be assessed in a sport-specific manner. The ingestion of CAF resulted in a significant improvement in cycling performance (2.0 (2.0)%) compared to PLA, which was due to the increased PO during the first and last two km. On the other hand, it failed to significantly improve handcycling performance (1.8 (3.0)%) and there was large intra-individual variability. The small effect sizes (-0.4 and -0.34 for cycling and handcycling, respectively) reflect the large standard deviations for both sets of results. Individual responses to caffeine supplementation have often been attributed to differing rates of caffeine metabolism, which may in turn be linked to training status and body composition [32]. Unfortunately, the rate of caffeine absorption and metabolism were not measured in the current study. Participant three, who produced the greatest handcycling $\dot{V}_{peak}$ value of the group, improved handcycling TT performance by 8.3% following CAF, yet only improved cycling TT performance by 0.2%. Aside from the participant displaying a learning effect or having an unexplained good/bad performance, a further explanation for some of the inter-individual variability may therefore be an individual's training status. Despite a non-significant finding, some sports practitioners would argue that if a 1.8% improvement held true for individual elite handcyclists, caffeine could positively impact performance and ultimately influence finishing positions in a sport where winning margins are small (~0.5%) [33]. The ingestion of CAF resulted in higher post-TT (Bla) during both modes of exercise. This increase in (Bla) following the ingestion of caffeine is common in the literature during both LBE [28] and UBE [12]. The increase is understandable when seen in conjunction with improved performance such as during the current cycling trials, yet remains to be explained when a performance improvement is absent as seen during the handcycling trials. The metabolic responses to exercise differ in arm and leg muscles. Arm exercise is physiologically more stressful than leg exercise and can increase adrenaline concentration, which in turn is a potent stimulant for muscle glycogenolysis [34]. The arms also have a lower oxygen extraction capacity, which results in an earlier onset of anaerobic metabolism (~50% and 75% $\dot{V}_{max}$ during arm and leg exercise, respectively) [6]. Hence, the greater (Bla) seen in the current study during handcycling. Accumulation of (Bla) during the handcycling TT, which was further increased during CAF may have limited the participants' ability to improve performance.

Evidence from biopsies suggests that the triceps muscle (an important force producing muscle during synchronous handcycling) exhibits a greater proportion of type II muscle fibers than the legs (vastus lateralis) [17,18]. This may partly explain a lack of performance improvement during the endurance handcycling TT (~24 min) during which type I fibers would dominate. Furthermore, type II fibers have been shown (in vitro) to be less sensitive to caffeine compared to type I fibers [35]. Hence, performance gains may be less likely following the ingestion of caffeine during exercise which relies on the arms (with a lower proportion of type I fibers). Endurance training can improve the oxidative capacity of muscle fibers [20] and hence may help to explain the observed handcycling TT improvements following caffeine in those that had an above average mode-specific $\dot{V}_{peak}$ (Figure 2).

Previous research suggests caffeine increases muscular strength (maximal voluntary contraction) and motor unit recruitment in the knee extensors but not in the elbow flexors [15,16]. More and larger muscles are recruited during LBE compared to UBE and hence caffeine's influence on muscle contractility may enhance LBE performance to a greater extent. This potential mechanism is supported by the improvement in cycling but not handcycling TT performance in the current study.

Although RPE was not reduced following the cycling TT, PO was higher during CAF suggesting that participants were able to cycle at a higher PO with no change in RPE. This is in line with previous literature that has shown caffeine to increase the PO/RPE ratio during a TT [1,2]. It has previously been suggested that the limitation to maximal UBE is likely due to localized fatigue rather than central circulatory factors [36]. At the end of the handcycling preload (30 min) RPE_P was reduced by CAF but this reduction in perceived arm and shoulder effort did not translate to improvements in TT performance. It has been suggested that caffeine is unable to have a hypoalgesic effect during heavy-severe fixed intensity exercise [16], and the same study reported no change in RPE during a 10 min asynchronous UBE performance trial. The current study adds further evidence that the reduced RPE and hypoalgesic effects seen during submaximal synchronous UBE do not translate to improved performance during a maximal performance trial. It is likely that the nociceptive stimuli contributing to the peripheral muscle pain during handcycling may be too great for the antagonism of adenosine receptors to reduce RPE and pain, and hence are unlikely to translate to improved performance.

The $\dot{V}_{peak}$ achieved during handcycling was 64% of that achieved during cycling (range: 52%–83%), which is lower than previously reported values (~70%) [37]. This is likely due to the training status of the current participants who were not specifically trained in either cycling or handcycling. The use of recreationally trained participants helped to limit the potential difference in performance between the cycling modalities and yet meant that participants were unfamiliar with the pacing strategies required, especially during handcycling. It is worth noting that those with a handcycling $\dot{V}_{peak}$ above the mean improved their handcycling TT performance by 3.2%, whereas those below the mean had a 0.3% reduction (Figure 2). Hence, an individual's training status appears to affect how they respond to caffeine during UBE. This theory is supported by improvements in swimming velocity (during which a large proportion of the force is generated by the upper-body) following the ingestion of caffeine by trained but not untrained participants [38]. The authors suggested that the intra and/or extracellular adaptations resulting from specific training are necessary to benefit from caffeine during sprint performance [38]. The current results suggest that this holds true for endurance UBE performance also.

It has been suggested that one familiarization session is sufficient for reproducible results in recreationally active individuals (cycling $\dot{V}_{peak}$ = 3.9 compared to 3.6 L·min^{-1} in the current study) completing a preloaded cycling TT [39] but it is unknown whether this is also the case for handcycling. That said, there was no statistical evidence of a trial order effect on cycling or handcycling performance, which suggests that the results cannot be solely attributed to a learning effect.

5. Conclusions

Pre-exercise ingestion of caffeine (4 mg·kg^{-1}) significantly improved cycling 10 km TT performance but there was no statistical improvement in handcycling in habitual caffeine users. The positive effects of caffeine on cycling performance may be related to reductions in RPE during the preload. The lack of a statistical improvement during handcycling is possibly due to elevated (Bla) owing to both the mode of exercise and the ingestion of CAF. Furthermore, participants' training status appears to influence the ability of caffeine to improve UBE performance.

Acknowledgments: The authors would like to thank all the participants for their effort and commitment to the study. Thanks to Elliot Owen and Xavi Lee for their help during data collection. The authors would also like to thank Clyde Williams for his guidance during the preparation of the manuscript and Keith Tolfrey for his assistance with the statistical analysis. The authors would also like to thank The Peter Harrison Centre for Disability Sport for the financial assistance.

Author Contributions: T.G.-P., C.P. and V.G.-T. conceived and designed the study; T.P. performed the experiments and analyzed the data; and all authors contributed to and proofread the paper.

Conflicts of Interest: The authors declare no conflict of interest.

Abbreviations

The following abbreviations are used in this manuscript:

AB	Able-bodied
(Bla)	Blood lactate concentration
CAF	Caffeine
CNS	Central nervous system
HR	Heart rate
LBE	Lower-body exercise
PO	Power output
PLA	Placebo
RPE	Rating of perceived exertion
RPE_C	Central rating of perceived exertion
RPE_O	Overall rating of perceived exertion
RPE_P	Peripheral rating of perceived exertion
SD	Standard deviation
TT	Time trial
UBE	Upper-body exercise
$\dot{V}$	Oxygen uptake
$\dot{V}_{peak}$	Peak oxygen uptake

References

1. Astorino, T.A.; Cottrell, T.; Lozano, A.T.; Aburto-Pratt, K.; Duhon, J. Effect of caffeine on RPE and perceptions of pain, arousal, and pleasure/displeasure during a cycling time trial in endurance trained and active men. *Physiol. Behav.* **2012**, *106*, 211–217. [CrossRef] [PubMed]

2. Santos Rde, A.; Kiss, M.A.; Silva-Cavalcante, M.D.; Bertuzzi, R.; Bishop, D.J.; Lima-Silva, A.E. Caffeine alters anaerobic distribution and pacing during a 4000-m cycling time trial. *PLoS ONE* **2013**, *8*, e75399. [CrossRef] [PubMed]

3. Braun, H.; Koehler, K.; Geyer, H.; Kleinert, J.; Mester, J.; Schänzer, W. Dietary supplement use among elite young German athletes. *Int. J. Sport Nutr. Exerc. Metab.* **2009**, *19*, 97–109. [PubMed]

4. Erdman, K.A.; Fung, T.S.; Reimer, R.A. Influence of performance level on dietary supplementation in elite Canadian athletes. *Med. Sci. Sports Exerc.* **2006**, *38*, 349–356. [CrossRef] [PubMed]

5. Graham-Paulson, T.S.; Perret, C.; Smith, B.; Crosland, J.; Goosey-Tolfrey, V.L. Nutritional supplement habits of athletes with an impairment and their sources of information. *Int. J. Sport Nutr. Exerc. Metab.* **2015**, *25*, 387–395. [CrossRef] [PubMed]

6. Pendergast, D.R. Cardiovascular, respiratory, and metabolic responses to upper body exercise. *Med. Sci. Sports Exerc.* **1989**, *21*, 121–125. [CrossRef]

7. Davis, J.M.; Zhao, Z.; Stock, H.S.; Mehl, K.A.; Buggy, J.; Hand, G.A. Central nervous system effects of caffeine and adenosine on fatigue. *Am. J. Physiol. Regul. Integr. Comp. Physiol.* **2002**, *284*, 399–404. [CrossRef] [PubMed]

8. Fredholm, B.B.; Bättig, K.; Holmen, J.; Nehlig, A.; Zvartau, E.E. Actions of caffeine in the brain with special reference to factors that contribute to its widespread use. *J. Pharmacol. Exp. Ther.* **1999**, *51*, 83–133.

9. Doherty, M.; Smith, P.M. Effects of caffeine ingestion on rating of perceived exertion during and after exercise: A meta-analysis. *Scand. J. Med. Sci. Sports* **2005**, *15*, 69–78. [CrossRef] [PubMed]
10. Smit, H.J.; Rogers, P.J. Effects of low doses of caffeine on cognitive performance, mood, and thirst in low, moderate and higher caffeine users. *Psychopharmacology* **2000**, *152*, 167–173. [CrossRef] [PubMed]
11. Cureton, K.J.; Warren, G.L.; Millard-Stafford, M.L.; Wingo, J.E.; Trilk, J.; Buyckx, M. Caffeinated sports drink: Ergogenic effects and possible mechanisms. *Int. J. Sport Nutr. Exerc. Metab.* **2007**, *17*, 35–55. [PubMed]
12. Stadheim, H.K.; Kvamme, B.; Olsen, R. Caffeine increases performance in cross-country double-poling time trial exercise. *Med. Sci. Sports Exerc.* **2013**, *45*, 2175–2183. [CrossRef] [PubMed]
13. Motl, R.W.; O'Connor, P.J.; Tubandt, L.; Puetz, T.; Ely, M.R. Effect of caffeine on leg muscle pain during cycling exercise among females. *Med. Sci. Sports Exerc.* **2006**, *38*, 598–604. [CrossRef] [PubMed]
14. O'Connor, P.J.; Motl, R.W.; Broglio, S.P.; Ely, M.R. Dose-dependent effect of caffeine on reducing leg muscle pain during cycling exercise is unrelated to systolic blood pressure. *Pain* **2004**, *109*, 291–298. [CrossRef] [PubMed]
15. Warren, G.L.; Park, N.D.; Maresca, R.S.; Mckibans, K.I.; Millard-Stafford, M.L. Effect of caffeine ingestion on muscular strength and endurance: A meta-analysis. *Med. Sci. Sports Exerc.* **2010**, *42*, 1375–1387. [CrossRef] [PubMed]
16. Black, C.D.; Waddell, D.E.; Gonglach, A.R. Caffeine's ergogenic effects on cycling: Neuromuscular and perceptual factors. *Med. Sci. Sports Exerc.* **2015**, *47*, 1145–1158. [CrossRef] [PubMed]
17. Mizuno, M.; Juel, C.; Bro-Rasmussen, T.; Mygind, E.; Schibye, B.; Rasmussen, B.; Saltin, B. Limb skeletal muscle adaptation in athletes after training at altitude. *J. Appl. Physiol.* **1990**, *68*, 496–502. [PubMed]
18. Mygind, E. Fibre characteritics and enzyme levels of arm and leg muscles in elite cross-country skiers. *Scand. J. Med. Sci. Sports* **1995**, *5*, 76–80. [CrossRef] [PubMed]
19. Cerretelli, P.; Pendergast, D.P.; Paganelli, W.C.; Rennie, D.W. Effects of specific muscle training on V̇ on-response and early blood lactate. *J. Appl. Physiol.* **1979**, *47*, 761–769.
20. Gollnick, P.D.; Armstrong, R.B.; Saubert, C.W.; Piehl, K.; Saltin, B. Enzyme activity and fiber composition in skeletal muscle of untrained and trained men. *J. App. Physiol.* **1972**, *33*, 312–319.
21. Aedma, M.; Timpmann, S.; Ööpik, V. Effect of caffeine on upper body anaerobic performance in wrestlers in simulated competition day conditions. *Int. J. Sport. Nutr. Exerc. Metab.* **2013**, *23*, 601–609. [PubMed]
22. Drust, B.; Waterhouse, J.; Atkinson, G.; Edwards, B.; Reilly, T. Circadian rhythms in sports performance-an update. *Chronobiol. Int.* **2005**, *22*, 21–44. [CrossRef] [PubMed]
23. Skinner, T.L.; Jenkins, D.G.; Coombes, J.S.; Taafe, D.R.; Leveritt, M.D. Dose response of caffeine on 2000-m rowing performance. *Med. Sci. Sports Exerc.* **2010**, *42*, 571–576. [CrossRef] [PubMed]
24. Spendiff, O.; Campbell, I.G. The effect of glucose ingestion on endurance upper-body exercise and performance. *Int. J. Sports Med.* **2002**, *23*, 142–147. [CrossRef] [PubMed]
25. Astorino, T.A.; Cottrell, T.; Lozano, A.T.; Aburto-Pratt, K.; Duhon, J. Increases in cycling performance in response to caffeine ingestion are repeatable. *Nutr. Res.* **2012**, *32*, 78–84. [CrossRef] [PubMed]
26. Borg, G. *Borg's Perceived Exertion and Pain Scales*; Human Kinetics Publishers: Champaign, IL, USA, 1998.
27. McNaughton, L.R.; Lovell, R.J.; Siegler, J.; Midgley, A.W.; Moore, L.; Bentley, D.J. The effects of caffeine ingestion on time trial cycling performance. *Int. J. Sports Physiol. Perf.* **2008**, *3*, 157–163.
28. Bell, D.G.; McLellan, T.M. Effect of repeated caffeine ingestion on repeated exhaustive exercise endurance. *Med. Sci. Sports Exerc.* **2003**, *35*, 1348–1354. [CrossRef] [PubMed]
29. Greer, F.; Friars, D.; Graham, T.E. Comparison of caffeine and theophylline ingestion: exercise metabolism and endurance. *J. Appl. Physiol.* **2000**, *89*, 1837–1844. [PubMed]
30. Ganio, M.S.; Klau, J.F.; Casa, D.J.; Armstrong, L.E.; Maresh, C.M. Effect of caffeine on sport-specific endurance performance: a systematic review. *J. Strength Cond. Res.* **2009**, *23*, 315–324. [CrossRef] [PubMed]
31. Graham, T.E. Caffeine and exercise: Metabolism, endurance and performance. *Sports Med.* **2001**, *31*, 785–807. [CrossRef] [PubMed]
32. Skinner, T.L.; Jenkins, D.G.; Leverett, M.D.; McGorm, A.; Bolam, K.A.; Coombes, J.S.; Taafe, D.R. Factors influencing serum caffeine concentrations following caffeine ingestion. *J. Sci. Med. Sport* **2014**, *17*, 516–520. [CrossRef] [PubMed]
33. Perret, C. Elite-adapted wheelchair sports performance: A systematic review. *Disabil. Rehabil.* **2015**, *27*, 1–9. [CrossRef] [PubMed]

34. Hooker, S.P.; Wells, C.L.; Manore, M.M.; Philip, S.A.; Martin, N. Differences in epinephrine and substrate responses between arm and leg exercise. *Med. Sci. Sports Exerc.* **1990**, *22*, 779–784. [CrossRef] [PubMed]

35. Mitsumoto, H.; DeBoer, G.E.; Bunge, G.; Andrish, J.T.; Tetzlaff, J.E.; Cruse, P. Fiber-type specific caffeine sensitivities in normal human skinned muscle fibers. *Anesthesiology* **1990**, *72*, 50–54. [CrossRef] [PubMed]

36. Price, M.J.; Campbell, I.G. Determination of peak oxygen uptake during upper body exercise. *Ergonomics* **1997**, *40*, 491–499. [CrossRef] [PubMed]

37. Sawka, M.; Pandolf, K. Upper body exercise: physiology and training application for human presence in space. *SAE Tech. Paper* **1991**. [CrossRef]

38. Collomp, K.; Ahmaidi, S.; Chatard, J.C.; Audran, M.; Préfaut, C. Benefits of caffeine ingestion on sprint performance in trained and untrained swimmers. *Eur. J. Appl. Physiol.* **1992**, *64*, 377–380. [CrossRef]

39. Sewell, D.A.; McGregor, R.A. Evaluation of a cycling time trial protocol in recreationally active humans. *Eur. J. Appl. Physiol.* **2008**, *102*, 615–621. [CrossRef] [PubMed]

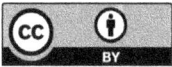

nutrients

MDPI

Article

The Effects of Montmorency Tart Cherry Concentrate Supplementation on Recovery Following Prolonged, Intermittent Exercise

Phillip G. Bell [1,2], Emma Stevenson [3], Gareth W. Davison [4] and Glyn Howatson [1,5,*]

[1] Department of Sport, Exercise and Rehabilitation, Faculty of Health and Life Sciences,
    Northumbria University, Newcastle upon Tyne NE1 8ST, UK; phillip.g.bell@northumbria.ac.uk
[2] GSK Human Performance Lab., Brentford, Middlesex TW8 9GS, UK
[3] Human Nutrition Research Centre, Institute of Cellular Medicine, Faculty of Medical Sciences,
    Newcastle University, Newcastle upon Tyne NE2 4HH, UK; emma.stevenson@ncl.ac.uk
[4] Sport and Exercise Sciences Research Institute, Ulster University, Jordanstown,
    Newtownabbey BT37 0QB, UK; gw.davison@ulster.ac.uk
[5] Water Research Group, School of Environmental Sciences and Development, Northwest University,
    Potchefstroom 2520, South Africa
*   Correspondence: glyn.howatson@northumbria.ac.uk; Tel.: +44-191-227-3575; Fax: +44-191-227-4515

Received: 22 June 2016; Accepted: 14 July 2016; Published: 22 July 2016

Abstract: This study investigated Montmorency tart cherry concentrate (MC) supplementation on markers of recovery following prolonged, intermittent sprint activity. Sixteen semi-professional, male soccer players, who had dietary restrictions imposed for the duration of the study, were divided into two equal groups and consumed either MC or placebo (PLA) supplementation for eight consecutive days (30 mL twice per day). On day 5, participants completed an adapted version of the Loughborough Intermittent Shuttle Test (LIST$_{ADAPT}$). Maximal voluntary isometric contraction (MVIC), 20 m Sprint, counter movement jump (CMJ), agility and muscle soreness (DOMS) were assessed at baseline, and 24, 48 and 72 h post-exercise. Measures of inflammation (IL-1-β, IL-6, IL-8, TNF-α, hsCRP), muscle damage (CK) and oxidative stress (LOOH) were analysed at baseline and 1, 3, 5, 24, 48 and 72 h post-exercise. Performance indices (MVIC, CMJ and agility) recovered faster and muscle soreness (DOMS) ratings were lower in the MC group ($p < 0.05$). Additionally, the acute inflammatory response (IL-6) was attenuated in the MC group. There were no effects for LOOH and CK. These findings suggest MC is efficacious in accelerating recovery following prolonged, repeat sprint activity, such as soccer and rugby, and lends further evidence that polyphenol-rich foods like MC are effective in accelerating recovery following various types of strenuous exercise.

Keywords: recovery; strenuous exercise; muscle damage; prunus cerasus; functional foods

1. Introduction

Prolonged, field-based, intermittent sprint sports are popular across the world at both elite and recreational levels [1]. Sports, such as soccer, field hockey and rugby, require a high volume of energy turnover and eccentric muscle actions resulting in metabolic and mechanically induced stress. Indeed, soccer play results in elevated post-match inflammatory [2,3], oxidative stress [2,4,5] and muscle damage [2,4] markers, as well as decrements in physical performance [2,4,5]. The Loughborough Intermittent Shuttle Test (LIST), which closely simulates activity patterns, and the physiological and metabolic demands of soccer [6], has been shown to incur similar stress responses [7–9], and, thus, provides a tool to induce similar physiological stress to game-play, but in a controlled environment. In light that athlete schedules require training or competition on multiple occasions within a few days, the importance of recovery strategies when preparing for the next game or training session is critical [10]. This is especially pertinent given that recovery is incomplete at 48 h following actual [2,11] and simulated [9] match-play.

Montmorency tart cherries have been shown on numerous occasions to be of benefit in exercise recovery [12–16], which have been proposed to be as a result of the high concentrations of phytochemicals, and in particular, the flavanoids anthocyanins [14,17–19]. These compounds can reduce oxidative stress and been shown to be a cyclooxygenase inhibitor (COX), to a similar extent as NSAIDs [20,21]. A series of studies have investigated the use of Montmorency cherries in influencing recovery from running [14,22], heavy eccentric contractions [15,16] and cycling [12,13]. Collectively, these lines of investigation suggest that Montmorency cherries could also be applied to aiding recovery following high intensity concurrent sports that incorporate and very high metabolic component that is accompanied by high intensity eccentric contractions.

Given that Montmorency cherries have been shown to be of benefit in exercise recovery following high intensity eccentric contractions and metabolically challenging exercise, it makes the expectation tenable that it could be applied to sports of a concurrent nature. Therefore the aim of this study was to investigate the effect of Montmorency cherries on recovery indices following a protocol designed to replicate the physiological demands of prolonged intermittent sprint activity such as those seen in field based sports. It was hypothesised that MC supplementation would attenuate post-exercise inflammatory and oxidative stress responses, and aid the return of functional performance.

2. Methods

2.1. Participants

Sixteen semi-professional (step 5 and above in the Football Association National pyramid, UK), male soccer players (mean $\pm$ SD age, height, mass, predicted $\dot{V}O_{2max}$ was 25 $\pm$ 4 years; 180.8 $\pm$ 7.4 cm, 81.9 $\pm$ 6.6 kg, 54.9 mL$\cdot$ kg$^{-1}\cdot$ min^{-1}, respectively) volunteered to take part in the study. All procedures were granted Ethical clearance by the University's Research Ethics Committee prior to testing and were conducted in accordance with the Helsinki Declaration. Inclusion criteria required participants to have trained in soccer consistently across the preceding 3 years and be free of any lower limb injury for the preceding 6 months. This was assessed through the completion of training history and health screening questionnaires. Following both verbal and written briefings on the requirements of the study, written informed consent was collected from all participants.

2.2. Study Design

A double blind, placebo controlled design with independent groups design was employed. Participants attended the laboratory on six separate occasions across a period of no longer than 15 days (Figure 1). On visit 1, participants completed a multi-stage shuttle test [23] in order to predict VO_{2max}, which was followed by familiarisation with a battery of functional performance tests and one 15 min section of the Loughborough Intermittent Shuttle Test Part A (LIST) [6]. Participants were then randomly but equally assigned to either a Montmorency cherry (MC) or placebo (PLA) group, matched by predicted VO_{2max} score (54.3 vs. 55.4 mL$\cdot$ kg$^{-1}\cdot$ min^{-1}).

Participants returned to the laboratory for visit 2 within 5 days to complete the battery of baseline functional measures that followed a standardised warm up; these were countermovement jump height (CMJ), 20 m sprint time (20 m), MVIC of the knee extensors, agility (5-0-5), which were preceded by assessment of active muscle soreness (DOMS). Participants were then provided with 24 MC or PLA beverages in a double blind manner along with verbal and written instructions on how to consume the beverages. They were also provided with a diet record diary and a list of foods to avoid throughout the 4 days prior to and during the trial period. During the 4 day period leading up to the trial day, participants were contacted and instructed to begin supplementation and dietary restrictions.

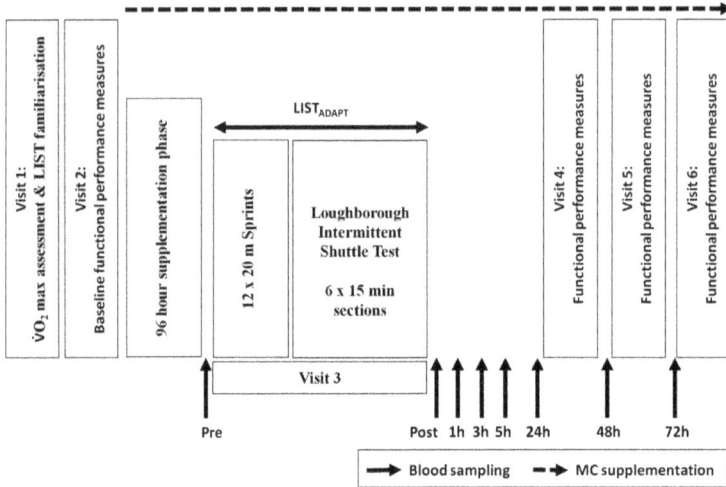

Figure 1. Timeline of study protocol including visit requirements, sampling point and supplementation period.

Visits 3–6 commenced at 8:00 a.m. in order to account for diurnal variation. On visit 3, participants were required to complete an adapted version of the LIST (LIST$_{ADAPT}$). Following the standardised warm-up, participants completed a series of 12×20 m sprints with a 10 m 'stopping zone', departing every 60 s. This addition was included because (1) the LIST protocol does not account for the many bounding, leaping and directional changes that are associated with team sports play; and (2) previous work from our laboratory has shown only moderate responses with regards to the magnitude of stress response following the LIST [9]. A secondary adaptation to the LIST protocol was the completion of 6×15 min sections from the LIST Part A, as opposed to 5×15 min sections detailed in the original protocol [6]. This section was included to standardise the distance covered by the two groups (in the original protocol, LIST Part B required a run to exhaustion, potentially resulting in group differences). During the LIST$_{ADAPT}$ participants were provided with water ad libitum.

Visits 4–6 took place at 24, 48 and 72 h following the start of visit 3 and required participants to complete the functional performance test battery outlined in visit 2. Venous blood samples were collected at baseline (prior to muscle soreness and performance test), immediately pre-trial, immediately post-trial and 1, 3, 5, 24, 48 and 72 h post-trial for markers of inflammation, oxidative stress and muscle damage.

2.3. Supplementation

The MC or PLA supplementation was provided to participants after the initial visit along with instructions detailing the dosing schedule (30 mL twice per day, (8:00 a.m., 6:00 p.m.), 7 consecutive days (4 days pre- and on each trial day [13])). Supplements were prepared by mixing each dose with 100 mL of water prior to consumption. The MC was a commercially available Montmorency cherry concentrate (CherryActive, Sunbury, UK); previous work from our laboratory has shown that the MC used in this study contains a total anthocyanin content of 73.5 mg· L^{-1} of cyanidin-3-glucoside, a total phenolic content of 178.8 gallic acid equivalent· L^{-1} and an antioxidant capacity (TEAC) of 0.58 trolox equivalents· L^{-1} [24]. A commercially available, less than 5% fruit, cordial, mixed with water and maltodextrin (MyProtein Ltd, Northwich, UK) until matched for energy content of the MC (102 kcal) was used for the PLA supplement. All supplements were prepared by an independent member of the department prepared in opaque bottles in order to maintain the double blind design.

2.4. Dietary and Exercise Restrictions

Participants were instructed to follow a low polyphenolic diet in the 48 h prior to the beginning of each MC or PLA supplementation and throughout the experimental phase of each study. A list of foods to avoid was provided and compliance was assessed through the completion of daily food diaries which has been successfully implemented in previous research [25]. This control measure was used to provide a washout period of polyphenols to enable the efficacy of the phenolic-rich cherry concentrate intervention. In addition, participants were instructed to abstain from any exercise that was not a part of the protocol, throughout the same time periods. Lastly, participants attended all exercise trials following an overnight fast. These measures ensured that dependant variable changes from baseline were likely to be in response to the supplementation and the exercise trials implemented within each study.

2.5. Functional Performance Tests

The functional performance test battery was performed in the following order on each occasion: Active muscle soreness assessment (DOMS), 20 m sprint, 5-0-5 agility (CV 2.8% [26]), countermovement jump (CV 1.9%), knee extensors (repeatability in Chapter 3.4). Timings were kept consistent throughout all functional performance tests, each test was performed 3 times (excluding DOMS), with a 1 min rest between repetitions and 3 min rest between tests.

Delayed onset of muscle soreness (DOMS) in the lower limbs was assessed using a 200 mm visual analogue scale (VAS) with 'no soreness' at one end and 'unbearably painful' at the other. On each occasion the VAS was used, participants were instructed to place their hands on hips, squat down to ~90°, before standing up and immediately making a mark on the scale consistent with their perceived soreness.

Sprint performance (20 m; coefficient of variation (CV) 0.9%) and the 5-0-5 agility test [27,28] (CV 2.8%) were assessed using wireless telemetry and infra-red timing gates (Brower Timing Systems, Draper, UT, USA) on an indoor athletics track. Countermovement jump height (CV 1.9%) was assessed using a jump mat (Just Jump, Probotics Inc., Huntsville, AL, USA); participants were instructed to stand on the jump mat with their feet parallel and approximately shoulder width apart. Following this, participants completed a maximal vertical jump whilst maintaining hands on hips through flight and landing. MVIC of the dominant knee extensors was determined using a strain gauge (MIE Medical Research Ltd., Leeds, UK) using the methods described previously [13]. The peak performance from each trial was used for data analysis.

2.6. Blood Sampling

Blood samples (35 mL) were collected from a forearm vein located in the antecubital fossa region in order to assess for markers of muscle damage (creatine kinase [CK]), inflammation (interleukin-1-beta (IL-1-β), interleukin-6 (IL-6), tumour necrosis factor-alpha (TNF-α), high-sensitivity C-reactive protein (hsCRP)) and oxidative stress (lipid hydroperoxides (LOOH)) using previously described methods [12,13]; intra-sample CVs ranged from 0.7% to 6.8%. Samples were collected into serum gel, ethylenediaminetetraacetic acid (EDTA) or sodium heparin treated tubes (Vacutainer®BD UK Ltd., Oxford, UK). Samples were then immediately centrifuged (Allegra X-22 Centrifuge, Beckman Coulter, Bucks, UK) at $2400 \times g$ at 4 °C for 15 min before having the supernatant removed and stored in aliquots. Aliquots were then immediately stored at -80 °C and subsequently analysed for the respective indices in each study.

2.7. Statistical Analysis

All data analyses were conducted using IBM SPSS Statistics 20 for Windows (Surrey, UK) and are reported as mean ± standard deviation. All data was confirmed as parametric via a Shapiro-Wilk test for normality. Differences between blood marker variables were analysed by using a group

(MC vs. PLA) by time-point (Pre-supplement, Post-supplement, 1, 3, 5, 24, 48 and 72 h) mixed model ANOVA. Functional performance measures were analysed using the same model, however with four fewer levels (Pre-supplement, Post-supplement, 24, 48 and 72 h). Where significant group baseline differences were apparent (MVIC, CMJ, 5-0-5 agility, 20 m sprint, DOMS) results were normalised to baseline values prior to subsequent statistical analysis. Mauchley's Test of Sphericity was used to assess homogeneity of data and where violations were present, Greenhouse-Geiser adjustments were made. Where necessary, interaction effects were assessed using LSD post hoc analysis. Prior to all analyses, a significance level of $p < 0.05$ was set.

3. Results

MVIC (Figure 2) showed significant time ($F_{(1,4)} = 6.586$, $p = 0.001$, $\eta^2 = 0.320$), group ($F_{(1,2)} = 19.445$, $p = 0.001$, $\eta^2 = 0.582$) and interaction ($F_{(1,4)} = 8.970$, $p < 0.001$, $\eta^2 = 0.391$) effects when data was normalised to baseline values. The decline in MIVC performance was not evident in the MC group whereas as function had not returned to basal levels at 72 h in the PLA. The peak difference occurred at 48 h where MVIC scores in the MC group were found to be 19% higher.

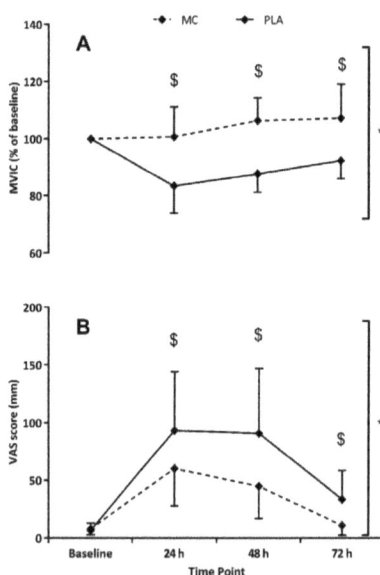

Figure 2. Changes in maximum voluntary isometric contraction (MVIC; Panel (**A**)) and delayed onset muscle soreness (DOMS; Panel (**B**)) in response to Montmorency cherry (MC) or placebo (PLA) supplementation. * Group effect; $ Interaction effect ($p < 0.05$).

When data was normalised to baseline values, CMJ also showed significant time ($F_{(1,4)} = 30.320$, $p < 0.001$, $\eta^2 = 0.684$), group ($F_{(1,2)} = 7.336$, $p = 0.017$, $\eta^2 = 0.345$) and interaction ($F_{(1,4)} = 3.334$, $p = 0.028$, $\eta^2 = 0.193$) effects (Figure 3). Both MC and PLA groups demonstrated reduced CMJ (vs. baseline) in the 72 h post-trial period, although the CMJ decrease in the MC group was significantly attenuated at 24 h (5%, $p = 0.022$) and 48 h (6%, $p = 0.017$) versus placebo. Significant time ($F_{(1,4)} = 12.988$, $p < 0.001$, $\eta^2 = 0.481$) and group ($F_{(1,2)} = 7.963$, $p = 0.015$, $\eta^2 = 0.355$) effects were found for the 5-0-5 agility test. MC times for the 5-0-5 agility were on average 3% faster (vs. PLA) across the 72 h post-trial testing period. For the last of the performance measures, 20 m sprint time, significant time ($F_{(1,4)} = 9.681$, $p = 0.001$, $\eta^2 = 0.409$) and interaction ($F_{(1,4)} = 3.145$, $p = 0.035$, $\eta^2 = 0.183$) effects were apparent, with both MC and PLA groups demonstrating slower times in all three post-trial tests. At 48 h in the MC group, 20 m sprint times were significantly ($p = 0.043$) faster (4%) than PLA. DOMS was significantly increased in both groups across the 72 h post-trial period ($F_{(1,4)} = 37.206$, $p < 0.001$). A significant group effect ($F_{(1,2)} = 8.486$, $p = 0.011$, $\eta^2 = 0.377$) showed that DOMS ratings were lower in the MC group (vs. PLA), which were mirrored by interaction effects ($F_{(1,4)} = 4.069$, $p = 0.013$, $\eta^2 = 0.225$) at 24 ($p = 0.044$), 48 ($p = 0.018$) and 72 h ($p = 0.007$), which showed almost complete recovery of at 72 h.

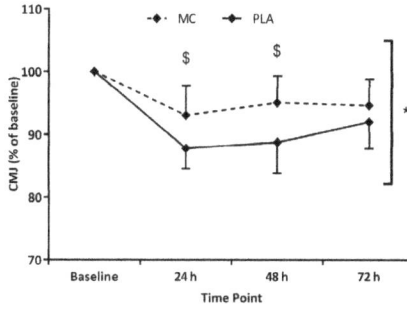

Figure 3. Comparison of countermovement jump (CMJ) height with Montmorency cherries (MC) or placebo (PLA) supplementation. * Group effect; $ Interaction effect ($p < 0.05$).

With regards to inflammatory markers, IL-6 (Figure 4) was found to be elevated in both groups following the trial ($F_{(1,8)} = 52.180$, $p < 0.001$, $\eta^2 = 0.788$). Group comparisons ($F_{(1,2)} = 10.223$, $p = 0.006$, $\eta^2 = 0.422$) demonstrated an overall significantly attenuated IL-6 response to the trial in MC (vs. PLA), with significant interaction effects ($F_{(1,8)} = 3.313$, $p = 0.003$, $\eta^2 = 0.191$) showing peak differences of 3.10 pg· mL^{-1} occurring immediately post-exercise ($p = 0.03$). Further inflammatory marker data for plasma IL-8 ($F_{(1,8)} = 4.905$, $p = 0.010$, $\eta^2 = 0.259$), TNF-α ($F_{(1,8)} = 6.343$, $p < 0.001$, $\eta^2 = 0.312$) and hsCRP ($F_{(1,8)} = 20.298$, $p < 0.001$, $\eta^2 = 0.592$) revealed significant increases in each variable in the 72 h following the trial, however, group and interaction comparisons failed to identify differences. IL-1-β was not found to be increased at any measurement point across the trial period. The trial significantly increased CK in both groups ($F_{(1,4)} = 10.243$, $p = 0.004$, $\eta^2 = 0.423$), although no group or interaction effects were found. Peaks values of 1200 IU/L were attained at 24 h (Table 1).

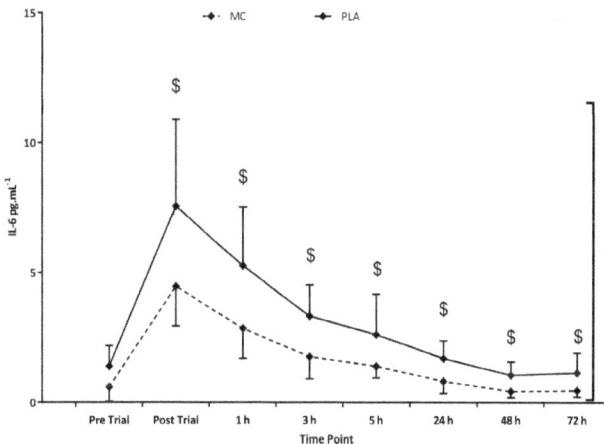

Figure 4. Interleukin-6 (IL-6) responses in the Montmorency cherry (MC) and placebo (PLA) groups to the adapted Loughborough Intermittent Shuttle Test (LIST$_{ADAPT}$) exercise. * Group effect; $ Interaction effect ($p < 0.05$).

Table 1. Summary of other performance, inflammatory and oxidative stress data.

	Pre-Trial		Post-Trial		1 h		3 h		5 h		24 h		48 h		72 h	
	Mean	SD	Mean	SD	Mean	SD	Mean	SD	Mean	SD	Mean	SD	Mean	SD	Mean	SD
5-0-5 Agility (s) *,§																
MC	2.34	0.11									2.42	0.17	2.38	0.10	2.35	0.12
PLA	2.30	0.13									2.41	0.17	2.43	0.17	2.37	0.18
20 m Sprint (s) *																
MC	3.11	0.14									3.17	0.15	3.14	0.12	3.12	0.15
PLA	3.05	0.12									3.18	0.18	3.23	0.24	3.17	0.19
DOMS (mm) *,§																
MC	8	5									60 [+]	32	44 [+]	28	10 [+]	8
PLA	7	6									93 [+]	51	90 [+]	56	33 [+]	25
IL-1-β (pg·mL^{-1})																
MC			0.04	0.08	0.03	0.06	0.02	0.04	0.11	0.13	0.03	0.05	0.06	0.14	0.01	0.01
PLA			0.02	0.05	0.36	1.00	0.02	0.05	0.02	0.02	0.01	0.02	0.01	0.04	0.03	0.03
IL-8 (pg·mL^{-1}) *																
MC			4.37	0.93	3.77	0.87	3.04	1.13	3.29	0.79	2.23	0.53	1.90	0.64	2.18	0.70
PLA			4.69	1.78	3.67	0.99	3.03	0.74	3.25	0.86	2.50	0.76	2.25	0.63	2.49	0.92
TNF-α (pg·mL^{-1}) *																
MC			1.23	0.42	1.18	0.29	1.16	0.32	1.11	0.35	1.36	0.39	1.22	0.38	1.36	0.52
PLA			1.96	0.84	1.76	0.69	1.73	0.77	1.60	0.77	1.83	0.90	1.78	0.80	1.88	0.97
CK (IU·L^{-1}) *																
MC	293	228	691	365	885	504	1243	1004	1538	1317	1551	1473	959	822	560	386
PLA	197	143	439	310	535	401	744	625	989	946	1034	1096	652	603	403	319
hsCRP (pg·mL^{-1}) *																
MC	0.70	0.86	0.70	0.82	0.69	0.83	0.69	0.75	0.90	0.69	1.94	0.88	1.39	0.63	1.00	0.54
PLA	1.24	1.38	1.36	1.36	1.40	1.48	1.40	1.47	1.55	1.60	2.93	2.73	2.29	1.63	1.73	1.22
LOOH (mmol·mL^{-1}) *																
MC	1.37	0.10	1.59	0.29	1.37	0.25	1.62	0.34	1.60	0.28	1.25	0.14	1.26	0.16	1.25	0.17
PLA	1.37	0.21	1.61	0.33	1.41	0.27	1.96	1.34	2.15	1.44	1.24	0.15	1.29	0.24	1.23	0.16

* Significant main effect for time ($p < 0.001$); § group $\times$ time interaction. DOMS, Delayed Onset Muscle Soreness; IL-1-β, Interleukin-1-beta; IL-8, Interleukin-8; TNF-α, Tumour Necrosis Factor-Alpha; CK, Creatine Kinase; hsCRP, high-sensitivity C-Reactive Protein; LOOH, Lipid Hydroperoxides.

Lipid hydroperoxides were increased in the 72 h post-exercise period as indicated by a significant time effect ($F_{(1,8)} = 5.973$, $p < 0.001$, $\eta^2 = 0.289$). Peak increases of 35% above baseline occurred at 5 h. Although there was a tendency for higher PLA group values, no significant group or interaction effects were found. A summary of variables is reported in Table 1.

In order to identify any group differences in LIST$_{ADAPT}$ performance, a comparison of sprint times during the LIST$_{ADAPT}$ protocol was performed using Student's *T*-test. No group differences in LIST$_{ADAPT}$ sprint performance were found ($t = 1.511$, $p = 0.153$).

4. Discussion

The main finding of this study was that participants supplemented with MC were able to maintain greater functional performance than PLA counterparts following prolonged intermittent sprint activity. More specifically, MVIC, CMJ, 20 m sprint and 5-0-5 agility performances were superior in the 72 h post-exercise with MC (vs. PLA). In addition, DOMS and IL-6 were lower in the MC group throughout the post-trial period.

The attenuated declines in muscle performance are consistent with the findings of previous studies investigating MC as a recovery aid [12–16] and additionally the magnitude of MVIC decline following the LIST$_{ADAPT}$ was comparative to previous work utilising a similar protocol [29]. The MVIC performance was on average 17%, superior in the MC group (vs. PLA). MC supplementation also resulted in better (vs. PLA) CMJ performance at 24 and 48 h. Sprint times in both groups were slower in the 72 h post-exercise period, however at 48 h the MC group was significantly faster. Agility (5-0-5) times were also faster in the MC group by an average of 3% across the 72 h post-trial period. Interestingly, the MVIC results in the 72 h following exercise suggests MC supplementation abolishes declines in this performance measure—a result that has been previously reported [13].

These data support the idea that supplementation with MC protect declines in muscle function following strenuous exercise, specifically in activity akin to repeated sprint sports and games play such as rugby, soccer and field hockey. A reduction in post-exercise IL-6 suggests a lower acute inflammatory response to the exercise bout that might contribute to the performance differences between groups. The COX, prostaglandin, IL-6 pathway, which are activated during the secondary inflammatory response to cellular disruption, has been associated with proteolytic and lipolytic processes [30] and subsequently muscular performance could be inhibited. Seemingly, MC supplementation reduced (but did not abolish) this process and allowed for greater maintenance of muscular performance in the recovery period. Conversely, there were no group differences in hsCRP. This is unexpected given that IL-6 is implicated as a signalling molecule for the expression of hsCRP [31,32]. We are unable to resolve the discrepancy between IL-6 and hsCRP and therefore suggest further work is needed to identify the mechanism by which MC might exert its anti-inflammatory responses in response to strenuous exercise.

In contrast to previous work [12] that examined repeated days cycling exercise, there were no differences in LOOH between groups. The obvious discrepancy between study findings may be attributed to single versus repeated days exercise. Unlike Bell et al. [12], where repeated days cycling exercise (metabolic challenge) were used, the current study investigated a single bout of strenuous exercise that incorporated both a metabolic and mechanical exercise stress. Conceptually, the accumulated stress response from repeated day's exercise would be greater than a single bout, but of course the modalities, cycling versus simulated concurrent exercise, pose very different exercise challenges and hence the redox response may also differ considerably between exercise stimuli.

In agreement with previous work [16,22], the lower post-exercise DOMS in the MC group provide further evidence for the protective effect of cherries. Despite this, previous work from our lab [13] using MC has not shown this positive effect. This discrepancy may be attributed to the different modes of exercise employed to induce stress. Whilst muscle actions during cycling are almost exclusively concentric [33], the repeated sprints and decelerations during the LIST$_{ADAPT}$ protocol in the present study, place a heavy eccentric load on the same muscle groups and as a result are likely to incur greater mechanical stress. Indeed, DOMS ratings from the present study were consistently higher than those in the cycling studies [12,13]. In further support of this supposition, CK (an index of cellular disruption following damaging exercise) was considerably higher than the aforementioned cycling studies. However, the CK response reported in previous work [14,15] using protocols that also incorporate a heavy eccentric component, showed no evidence for a protective effect of MC.

The high-intensity, prolonged, intermittent nature of soccer and other repeated sprint sports places a high degree of both mechanical and metabolic stress [2], which is reflected by the increase in the appearance of physiological stress responses in the present study. Whilst this is not the first study to demonstrate accelerated recovery of functional performance with MC supplementation, it is the first to do so following simulated games play and therefore represents an important wider application of this intervention to aid exercise recovery in sports of an intermittent sprint nature, such as soccer, rugby, field hockey and basketball. Collectively, there is a growing body of evidence suggesting that MC has the ability to facilitate exercise recovery—perhaps by modulating inflammation and/or oxidative stress. The exact mechanisms behind these promising data are not clear, so it seems prudent to explore further; perhaps by using animal, cellular and molecular techniques to provide a greater understanding of the application of MC and other phenolic-rich foods.

In summary, this study provides further evidence for the use of MC as a recovery aid. For the first time, MC supplementation has been shown to accelerate the recovery of a number of functional performance measures following prolonged intermittent sprint activity and suggest that some dampening of the post-exercise inflammatory processes might be responsible. With regards to application, the dampening of such responses could be highly advantageous in sports requiring athletes to complete high volumes of training whilst 'in-season', or athletes competing in tournament scenario's that require multiple performances within a short time period and the ability to recover in sufficient time is a challenge. Additionally, although dietary restrictions were imposed throughout the study period, the results suggest that sports requiring sprinting or high intensity directional changes might benefit from MC supplementation when playing schedules are congested and recovery time is limited between games. Finally, the issue of modulating the post-exercise oxidative stress and inflammatory response has raised concerns; insofar as these stressors are implicated in the adaptive response. Although there is no evidence that the adaptive response is affected by functional foods, this question should be addressed in order to determine if periodiation of these sorts of supplements is warranted.

Author Contributions: P.G.B., E.S. and G.H. conceived and designed the experiments; P.G.B. performed the experiments; P.G.B., G.W.D. and G.H. analyzed the data; G.W.D. contributed reagents/materials/analysis tools; P.G.B., E.S. and G.H. wrote the paper.

Conflicts of Interest: The authors declare no conflict of interest.

References

1. Spencer, M.; Bishop, D.; Dawson, B.; Goodman, C. Physiological and metabolic responses of repeated-sprint activities: Specific to field-based team sports. *Sports Med.* **2005**, *35*, 1025–1044. [CrossRef] [PubMed]
2. Ispirlidis, I.; Fatouros, I.G.; Jamurtas, A.Z.; Nikolaidis, M.G.; Michailidis, I.; Douroudos, I.; Margonis, K.; Chatzinikolaou, A.; Kalistratos, E.; Katrabasas, I.; et al. Time-course of changes in inflammatory and performance responses following a soccer game. *Clin. J. Sport Med.* **2008**, *18*, 423–431. [CrossRef] [PubMed]
3. Andersson, H.; Bøhn, S.K.; Raastad, T.; Paulsen, G.; Blomhoff, R.; Kadi, F. Differences in the inflammatory plasma cytokine response following two elite female soccer games separated by a 72-h recovery. *Scand. J. Med. Sci. Sports* **2010**, *20*, 740–747. [CrossRef] [PubMed]
4. Ascensão, A.; Rebelo, A.; Oliveira, E.; Marques, F.; Pereira, L.; Magalhães, J. Biochemical impact of a soccer match—Analysis of oxidative stress and muscle damage markers throughout recovery. *Clin. Biochem.* **2008**, *41*, 841–851.
5. Fatouros, I.G.; Chatzinikolaou, A.; Douroudos, I.I.; Nikolaidis, M.G.; Kyparos, A.; Margonis, K.; Michailidis, Y.; Vantarakis, A.; Taxildaris, K.; Katrabasas, I.; et al. Time-course of changes in oxidative

stress and antioxidant status responses following a soccer game. *J. Strength Cond. Res.* **2010**, *24*, 3278–3286. [CrossRef] [PubMed]

6. Nicholas, C.W.; Nuttall, F.E.; Williams, C. The loughborough intermittent shuttle test: A field test that simulates the activity pattern of soccer. *J. Sports Sci.* **2000**, *18*, 97–104. [CrossRef] [PubMed]

7. Cockburn, E.; Bell, P.G.; Stevenson, E. Effect of milk on team sport performance following exercise-induced muscle damage. *Med. Sci. Sports Exerc.* **2013**, *45*, 1585–1592. [CrossRef] [PubMed]

8. Magalhaes, J.; Rebelo, A.; Oliveira, E.; Silva, J.R.; Marques, F.; Ascensao, A. Impact of loughborough intermittent shuttle test versus soccer match on physiological, biochemical and neuromuscular parameters. *Eur. J. Appl. Physiol.* **2010**, *108*, 39–48. [CrossRef] [PubMed]

9. Leeder, J.; van Someren, K.A.; Gaze, D.; Jewell, A.; Deshmukh, N.; Shah, I.; Howatson, G. Recovery and adaptation from repeated intermittent-sprint exercise. *Int. J. Sports Physiol. Perform.* **2014**, *9*, 489–496. [CrossRef] [PubMed]

10. Reilly, T.; Ekblom, B. The use of recovery methods post-exercise. *J. Sports Sci.* **2005**, *23*, 619–627. [CrossRef] [PubMed]

11. Russell, M.; Northeast, J.; Atkinson, G.; Shearer, D.A.; Sparkes, W.; Cook, C.J.; Kilduff, L. The between-match variability of peak power output and creatine kinase responses to soccer match-play. *J. Strength Cond. Res.* **2015**, *29*, 2079–2085. [CrossRef] [PubMed]

12. Bell, P.G.; Walshe, I.H.; Davison, G.W.; Stevenson, E.; Howatson, G. Montmorency cherries reduce the oxidative stress and inflammatory responses to repeated days high-intensity stochastic cycling. *Nutrients* **2014**, *6*, 829–843. [CrossRef] [PubMed]

13. Bell, P.G.; Walshe, I.W.; Davison, G.W.; Stevenson, E.J.; Howatson, G. Recovery facilitation with montmorency cherries following high-intensity, metabolically challenging exercise. *Appl. Physiol. Nutr. Metab.* **2014**, *40*, 414–423. [CrossRef] [PubMed]

14. Howatson, G.; McHugh, M.P.; Hill, J.A.; Brouner, J.; Jewell, A.P.; Van Someren, K.A.; Shave, R.E.; Howatson, S.A. Influence of tart cherry juice on indices of recovery following marathon running. *Scand. J. Med. Sci. Sports* **2010**, *20*, 843–852. [CrossRef] [PubMed]

15. Bowtell, J.L.; Sumners, D.P.; Dyer, A.; Fox, P.; Mileva, K. Montmorency cherry juice reduces muscle damage caused by intensive strength exercise. *Med. Sci. Sports Exerc.* **2011**, *43*, 1544–1551. [CrossRef] [PubMed]

16. Connolly, D.A.J.; McHugh, M.P.; Padilla-Zakour, O.I. Efficacy of a tart cherry juice blend in preventing the symptoms of muscle damage. *Br. J. Sports Med.* **2006**, *40*, 679–683. [CrossRef] [PubMed]

17. McCune, L.M.; Kubota, C.; Stendell-Hollis, N.R.; Thomson, C.A. Cherries and health: A review. *Crit. Rev. Food Sci. Nutr.* **2011**, *51*, 1–12. [CrossRef] [PubMed]

18. Bell, P.G.; Gaze, D.C.; Davison, G.W.; George, T.W.; Scotter, M.J.; Howatson, G. Montmorency tart cherry (prunus cerasus l.) concentrate lowers uric acid, independent of plasma cyanidin-3-*O*-glucosiderutinoside. *J. Funct. Foods* **2014**, *11*, 82–90. [CrossRef]

19. Keane, K.M.; Bell, P.G.; Lodge, J.K.; Constantinou, C.L.; Jenkinson, S.E.; Bass, R.; Howatson, G. Phytochemical uptake following human consumption of montmorency tart cherry (L. *Prunus cerasus*) and influence of phenolic acids on vascular smooth muscle cells in vitro. *Eur. J. Nutr.* **2016**, *55*, 1695–1705. [CrossRef] [PubMed]

20. Wang, H.; Nair, M.G.; Strasburg, G.M.; Chang, Y.-C.; Booren, A.M.; Gray, J.I.; DeWitt, D.L. Antioxidant and antiinflammatory activities of anthocyanins and their aglycon, cyanidin, from tart cherries. *J. Nat. Prod.* **1999**, *62*, 294–296. [CrossRef] [PubMed]

21. Seeram, N.P.; Momin, R.A.; Nair, M.G.; Bourquin, L.D. Cyclooxygenase inhibitory and antioxidant cyanidin glycosides in cherries and berries. *Phytomedicine* **2001**, *8*, 362–369. [CrossRef] [PubMed]

22. Kuehl, K.; Perrier, E.; Elliot, D.; Chesnutt, J. Efficacy of tart cherry juice in reducing muscle pain during running: A randomized controlled trial. *J. Int. Soc. Sports Nutr.* **2010**, *7*, 17. [CrossRef] [PubMed]

23. Léger, L.A.; Lambert, J. A maximal multistage 20-m shuttle run test to predict VO2 max. *Eur. J. Appl. Physiol. Occup. Physiol.* **1982**, *49*, 1–12.

24. Keane, K.M.; George, T.W.; Constantinou, C.L.; Brown, M.A.; Clifford, T.; Howatson, G. Effects of montmorency tart cherry (*Prunus cerasus* L.) consumption on vascular function in men with early hypertension. *Am. J. Clin. Nutr.* **2016**, *103*, 1531–1539. [CrossRef] [PubMed]

25. Howatson, G.; Bell, P.G.; Tallent, J.; Middleton, B.; McHugh, M.P.; Ellis, J. Effect of tart cherry juice (*Prunus cerasus*) on melatonin levels and enhanced sleep quality. *Eur. J. Nutr.* **2012**, *51*, 909–916. [CrossRef] [PubMed]
26. Sayers, M.; Kilip, J.V. Reliability and validity of the 5-0-5 agility test. In Proceedings of the 4th Evolution of the Athlete Coach Education Conference, Brisbane, Australia, 25–26 October 2010.
27. Davies, V.; Thompson, K.G.; Cooper, S.M. The effects of compression garments on recovery. *J. Strength Cond. Res.* **2009**, *23*, 1786–1794. [CrossRef] [PubMed]
28. Houghton, L.A.; Dawson, B.T.; Rubenson, J. Effects of plyometric training on achilles tendon properties and shuttle running during a simulated cricket batting innings. *J. Strength Cond. Res.* **2013**, *27*, 1036–1046. [CrossRef] [PubMed]
29. Leeder, J.D.; Van Someren, K.A.; Bell, P.G.; Spence, J.R.; Jewell, A.P.; Gaze, D.; Howatson, G. Effects of seated and standing cold water immersion on recovery from repeated sprinting. *J. Sports Sci.* **2015**, *33*, 1544–1552. [CrossRef] [PubMed]
30. Trappe, T.A.; Standley, R.A.; Jemiolo, B.; Carroll, C.C.; Trappe, S.W. Prostaglandin and myokine involvement in the cyclooxygenase-inhibiting drug enhancement of skeletal muscle adaptations to resistance exercise in older adults. *Am. J. Physiol. Regul. Integr. Comp. Physiol.* **2013**, *304*, R198–R205. [CrossRef] [PubMed]
31. Petersen, A.M.; Pedersen, B.K. The anti-inflammatory effect of exercise. *J. Appl. Physiol.* **2005**, *98*, 1154–1162. [CrossRef] [PubMed]
32. Pepys, M.B.; Hirschfield, G.M. C-reactive protein: A critical update. *J. Clin. Investig.* **2003**, *111*, 1805–1812. [CrossRef] [PubMed]
33. Bijker, K.; de Groot, G.; Hollander, A. Differences in leg muscle activity during running and cycling in humans. *Eur. J. Appl. Physiol.* **2002**, *87*, 556–561. [PubMed]

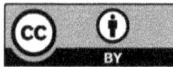

nutrients

MDPI

Article

Vitamin D Status and Supplementation Practices in Elite Irish Athletes: An Update from 2010/2011

Joshua Todd [1], Sharon Madigan [2], Kirsty Pourshahidi [1], Emeir McSorley [1], Eamon Laird [3], Martin Healy [4] and Pamela Magee [1,*]

[1] Northern Ireland Centre for Food and Health, University of Ulster, Coleraine, Londonderry BT52 1SA, Northern Ireland, UK; todd-j10@email.ulster.ac.uk (J.T.); k.pourshahidi@ulster.ac.uk (K.P.); em.mcsorley@ulster.ac.uk (E.M.)

[2] Irish Institute of Sport, Sports Campus Ireland, Abbotstown, Dublin 15, Republic of Ireland; smadigan@instituteofsport.ie

[3] School of Biochemistry and Immunology, Trinity College Dublin, Dublin 2, Republic of Ireland; lairdea@tcd.ie

[4] Department of Biochemistry, Central Pathology Laboratory, St. James's Hospital, Dublin 8, Republic of Ireland; mhealy@stjames.ie

* Correspondence: pj.magee@ulster.ac.uk; Tel.: +44-28-7012-4360

Received: 24 May 2016; Accepted: 3 August 2016; Published: 9 August 2016

Abstract: Vitamin D deficiency is a global health concern that is prevalent in Ireland. The vitamin D status of elite Irish athletes following implementation of a revised supplementation policy in 2010/2011 has not been explored to date. This study aimed to assess the vitamin D status of elite Irish athletes participating in high-profile sports and establish if equatorial travel, supplementation and/or sunbed use predict vitamin D status. Across Ireland, blood samples ($n = 92$) were obtained from cricketers ($n = 28$), boxers ($n = 21$) and women's rugby sevens players ($n = 43$) between November 2013 and April 2015. Total 25-hydroxyvitamin D (25(OH)D) concentrations were quantified using LC-MS/MS. Parathyroid hormone and adjusted calcium concentrations were measured by clinical biochemistry. Athletes completed a questionnaire that queried equatorial travel, supplementation and sunbed use. Vitamin D sufficiency (25(OH)D >50 nmol/L) was evident in 86% of athletes. Insufficiency (31–49 nmol/L) and deficiency (<30 nmol/L) was present in only 12% and 2% of athletes respectively. On average, athletes from all sport disciplines were vitamin D sufficient and 25% reported vitamin D supplementation which was a significant positive predictor of vitamin D status, (OR 4.31; 95% CI 1.18–15.75; $p = 0.027$). Equatorial travel and sun bed use were reported in 47% and 16% of athletes respectively however these factors did not predict vitamin D status (both $p > 0.05$). Although different cohorts were assessed, the overall prevalence of vitamin D insufficiency/deficiency was 55% in 2010/2011 compared with only 14% in 2013/2015. Targeted supplementation is highly effective in optimising vitamin D status, negating the need for blanket-supplementation in elite cohorts.

Keywords: Elite athletes; vitamin D; supplementation

1. Introduction

In Ireland, vitamin D insufficiency and deficiency, defined by the U.S Institute of Medicine as a total 25-hydroxyvitamin D (25(OH)D) concentration below 50 nmol/L and 30 nmol/L respectively [1], is pervasive in athletes, thus raising concern of potential skeletal and extra-skeletal health implications [2]. Chronic vitamin D deficiency (25(OH)D <30 nmol/L) clinically manifests as rickets in children and osteomalacia in adults, debilitating conditions characterised by a bow-legged posture and an increased risk of fracture [3]. Emerging research also suggests that vitamin D may be important in maintaining a healthy immune system, particularly with respect to upper respiratory tract infections which are commonly reported in athletes [4,5]. It has been suggested that a total 25(OH)D concentration of >75 or even >120 nmol/L may be considered optimal for achieving the proposed extra-skeletal health benefits of vitamin D [6,7] however there is currently insufficient evidence from randomised controlled trials to support such thresholds for athletes.

The primary source of vitamin D is cutaneous synthesis driven by ultraviolet-B radiation, at a wavelength of 290–315 nm, interacting with 7-dehydrocholesterol and forming pre-vitamin D in cells of the upper epidermis [8]. Due to Ireland's northerly latitude (51°N–55°N), sunlight is only of sufficient strength to trigger cutaneous vitamin D synthesis for 6 months of the year (April to September); resulting in seasonal fluctuation in vitamin D status [9]. As such, geographical location is the major factor contributing to poor vitamin D status in Irish athletes as well as the general population [10,11]. In addition, indoor, early-morning and late-evening training sessions may also contribute to the prevalence of vitamin D insufficiency/deficiency in athletes [12]. Compounding this issue is the limited availability and consumption of vitamin D-rich foods by Irish athletes such as fatty fish and liver [10,13].

Previous studies conducted by our research group have identified a particularly high prevalence of vitamin D insufficiency/deficiency in Gaelic footballers, Paralympians and boxers competing at both the collegiate and elite-level [10,13]. Based on these findings the Irish Institute of Sport revised their vitamin D supplementation policy; aiming to ensure that identified cases of vitamin D insufficiency/deficiency were dealt with appropriately. It is not known, however, if the extent of this health concern extends to elite athletes competing in other high-profile sports in Ireland such as those within international cricket and rugby teams. This study therefore aimed to assess the vitamin D status of elite Irish athletes participating in a range of high-profile sports and establish if equatorial travel, supplement use and/or sunbed use are predictors of vitamin D status.

2. Materials and Methods

2.1. Recruitment

This observational study took place between November 2013 and April 2015 at training locations across the island of Ireland. The study was approved by the University Research Ethics Committee (REC/13/0235) and conducted in accordance with the declaration of Helsinki. A total of 64 elite athletes, that were actively competing internationally, were recruited through the teams' performance dietitian and provided with an information sheet detailing the study procedures prior to obtaining informed consent. Overall, 92 blood samples were obtained from male cricketers ($n = 28$), male and female boxers ($n = 18$ and $n = 3$ respectively), and female rugby seven players ($n = 43$) across multiple time points. Samples were obtained in the months of February (cricket $n = 14$); March (rugby $n = 7$); April (boxing $n = 18$); May (cricket $n = 15$); September (cricket $n = 13$) and November (rugby $n = 22$ and boxing $n = 3$).

2.2. Blood Collection and Processing

Trained phlebotomists obtained blood samples from the antecubital fossa; using a 21-gauge butterfly needle and 8 mL serum and 9 mL ethylenediaminetetraacetic (EDTA) plasma tubes (Greiner Bio-One GmbH, Kremsmünster, Austria). Following inversion, serum tubes were left at room temperature for up to 60 min and EDTA plasma tubes placed in refrigeration or on ice until processing. Within 3 h of collection, tubes were centrifuged at 2200 rpm for 15 min at 4 °C. Following separation, serum and plasma samples were pipetted into 0.5 mL aliquots and stored at −80 °C until further analysis.

2.3. Blood Analyses

All analyses were run in duplicate. Liquid chromatography-tandem mass spectrometry (LC-MS/MS) (API 4000; AB SCIEX) was used to quantify serum $25(OH)D_2$ and $25(OH)D_3$ concentrations, using a commercially available assay (Chromsystems Instruments and Chemicals GmbH; MassChrom 25-OH-Vitamin D3/D2). This analysis was undertaken at the biochemistry department of St James' Hospital Dublin; a laboratory that complies with the Vitamin D External Quality Assessment Scheme and use of the National Institute of Standards and Technology 972 vitamin D standard reference material. The respective inter- and intra-assay coefficients of variation were 6.5% and 7.5%. Serum calcium concentrations (adjusted for serum albumin) were determined using an ILab 650 clinical biochemistry analyser at the University of Ulster, Coleraine. Plasma parathyroid hormone (PTH) concentration was quantified at Altnagelvin area hospital using a Cobas 4000 clinical biochemistry analyser (Roche Diagnostics Ltd., Burgess Hill, UK).

2.4. Lifestyle Questionnaire

In the presence of a researcher, a self-reported lifestyle questionnaire was completed by each athlete in order to estimate use of dietary supplements containing vitamin D, sunbed use and equatorial travel in the 6 months prior to sampling.

2.5. Statistical Analysis

An a priori power calculation with significance set at $p < 0.05$ and statistical power at 95% determined that 27 athletes were required in order to detect a 31.4 nmol/L difference in total 25(OH)D concentration between sport disciplines (GPower Version 3.1) [10]. The Statistical Package for the Social Sciences (SPSS) was used for all further analyses (IBM SPSS Statistics for Windows, Version 21.0, IBM Corp., Armonk, NY, USA). Data distribution was assessed using the Shapiro-Wilk test. All measures had a skewed data distribution and were therefore log-transformed prior to hypothesis testing. For continuous variables, differences in outcome measures between sport disciplines were identified using analysis of variance (ANOVA) with Bonferroni post-hoc test. *p*-values were adjusted using the Bonferroni correction for multiple comparisons. A Chi square test was used to identify if vitamin D status varied according to season of sampling (Spring/Summer (March–August) versus Autumn/Winter (September–February)). A Chi squared test was also used to determine seasonal variation in sampling according to sex. Differences in questionnaire responses, between sport disciplines, were determined using a Chi-square test with *post-hoc* analysis comparing standardised residuals [14]. A logistic regression model was used to identify if vitamin D supplementation, sunbed use or travel to an equatorial location were significant predictors of vitamin D status. As only 2 athletes exhibited vitamin D deficiency (total 25(OH)D concentration <30 nmol/L); vitamin D status was defined as sufficiency (>50 nmol/L) and insufficiency/deficiency (<50 nmol/L).

3. Results

Physical and biochemical characteristics of elite athletes are detailed in Table 1.

As expected, there was a significant difference in the distribution of male and female athletes recruited from each sport discipline (rugby $n = 43$ females; boxing $n = 18$ males and $n = 3$ females; cricket $n = 28$ males) $p < 0.001$. The vitamin D status of athletes is outlined in Figure 1 and this did not vary according to season of sampling, $p = 0.548$.

Table 1. Physical and biochemical characteristics of elite athletes presented as mean $\pm$ SD.

Measure	Total Samples ($n = 92$)	Rugby ($n = 43$)	Boxing ($n = 21$)	Cricket ($n = 28$)	p [a]
Age, y	25 $\pm$ 5	25 $\pm$ 4	23 $\pm$ 4 [d]	28 $\pm$ 7 [c]	0.021
Height, cm	175 $\pm$ 9	168 $\pm$ 6 [c,d]	179 $\pm$ 10 [b]	182 $\pm$ 6 [b]	0.003
Weight, kg	75.79 $\pm$ 14.12	68.05 $\pm$ 6.64 [d]	74.52 $\pm$ 16.87 [d]	88.64 $\pm$ 11.16 [b,c]	0.003
BMI, kg/m^2	24.55 $\pm$ 2.95	23.83 $\pm$ 1.67 [d]	22.96 $\pm$ 2.88 [d]	26.85 $\pm$ 3.25 [b,c]	0.003
25(OH)D$_2$, nmol/L	2.02 $\pm$ 1.54	2.05 $\pm$ 1.36	2.76 $\pm$ 1.76 [d]	1.42 $\pm$ 1.43 [c]	0.006
25(OH)D$_3$, nmol/L	74.48 $\pm$ 27.54	64.16 $\pm$ 24.73 [d]	81.27 $\pm$ 34.46	85.24 $\pm$ 20.00 [c]	0.003
Total 25(OH)D, nmol/L	76.50 $\pm$ 27.00	66.20 $\pm$ 24.44 [c,d]	84.03 $\pm$ 33.20 [b]	86.66 $\pm$ 19.78 [b]	0.003
Adjusted calcium, mmol/L	2.30 $\pm$ 0.17	2.26 $\pm$ 0.13	2.33 $\pm$ 0.08	2.32 $\pm$ 0.10	0.060
PTH, pg/mL	32.71 $\pm$ 11.54	34.69 $\pm$ 12.82	31.08 $\pm$ 12.18	30.84 $\pm$ 8.49	1.000

[a] Differences between sport disciplines, ANOVA with Bonferroni post-hoc test. p value corrected for multiple comparisons; [b] Significantly different from rugby, $p < 0.05$; [c] Significantly different from boxing, $p < 0.05$; [d] Significantly different from cricket, $p < 0.05$.

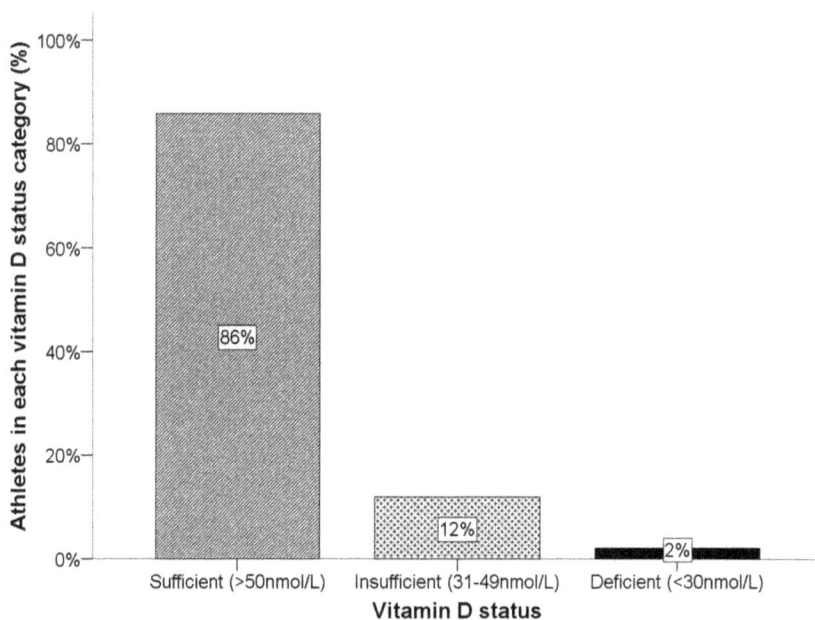

Figure 1. Vitamin D status of athletes. Overall, 86% of athletes were vitamin D sufficient; 12% of athletes were vitamin D insufficient (31–49 nmol/L) and 2% vitamin D deficient (<30 nmol/L).

Rugby players had a significantly lower mean total 25(OH)D concentration compared to boxers and cricketers. Overall, females exhibited a significantly lower mean total 25(OH)D concentration compared to males (65.37 $\pm$ 24.91 versus 88.24.04 nmol/L respectively, $p < 0.001$). A significantly greater proportion of female athletes were sampled during the autumn/winter compared to male athletes ($n = 36$ and $n = 16$ respectively, $p < 0.001$). In total, 25% of athletes reported consuming vitamin D supplements in the 6 months prior to sampling. There was no difference in the ratio of athletes reporting/not reporting vitamin D supplement use between sport disciplines, Table 2.

Table 2. Number of athletes reporting equatorial travel, vitamin D supplementation and sunbed use in the 6 months prior to sampling.

	Total Cohort (n = 92)	Rugby (n = 43)	Boxing (n = 21)	Cricket (n = 28)	p [a]
Measure	Yes/No	Yes/No	Yes/No	Yes/No	
Equatorial travel	43:48	24:19 [b]	2:18	17:11 [b]	0.006
Vitamin D supplement use	23:68	12:31	6:14	5:23	1.00
Sun bed use	15:76	8:35 [c]	7:13 [c]	0:28	0.030

[a] Chi-square test with Bonferroni post-hoc test. *p* value corrected for multiple comparisons; [b] Yes/No responses were significantly different from boxing, *p* < 0.05; [c] Yes/No responses were significantly different from cricket, *p* < 0.05.

Vitamin D supplementation was a significant positive predictor of vitamin D status (Table 3).

Table 3. Logistic regression model predicting likelihood of athletes having a total 25(OH)D concentration above 50 nmol/L.

Predictor	β	S.E	Wald	p	Odds Ratio	95.0% C.I. for Odds Ratio	
						Lower	Upper
Vitamin D supplementation	1.46	0.66	4.88	0.027 [a]	4.31	1.18	15.75
Equatorial travel	0.23	0.65	0.13	0.720	1.26	0.35	4.49
Sunbed use	−1.18	1.12	1.12	0.291	0.29	0.03	2.75

[a] Statistically significant predictor of a total 25(OH)D concentration above 50 nmol/L, *p* < 0.05.

Equatorial travel and sunbed use were reported in 47% and 16% of athletes respectively. A higher ratio of rugby players and cricketers reported equatorial travel compared to boxers and a higher ratio of rugby players and boxers reported sunbed use compared to cricketers (Table 2), but these factors did not predict vitamin D status (Table 3).

4. Discussion

The terminology pertaining to deficient/insufficient/sufficient vitamin D status remains a topic of ongoing debate, with no widely accepted guidelines in place for athletes [12]. According to U.S Institute of Medicine guidelines, 14% of athletes in the current study exhibited vitamin D insufficiency/deficiency; a stark difference from 55% when elite Irish athletes were tested in 2010/2011, albeit not in the same cohort [10]. Elite boxers were tested in both studies and, in this group specifically, the prevalence of vitamin D insufficiency/deficiency has decreased from 29% to 10% since 2010/2011. On average, athletes from all sport disciplines were vitamin D sufficient. Although rugby seven players had a lower mean total 25(OH)D concentration than those from other sport disciplines, this is unlikely to be clinically meaningful; certainly with respect to bone health. Furthermore, this difference can likely be attributed to a greater proportion of female athletes being sampled during autumn/winter than male athletes.

Whilst studies around the globe have demonstrated that vitamin D insufficiency/deficiency is a health concern affecting athletes [2]; not all elite cohorts have exhibited clinical deficiency, in support of the current findings [15–22]. Unlike the majority of athletes, those competing at the elite level have access to a support network of dietitians that regularly monitor dietary intake and nutrient status by analysis of food diaries and blood screening. Since the findings of Magee and colleagues [10], total 25(OH)D concentrations have been included as part of routine blood screening for elite athletes in Ireland; thereby enabling targeted supplementation practices. Vitamin D supplement use was confirmed as a positive predictor of vitamin D status in the current study. This finding reinforces the important role that vitamin D supplementation has to play in the optimisation of elite athletes vitamin D status. Elite Irish athletes are routinely screened during the late autumn/early winter (October onward) when ultraviolet B radiation is no longer able to trigger dermal vitamin D synthesis and risk of deficiency increases concomitantly [23]. This marks a change in strategy from pre-2010/2011 when vitamin D screening and supplementation was uncommon. Athletes that exhibit a total 25(OH)D concentration below 125 nmol/L are currently assigned to a supplementation protocol based upon their initial total 25(OH)D concentration. This targeted approach likely decreases the risk of inadvertent vitamin D toxicity (total 25(OH)D concentration $\approx$ 250 nmol/L) through excessive supplementation when it is not required [24]. Total 25(OH)D is quantified in athlete's serum using liquid chromatography-tandem mass spectrometry (LC-MS/MS); a method that is widely regarded as the current gold-standard [25]. Alternative analytical methods, such as immunoassay, can overestimate 25(OH)D concentrations leading to misdiagnosis [26].

There is growing evidence that vitamin D_3 (cholecalciferol) has superior bioavailability compared to vitamin D_2 (ergocalciferol) as a result of stronger association to vitamin D binding protein [27]. This concept has been corroborated by several randomised controlled trials demonstrating that vitamin D_3 can be up to 70% more effective than vitamin D_2 at increasing total 25(OH)D [28,29]. As such, elite Irish athletes are supplemented with vitamin D_3.

The Irish Sports Council promotes a 'food-first' approach with regard to dietary supplements [30]. This is a precautionary stance consistent with other National Governing Body policies worldwide owing to numerous reports of supplement contamination with World Anti-Doping Agency (WADA)-banned substances [31–35]. Although there are a growing number of vitamin D-fortified products available in Ireland [36,37], there are few naturally-occurring dietary sources of vitamin D and intake of such foods is low in the typical Western diet [38,39]. It therefore remains challenging for athletes to attain the current UK reference nutrient intake of 10 μg/day from diet alone [10,13]. In the absence of widespread vitamin D fortification; this conundrum may be best resolved through athlete's consultation with the team dietitian and provision of batch-tested supplements that are confirmed to be free of contaminants. In the United Kingdom and Ireland, vitamin D_3 supplements certified as contaminant-free by Informed Sport are currently available in doses ranging from 1000 IU (25 μg) to 5000 IU (125 μg) [40–42]. It should be noted however that the tolerable upper intake limit for vitamin D has been set at 4000 IU (100 μg)/day by the European Food Safety Authority [43].

Strengths of this study include the large sample size and recruitment of both male and female athletes from several high-profile sport disciplines. A potential limitation is the self-reported measure of equatorial travel. Although 47% of athletes reported equatorial travel, this was not deemed a significant predictor of vitamin D status. Although this may seem surprising owing to the unequivocal role of UVB exposure in vitamin D synthesis [44]; one should not assume that equatorial travel for training/competition invariably results in an enhanced vitamin D status. It is plausible to suggest that effective application of high sun protection factor cream and indoor training, to avoid excessive heat exposure during peak sunlight hours, may limit vitamin D synthesis despite an equatorial location [45]. The lifestyle questionnaire in the current study had not been previously validated and therefore this could be deemed a potential limitation. Future studies may wish to consider assessing the habitual dietary intake of vitamin D-containing foods by elite athletes, albeit expected to make a negligible contribution to overall vitamin D status [10,13] and using dosimeters to quantify UVB exposure of athletes whilst away on training camps and competition. In summary, vitamin D sufficiency is now commonplace in elite Irish athletes. This finding demonstrates the efficacy of targeted supplementation in elite sport and suggests that blanket-supplementation of elite Irish athletes may therefore not be appropriate.

Acknowledgments: The authors would like to thank all athletes that participated in the study and the Department of Employment and Learning for supporting this research. The authors would also like to acknowledge Mark Lynch, Ruth Wood-Martin RD, John Cleary, Brendan Connor, Ciara Beggan, Laura Beggan and Neil Dennison for their assistance throughout the study.

Author Contributions: J.T., S.M., E.M., K.P. and P.M. conceived and designed the experiments; J.T., K.P., E.L. and M.H. performed laboratory analyses; J.T. analyzed the data and wrote the paper. All authors reviewed and approved the final manuscript.

Conflicts of Interest: Magee reports grants from the Irish Amateur Boxing Association, Cricket Ireland and the Irish Rugby Football Union, during the conduct of the study; and Sharon Madigan is employed by the Irish Institute of Sport. The Irish Institute of Sport oversees the monitoring of athletes from the above mentioned teams involved in this study.

Abbreviations

BMI	body mass index
25(OH)D$_2$	25-hydroxyvitamin D$_2$
25(OH)D$_3$	25-hydroxyvitamin D$_3$
PTH	parathyroid hormone

References

1. IOM (Institute of Medicine). *Dietary Reference Intakes for Calcium and Vitamin D*; The National Academies Press: Washington, DC, USA, 2011.
2. Farrokhyar, F.; Tabasinejad, R.; Dao, D.; Peterson, D.; Ayeni, O.; Hadioonzadeh, R.; Bhandari, M. Prevalence of vitamin D inadequacy in athletes: A systematic-review and meta-analysis. *Sports Med.* **2015**, *45*, 365–378. [CrossRef] [PubMed]
3. Christodoulou, S.; Goula, T.; Ververidis, A.; Drosos, G. Vitamin D and bone disease. *BioMed. Res. Int.* **2013**, 396541. [CrossRef] [PubMed]
4. Baeke, F.; Etten, E.V.; Overbergh, L.; Mathieu, C. Vitamin D$_3$ and the immune system: Maintaining the balance in health and disease. *Nutr. Res. Rev.* **2007**, *20*, 106–118. [CrossRef] [PubMed]
5. He, C.; Handzlik, M.; Fraser, W.D.; Muhamad, A.; Preston, H.; Richardson, A.; Gleeson, M. Influence of vitamin D status on respiratory infection incidence and immune function during 4 months of winter training in endurance sport athletes. *Exerc. Immunol. Rev.* **2013**, *19*, 86–101. [PubMed]
6. Barker, T.; Martins, T.B.; Hill, H.R.; Kjeldsberg, C.R.; Dixon, B.M.; Schneider, E.D.; Henriksen, V.T.; Weaver, L.K. Circulating pro-inflammatory cytokines are elevated and peak power output correlates with 25-hydroxyvitamin D in vitamin D insufficient adults. *Eur. J. Appl. Physiol.* **2013**, *113*, 1523–1534. [CrossRef] [PubMed]
7. Heaney, R.P. Assessing vitamin D status. *Curr. Opin. Clin. Nutr. Metab. Care* **2011**, *14*, 440–444. [CrossRef] [PubMed]
8. Webb, A.R. Who, what, where and when-influences on cutaneous vitamin D synthesis. *Prog. Biophys. Mol. Biol.* **2006**, *92*, 17–25. [CrossRef] [PubMed]
9. Cashman, K.D.; Muldowney, S.; McNulty, B.; Nugent, A.; FitzGerald, A.P.; Kiely, M.; Walton, J.; Gibney, M.J.; Flynn, A. Vitamin D status of Irish adults: Findings from the National Adult Nutrition Survey. *Br. J. Nutr.* **2013**, *209*, 1248–1256. [CrossRef] [PubMed]
10. Magee, P.J.; Pourshahidi, L.K.; Wallace, J.M.W.; Cleary, J.; Conway, J.; Harney, E.; Madigan, S.M. Vitamin D status and supplementation in elite Irish athletes. *Int. J. Sport Nutr. Exerc. Metab.* **2013**, *23*, 441–448. [PubMed]
11. Hill, T.R.; McCarthy, D.; Jakobsen, J.; Lamberg-Allard, C.; Kiely, M.; Cashman, K.D. Seasonal changes in vitamin D status and bone turnover in healthy Irish postmenopausal women. *Int. J. Vitam. Nutr. Res.* **2007**, *77*, 320–325. [CrossRef] [PubMed]
12. Todd, J.J.; Pourshahidi, L.K.; McSorley, E.M.; Madigan, S.M.; Magee, P.J. Vitamin D: Recent advances and implications for athletes. *Sports Med.* **2015**, *45*, 213–219. [CrossRef] [PubMed]
13. Todd, J.J.; McSorley, E.M.; Pourshahidi, L.K.; Madigan, S.M.; Laird, E.; Healy, M.; Magee, P.J. Vitamin D$_3$ supplementation using an oral spray solution resolves deficiency but has no effect on VO$_2$ max in Gaelic footballers: Results from a randomised, double-blind, placebo-controlled trial. *Eur. J. Nutr.* **2016**. in press. [CrossRef] [PubMed]
14. Beasley, M.T.; Schumacker, R.R. Multiple regression approach to analyzing contingency tables: Post hoc and planned comparison procedures. *J. Exp. Educ.* **1995**, *64*, 79–93. [CrossRef]

15. Maroon, J.C.; Mathyssek, C.M.; Bost, J.W.; Amos, A.; Winkelman, R.; Yates, A.P.; Duca, M.A.; Norwig, J.A. Vitamin D profile in national football league players. *Am. J. Sports Med.* **2015**, *43*, 1241–1245. [CrossRef] [PubMed]

16. Sghaier-Ayadi, A.; Feki, M.; Ayed, I.B.; Abene, O.; Fredj, M.B.; Kaabachi, K.; Chaouachi, A. Vitamin D status and determinants of deficiency in non-supplemented athletes during the winter months in Tunisia. *Biol. Sport* **2015**, *32*, 281–287. [CrossRef] [PubMed]

17. Wentz, L.M.; Liu, P.Y.; Ilich, J.Z.; Haymes, E.M. Female distance runners training in Southeastern United States have adequate vitamin D status. *Int. J. Sport Nutr. Exerc. Metab.* **2015**. in press. [CrossRef] [PubMed]

18. Allison, R.J.; Close, G.L.; Farooq, A.; Riding, N.R.; Salah, O.; Hamilton, B. Severely vitamin D-deficient athletes present smaller hearts than sufficient athletes. *Eur. J. Prev. Cardiol.* **2015**, *22*, 535–542. [CrossRef] [PubMed]

19. Caroli, B.; Pasin, F.; Aloe, R.; Gnocchi, C.; Dei Cas, A.; Galli, C.; Passeri, G. Characterization of skeletal parameters in a cohort of North Italian rugby players. *J. Endocrinol. Invest.* **2014**, *37*, 609–617. [CrossRef] [PubMed]

20. Solarz, K.; Kopeć, A.; Pietraszewska, J.; Majda, F.; Słowińska-Lisowska, M.; Mędraś, M. An evaluation of the levels of 25-hydroxyvitamin D_3 and bone turnover markers in professional football players and in physically inactive men. *Physiol. Res.* **2014**, *63*, 237–243. [PubMed]

21. Kopeć, A.; Solarz, K.; Majda, F.; Słowińska-Lisowska, M.; Mędraś, M. An evaluation of the levels of vitamin D and bone turnover markers after the summer and winter periods in polish professional soccer players. *J. Hum. Kinet.* **2013**, *38*, 135–140. [CrossRef] [PubMed]

22. Valtueña, J.; Dominguez, D.; Til, L.; González-Gross, M.; Drobnic, F. High prevalence of vitamin D insufficiency among elite Spanish athletes the importance of outdoor training adaptation. *Nutr. Hosp.* **2014**, *30*, 124–131. [PubMed]

23. Hyppönen, E.; Power, C. Hypovitaminosis D in British adults at age 45 years: Nationwide cohort study of dietary and lifestyle predictors. *Am. J. Clin. Nutr.* **2007**, *85*, 860–868. [PubMed]

24. Jones, G. Pharmacokinetics of vitamin D toxicity. *Am. J. Clin. Nutr.* **2008**, *88*, 582S–586S. [PubMed]

25. Lai, J.K.; Lucas, R.M.; Clements, M.S.; Harrison, S.L.; Banks, E. Assessing vitamin D status: Pitfalls for the unwary. *Mol. Nutr. Food Res.* **2010**, *54*, 1062–1071. [CrossRef] [PubMed]

26. Lai, J.K.; Lucas, R.M.; Banks, E.; Ponsonby, A. Variability in vitamin D assays impairs clinical assessment of vitamin D status. *Intern. Med. J.* **2012**, *42*, 43–50. [CrossRef] [PubMed]

27. Houghton, L.A.; Vieth, R. The case against ergocalciferol (vitamin D_2) as a vitamin supplement. *Am. J. Clin. Nutr.* **2006**, *84*, 694–697. [PubMed]

28. Tripkovic, L.; Lambert, H.; Hart, K.; Smith, C.P.; Bucca, G.; Penson, S.; Chope, G.; Hyppönen, E.; Berry, J.; Vieth, R.; et al. Comparison of vitamin D_2 and vitamin D_3 supplementation in raising serum 25-hydroxyvitamin D status: A systematic review and meta-analysis. *Am. J. Clin. Nutr.* **2012**, *95*, 1357–1364. [CrossRef] [PubMed]

29. Lehmann, U.; Hirchem, F.; Stangl, G.I.; Hinz, K.; Westphal, S.; Dierkes, J. Bioavailability of vitamin D_2 and D_3 in healthy volunteers, a randomized placebo-controlled trial. *J. Clin. Endocrinol. Metab.* **2013**, *98*, 4339–4345. [CrossRef] [PubMed]

30. Irish Sports Council. *Irish Sports Council Supplements and Sports Food Policy*; Irish Sports Council: Dublin, Republic of Ireland, 2012.

31. Maughan, R.J. Contamination of dietary supplements and positive drug tests in sport. *J. Sports Sci.* **2005**, *23*, 883–889. [CrossRef] [PubMed]

32. Kamber, M.; Baume, N.; Saugy, M.; Rivier, L. Nutritional supplements as a source for positive doping cases? *Int. J. Sport Nutr. Exerc. Metab.* **2001**, *11*, 258–263. [PubMed]

33. British Athletics. UK Athletics' Supplements Position Statement. Available online: http://www.britishathletics.org.uk/anti-doping/supplements-and-nutrition/ (accessed on 16 May 2016).

34. Australian Rugby. Australian Rugby Union Sports Supplements Policy. Available online: http://www.rugby.com.au/ARUHQ/ARUSportsSupplementsPolicy.aspx (accessed on 16 May 2016).

35. Catlin, D.H.; Leder, B.Z.; Ahrens, B.; Starcevic, B.; Hatton, C.K.; Green, G.A.; Finkelstein, J.S. Trace contamination of over-the-counter androstenedione and positive urine test results for a nandrolone metabolite. *JAMA* **2000**, *284*, 2618–2621. [CrossRef] [PubMed]

36. Monterey Mushrooms Mushroom Nutritional Chart. Available online: http://www.montereymushrooms.com/nutrition/mushroom-nutrition (accessed on 16 May 2016).

37. Avonmore Whole Super Milk. Available online: http://www.avonmore.ie/our-range/our-products-milk/avonmore-whole-super-milk (accessed on 16 May 2016).

38. Spiro, A.; Buttriss, J. Vitamin D: An overview of vitamin D status and intake in Europe. *Nutr. Bull.* **2014**, *39*, 322–350. [CrossRef] [PubMed]

39. Black, L.J.; Walton, J.; Flynn, A.; Cashman, K.D.; Kiely, M. Small increments in vitamin D intake by Irish adults over a decade show that strategic initiatives to fortify the food supply are needed. *J. Nutr.* **2015**, *145*, 969–976. [CrossRef] [PubMed]

40. Proto-Col Vitamin D Tablets 5000 IU. Available online: http://www.proto-col.com/vitamin-d.html (accessed on 16 May 2016).

41. Healthspan Elite Vitamin D3 1000 IU. Available online: http://www.healthspan.co.uk/elite/elite-high-strength-vitamin-D3 (accessed on 16 May 2016).

42. Informed Sport Registered Product Search. Available online: http://www.informed-sport.com/supplement_search?s=vitamin+d (accessed on 16 May 2016).

43. Agostoni, C.; Bresson, J.L.; Fairweather-Tait, S. *Scientific Opinion on the Tolerable Upper Intake Level of Vitamin D*; European Food Safety Authority (EFSA): Parma, Italy, 2012. [CrossRef]

44. Holick, M.F. Sunlight and vitamin D for bone health and prevention of autoimmune diseases, cancers, and cardiovascular disease. *Am. J. Clin. Nutr.* **2004**, *6*, 1678S–1688S.

45. Holick, M.; Chen, T. Vitamin D deficiency: A worldwide problem with health consequences. *Am. J. Clin. Nutr.* **2008**, *87*, 1080S–1086S. [CrossRef] [PubMed]

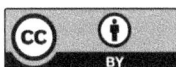

nutrients

MDPI

Article

Effects of Beetroot Juice on Recovery of Muscle Function and Performance between Bouts of Repeated Sprint Exercise

Tom Clifford [1], Bram Berntzen [2], Gareth W. Davison [3], Daniel J. West [4], Glyn Howatson [1,5,]* and Emma J. Stevenson [4]

[1]   Faculty of Health and Life Sciences, Department of Sport, Exercise & Rehabilitation,
     Northumbria University, Newcastle NE1 8ST, UK; tom.clifford@northumbria.ac.uk
[2]   Faculty of Health Medicine and Life Sciences, Maastricht University, Maastricht 6211 LK, The Netherlands;
     bram.berntzen@student.maastrichtuniversity.nl
[3]   Sport and Exercise Sciences Research Institute, Ulster University, Ulster BT52 1SA, Northern Ireland, UK;
     gw.davison@ulster.ac.uk
[4]   Human Nutrition Research Centre, Institute of Cellular Medicine, Newcastle University,
     Newcastle NE2 4HH, UK; daniel.west@newcastle.ac.uk (D.J.W.); emma.stevenson@newcastle.ac.uk (E.J.S.)
[5]   Water Research Group, School of Environmental Sciences and Development, Northwest University,
     Potchefstroom 2520, South Africa
*   Correspondence: glyn.howatson@northumbria.ac.uk; Tel.: +44-0191-227-3573

Received: 27 July 2016; Accepted: 15 August 2016; Published: 18 August 2016

Abstract: This study examined the effects of beetroot juice (BTJ) on recovery between two repeated-sprint tests. In an independent groups design, 20 male, team-sports players were randomized to receive either BTJ or a placebo (PLA) (2 × 250 mL) for 3 days after an initial repeated sprint test (20 × 30 m; RST1) and after a second repeated sprint test (RST2), performed 72 h later. Maximal isometric voluntary contractions (MIVC), countermovement jumps (CMJ), reactive strength index (RI), pressure-pain threshold (PPT), creatine kinase (CK), C-reactive protein (hs-CRP), protein carbonyls (PC), lipid hydroperoxides (LOOH) and the ascorbyl free radical ($A^{\bullet-}$) were measured before, after, and at set times between RST1 and RST2. CMJ and RI recovered quicker in BTJ compared to PLA after RST1: at 72 h post, CMJ and RI were 7.6% and 13.8% higher in BTJ vs. PLA, respectively ($p < 0.05$). PPT was 10.4% higher in BTJ compared to PLA 24 h post RST2 ($p = 0.012$) but similar at other time points. No group differences were detected for mean and fastest sprint time or fatigue index. MIVC, or the biochemical markers measured ($p > 0.05$). BTJ reduced the decrement in CMJ and RI following and RST but had no effect on sprint performance or oxidative stress.

Keywords: beetroot juice; muscle damage; exercise recovery; repeated sprint exercise

1. Introduction

Repeated sprint exercise (RSE), in which a number of short-duration maximal effort sprints (2–6 s) are completed intermittently with brief recovery periods ($\leq$60 s), places a great deal of stress on the physiological and musculoskeletal systems [1]. The high energy turnover during RSE induces significant metabolic stress, triggering rapid perturbations in the nervous, immune, and endocrine systems [1], as well as an increased formation of reactive oxygen species (ROS) [2]. In addition, the high-force eccentric muscle contractions required to accelerate and decelerate during RSE places a great deal of mechanical stress on the musculoskeletal system, particularly the quadriceps and hamstring muscle groups [3]. It is therefore not surprising that team-sport players, who routinely engage in RSE in training sessions and matches, often display symptoms of muscle damage (i.e., muscle soreness and reduced muscle function) that can persist for several days [4–6].

Because the typical time between training sessions and or matches is often not sufficient for full recovery ($\leq$72 h) athletes and coaches are continually seeking strategies that could help minimise the negative effects of muscle damage [7,8].

The exact mechanisms to explain the causes of muscle damage after RSE are not fully understood, but a host of factors such as muscle membrane damage, sarcomere disorganization, excitation-contraction coupling dysfunction, contractile protein degradation and inflammation are all likely to play a role [9,10]. Furthermore, it has been suggested that the generation of ROS in the days post-exercise, likely a consequence of inflammatory mediated repair processes, might exacerbate the existing muscle damage by degrading components of the cytosol that are integral to force production [11–13]. A number of studies have provided evidence of oxidative stress in the hours and days following RSE [2,6,14], suggesting that the endogenous antioxidant system is unable to cope with excess ROS production under these conditions. Thus, it would be reasonable to assume that the prolonged decrement in muscle function might be, at least in part, attributable to oxidative stress. This also makes the expectation tenable that interventions attempting to combat the excess production of ROS and control oxidative stress, such as antioxidants, could help accelerate the rate of muscle recovery following RSE.

While the nutritional antioxidants vitamin C and E have proven largely ineffective at attenuating muscle damage [15–17], there is growing support for the use of antioxidant-rich fruit and vegetable beverages as recovery aids [18]. Recently, we showed that supplementation with beetroot juice (BTJ) attenuated some aspects of muscle damage following high intensity plyometric exercise [19]. We proposed that one of the potential mechanisms by which of BTJ might have attenuated EIMD in this study was via its antioxidant effects. Although the antioxidant effects of BTJ has received little attention in the literature, findings from our previous work [20] and others [21,22] suggest that its antioxidant capacity is markedly higher than other vegetable juices, such as tomato and carrot juice, and also than several other drinks considered to have a high antioxidant capacity such as green tea, apple, cherry and cranberry juice [20,23,24]. The high antioxidant capacity of BTJ is due to the fact that several of the phytonutrient compounds it contains have been shown to scavenge ROS production in vitro and in vivo and subsequently limit cellular injury [25–27]. The most potent antioxidant molecules in BTJ are thought to be the betalain pigments, which are responsible for beetroot's violet colour [28]. The betalains, and betanin in particular, are very effective electron donors that have been shown to not only attenuate ROS mediated injury but also to upregulate endogenous antioxidant enzymes and stimulate host defence [29–32]. In addition, BTJ is rich in nitrate, which, via its reduction to nitric oxide (NO) might have indirect antioxidant effects by supressing the accumulation of leukocytes [33], which are thought to be the main producers of ROS after muscle-damaging exercise [34]. Nonetheless, we failed to quantify oxidative stress in our aforementioned experiment [19] to confirm or refute this posit. Furthermore, the aforementioned findings were in recreationally active participants and therefore these results might not be directly transferable to better trained athletic populations.

To our knowledge, the effects of BTJ on muscle damage and recovery after activity incorporating RSE has not been investigated. Additionally, the effectiveness of such an intervention on subsequent performance has not been considered. Therefore, the main aim of this study was to examine whether BTJ can attenuate losses in muscle function and performance between two sport-specific repeated sprint tests (RST) performed 72 h apart. We also examined the effects of BTJ on biochemical markers associated with muscle damage, specifically oxidative stress, to try and discern what role (if any) the antioxidant potential of BTJ has on attenuating EIMD. Based on our previous findings [19], we hypothesized that: (1) BTJ would attenuate muscle function deficits and oxidative stress between and after the two repeated sprint tests; and (2) that performance during the second sprint test would be preserved with BTJ compared to a placebo.

2. Materials and Methods

2.1. Participants

Twenty male participants gave written informed consent for participation in this study (characteristics presented in Table 1). The sample size for this study was based on a priori power calculation. Based on a previous study [19], with a power of 0.80 and two tailed α level set at 0.05, the minimum number of participants required to detect an 8% difference in counter movement jump (CMJ) performance between groups (SD: 6%) was estimated as 10 per group. We selected CMJ as our primary outcome measure because it is believed to be the most sensitive test for detecting reductions in neuromuscular function after RSE [35]. Our secondary outcomes included other markers of neuromuscular function, repeated sprint performance, muscle pain, and biochemical markers of inflammation, oxidative stress and muscle damage (specific details in relevant sections below). All participants were collegiate team-sports players, competing in either soccer ($n = 10$), rugby ($n = 5$), basketball ($n = 2$) hockey ($n = 2$) or handball ($n = 1$) on a regular basis; all testing was performed at the end of the competitive season (between March 2015 and June 2015). Participant's eligibility was assessed with a health screening questionnaire. None had any known food allergies, were suffering from a musculoskeletal injury, or had previous history of renal, gastrointestinal or cardiovascular complications or any other contraindication to the study procedures. For the 48 h prior to and throughout data collection, participants were prohibited from consuming alcoholic beverages, and instructed to avoid any strenuous exercise outside of the trial requirements. The study protocol received ethical approval from the Faculty of Health and Life Sciences ethics committee at Northumbria University. Approval was granted on the 26 February 2015 and assigned the following project identification code: HLSTC200115.

Table 1. Descriptive data for participants in the beetroot juice (BTJ) and placebo (PLA) groups.

Group	Age (Years)	Height (m)	Mass (kg)
BTJ	23 ± 3	1.83 ± 0.90	76.8 ± 9.5
PLA	21 ± 2	1.77 ± 0.51	73.4 ± 12.4

Values are mean $\pm$ SD ($n = 10$ per group). No significant differences were detected between groups for any variable ($p > 0.05$).

2.2. Experimental Design

This study employed a double-blind, placebo controlled, independent groups design. Participants were required to attend the laboratory for 6 visits over a 2 week period. The first visit was to familiarise the participants with the study procedures and randomly allocate them to either a beetroot juice (BTJ) or an isocaloric placebo (PLA) group. Their baseline maximal isometric voluntary contraction (MIVC) was used to match the groups. The principal investigator was responsible for the randomizing procedures. The next five visits were performed on consecutive days in the same laboratory at the same time of day and were preceded by an overnight fast. For the main trials, participants performed two repeated sprint tests separated by 72 h (visit 2 = RST1 and visit 5 = RST2) (see Figure 1 for schematic outline). A range of dependent variables were taken pre, 30-min post, 24, 48 and 72 h after RST1, and 30-min post and 24 h after RST2 to monitor recovery. On each occasion, dependent variables were performed in the following order: pressure-pain threshold (PPT), venous blood draw, CMJ, reactive strength index (RI) and MIVC. After completing the post-exercise measures participants consumed 1 serving of their allocated treatment, and returned to the lab 2.5 h post ingestion for a further blood sample. Another treatment was taken with an evening meal, and then at the same points (with breakfast and with an evening meal) for the following 3 days. All data collection took place in the exercise laboratories at Northumbria University.

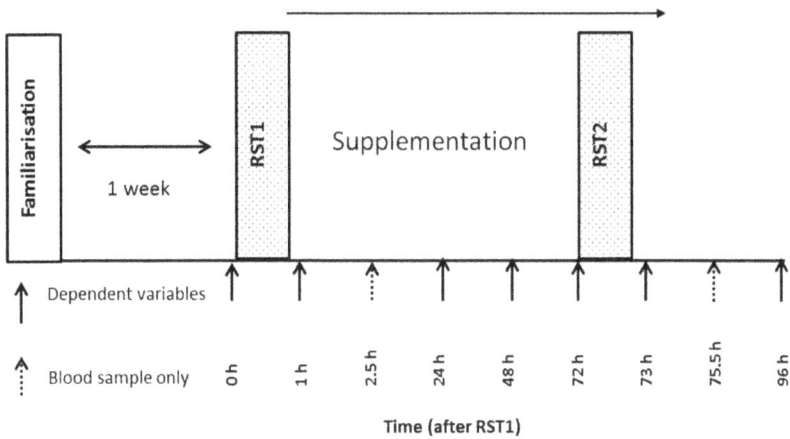

Figure 1. Schematic outline of study procedures.

2.3. Repeated Sprint Test

The RST consisted of 20 maximal-effort 30 m sprints, interspersed by 30 s of passive recovery. A 10 m deceleration zone was marked out at the end of each 30 m sprint, in which participants were required to stop within; the 30 s rest period commenced when participants had come to a halt. The RST was adapted from previous studies that showed repeated sprints with forced decelerations induce substantial muscle damage and fatigue in team-sport trained participants [3,36,37]. Furthermore, the muscle damage induced by an analogous RST seems to cause reductions in muscle function not different to those observed after intermittent sport simulations [38] and competitive matches [39]. Before performing each RST, participants undertook a standardized warm up as previously described [3]. Briefly, participants completed 400 m of self-selected jogging, a series of dynamic stretches, and sprints at 60% and 80% of maximal effort. Participants were then given a further 5 min to complete their own stretching. Timing gates (Brower Timing Systems, Draper, UT, USA) were positioned at 0 and 30 m to record sprint times. Participants were instructed to give maximal-effort for each sprint and were provided with strong verbal encouragement throughout. All testing took place in an air conditioned sprint track in similar environmental conditions.

2.4. Maximal Isometric Voluntary Contractions

MIVC of the right knee extensors was assessed as previously described [3,19]. Participants were seated and fitted to a portable strain gauge (MIE Medical Research Ltd., Leeds, UK) via a plinth placed just above the malleoli of the right ankle. In this positon, joint angle was adjusted to 90° of knee flexion using a goniometer and marked to ensure consistency across visits. Participants performed 3 maximal effort isometric contractions, each lasting 3 s, and separated by 60 s seated rest. The peak value in Newton's (N) was used for analysis. Coefficient of variation (CV) for this protocol in our lab was calculated as 1.1%.

2.5. Counter Movement Jump

CMJ height was determined from flight time using an optical measurement system (Optojump next, Bolzano, Italy). Participants started the movement upright with hands fixed to their hips and after a verbal cue, descended into a squat prior to performing a maximal effort vertical jump. Participants performed 3 maximal efforts, separated by 30 s standing recovery. Mean height (cm) was used for analysis. The CV for this protocol in our lab was calculated as 2.1%.

2.6. Reactive Strength Index

Reactive strength index (RI) was used to measure the impact of muscle damaging exercise on participant's ability to utilize the stretch shortening cycle and perform explosive actions. In a similar fashion to previous studies [40], participants performed a drop jump from a 30 cm box and, upon landing, immediately jumped vertically, with instructions to minimise ground contact time while maximising jump height. RI was calculated as jump height divided by ground contact time (cm/ms) recorded from an optical measurement system (Optojump next). Participants performed 3 maximal efforts separated by 30 s of passive (standing recovery) with the mean height of the 3 jumps used for analysis. The CV for this protocol was calculated as 1.9% in our lab.

2.7. Treatments and Dietary Control

Participants consumed 2 bottles (250 mL per bottle) of their assigned treatment (BTJ or PLA) on the day, 24, and 48 h after RST1 and 30-min post RST2, equating to 8 servings in total. One bottle was consumed 30-min after each trial, and one with an evening meal. The BTJ was supplied by Gs Fresh Ltd., (Cambridgeshire, UK) and consisted of 99% beetroot juice concentrate, nitrate and other phytonutrients; specific details of the antioxidant capacity and phytonutrient content of this drink can be found elsewhere [20]. The PLA consisted of a low fruit containing (<1%) squash (Kia Ora, Coca Cola Enterprises, Uxbridge, UK), flavourless protein powder (Arla Foods, Amba, Denmark) and maltodextrin powder (Myprotein, Manchester, UK) providing a negligible amount of phytochemicals and nitrate. Treatments were closely matched for volume, macro-nutrient and energy content, but differed in antioxidant capacity and nitrate content (see Table 2). Participants were provided with food dairies to record their intake 24 h prior to RST1 up until data collection was complete (24 h post RST2; 5 days in total). Average energy and macronutrient intake for each group is presented in Table 3. To comply with the double-blind, randomized design, drinks were provided in identically masked bottles, only distinguished by a single letter code. These were prepared by an individual not involved in data collection. As detailed in a previous study [19], due to the distinct taste of BTJ, the PLA was not matched for taste and texture, only energy content. While others have used nitrate depleted BTJ as a PLA so that the taste is the same, this is not a true PLA because it will still contain many other bioactive constituents (i.e., phenolics and betalains) that, as outlined in the introduction, could favourably affect recovery. Thus, this would not have been plausible in the present study. Rather, in an attempt to overcome this, the participants were not informed of what the specific drinks being investigated were. The only information they received was that they were antioxidant-containing drinks used for recovery. This ensured that the participants did not know the overall aim of the study, eliminating any bias based on pre-conceptions regarding BTJs potential ergogenic effects. Additionally, because we employed an independent groups design, participants were never aware of the taste/texture of the other treatment under investigation.

Table 2. Energy and macronutrient content, trolox equivalence antioxidant capacity (TEAC) and nitrate content of the beetroot juice (BTJ) and placebo (PLA) supplements.

Treatment	BTJ	PLA
Energy (Kcals)	81	77
Volume (mL)	250	250
Carbohydrate (g)	16.4	16.4
Protein (g)	2.8	2.8
Fat (g)	0.4	Trace
Nitrate (mg)	≥ 143	Trace
TEAC * (mmol·L^{-1})	11.4 ± 0.2	0.25 ± 0.02

* Estimation based on previous analyses [20].

Table 3. Average intake and macro nutrient composition of participants diets (average of 5 days).

	Mean Dietary Intake (5 Days)	
	BTJ	**PLA**
Energy (Kcal)	2554 ± 682	2448 ± 390
Carbohydrates (%)	41 ± 5	43 ± 6
Protein (%)	21 ± 3	24 ± 7
Fat (%)	38 ± 7	33 ± 9

Values are mean ± SD (n = 10 per group). No significant differences were detected between groups for any variable ($p > 0.05$).

2.8. Muscle Soreness

Site specific muscle soreness was assessed with a handheld algometer (Wagner Instruments, Greenwich, CT, USA). A cylindrical flat headed pad (1 cm diameter) was applied with increasing pressure on the muscle belly at three pre-marked sites: vastus lateralis, mid-way between the superior aspect of the greater trochanter and head of the tibia, rectus femoris, mid-way between the anterior patella and inguinal fold, and gastrocnemius, most medial aspect of the calf at relaxed maximum girth. The point at which the participant signified they felt pain was recorded in N^2 as pressure pain threshold (PPT). Sites were re-marked on each visit to ensure consistency between recordings. The average of two values from each site was used for analysis, unless the difference between the two values was >10 N^2 apart, in which case a third recording was taken, and the average of the two closest values used for analysis.

2.9. Blood Sampling

Venous blood was obtained via venepuncture from a branch of the basilica vein at the antecubital fossa. Samples were collected into di-potassium ethylene diamine tetra-acetic acid (EDTA) (1 × 10 mL) and serum vacutainers (1 × 10 mL). EDTA tubes were immediately centrifuged at 3000× g (4°) for 10 min, while serum tubes were allowed to clot for 45 min before centrifugation. Plasma and serum supernatant was aspirated into a series of aliquots and stored at −80 °C for later analysis.

2.10. Biochemical Analysis

High sensitivity C-reactive protein (hs-CRP) and creatine kinase (CK) were measured in serum using an automated system based on an electrochemiluminescence method (Roche Modular, Roche Diagnostics, Indianapolis, IN, USA. The typical CV for this method is <2%. Plasma protein carbonyls were measured using a commercially available assay kit (Cayman Chemical, Ann Arbor, MI, USA). Lipid hyroperoxides (LOOH) were measured in serum using the ferrous iron/xylenol orange (FOX) assay (Wolff 1994). The FOX assay determines the susceptibility to iron-induced LOOH formation in blood; consequently, the presence of iron ions in the assay protocol might lead to slightly higher LOOH values compared with other methods. Absorbance was read at 560 nm using a spectrophotometer (U-2001, Hitachi, Berkshire, UK) (range 0–5 μmol·L^{-1}).

Ascorbyl free radical determination was quantified at room temperature using a Bruker EMX series X-band EPR spectrometer (Bruker, Karlsruhe, Germany). 1 mL of plasma was mixed thoroughly with 1 mL of dimethyl sulfoxide (DMSO) and slowly flushed into an aqua X multiple bore cavity cell. The EMX parameter settings were frequency, 9.785 GHz; microwave power, 20 mW; modulation frequency, 100 kHz and modulation amplitude, 1.194 G. All EPR spectra were subjected to 3 scans identically filtered and analysed using WinEPR software (Version 3.2, Bruker WinEPR, Coventry, UK). The average spectral peak-to-trough line amplitude was used to determine free radical concentration.

2.11. Data Analysis

All data are expressed as mean $\pm$ standard deviation (SD) and were analysed using IBM SPSS Statistics 22 for Windows (Surrey, UK). Participant's food diaries (5 days) were analysed for macronutrient content using dietary analysis software (Nutritics LTD, Dublin, Ireland). Differences between participant group characteristics were analysed with an independent samples *t*-test. CMJ, RI, MIVC and PPT were measured using a mixed model ANOVA; 2 group levels (BTJ vs. PLA) by 7 time levels (pre, post, 24, 48, 72, 73 and 96 h post RST1). The same ANOVA was use to analyse all blood indices but with 2 additional time levels (2.5 h post RST1 and 2.5 h post RS2). A separate ANOVA was used to measure for differences between RST1 and RST2; 2 group levels (BTJ vs. PLA) by 2 time levels (pre and post). In the event of a significant interaction effect (group * time) Fisher LSD *post hoc* analysis was performed to locate where the significant differences occurred. Statistical significance was set at $p < 0.05$ prior to analyses. To estimate the magnitude of the supplements effects, Cohen's *d* effect sizes (ES) were calculated with the magnitude of effects considered either small (0.20–0.49), medium (0.50–0.79) and large (>0.80).

3. Results

There were no between group differences in age, height, mass or baseline MIVC strength (Table 1; $p > 0.05$), indicating that the groups were well matched prior to testing. Furthermore, there were no differences in participant's energy and macronutrient intake 24 h prior to and throughout the duration of the study (Table 3; $p > 0.05$). No adverse effects were reported by the participants throughout the trial.

3.1. Repeated Sprints

RPE showed no bout ($p = 0.925$) or interaction effects ($p = 0.584$) between RST1 and RST2, indicating that perceived exertion was not different for both bouts (Table 4). This was reflected in the sprint data, as fastest sprint time and fatigue index were not different between repeated sprint bouts, showing no main effects of time, bout, or bout * group interactions ($p > 0.05$). No group or group * bout interaction effects were present ($p > 0.05$).

Table 4. Sprint and RPE data for the beetroot juice (BTJ) and placebo (PLA) groups in the first and second repeated sprint tests (RST1 and RST2, respectively).

Group	Average Sprint Time (s)	Fastest Sprint Time (s)	Fatigue Index (%)	RPE
BTJ				
RST1	4.65 ± 0.25	4.41 ± 0.23	5.60 ± 2.13	15 ± 1
RST2	4.66 ± 0.24	4.38 ± 0.17	6.48 ± 2.66	15 ± 1
PLA				
RST1	4.70 ± 0.15	4.48 ± 0.14	4.91 ± 1.51	14 ± 2
RST2	4.77 ± 0.20	4.53 ± 0.15	5.19 ± 3.21	14 ± 2

3.2. Functional Measures

All tests of neuromuscular function (CMJ, MIVC, RI), and PPT, showed main effects for time ($p < 0.05$), indicating that the RST induced muscle damage. Immediately post RST1, CMJ height was reduced by 11.8% $\pm$ 8.9% and 9.6% $\pm$ 4.8% (of baseline values) in the BTJ and PLA groups, respectively. A group effect showed that CMJ height appeared to recover quicker in BTJ vs. PLA throughout the remainder of the testing period ($p = 0.048$; Figure 2). Although no group*time interaction effects were present ($p = 0.176$), there was a large effect size (1.86) at 72 h post RST1 whereby CMJ height in the BTJ group was 7.6% higher than the PLA group. A group effect for RI ($p = 0.030$) showed that the maintenance of RI performance was also greater in BTJ vs. PLA throughout the trial (Figure 3). As with

CMJ, a large effect size (1.43) was evident at 72 h post RST1 where RI had returned to 95.8% ± 9.5% of baseline values in BTJ compared to 82% ± 9.5% in PLA. There were no group effects for PPT (p = 0.368); however, an interaction effect was observed (p = 0.013; Figure 4). *Post-hoc* analysis revealed a group difference at 96 h post RST1 (p = 0.012; ES = 0.57); in the BTJ group, PPT had recovered to 104.7% ± 12.5% of baseline values, while in the PLA group, PPT was 94.3% ± 18% of baseline values. There were no significant group or interaction effects for MIVC (p > 0.05).

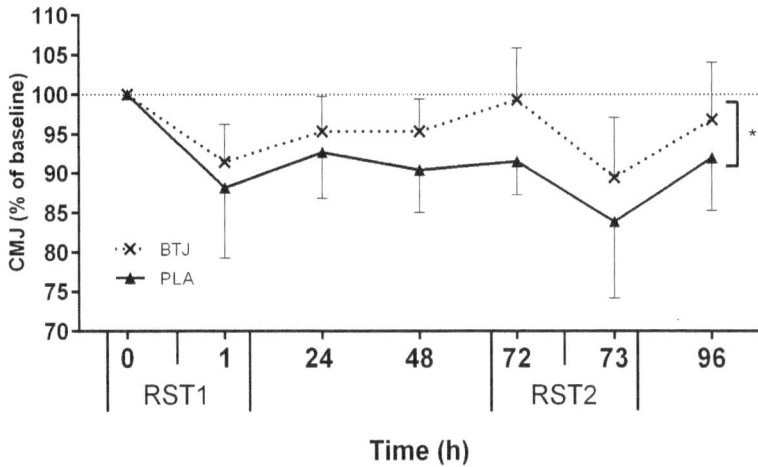

Figure 2. Percentage changes in counter movement jump (CMJ) height between repeated sprint tests (RST1 and RST2). * Represents group difference (beetroot juice (BTJ) vs. placebo (PLA); p < 0.05). Values are mean ± SD (n = 10 per group).

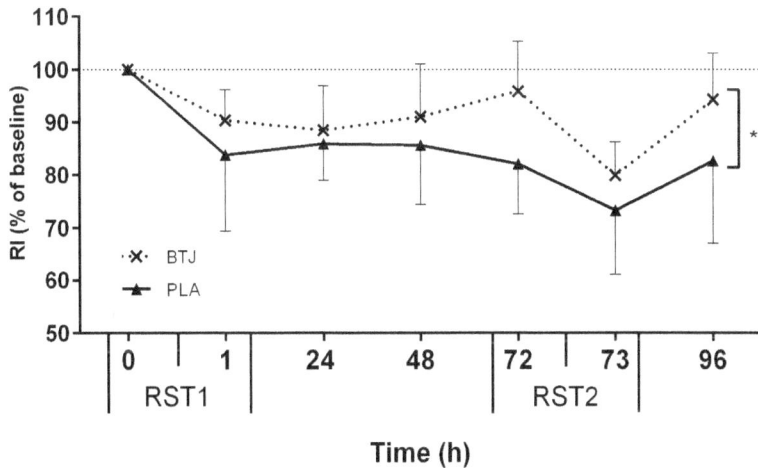

Figure 3. Percentage changes in reactive strength index (RI) between repeated sprint tests (RST1 and RST2). * Represents group difference (beetroot juice (BTJ) vs. placebo (PLA); p < 0.05). Values are mean ± SD (n = 10 per group).

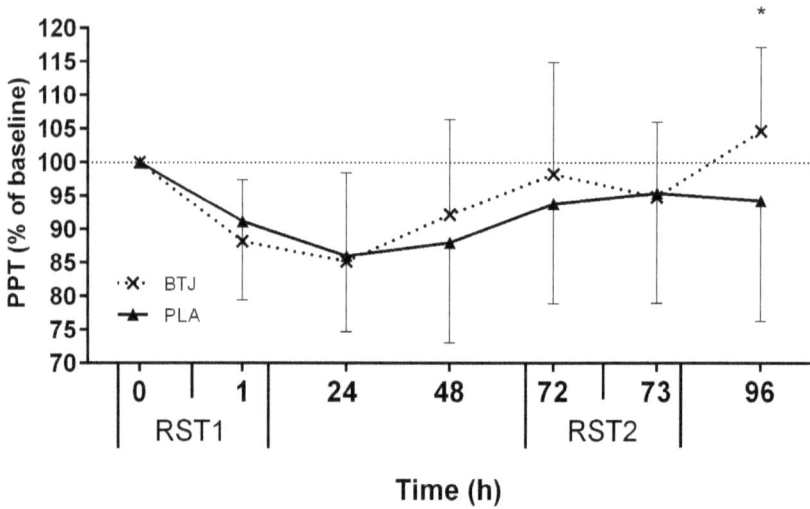

Figure 4. Percentage changes in pressure pain threshold (PPT) between repeated sprint tests (RST1 and RST2). Values presented are average of the three sites measured (calf (CF), rectus femoris (RF) and vastus laterialis (VL). * Indicates interaction effect (beetroot juice (BTJ) vs. placebo (PLA); $p < 0.05$). Values are mean ± SD ($n = 10$ per group).

3.3. Biochemical Indices

Serum concentrations of hs-CRP remained close to baseline values throughout the trial, showing no time, group or interaction effects ($p > 0.05$). Serum CK showed main effects for time ($p < 0.001$), with the greatest increases observed 2.5 and 24 h post RST1 and RST2 in both groups ($p > 0.05$; Table 5). However, no group of interaction effects were observed ($p > 0.05$). A main effect for time was observed for serum LOOH ($p < 0.001$); LOOH was elevated immediately and at 2.5 h post-RST1 in both groups before returning to baseline 24 h post. A transient increase in LOOH was also evident at 75 h (2.5 h post RST2) but by 96 h had recovered to pre-exercise values. No group or interaction effects were present for LOOH ($p > 0.05$). Protein carbonyls, a common measure of protein oxidation, remained largely unchanged after both sprint bouts and showed no group or interaction effects ($p > 0.05$). Likewise, $A^{\bullet-}$, as measured by EPR, showed no time, group or interaction effects throughout the trial ($p > 0.05$).

Table 5. Maximal isometric voluntary contractions (MIVC), high sensitivity-C-reactive protein (hs-CRP), creatine kinase (CK), lipid hydroperoxides (LOOH), protein carbonyls (PC) and plasma ascorbate free radical ($A^{\bullet-}$) for the beetroot juice (BTJ) and placebo (PLA) group's pre-RST1 (0 h)—96 h post.

	0 h	1 h	2.5 h	24 h	48 h	72 h	73 h	75.5 h	96 h
					MIVC (N) *				
BTJ	601 ± 89	554 ± 75		545 ± 92	558 ± 94	579 ± 121	516 ± 101		558 ± 75
PLA	590 ± 123	541 ± 128		535 ± 120	544 ± 130	540 ± 126	509 ± 124		537 ± 122
					hsCRP (mg·L^{-1})				
BTJ	0.6 ± 0.72	0.61 ± 0.75	0.57 ± 0.69	0.64 ± 0.56	0.64 ± 0.58	0.52 ± 0.52	0.52 ± 0.49	0.46 ± 0.50	0.48 ± 0.50
PLA	0.44 ± 0.39	0.45 ± 0.45	0.44 ± 0.42	0.52 ± 0.52	0.4 ± 0.25	0.34 ± 0.21	0.35 ± 0.21	0.38 ± 0.22	0.38 ± 0.24
					CK (IU·L^{-1}) *				
BTJ	188 ± 62	219 ± 68	383 ± 197	542 ± 461	406 ± 252	310 ± 145	349 ± 163	474 ± 246	516 ± 210
PLA	318 ± 145	362 ± 154	518 ± 274	592 ± 321	435 ± 255	387 ± 273	433 ± 290	623 ± 423	749 ± 423
					LOOH (mmol·mL^{-1}) *				
BTJ	1.49 ± 0.25	1.68 ± 0.23	1.69 ± 0.37	1.33 ± 0.36	1.46 ± 0.19	1.47 ± 0.17	1.53 ± 0.40	1.74 ± 0.31	1.44 ± 0.21
PLA	1.53 ± 0.14	1.79 ± 0.23	1.77 ± 0.40	1.54 ± 0.16	1.57 ± 0.14	1.53 ± 0.12	1.69 ± 0.23	1.94 ± 0.75	1.44 ± 0.14
					PC (µmol·L^{-1})				
BTJ	14 ± 6	15 ± 0	15 ± 6	17 ± 5	18 ± 7	14 ± 5	16 ± 5	17 ± 10	15 ± 6
PLA	16 ± 8	19 ± 6	14 ± 6	13 ± 5	14 ± 5	18 ± 9	16 ± 7	15 ± 5	15 ± 4
					$A^{\bullet-}$ (AU)				
BTJ	5567 ± 1898	6111 ± 2145	5883 ± 2044	6247 ± 1846	6202 ± 1911	5809 ± 2238	5752 ± 1854	5422 ± 2002	5862 ± 1802
PLA	6372 ± 1454	6730 ± 1337	6559 ± 2027	5674 ± 1716	5225 ± 1088	6013 ± 671	5433 ± 1521	6354 ± 1315	5819 ± 975

AU = Arbitrary unit; * denotes time effect ($p < 0.05$).

4. Discussion

The main finding of the present study was that beetroot juice, when compared to a placebo, was able to accelerate the recovery of CMJ and RI performance and reduce pain after a muscle-damaging RST, but had no influence on sprint performance. Markers of systemic oxidative stress or other biochemical indices associated with muscle damage were unaffected by beetroot juice supplementation.

In both the BTJ and PLA groups CMJ and RI significantly decreased after RST1, indicating the presence of muscle damage; however, both CMJ and RI recovered quicker with BTJ (vs. PLA) during the following +96 h (Figures 2 and 3, respectively). This was most evident at 72 h after the first sprint bout (RST1), whereby CMJ and RI were still significantly lower than baseline values, but restored close to pre-exercise values in BTJ group. These findings are consistent with our previous work, in which we reported 3 days of BTJ supplementation enhanced the recovery of CMJ performance 72 h after plyometric activity [19].

Interestingly, although BTJ appeared to enhance the recovery of the dynamic muscle function (CMJ and RI), isometric strength (MIVC) was unaffected by BTJ supplementation. As previously suggested [19], perhaps this discrepancy can be explained by the different movement patterns (i.e., static vs. dynamic function) and specific abilities each test measures (power vs. isometric strength). Both CMJ and RI are arguably more ecologically valid tests of functional recovery than MIVC, particularly for team-sports players as their movement patterns more closely reflect the activity required for performance [35]. We initially hypothesized that sprint performance would be reduced in RST2 compared to RST1; a consequence of muscle damage, and that this reduction would be attenuated with BTJ supplementation. However, contrary to our hypothesis, aside from a non-significant decrease in average sprint time (Table 3), sprint performance was largely unaffected in RST2 compared to RST1. The reductions in muscle function were not different ≤24 h after both sprints tests though, suggesting that the participants did not become accustomed to the sprint test after the first bout. Additionally, BTJ had no influence on any aspect of sprint performance, although perhaps our ability to detect any differences between groups was limited by the lack of change in performance between the two sprint tests. Nonetheless, the fact that sprint performance was unchanged seems to contrast with other studies who reported sprint times to still be slower than pre-exercise values up to 72 h after an RST similar to the present study [36,41,42]. Because the muscle-damaging RST was fairly similar between these studies (in fact, the one in the present study was designed to be more challenging), perhaps the divergent findings between these studies and the present one is due, in large part, to the different training status of the participants. The participants in the present study were experienced team-sports players who regularly perform RSE as part of training and matches and, thus, may have been less vulnerable to prolonged decrements in sprint performance than recreationally active participants tested in some of the other studies [41,42].

In addition, the fact that CMJ and RI were still significantly depressed at 72 h post RST1, but sprint performance was not, suggests that there is dissociation between these tests of dynamic muscle function (CMJ and RI) and repeated sprint ability. Indeed, previous literature appears to be equivocal on how well sprint and jump tests correlate. Some studies demonstrate that the time course of recovery for CMJ and sprint performance are not different after muscle-damaging RSE [36,41,42], while others agree with the present study [35,39,43], and have found that reductions in CMJ are more prolonged than sprint decrements. A recent study attempted to address this issue by comparing CMJ, drop jumps (DJ) and a 20 m sprint test after intermittent exercise and concluded that sprint performance seemed to recover more rapidly than both CMJ and DJ performance, both of which were still below pre-exercise values 72 h post-exercise [35]. This led the authors to suggest that CMJ and DJ are more sensitive tests of prolonged changes in neuromuscular function, which could provide and explanation for the dissociation between the jump and sprint tests in the present study.

Due to the fact that oxidative stress has been associated with muscle damage after eccentric-heavy exercise [14,44], and that beetroot and its constituents have been shown to act as antioxidants [25,29], we hypothesized that BTJ could attenuate muscle damage by protecting cells against oxidative stress.

However, our findings do not support this contention. We found no evidence that BTJ attenuated oxidative stress as both indirect markers (LOOH and PC) and a direct marker of free radical production ($A^{\bullet-}$) were not different between the BTJ and PLA groups at all-time points (Table 5). These data are in contrast to a number of previous studies that found antioxidant-rich food supplements reduced oxidative stress after high intensity sprint exercise [14,45,46]. However, unlike these studies, we did not find any evidence of oxidative stress throughout the trial, apart from an increase in LOOH immediately post and 2.5 h post both sprint tests (Table 5). The modest increase in these markers was unexpected, as previous studies reported large systemic elevations in oxidative stress up to 48 h after high intensity intermittent cycling exercise [2,14] an activity which, in comparison to running, typically results in less oxidative stress because of the absence of an extensive eccentric component [34]. The divergent findings in oxidative stress response between the present and aforementioned studies could, therefore, be explained by the different biochemical markers examined and/or analytical techniques used. Jowko and colleagues [14] for instance, noted systemic increases in total antioxidant capacity (TAC), superoxide dismutase and glutathione peroxidase (GPX) 24 h after exercise and Bogdanis and colleagues [2] noted increases in TAC, PC and GPX; thus, neither study measured LOOH or $A^{\bullet-}$ formation, as in the present study. Although this study and [2] both measured PC, different analytical methods were used, which could account for the discrepant results. Nonetheless, EPR spectroscopy is considered a valid and sensitive method for direct detection of excessive free radical production [47,48], and the fact that we found no evidence of an increase in our data perhaps draws into question the reliability of the indirect biomarkers in other studies using a similar protocol.

The fact that muscle damage was clearly evident in the days after both RST tests but oxidative stress was not, suggests that muscle damage occurred independent of any systemic changes in oxidative stress. This would perhaps suggest that ROS have a limited role in the muscle damage process post-exercise. However, it cannot be ruled out that oxidative stress occurred, but was confined predominately to muscle cells and surrounding tissues. Unfortunately, we did not measure muscle samples in our study, and as such, this supposition is speculative. A recent review however, concluded that skeletal muscle is a prime producer of ROS following exercise; so, intuitively, oxidative stress would be expected to be greater in muscle than perhaps the circulation [49]. We recognize that the inability to obtain muscle biopsy samples for oxidative stress measures could be considered a limitation of this study. Alternatively, the muscle damage we observed could have been unrelated to oxidative stress. Instead, the muscle damage could have been caused by other biochemical changes within muscle, such as increased inflammation and calpain activity [50,51] or damage to components involved in the excitation-contraction coupling pathway, as previously suggested [52].

Serum CK concentrations, incorporated as a surrogate marker of sarcolemma damage, were not different in both groups after exercise (Table 5). The increase in CK after the RST was similar to previous reports [3,42], as was the lack of a suppressive effect with an antioxidant-rich food beverage [19,23,45]. These data suggest that improved sarcolemma integrity cannot explain the enhanced rate of recovery by BTJ in this study.

Because we found no changes in oxidative stress between groups, the beneficial effects of BTJ on the recovery of CMJ and RI cannot be attributed to an antioxidant effect of the juice. This suggests that mechanisms other than antioxidant effects were possibly involved. It was beyond the scope of this study to examine the role of other mechanisms by which BTJ could attenuate muscle damage, but owing to the seemingly pleotropic nature of phenolic and betalainic compounds and NO, there are a number of possible candidates. For instance, other effects associated with phenolic compounds and NO donors akin to BTJ are anti-inflammatory [25,33] and regenerative, in so far as they appear to have a regulatory role in phagocytosis and promote satellite cell proliferation in skeletal muscle [53–55]. Increasing in vivo NO availability has also demonstrated additional biochemical effects that, conceivably, could contribute to improved functional recovery after exercise, such as reduced calpain activity [56], increased muscle blood flow [57,58], and enhanced muscle power potential,

Nutrients **2016**, *8*, 506

possibly via improved Ca^{2+} handing [59,60]. Thus, there are a number of potential mechanisms that could explain why BTJ supplementation was able to enhance the recovery of muscle function, independent of antioxidant effects. However, since none of these mechanisms were measured *per se*, we can only speculate the role, if any, that they may have had in the present study's findings. The potential role and their relative contributory effects require further exploration.

Participants in the BTJ group reported a significantly higher PPT than the PLA group 24 h after the second sprint test (Figure 4). Reduced muscle pain when antioxidant-rich food supplements are taken after muscle-damaging exercise has been reported by our group [19] and others [61]. The mechanism by which BTJ might attenuate muscle pain is unclear however. Previous reports suggest that the betalains in beetroot are responsible for its analgesic effects, most likely via an anti-inflammatory related mechanism [26,62]. The possibility that an anti-inflammatory mechanism would be involved is supported by data that suggests muscle pain after exercise may stem from the release of inflammatory and noxious stimuli (i.e., bradykin and nerve growth factor) due to tears at the extracellular matrix [63,64]. Perhaps BTJ acts to dampen inflammatory responses or desensitize pain receptors, as has been suggested with ginger [65] and curcumin supplements [66]; however, whatever the precise mechanisms, they are likely to occur at the skeletal muscle level.

It is also unclear why BTJ only improved PPT 24 h after RST2 in the present study and not at earlier time points, as was shown in our earlier work [19]. A previous study did observe greater reductions in pain scores after participants took betalain-rich beetroot supplements for 5–10 days compared to 1 day [26], which, coupled with our data, suggests that the analgesic effects of BTJ might be augmented with longer-term dosage regimens. Such a possibility needs to be investigated in future studies.

In conclusion, this study demonstrates that consuming BTJ for 4 days after a muscle damaging RST attenuated muscle pain and decrements in dynamic muscle function, as measured by CMJ and RI. These effects did not translate to improved recovery of isometric strength or sprint performance however. These data suggest BTJ could be applied as a post-exercise recovery strategy to attenuate losses in some aspects of dynamic muscle function in team-sports players between bouts of repeated sprint exercise; however, because sprint performance was unchanged, how transferable these findings are to real-world team-sport competition is unclear. Future studies are needed to clarify the underlying cellular mechanisms, as the beneficial effects of BTJ were shown to be unrelated to systemic changes in oxidative stress or other biochemical markers of muscle damage.

Acknowledgments: The authors wish to thank all the participants for their hard work and commitment displayed throughout testing.

Author Contributions: T.C., G.H., D.J.W., E.J.S. conceived and designed the experiments; T.C. and B.B. performed the experiments; T.C. and B.B. analyzed the data; G.W.D. performed biochemical analysis; T.C., G.H., D.J.W., E.J.S., G.W.D. wrote the paper.

Conflicts of Interest: This study was funded as part of a doctoral degree that receives financial support from Gs Fresh Ltd. The funders supplied the supplements used in this study but had no role in the conception of the study, its design, preparation, analysis and writing of the manuscript. The authors declare no conflict of interest.

References

1. Girard, O.; Mendez-Villanueva, A.; Bishop, D. Repeated-sprint ability—Part I: Factors contributing to fatigue. *Sports Med.* **2011**, *41*, 673–694. [CrossRef] [PubMed]
2. Bogdanis, G.C.; Stavrinou, P.; Fatouros, I.G.; Philippou, A.; Chatzinikolaou, A.; Draganidis, D.; Ermidis, G.; Maridaki, M. Short-term high-intensity interval exercise training attenuates oxidative stress responses and improves antioxidant status in healthy humans. *Food Chem. Toxicol.* **2013**, *61*, 171–177. [CrossRef] [PubMed]
3. Howatson, G.; Milak, A. Exercise-induced muscle damage following a bout of sport specific repeated sprints. *J. Strength Cond. Res.* **2009**, *23*, 2419–2424. [CrossRef] [PubMed]
4. Duffield, R.; Cannon, J.; King, M. The effects of compression garments on recovery of muscle performance following high-intensity sprint and plyometric exercise. *J. Sci. Med. Sport* **2010**, *13*, 136–140. [CrossRef] [PubMed]

5. Howatson, G.; van Someren, K.A. The prevention and treatment of exercise-induced muscle damage. *Sports Med.* **2008**, *38*, 483–503. [CrossRef] [PubMed]
6. Mohr, M.; Draganidis, D.; Chatzinikolaou, A.; Barbero-Alvarez, J.C.; Castagna, C.; Douroudos, I.; Avloniti, A.; Margeli, A.; Papassotiriou, I.; Flouris, A.D.; et al. Muscle damage, inflammatory, immune and performance responses to three football games in 1 week in competitive male players. *Eur. J. Appl. Physiol.* **2016**, *116*, 179–193. [CrossRef] [PubMed]
7. Barnett, A. Using recovery modalities between training sessions in elite athletes—Does it help? *Sports Med.* **2006**, *36*, 781–796. [CrossRef] [PubMed]
8. Nedelec, M.; McCall, A.; Carling, C.; Legall, F.; Berthoin, S.; Dupont, G. Recovery in soccer: Part II—Ecovery strategies. *Sports Med.* **2013**, *43*, 9–22. [CrossRef] [PubMed]
9. Clarkson, P.M.; Hubal, M.J. Exercise-induced muscle damage in humans. *Am. J. Phys. Med. Rehabil.* **2002**, *81*, S52–S69. [CrossRef] [PubMed]
10. Hyldahl, R.D.; Hubal, M.J. Lengthening our perspective: Morphological, cellular, and molecular responses to eccentric exercise. *Muscle Nerve* **2014**, *49*, 155–170. [CrossRef] [PubMed]
11. Brickson, S.; Ji, L.L.; Schell, K.; Olabisi, R.; St Pierre Schneider, B.; Best, T.M. M1/70 attenuates blood-borne neutrophil oxidants, activation, and myofiber damage following stretch injury. *J. Appl. Physiol.* **2003**, *95*, 969–976. [CrossRef] [PubMed]
12. Pizza, F.X.; Peterson, J.M.; Baas, J.H.; Koh, T.J. Neutrophils contribute to muscle injury and impair its resolution after lengthening contractions in mice. *J. Physiol.* **2005**, *562*, 899–913. [CrossRef] [PubMed]
13. Toumi, H.; Best, T.M. The inflammatory response: Friend or enemy for muscle injury? *Br. J. Sports Med.* **2003**, *37*, 284–286. [CrossRef] [PubMed]
14. Jowko, E.; Dlugolecka, B.; Makaruk, B.; Cieslinski, I. The effect of green tea extract supplementation on exercise-induced oxidative stress parameters in male sprinters. *Eur. J. Nutr.* **2015**, *54*, 783–791. [CrossRef] [PubMed]
15. Bailey, D.M.; Williams, C.; Betts, J.A.; Thompson, D.; Hurst, T.L. Oxidative stress, inflammation and recovery of muscle function after damaging exercise: Effect of 6-week mixed antioxidant supplementation. *Eur. J. Appl. Physiol.* **2011**, *111*, 925–936. [CrossRef] [PubMed]
16. Nikolaidis, M.G.; Kerksick, C.M.; Lamprecht, M.; McAnulty, S.R. Does vitamin C and E supplementation impair the favorable adaptations of regular exercise? *Oxid. Med. Cell. Longev.* **2012**, *2012*, 707941. [CrossRef] [PubMed]
17. Close, G.L.; Ashton, T.; Cable, T.; Doran, D.; Holloway, C.; McArdle, F.; MacLaren, D.P. Ascorbic acid supplementation does not attenuate post-exercise muscle soreness following muscle-damaging exercise but may delay the recovery process. *Br. J. Nutr.* **2006**, *95*, 976–981. [CrossRef] [PubMed]
18. Sousa, M.; Teixeira, V.H.; Soares, J. Dietary strategies to recover from exercise-induced muscle damage. *Int. J. Food Sci. Nutr.* **2014**, *65*, 151–163. [CrossRef] [PubMed]
19. Clifford, T.; Bell, O.; West, D.J.; Howatson, G.; Stevenson, E.J. The effects of beetroot juice supplementation on indices of muscle damage following eccentric exercise. *Eur. J. Appl. Physiol.* **2016**, *116*, 353–362. [CrossRef] [PubMed]
20. Clifford, T.; Constantinou, C.M.; Keane, K.M.; West, D.J.; Howatson, G.; Stevenson, E.J. The plasma bioavailability of nitrate and betanin from beta vulgaris rubra in humans. *Eur. J. Nutr.* **2016**. [CrossRef] [PubMed]
21. Wootton-Beard, P.C.; Moran, A.; Ryan, L. Stability of the total antioxidant capacity and total polyphenol content of 23 commercially available vegetable juices before and after in vitro digestion measured by frap, dpph, abts and folin–ciocalteu methods. *Food Res. Int.* **2011**, *44*, 217–224. [CrossRef]
22. Ryan, L.; Prescott, S.L. Stability of the antioxidant capacity of twenty-five commercially available fruit juices subjected to an in vitro digestion. *Int. J. Food Sci. Technol.* **2010**, *45*, 1191–1197. [CrossRef]
23. Howatson, G.; McHugh, M.P.; Hill, J.A.; Brouner, J.; Jewell, A.P.; van Someren, K.A.; Shave, R.E.; Howatson, S.A. Influence of tart cherry juice on indices of recovery following marathon running. *Scand. J. Med. Sci. Sports* **2010**, *20*, 843–852. [CrossRef] [PubMed]
24. Seeram, N.P.; Aviram, M.; Zhang, Y.; Henning, S.M.; Feng, L.; Dreher, M.; Heber, D. Comparison of antioxidant potency of commonly consumed polyphenol-rich beverages in the United States. *J. Agric. Food Chem.* **2008**, *56*, 1415–1422. [CrossRef] [PubMed]

25. El Gamal, A.A.; AlSaid, M.S.; Raish, M.; Al-Sohaibani, M.; Al-Massarani, S.M.; Ahmad, A.; Hefnawy, M.; Al-Yahya, M.; Basoudan, O.A.; Rafatullah, S. Beetroot (*Beta vulgaris* L.) extract ameliorates Gentamicin-induced nephrotoxicity associated oxidative stress, inflammation, and apoptosis in rodent model. *Mediat. Inflamm.* **2014**, *2014*, 983952. [CrossRef] [PubMed]
26. Pietrzkowski, Z.; Nemzer, B.; Spórna, A.; Stalica, P.; Tresher, W.; Keller, R.; Jimenez, R.; Michałowski, T.; Wybraniec, S. Influence of betalain-rich extract on reduction of discomfort associated with osteoarthritis. *New Med.* **2010**, *1*, 12–17.
27. Vulic, J.J.; Cebovic, T.N.; Canadanovic, V.M.; Cetkovic, G.S.; Djilas, S.M.; Canadanovic-Brunet, J.M.; Velicanski, A.S.; Cvetkovic, D.D.; Tumbas, V.T. Antiradical, antimicrobial and cytotoxic activities of commercial beetroot pomace. *Food Funct.* **2013**, *4*, 713–721. [CrossRef] [PubMed]
28. Wootton-Beard, P.C.; Ryan, L. A beetroot juice shot is a significant and convenient source of bioaccessible antioxidants. *J. Funct. Foods* **2011**, *3*, 329–334. [CrossRef]
29. Esatbeyoglu, T.; Wagner, A.E.; Motafakkerazad, R.; Nakajima, Y.; Matsugo, S.; Rimbach, G. Free radical scavenging and antioxidant activity of betanin: Electron spin resonance spectroscopy studies and studies in cultured cells. *Food Chem. Toxicol.* **2014**, *73*, 119–126. [CrossRef] [PubMed]
30. Esatbeyoglu, T.; Wagner, A.E.; Schini-Kerth, V.B.; Rimbach, G. Betanin-a food colorant with biological activity. *Mol. Nutr. Food Res.* **2015**, *59*, 36–47. [CrossRef] [PubMed]
31. Krajka-Kuzniak, V.; Paluszczak, J.; Szaefer, H.; Baer-Dubowska, W. Betanin, a beetroot component, induces nuclear factor erythroid-2-related factor 2-mediated expression of detoxifying/antioxidant enzymes in human liver cell lines. *Br. J. Nutr.* **2013**, *110*, 2138–2149. [CrossRef] [PubMed]
32. Szaefer, H.; Krajka-Kuzniak, V.; Ignatowicz, E.; Adamska, T.; Baer-Dubowska, W. Evaluation of the effect of beetroot juice on DMBA-induced damage in liver and mammary gland of female sprague-dawley rats. *Phytother. Res.* **2014**, *28*, 55–61. [CrossRef] [PubMed]
33. Jadert, C.; Petersson, J.; Massena, S.; Ahl, D.; Grapensparr, L.; Holm, L.; Lundberg, J.O.; Phillipson, M. Decreased leukocyte recruitment by inorganic nitrate and nitrite in microvascular inflammation and nsaid-induced intestinal injury. *Free Radic. Biol. Med.* **2012**, *52*, 683–692. [CrossRef] [PubMed]
34. Nikolaidis, M.G.; Jamurtas, A.Z.; Paschalis, V.; Fatouros, I.G.; Koutedakis, Y.; Kouretas, D. The effect of muscle-damaging exercise on blood and skeletal muscle oxidative stress: Magnitude and time-course considerations. *Sports Med.* **2008**, *38*, 579–606. [CrossRef] [PubMed]
35. Gathercole, R.J.; Sporer, B.C.; Stellingwerff, T.; Sleivert, G.G. Comparison of the capacity of different jump and sprint field tests to detect neuromuscular fatigue. *J. Strength Cond. Res.* **2015**, *29*, 2522–2531. [CrossRef] [PubMed]
36. Keane, K.M.; Salicki, R.; Goodall, S.; Thomas, K.; Howatson, G. Muscle damage response in female collegiate athletes after repeated sprint activity. *J. Strength Cond. Res.* **2015**, *29*, 2802–2807. [CrossRef] [PubMed]
37. Lakomy, J.; Haydon, D.T. The effects of enforced, rapid deceleration on performance in a multiple sprint test. *J. Strength Cond. Res.* **2004**, *18*, 579–583. [CrossRef] [PubMed]
38. Thompson, D.; Nicholas, C.W.; Williams, C. Muscular soreness following prolonged intermittent high-intensity shuttle running. *J. Sports Sci.* **1999**, *17*, 387–395. [CrossRef] [PubMed]
39. Andersson, H.; Raastad, T.; Nilsson, J.; Paulsen, G.; Garthe, I.; Kadi, F. Neuromuscular fatigue and recovery in elite female soccer: Effects of active recovery. *Med. Sci. Sports Exerc.* **2008**, *40*, 372–380. [CrossRef] [PubMed]
40. Cockburn, E.; Robson-Ansley, P.; Hayes, P.R.; Stevenson, E. Effect of volume of milk consumed on the attenuation of exercise-induced muscle damage. *Eur. J. Appl. Physiol.* **2012**, *112*, 3187–3194. [CrossRef] [PubMed]
41. Brown, M.A.; Howatson, G.; Keane, K.; Stevenson, E.J. Exercise-induced muscle damage following dance and sprint specific exercise in females. *J. Sports Med. Phys. Fit.* **2015**, in press.
42. Woolley, B.P.; Jakeman, J.R.; Faulkner, J.A. Multiple sprint exercise with a short deceleration induces muscle damage and performance impairment in young, physically active males. *J. Athl. Enhanc.* **2014**, *3*. [CrossRef]
43. Semark, A.; Noakes, T.D.; St Clair Gibson, A.; Lambert, M.I. The effect of a prophylactic dose of flurbiprofen on muscle soreness and sprinting performance in trained subjects. *J. Sports Sci.* **1999**, *17*, 197–203. [CrossRef] [PubMed]

44. Close, G.L.; Ashton, T.; Cable, T.; Doran, D.; MacLaren, D.P. Eccentric exercise, isokinetic muscle torque and delayed onset muscle soreness: The role of reactive oxygen species. *Eur. J. Appl. Physiol.* **2004**, *91*, 615–621. [CrossRef] [PubMed]

45. Bell, P.G.; Walshe, I.H.; Davison, G.W.; Stevenson, E.; Howatson, G. Montmorency cherries reduce the oxidative stress and inflammatory responses to repeated days high-intensity stochastic cycling. *Nutrients* **2014**, *6*, 829–843. [CrossRef] [PubMed]

46. Goldfarb, A.H.; Garten, R.S.; Cho, C.; Chee, P.D.; Chambers, L.A. Effects of a fruit/berry/vegetable supplement on muscle function and oxidative stress. *Med. Sci. Sports Exerc.* **2011**, *43*, 501–508. [CrossRef] [PubMed]

47. Buettner, G.R.; Jurkiewicz, B.A. Ascorbate free-radical as a marker of oxidative stress—An EPR study. *Free Radic. Biol. Med.* **1993**, *14*, 49–55. [CrossRef]

48. Pietri, S.; Seguin, J.R.; Darbigny, P.; Culcasi, M. Ascorbyl free-radical—A noninvasive marker of oxidative stress in human open-heart-surgery. *Free Radic. Biol. Med.* **1994**, *16*, 523–528. [CrossRef]

49. Jackson, M.J.; Vasilaki, A.; McArdle, A. Cellular mechanisms underlying oxidative stress in human exercise. *Free Radic. Biol. Med.* **2016**, *98*, 13–17. [CrossRef] [PubMed]

50. Belcastro, A.N.; Shewchuk, L.D.; Raj, D.A. Exercise-induced muscle injury: A calpain hypothesis. *Mol. Cell. Biochem.* **1998**, *179*, 135–145. [CrossRef] [PubMed]

51. Paulsen, G.R.; Benestad, H.B.; Strom-Gundersen, I.; Morkrid, L.; Lappegard, K.T.; Raastad, T. Delayed leukocytosis and cytokine response to high-force eccentric exercise. *Med. Sci. Sports Exerc.* **2005**, *37*, 1877–1883. [CrossRef] [PubMed]

52. Warren, G.L.; Ingalls, C.P.; Lowe, D.A.; Armstrong, R.B. What mechanisms contribute to the strength loss that occurs during and in the recovery from skeletal muscle injury? *J. Orthop. Sports Phys. Ther.* **2002**, *32*, 58–64. [CrossRef] [PubMed]

53. Rigamonti, E.; Touvier, T.; Clementi, E.; Manfredi, A.A.; Brunelli, S.; Rovere-Querini, P. Requirement of inducible nitric oxide synthase for skeletal muscle regeneration after acute damage. *J. Immunol.* **2013**, *190*, 1767–1777. [CrossRef] [PubMed]

54. Sakurai, T.; Kashimura, O.; Kano, Y.; Ohno, H.; Ji, L.L.; Izawa, T.; Best, T.M. Role of nitric oxide in muscle regeneration following eccentric muscle contractions in rat skeletal muscle. *J. Physiol. Sci.* **2013**, *63*, 263–270. [CrossRef] [PubMed]

55. Kruger, M.J.; Smith, C. Postcontusion polyphenol treatment alters inflammation and muscle regeneration. *Med. Sci. Sports Exerc.* **2012**, *44*, 872–880. [CrossRef] [PubMed]

56. Lomonosova, Y.N.; Shenkman, B.S.; Kalamkarov, G.R.; Kostrominova, T.Y.; Nemirovskaya, T.L. L-arginine supplementation protects exercise performance and structural integrity of muscle fibers after a single bout of eccentric exercise in rats. *PLoS ONE* **2014**, *9*, e94448. [CrossRef] [PubMed]

57. Ferguson, S.K.; Holdsworth, C.T.; Wright, J.L.; Fees, A.J.; Allen, J.D.; Jones, A.M.; Musch, T.I.; Poole, D.C. Microvascular oxygen pressures in muscles comprised of different fiber types: Impact of dietary nitrate supplementation. *Nitric Oxide* **2015**, *48*, 38–43. [CrossRef] [PubMed]

58. Ferguson, S.K.; Hirai, D.M.; Copp, S.W.; Holdsworth, C.T.; Allen, J.D.; Jones, A.M.; Musch, T.I.; Poole, D.C. Effects of nitrate supplementation via beetroot juice on contracting rat skeletal muscle microvascular oxygen pressure dynamics. *Respir. Physiol. Neurobiol.* **2013**, *187*, 250–255. [CrossRef] [PubMed]

59. Hernandez, A.; Schiffer, T.A.; Ivarsson, N.; Cheng, A.J.; Bruton, J.D.; Lundberg, J.O.; Weitzberg, E.; Westerblad, H. Dietary nitrate increases tetanic $[ca^{2+}]_i$ and contractile force in mouse fast-twitch muscle. *J. Physiol.* **2012**, *590*, 3575–3583. [CrossRef] [PubMed]

60. Coggan, A.R.; Leibowitz, J.L.; Kadkhodayan, A.; Thomas, D.P.; Ramamurthy, S.; Spearie, C.A.; Waller, S.; Farmer, M.; Peterson, L.R. Effect of acute dietary nitrate intake on maximal knee extensor speed and power in healthy men and women. *Nitric Oxide* **2015**, *48*, 16–21. [CrossRef] [PubMed]

61. Connolly, D.A.; McHugh, M.P.; Padilla-Zakour, O.I.; Carlson, L.; Sayers, S.P. Efficacy of a tart cherry juice blend in preventing the symptoms of muscle damage. *Br. J. Sports Med.* **2006**, *40*, 679–683. [CrossRef] [PubMed]

62. Reyes-Izquierdo, T.; Pietrzkowski, Z.; Argumedo, R.; Shu, C.; Nemzer, B.; Wybraniec, S. Betalain-rich red beet concentrate improves reduced knee discomfort and joint function: A double blind, placebo-controlled pilot clinical study. *Nutr. Diet. Suppl.* **2014**, *2014*, 9–10. [CrossRef]

63. Crameri, R.M.; Aagaard, P.; Qvortrup, K.; Langberg, H.; Olesen, J.; Kjaer, M. Myofibre damage in human skeletal muscle: Effects of electrical stimulation versus voluntary contraction. *J. Physiol.* **2007**, *583*, 365–380. [CrossRef] [PubMed]

64. Murase, S.; Terazawa, E.; Queme, F.; Ota, H.; Matsuda, T.; Hirate, K.; Kozaki, Y.; Katanosaka, K.; Taguchi, T.; Urai, H.; et al. Bradykinin and nerve growth factor play pivotal roles in muscular mechanical hyperalgesia after exercise (delayed-onset muscle soreness). *J. Neurosci.* **2010**, *30*, 3752–3761. [CrossRef] [PubMed]

65. Wilson, P.B. Ginger (zingiber officinale) as an analgesic and ergogenic aid in sport: A systemic review. *J. Strength Cond. Res.* **2015**, *29*, 2980–2995. [CrossRef] [PubMed]

66. Drobnic, F.; Riera, J.; Appendino, G.; Togni, S.; Franceschi, F.; Valle, X.; Pons, A.; Tur, J. Reduction of delayed onset muscle soreness by a novel curcumin delivery system (meriva®): A randomised, placebo-controlled trial. *J. Int. Soc. Sports Nutr.* **2014**, *11*, 31. [CrossRef] [PubMed]

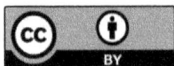

nutrients

MDPI

Article

Comparison of Watermelon and Carbohydrate Beverage on Exercise-Induced Alterations in Systemic Inflammation, Immune Dysfunction, and Plasma Antioxidant Capacity

R. Andrew Shanely [1,2,*], David C. Nieman [1,2], Penelope Perkins-Veazie [3], Dru A. Henson [4], Mary P. Meaney [1,2], Amy M. Knab [5] and Lynn Cialdell-Kam [6]

1   Human Performance Laboratory, Appalachian State University, North Carolina Research Campus, Kannapolis, NC 28081, USA; niemandc@appstate.edu (D.C.N.); meaneymp@appstate.edu (M.P.M.)
2   Department of Health and Exercise Science, Appalachian State University, Boone, NC 28608, USA
3   Plants for Human Health Institute, North Carolina State University, Department of Horticulture Science, North Carolina Research Campus, 600 Laureate Way, Kannapolis, NC 28081, USA; penelope_perkins@ncsu.edu
4   Department of Biology, Appalachian State University, Boone, NC 28608, USA; hensonda@appstate.edu
5   Kinesiology Department, Queens University of Charlotte, Charlotte, NC 28274, USA; knaba@queens.edu
6   Department of Nutrition, Case Western Reserve University, Cleveland, OH 44106, USA; lak99@case.edu
*   Correspondence: shanelyra@appstate.edu; Tel.: +1-828-262-6339

Received: 8 July 2016; Accepted: 18 August 2016; Published: 22 August 2016

Abstract: Consuming carbohydrate- and antioxidant-rich fruits during exercise as a means of supporting and enhancing both performance and health is of interest to endurance athletes. Watermelon (WM) contains carbohydrate, lycopene, L-citrulline, and L-arginine. WM may support exercise performance, augment antioxidant capacity, and act as a countermeasure to exercise-induced inflammation and innate immune changes. Trained cyclists ($n = 20$, 48 ± 2 years) participated in a randomized, placebo controlled, crossover study. Subjects completed two 75 km cycling time trials after either 2 weeks ingestion of 980 mL/day WM puree or no treatment. Subjects drank either WM puree containing 0.2 gm/kg carbohydrate or a 6% carbohydrate beverage every 15 min during the time trials. Blood samples were taken pre-study and pre-, post-, 1 h post-exercise. WM ingestion versus no treatment for 2-weeks increased plasma L-citrulline and L-arginine concentrations ($p < 0.0125$). Exercise performance did not differ between WM puree or carbohydrate beverage trials ($p > 0.05$), however, the rating of perceived exertion was greater during the WM trial ($p > 0.05$). WM puree versus carbohydrate beverage resulted in a similar pattern of increase in blood glucose, and greater increases in post-exercise plasma antioxidant capacity, L-citrulline, L-arginine, and total nitrate (all $p < 0.05$), but without differences in systemic markers of inflammation or innate immune function. Daily WM puree consumption fully supported the energy demands of exercise, and increased post-exercise blood levels of WM nutritional components (L-citrulline and L-arginine), antioxidant capacity, and total nitrate, but without an influence on post-exercise inflammation and changes in innate immune function.

Keywords: endurance exercise performance; L-citrulline; L-arginine; total nitrate; ferric reducing ability of plasma (FRAP); oxygen radical absorbance capacity (ORAC)

1. Introduction

The importance of ingesting carbohydrate to maintain blood glucose levels during prolonged, vigorous exercise was recognized at the Boston Marathon in the early 1920s [1,2]. Carbohydrate intake improves endurance performance 2%–6%, lowers perceived exertion, and attenuates post-exercise inflammation 25%–40% [3–6]. The consumption of multiple transportable carbohydrates (e.g., a mixture of glucose and fructose) during exercise improves the rate of carbohydrate oxidation [7], due to absorption of the carbohydrates by multiple transporters including the sodium-glucose transporter 1 (SGLT1), the universal glucose and fructose transporter (GLUT2), and the fructose transporter (GLUT5) [8]. Data support the use of solutions with a fructose:glucose ratio of 0.8:1 and a consumption rate up to 1.7 g/min [9] to support performance.

Consumption of fruit and fruit juice during endurance exercise as a means of sustaining performance and health is of interest to those desiring natural sources of exogenous carbohydrate. Use of raisins (fructose:glucose ratio of 1.1:1) as the carbohydrate source before and during exercise produced greater rates of carbohydrate oxidation and performance compared to water only [10]. Consuming bananas (fructose:glucose ratio of 1:1) maintained blood glucose during endurance exercise and significantly increased time to exhaustion compared to placebo [11]. Recently, we demonstrated that consuming bananas during a simulated mountainous 75 km cycling time trial resulted in equal performance, maintenance of blood glucose levels, elevated antioxidant capacity, and similar post-exercise inflammation compared to a standard 6% carbohydrate sports drink [12]. These findings were confirmed and extended in a comparison of banana or pear (fructose:glucose ratio of 1:0.44) consumption versus water only during a cycling time trial [13]. Pear consumption during exercise supported performance nearly as well as banana consumption, and both carbohydrate sources resulted in higher blood glucose and carbohydrate oxidation rates, elevated antioxidant capacity, and attenuated post-exercise inflammation compared to water [13]. These data indicate that fruit consumption supports the carbohydrate requirements of prolonged vigorous endurance exercise with the added advantage of augmenting antioxidant capacity.

Watermelon (*Citrullus lanatus*) is a member of the Cucurbitaceae family of gourds and is related to the cucumber, squash, and pumpkin. Watermelon flesh (WM) is ~91% water by weight, and is a rich source of bioavailable compounds including lycopene and other carotenoids, vitamins A and C, and the non-essential amino acid L-citrulline, and is about 6% sugar by weight (fructose:glucose ratio of 1:0.55) [14,15].

Carotenoids are natural fat-soluble compounds that exert antioxidant, anti-inflammatory, and anti-carcinogenic effects [16,17]. Lycopene is the pigment principally responsible for the characteristic deep-red color of watermelon (4532 µg/100 g), and is a highly efficient singlet oxygen quencher [18]. American adults consume 4.5–6.5 mg/day lycopene, of which approximately one-fourth is absorbed in the small intestine, achieving a maximal plasma concentration after about two days with a half-life of nine days [19]. Limited human evidence suggest that lycopene-rich tomato extracts may counter inflammation and oxidative stress following short-term, intensive exercise [20,21].

The amino acid L-citrulline is an endogenous precursor of L-arginine, and nearly all dietary L-citrulline is converted into L-arginine in animals [22]. Nitric oxide (NO) is synthesized from L-arginine by tetrahydrobiopterin (BH4)-dependent NO synthase [22] and L-citrulline supplementation increases NO synthesis [23]. NO increases glucose transporter type 4 (GLUT4) translocation and thus glucose flux, which may enhance performance [24]. Acute WM consumption significantly increases L-citrulline and L-arginine plasma levels [25] and chronic WM consumption significantly increases fasting L-arginine plasma levels, but not L-citrulline [26]. The degree to which WM supplementation increases NO levels before and after exercise is currently unknown. Increased fruit ingestion has been linked in several studies to increased antioxidant capacity [27]. Watermelon contains the antioxidants L-citrulline, lycopene, β-carotene, and vitamin C [18,28–31], and has the potential to increase plasma antioxidant capacity and decrease oxidative stress before and after exercise. To date, two studies using short duration, high intensity exercise protocols have examined the possible ergogenic effects of WM. Acute WM consumption providing ~1.2 g of L-citrulline attenuated moderate muscle soreness in untrained healthy subjects participating in high-intensity exercise intervals, but did not improve performance [32]. Similarly, time to exhaustion during a graded exercise test was not improved following acute consumption of watermelon juice containing ~1 g L-cirulline [33].

Long duration, high-intensity exercise induces significant physiological stress. Given the unique nutritional components in watermelon, we tested the efficacy of WM supplementation before (2 weeks) and during a 75 km cycling time-trial on performance and antioxidant capacity, and as a countermeasure to exercise-induced inflammation and innate immune changes compared to a standard 6% carbohydrate sports beverage.

2. Materials and Methods

2.1. Subjects

Twenty male cyclists with competitive road racing and time trial experience were recruited from local racing teams. Subjects agreed to train normally, remain weight-stable, and avoid the use of large-dose vitamin/mineral supplements (above 100% of recommended dietary allowances), herbs, and medications known to affect inflammation and immune function during the study. Informed consent was obtained from each subject and all study procedures were reviewed and approved by the Appalachian State University Institutional Review Board.

2.2. Study Design and Procedures

Two weeks prior to the first 75 km time trial, each subject completed study orientation and baseline testing in the North Carolina Research Campus Human Performance Laboratory operated by Appalachian State University. During study orientation subjects provided demographic information and training histories and were instructed to follow a diet moderate in carbohydrate (using a provided food list) during the 3 day period before each 75 km time trial.

During baseline testing, maximal cardiorespiratory fitness and body composition were measured. A cycle ergometry protocol (beginning at 150 W, 25 W increase per 2 min stage) was used to measure maximal power on a Lode cycle ergometer (Lode Excaliber Sport, Lode B.V., Groningen, The Netherlands) and peak oxygen consumption (VO_{2peak}) with a Cosmed Quark CPET metabolic cart (Rome, Italy) [12]. Heart rate was measured using a Polar Heart Rate Monitor (Polar Electro Inc., Woodbury, NY, USA). Body composition was measured with the BodPod system (Life Measurement, Concord, CA, USA). The environmental conditions were maintained at 19–20 °C and 45%–55% relative humidity; each subject had a fan directed on them to ensure consistent air flow during the time trial.

Subjects were randomized to either the watermelon (WM) or the 6% carbohydrate beverage (CHO) condition for the first 75 km time trial and then crossed over to the opposite condition for the second time trial with a 2-week washout period between trials. Subjects randomized to the WM trial were provided a 2-week supply of frozen WM puree. The subjects maintained the containers of the frozen WM in a standard freezer (−20 °C) and rapidly thawed each container of WM puree under hot running water prior to drinking it. Slowly thawing non-pasteurized WM results in a poor taste. However, thawing it quickly under hot water results in a more normal taste. The amount lycopene and L-citrulline do not change appreciably with a single freeze/thaw cycle. The subjects consumed 980 mL WM puree per day (equivalent of 60.7 g total sugar, 1.47 g L-citrulline, 0.465 g L-arginine, 44.4 mg lycopene, 5576 IU vitamin A, 0.44 IU vitamin B-6, and 79.4 IU vitamin C [15,26,34]) during the 2 weeks period prior to the WM trial. Watermelon puree for the study was prepared at Blue Ridge Venture Foods (Candler, NC, USA) from the seedless variety Crunchy Red harvested in eastern North Carolina. Watermelon flesh was pureed using a screw finisher with a 0.1 mm diameter stainless steel screen tube. The puree was bottled in 1 L capacity polyethylene containers and flash frozen without filtration or pasteurization. The frozen WM puree was maintained at −20 °C.

The morning of the 75 km time trial, subjects consumed the WM puree (980 mL) (or no WM puree) and then a standardized meal at 12:00 p.m. using Boost Plus at 10 kcal/kg (41.9 kJ/kg) (Boost Plus; Mead Johnson Nutritionals, Evansville, IN, USA). Subjects reported to the lab at 2:45 p.m. and then provided a blood sample. At 3:20 p.m., subjects ingested 0.4 g/kg carbohydrate from WM or from a standard 6% CHO beverage (Gatorade™, Chicago, IL, USA). Subjects ingested 0.2 g/kg of carbohydrates body weight every 15 min of WM or 6% CHO beverage during the 75 km time trials.

Subjects cycled (3:30 p.m. start) the mountainous 75 km time trial course [12] on their own bicycles on CompuTrainer Pro Model 8001 trainers (RacerMate, Seattle, WA, USA). Workload was continuously monitored using the CompuTrainer MultiRider software system (version 3.0, RacerMate, Seattle, WA, USA). Heart rate and rating of perceived exertion (RPE) were recorded every 30 min. Pre- and post-exercise fingertip capillary blood samples were drawn and analyzed using the YSI 2300 STAT Plus Glucose and Lactate analyzer (Yellow Springs, OH, USA). Blood samples were taken via venipuncture post-exercise and 1 h post-exercise. Subjects answered questions on digestive health using a 12-point Likert scale (1 relating to "none at all", 6 "moderate", and 12 "very high").

2.3. Analytical Measures

2.3.1. Complete Blood Count

Routine complete blood counts with white blood cell differential counts were made (Coulter Ac.T™ 5Diff Hematology Analyzer, Beckman Coulter, Inc., Miami, FL, USA) for the determination of plasma volume change and leukocyte subtypes for the immune function assay [35].

2.3.2. Plasma Cytokines

The total plasma concentration of six inflammatory cytokines (tumor necrosis factor α (TNFα), interleukins 6, 8, and 10 (IL-6, IL-8, IL-10), monocyte chemoattractant protein-1 (MCP-1), and granulocyte colony-stimulating factor (G-CSF)) was determined using an electrochemiluminescence based solid-phase sandwich immunoassay (Meso Scale Discovery, Gaithersburg, MD, USA) [12,36]. All samples and provided standards were analyzed in duplicate; the intra-assay CV ranged from 1.7% to 7.5% and the inter-assay CV ranged 2.4% to 9.6% for the cytokines measured. The minimum detectable concentration of IL-6 was 0.27 pg/mL, TNFα 0.50 pg/mL, GM-CSF 0.20 pg/mL, IFNγ 0.53 pg/mL, IL-1β 0.36 pg/mL, IL-2 0.35 pg/mL, IL-8 0.09 pg/mL, and IL-10 0.21 pg/mL. Pre- and post-exercise samples for the cytokines were analyzed on the same assay plate to decrease inter-kit assay variability.

2.3.3. Granulocyte and Monocyte Phagocytosis, Oxidative Burst Activity

Granulocyte and monocyte phagocytosis (GR-PHAG, MO-PHAG), oxidative burst activity (GR-OBA, MO-OBA) were assayed as previously described by Meaney et al. [37]. Briefly, phagocytosis was measured through the uptake of fluorescein isothiocyanate (FITC)-labeled *Staphylococcus aureus* bacteria and oxidative burst was measured through the oxidation of nonfluorescent hydroethidine (HE) to fluorescent ethidium bromide in cells stimulated with unlabeled bacteria. Samples were processed on a Q-Prep™ Workstation (Beckman Coulter, Inc.) and analysis was performed within 18 h of blood collection using a Beckman Coulter FC10 500 flow cytometer. After gating on the granulocyte and monocyte populations using forward scatter and side scatter, the mean fluorescence intensity (MFI; x-mean) and percent positive cells for FITC (FL1) and oxidized HE (FL2) were determined.

2.3.4. Plasma Antioxidant Capacity

Plasma antioxidant capacity was determined by two independent measures; the ferric reducing ability of plasma (FRAP) assay and the oxygen radical absorbance capacity (ORAC). The FRAP assay, a single electron transfer reaction, was conducted as previously described [30,36,38]. The FRAP assay utilizes water-soluble antioxidants native to the plasma collected from EDTA-treated blood to reduce ferric iron to the ferrous form subsequently producing a chromogen identifiable at 593 nm (Synergy H1 Hybrid Reader, BioTek Instruments Inc., Winooski, VT, USA). Samples and standards are expressed as ascorbate equivalents based on an ascorbate standard curve. Intra-assay and inter-assay coefficients of variation (CVs) were less than 5% and 7%, respectively. Plasma antioxidant power was also measured by the ORAC assay using methods previously described [36]. The ORAC assay depends on exogenous peroxyl radicals generated by 2,2'-azobis (2-methylpropionamide) dihydrochloride (AAPH) to oxidize fluorescein. Antioxidants in blood plasma delay oxidation of the fluorescent probe. Samples and standards are expressed as Trolox equivalents (μmol/L) based on a Trolox standard curve calculated by a fluorescence plate reader (Synergy H1 Hybrid Reader) as area under the curve. Intra and inter-assay CVs for ORAC were 4% and 7%, respectively.

2.3.5. Plasma Amino Acid Analysis

The amino acid concentration of plasma collected from heparin-treated blood was determined according to the methods of Wu and Meininger [39]. Briefly, 50 μL of plasma was mixed with 50 μL of 1.5 M $HClO_4$. To this, 1.125 mL of HPLC-grade water and 25 μL of 2 M K_2CO_3 were added. The mixture was centrifuged ($10,000 \times g$ for 1 min) and the supernatant was analyzed by HPLC using a Supelco C18 column (Supelco, Bellefonte, PA, USA) and a Waters HPLC system (Waters, Milford, MA, USA). Amino acids in samples were quantified on the basis of standards (Sigma Chemicals, St. Louis, MO, USA).

2.3.6. Total Nitrate

The total nitrate concentration of plasma collected from EDTA-treated blood was determined fluorometrically according to the manufacture's protocol (#780051; Cayman Chemical Company, Ann Arbor, MI, USA). Immediately prior to conducting the assay, the plasma was filtered according to the manufacturer's recommendation (#UFC801096, Millipore, Billerica, MA, USA). All samples and standards were analyzed in triplicate. The minimum detectable limit of the assay is 30 nM nitrite. Pre- and post-exercise samples were analyzed on the same assay plate to decrease inter-kit assay variability.

2.4. Statistical Analysis

All data are expressed as mean ± SEM. The biomarker data were analyzed using a 2 (condition) × 3 (time) repeated-measures ANOVA, within-subject design. When interaction effects were significant ($p \leq 0.05$), changes between baseline and each pre-exercise condition and pre-exercise, post-exercise, and 1 h post-exercise time points within Watermelon or CHO conditions were compared between trials using 2-tailed paired t-tests, with significance set after Bonferroni adjustment at $p \leq 0.0125$.

3. Results

Twenty subjects completed the study; subject characteristics are summarized in Table 1. Mean power (192 ± 9.2, 198 ± 9.1 watts; $p = 0.203$), heart rate ($87.2\% \pm 1.10\%$, $85.5\% \pm 1.13\%$ HR_{max}; $p = 0.111$), and total time (2.74 ± 0.35, 2.68 ± 0.36 h; $p = 0.192$) did not differ between WM and CHO 75 km time trials, respectively. Subjects reported a slightly higher rating of perceived exertion (16.8 ± 0.29, 16.2 ± 0.23 RPE units; $p = 0.030$) at the conclusion of the WM trial than the CHO trial, respectively. The pattern of increase in blood glucose (30.2%, 29.2%; interaction effect $p = 0.959$) and blood lactate (294%, 314%; interaction effect $p - 0.248$) did not differ between WM and CHO trials. Mean carbohydrate intake during the WM and CHO trials was 182 ± 9.79 grams and did not differ between trials ($p = 0.178$). The volume of WM puree consumed during the trial did not differ from volume of CHO beverage consumed (2.98 ± 0.17 L, 2.86 ± 0.16 L; $p = 0.098$). Compared to the CHO condition, subjects reported feeling fuller ($p = 0.0148$) but not more bloated ($p = 0.226$) after consuming WM during the time trial. Subjects lost more body mass during the WM condition (-0.60 ± 0.58 kg, -0.01 ± 0.60 kg; $p = 0.002$) than during the CHO condition, respectively, but the pre- to post-exercise change in plasma volume did not differ ($6.49\% \pm 4.08\%$, $6.30\% \pm 2.25\%$; $p = 0.970$).

The acute inflammatory response to completing the 75 km time trial did not differ appreciably between WM and CHO trials (Table 2). The pattern of increase in the plasma cytokine G-CSF was greater after the WM trial than the CHO trial (Table 2); however, post hoc analysis did not reveal differences ($p > 0.0125$). Exercise-induced changes in innate immune function did not differ between

WM and CHO trials (Table 2). The pattern of increase in GR-PHAG and MO-PHAG and GR-OBA and MO-OBA did not differ between WM and CHO (Table 2).

Table 1. Subject characteristics ($n = 20$).

Variable	Mean ± SEM
Age (year)	48.5 ± 2.3
Body mass (kg)	81.04 ± 2.2
% Body fat	19.6 ± 1.5
BMI (kg/m^2)	25.1 ± 0.7
Years cycling	10.95 ± 2.3
Watt$_{max}$	314 ± 9.8
Peak oxygen consumption (VO$_{2peak}$, mL·kg^{-1}·min^{-1})	51.5 ± 1.9

Data are means ± SEM; BMI = body mass index; W = watts.

Table 2. Inflammation and immune-function markers.

Variable	Baseline	Pre-Exercise	Post-Exercise	1-h Post-Exercise	Time; Interaction p Values
Inflammatory markers					
WBC (10^9/L)	6.2 ± 0.34				
CHO		5.74 ± 0.31	12.2 ± 0.96	10.9 ± 0.83	<0.001; 0.125
WM		5.58 ± 0.39	14.7 ± 1.01	12.4 ± 0.85	
TNF-α (pg/mL)	10.5 ± 1.03				
CHO		10.2 ± 0.92	12.8 ± 1.11	11.9 ± 1.14	0.005; 0.936
WM		10.2 ± 0.99	12.3 ± 1.29	12.1 ± 1.19	
IL-6 (pg/mL)	1.02 ± 0.28				
CHO		0.80 ± 0.13	10.2 ± 1.83	7.92 ± 1.58	<0.001; 0.921
WM		0.71 ± 0.14	9.98 ± 1.63	7.68 ± 1.56	
IL-8 (pg/mL)	3.21 ± 0.33				
CHO		3.26 ± 0.37	10.9 ± 1.01	12.2 ± 1.55	<0.001; 0.506
WM		3.59 ± 0.33	12.1 ± 1.52	11.4 ± 1.55	
IL-10 (pg/mL)	2.31 ± 0.44				
CHO		2.46 ± 0.48	10.5 ± 3.83	8.44 ± 2.82	0.002; 0.292
WM		2.93 ± 0.82	15.5 ± 5.68	16.0 ± 6.64	
MCP-1 (pg/mL)	194 ± 7.80				
CHO		188 ± 8.99	344 ± 23.8	333 ± 27.3	<0.001; 0.206
WM		188 ± 9.44	375 ± 21.1	338 ± 16.9	
G-CSF (pg/mL)	9.47 ± 0.56				
CHO		9.94 ± 0.97	16.2 ± 1.55	16.8 ± 1.53	<0.001; 0.041
WM		10.7 ± 0.96	18.7 ± 2.12	19.9 ± 1.94	
GR-PHAG (MFI)	49.7 ± 4.20				
CHO		32.7 ± 2.81	63.2 ± 8.83	75.3 ± 11.9	0.001; 0.635
WM		40.8 ± 6.75	72.2 ± 12.0	83.6 ± 16.3	
MO-PHAG (MFI)	26.5 ± 1.64				
CHO		20.1 ± 1.50	36.0 ± 3.46	44.4 ± 5.18	<0.001; 0.612
WM		23.9 ± 3.89	39.2 ± 4.87	44.4 ± 6.88	
GR-OBA (MFI)	23.3 ± 1.11				
CHO		16.3 ± 1.35	24.6 ± 2.08	26.3 ± 2.78	<0.001; 0.612
WM		18.5 ± 2.54	26.2 ± 3.28	23.8 ± 3.47	
MO-OBA (MFI)	11.8 ± 0.44				
CHO		9.70 ± 0.59	13.5 ± 0.73	14.7 ± 0.98	<0.001; 0.173
WM		10.6 ± 1.15	13.1 ± 1.09	13.0 ± 1.09	

Data are means ± SEM; WBC = Total blood leukocytes; TNF = Tumor Necrosis Factor; IL = interleukin; MCP = monocyte chemo attractant protein; granulocyte colony-stimulating factor = G - CSF; MFI = mean fluorescence intensity; GR = granulocyte; PHAG = phagocytosis; MO = monocyte; OBA = oxidative burst activity.

The exercise-induced patterns of change in plasma antioxidant capacity were greater in WM compared to CHO trials. In contrast to the CHO trial, WM consumption resulted in a significantly greater pre- to post-exercise and pre- to 1 h post-exercise increase in plasma FRAP (interaction effect $p < 0.001$) (Figure 1A). Similarly, the pre- to post-exercise pattern of increase in plasma ORAC was greater in WM than CHO (interaction effect $p < 0.001$) (Figure 1B).

The pattern of increase in plasma L-citrulline differed between WM and CHO trials (interaction effect $p < 0.001$) with differences measured between conditions after 2 weeks WM ingestion, immediately post-, and 1 h post-exercise (Figure 2A). The pattern of increase in plasma L-arginine differed between WM and CHO trials (interaction effect $p < 0.001$) with an increase from baseline, and differences measured between trials after 2 weeks WM ingestion, immediately post-, and 1 h post-exercise (Figure 2B). The pattern of increase in plasma total nitrate differed between WM and CHO trials (interaction effect $p = 0.004$) with differences measured between conditions immediately post-, and 1 h post-exercise (Figure 2C).

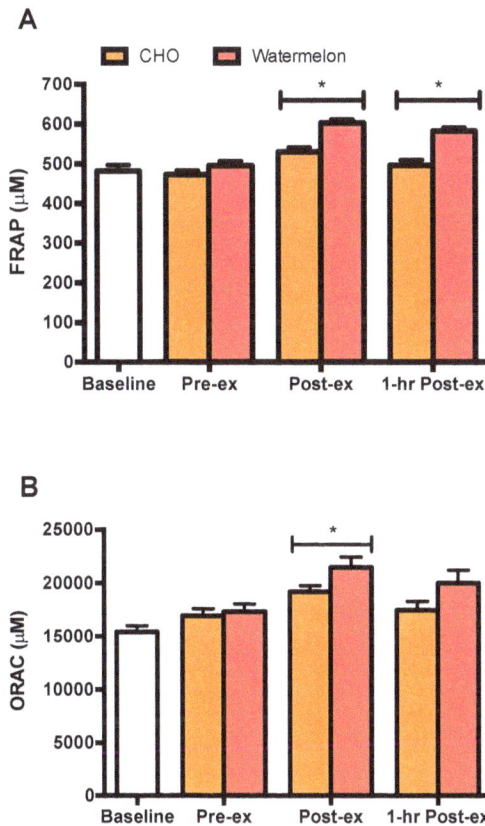

Figure 1. Watermelon consumption during exercise potentiates the exercise-induced increase in plasma antioxidant capacity. (**A**) Plasma FRAP = ferric reducing ability of plasma (expressed as ascorbate equivalents) and (**B**) plasma ORAC = oxygen radical absorbance capacity (expressed as trolox equivalents) were higher in WM compared to CHO following 75 km cycling (interaction effect, $p < 0.001$, each); * $p < 0.0125$ compared to time matched CHO.

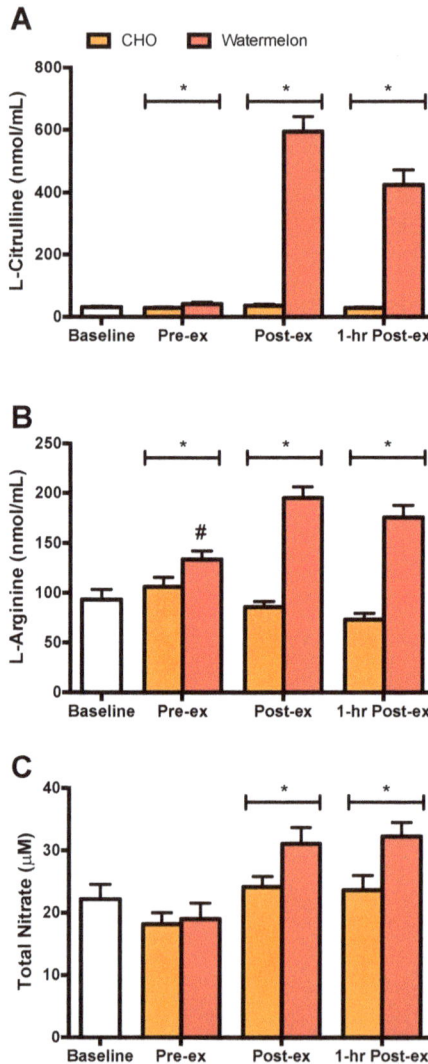

Figure 2. Watermelon consumption increases plasma L-citrulline (interaction effect $p < 0.001$), L-arginine (interaction effect $p < 0.001$), and total nitrate (interaction effect $p = 0.004$). Plasma concentrations of (**A**) L-citrulline; (**B**) arginine; and (**C**) total nitrate; # $p < 0.0125$ compared to baseline; * $p < 0.0125$ compared to time matched CHO.

4. Discussion

This randomized, crossover study investigated the effect of WM puree consumption for two weeks before and during a bout of vigorous exercise (relative to matched carbohydrate beverage ingestion) on exercise performance and antioxidant capacity, and as a countermeasure to exercise-induced inflammation and innate immune changes in trained cyclists. The 75 km cycling time trial was associated with the typical increases in plasma cytokines and granulocyte and monocyte phagocytosis (a marker of post-exercise inflammation) measured during previous trials with carbohydrate-fed athletes [12,40]. Despite significantly higher plasma antioxidant capacity, L-arginine, nitrate, and citrulline, WM ingestion was not associated with alterations in the pattern of change in inflammation and immune measures. Performance times were comparable between WM and CHO beverage ingestion, supporting previous findings in our lab that high-fructose fruit ingestion supports intensive, long duration exercise to the same degree as sports beverages [12,13].

WM benefits in attenuating post-exercise inflammation may be measurable during extended periods of heavy training and not after one exercise challenge event. The water content (91%) and unique combination of nutritional components found in WM are of interest to athletes seeking a natural whole food source for hydration and nutrition during physical activity. Lycopene is the major carotenoid (84%–97%) in red WM flesh, and one serving (280 g) contains 14–22 mg of lycopene [41]. WM is high in fructose, and each serving contains 3.4 g sucrose, 4.4 g glucose, and 9.4 g of fructose. Watermelon is one of the richest food sources of L-citrulline, a non-essential amino acid, and contains a small amount of L-arginine, an essential amino acid. Each serving of WM (286 g) provides 0.429 g of L-citrulline, 0.135 g of L-arginine, and small amounts of other amino acids [15,26,34]. WM has moderate amounts of potassium and vitamin C. In general, the distinctive mixture of nutritional components in WM led us to hypothesize that 2 weeks ingestion would alter post-exercise cytokine and immune measures, but these effects did not emerge within the context and limitations of this study. We have previously shown that carbohydrate compared to water ingestion during 75 km cycling trials results in muted post-exercise inflammation, and this study would have been strengthened had the research design included a water-only condition. Nonetheless, contrary to our hypothesis, WM ingestion did not add to the well-known anti-inflammatory effects associated with carbohydrate ingestion during exercise [13,40].

To our knowledge this is the first study to determine the effectiveness of WM to support the energy demands of vigorous endurance (>2 h) exercise. The amount and timing of the carbohydrate provided to our subjects was based on the American College of Sports Medicine recommendation, 30–60 g/h or 0.7 g/kg/h delivered every 15–20 min [42]. The fructose:glucose ratio of WM is 1:0.55 [14]. Although gut absorption [43], and thus the rate of oxidation [44], of exogenous fructose is lower than glucose, the blood glucose and lactate data and performance measures (time and average power output) indicate that the dose of WM utilized in this study prevented exercise-induced hypoglycemia and supported the energy demands of vigorous endurance cycling. The current data support our previous findings wherein providing exogenous carbohydrate via bananas and pears maintained blood glucose levels and supported the energy demands of vigorous cycling [12,13]. Tarazona-Diaz et al. [32] found that acute WM supplementation did not enhance anaerobic cycle ergometer work capacity. Cutrufello et al. [33] recently reported that a single acute dose of WM did not enhance strength, anaerobic threshold, time to exhaustion or VO_{2max}. These two WM studies utilized short-duration, high-intensity exercise bouts that are not limited by blood glucose or glycogen levels.

The rate and total volume of beverage consumed did not differ between trials. However, the subjects reported feeling significantly fuller during the WM trial. In our previous studies, we reported that subjects consuming bananas and pears felt fuller and more bloated, but without influencing RPE [12,13]. The fiber content of WM and fruit more than likely contributed to the perception of feeling fuller, and may have contributed to the small but significantly higher RPE during the WM trial. The subjects lost approximately 0.5 kg (0.62%) more body mass during the WM trial than the CHO trail; similar to what we previously reported when bananas were consumed during prolonged exercise [12]. The loss in body mass did not result in a greater pre- to post-exercise change in plasma volume between trials. For most individuals, a loss of >2% body mass may hinder aerobic performance due to dehydration [45]. Consuming WM puree, within the conditions employed in this study, met the hydration needs of the cyclists.

WM ingestion was associated with increases in both measures of plasma antioxidant capacity (FRAP and ORAC). These data support our previous findings with banana and pear [12,13]. The increase in plasma antioxidant capacity, especially post-exercise, may be attributed to an increase in the plasma concentration of uric acid [30,46]. During fatiguing exercise, active skeletal muscle oxidation of purines increases, thus increasing the efflux of uric acid from skeletal muscle into the blood compartment [47]. However, hydrogen peroxide is generated at two steps of this biochemical process, consequently, the exercise-induced increase in plasma uric acid may not be a mechanism of compensatory antioxidant enhancement as some speculate. Independent of the exercise-induced increase in plasma uric acid, the greater amount of fructose consumed during the WM trial may have resulted in a larger increase in hepatic uric acid production. In the liver, metabolism of fructose to fructose 1-phosphate through fructokinase results in production of uric acid [48]. While an acute decrease in uric acid does not exacerbate exercise-induced oxidative stress in the blood or hinder exercise performance [49], the benefit of WM-derived uric acid did not improve performance in this study. Consumption of L-citrulline, a hydroxyl scavenger, and other antioxidants present in WM (lycopene, β-carotene, and vitamin C), may have further contributed to the increased total antioxidant capacity of the plasma [18,28–31]. The performance benefit of acutely increasing the total antioxidant capacity of plasma is unclear [50] and remains an interesting area of study.

With the exception of G-CSF, the pattern of change in the markers of systemic inflammation and immune function differed little between the WM and CHO. The WM trial post-exercise and 1 h post-exercise increase in G-CSF was 15% and 18% greater, respectively. In response to intense exercise G-CSF mediates mobilization of progenitor cells [51] and prevents neutrophil apoptosis and stimulates neutrophil release [52,53]. The mechanism by which WM consumption potentiated the G-CSF response to exercise warrants further study. Watermelon provides a significant amount of L-citrulline and a previous report suggests that citrulline-malate modulates polymorphonuclear neutrophil function. Sureda et al. [23] supplemented competitive cyclists with 6 g of citrulline-malate prior to a competitive 3 h cycling race. Post-exercise polymorphonuclear neutrophils from subjects in the supplemented condition had significantly greater reactive oxygen species levels than baseline, indicating that acute citrulline-malate may attenuate exercise-induced immune dysfunction through an NO-dependent mechanism [23]. In the current study total nitrate, a proxy measure of NO production, significantly increased during the WM trial in similar fashion to the report by Sureda et al. [23], but without an effect on oxidative burst activity.

L-citrulline and L-arginine have been studied as potential ergogenic aids. Nitric oxide (NO) synthase, in conjunction with specific cofactors, converts L-arginine into NO and L-citrulline. Further, L-citrulline may be converted to L-arginine via argininosuccinate synthase [22]. Putatively, enhancing NO metabolism would improve performance through greater blood flow and increasing glucose uptake via enhance GLUT4 translocation in working skeletal muscle [24]. During the 2-week intervention period subjects consumed 980 mL of WM/ day, the equivalent of 1.47 g L-citrulline and 0.465 g L-arginine/day and approximately 4.39 g L-citrulline and 1.41 g L-arginine during the 75 km time trial. Plasma L-citrulline concentrations return to baseline values approximately 3–5 h after ingestion [54] and the small but non-significant elevation in pre-exercise plasma concentration is attributable to the 980 mL dose of WM consumed the morning of the WM trial. Following consumption of L-citrulline, plasma L-arginine concentrations take approximately 8 h to return to baseline [54]. The significant pre-exercise increase in plasma L-arginine is the result of consuming the WM during the previous supplementation period [26] and the morning of the WM time trial. Our baseline and pre-exercise plasma L-citrulline and L-arginine data are in agreement with Collins et al. [26] and Mandel et al. [25].

Subjects completed the WM trial in less than 3 h and consumed ~3 L of WM. This resulted in a 14-fold and a 32% increase in the pre- to post-exercise plasma concentration of L-citrulline and L-arginine, respectively. To our knowledge only one study has measured plasma L-citrulline and L-arginine concentrations after consuming one dose of WM [25]. In this study [25] subjects consumed a single 3.3 kg serving of WM. One hour post-WM consumption, plasma L-citrulline and L-arginine concentrations increased 27-fold and 3-fold, respectively, and returned to baseline by the 8-h time point. The smaller increase in plasma L-citrulline and L-arginine in our study was due to the smaller amount of WM consumed and the greater amount of time over which our subjects consumed the WM. Short-duration high-intensity exercise is not improved by a single dose of L-citrulline or L-citrulline supplemented over a 24 h period [33,55]. Recent evidence suggests that L-citrulline supplementation over a 1-week period can increase performance when exercising at a high percentage of the subject's VO_{2max} for approximately 10 min [56,57]. L-citrulline supplementation is postulated to improve performance by enhancing NO-dependent vasodilation, and thus blood flow, and increased mitochondrial respiration during exercise [56]. The plasma concentration of total nitrate, a proxy measure of NO production, increased significantly more during the WM trial compared to the CHO trial, 63% and 33%, respectively. The lack of improved performance during the WM trial, despite the apparent increase in NO production, suggests that NO-dependent mechanisms did not limit exercise performance in the current study.

5. Conclusions

Our data indicate that ingestion of watermelon (WM) puree is as effective as a 6% CHO beverage in supporting endurance exercise performance, with the added advantage of improving antioxidant capacity through increased intake of lycopene, L-citrulline, and vitamins A and C. While the RPE was greater during the WM trial this did not dampen time trial performance. Changes in blood glucose, lactate, inflammation, antioxidant capacity, and innate immune measures were comparable between WM puree and 6% CHO beverage 75 km cycling trials, and similar to what we have previously reported for CHO-fed athletes. WM puree ingestion during exercise increased plasma L-citrulline, L-arginine, and total nitrate, but without discernable acute effects on post-exercise inflammation and innate immune function relative to CHO.

Acknowledgments: This work and the funds for covering the costs to publish in open access were supported in part by a grant from the National Watermelon Promotion Board, Orlando, FL, USA.

Author Contributions: R.A.S., D.C.N., and P.P.V. conceived and designed the experiments; R.A.S., D.A.H., M.P.M., A.M.K., and L.C.K. performed the experiments; R.A.S., D.C.N. and A.M.K. analyzed the data; R.A.S. and D.C.N. wrote the manuscript.

Conflicts of Interest: R.A.S., D.C.N., D.A.H., M.P.M., A.M.K., L.C.K. declare no conflict of interest. P.P.V. is a science advisor to the National Watermelon Promotion Board, Orlando, FL, USA. The funding sponsors had no role in the design of the study; in the collection, analyses, or interpretation of data; in the writing of the manuscript, and in the decision to publish the results.

References

1. Levine, S.A.; Gordon, B.; Derick, C.L. Some changes in the chemical constituents of the blood following a marathon race: With special reference to the development of hypoglycemia. *J. Am. Med. Assoc.* **1924**, *82*, 1778–1779. [CrossRef]
2. Gordon, B.; Kohn, L.A.; Levine, S.A.; Matton, M.; Scriver, W.M.; Whiting, W.B. Sugar content of the blood in runners following a marathon race: With especial reference to the prevention of hypoglycemia: Further observations. *J. Am. Med. Assoc.* **1925**, *85*, 508–509. [CrossRef]
3. Coyle, E.F.; Hagberg, J.M.; Hurley, B.F.; Martin, W.H.; Ehsani, A.A.; Holloszy, J.O. Carbohydrate feeding during prolonged strenuous exercise can delay fatigue. *J. Appl. Physiol.* **1983**, *55*, 230–235. [PubMed]
4. Carter, J.; Jeukendrup, A.E.; Mundel, T.; Jones, D.A. Carbohydrate supplementation improves moderate and high-intensity exercise in the heat. *Pflug. Arch.* **2003**, *446*, 211–219. [CrossRef] [PubMed]
5. De Sousa, M.V.; Madsen, K.; Fukui, R.; Santos, A.; da Silva, M.E. Carbohydrate supplementation delays DNA damage in elite runners during intensive microcycle training. *Eur. J. Appl. Physiol.* **2012**, *112*, 493–500. [CrossRef] [PubMed]
6. Scharhag, J.; Meyer, T.; Auracher, M.; Gabriel, H.H.; Kindermann, W. Effects of graded carbohydrate supplementation on the immune response in cycling. *Med. Sci. Sports Exerc.* **2006**, *38*, 286–292. [CrossRef] [PubMed]
7. Jentjens, R.L.; Moseley, L.; Waring, R.H.; Harding, L.K.; Jeukendrup, A.E. Oxidation of combined ingestion of glucose and fructose during exercise. *J. Appl. Physiol.* **2004**, *96*, 1277–1284. [CrossRef] [PubMed]

8. Shi, X.; Summers, R.W.; Schedl, H.P.; Flanagan, S.W.; Chang, R.; Gisolfi, C.V. Effects of carbohydrate type and concentration and solution osmolality on water absorption. *Med. Sci. Sports Exerc.* **1995**, *27*, 1607–1615. [CrossRef] [PubMed]
9. O'Brien, W.J.; Stannard, S.R.; Clarke, J.A.; Rowlands, D.S. Fructose-maltodextrin ratio governs exogenous and other cho oxidation and performance. *Med. Sci. Sports Exerc.* **2013**, *45*, 1814–1824. [CrossRef] [PubMed]
10. Too, B.W.; Cicai, S.; Hockett, K.R.; Applegate, E.; Davis, B.A.; Casazza, G.A. Natural versus commercial carbohydrate supplementation and endurance running performance. *J. Int. Soc. Sports Nutr.* **2012**, *9*, 27–35. [CrossRef] [PubMed]
11. Murdoch, S.D.; Bazzarre, T.L.; Snider, I.P.; Goldfarb, A.H. Differences in the effects of carbohydrate food form on endurance performance to exhaustion. *Int. J. Sport Nutr.* **1993**, *3*, 41–54. [CrossRef] [PubMed]
12. Nieman, D.C.; Gillitt, N.D.; Henson, D.A.; Sha, W.; Shanely, R.A.; Knab, A.M.; Cialdella-Kam, L.; Jin, F. Bananas as an energy source during exercise: A metabolomics approach. *PLoS ONE* **2012**, *7*, e37479. [CrossRef] [PubMed]
13. Nieman, D.C.; Gillitt, N.D.; Sha, W.; Meaney, M.P.; John, C.; Pappan, K.L.; Kinchen, J.M. Metabolomics-based analysis of banana and pear ingestion on exercise performance and recovery. *J. Proteome Res.* **2015**, *14*, 5367–5377. [CrossRef] [PubMed]
14. U.S. Department of Agriculture. USDA National Nutrient Database for Standard Reference, Release 27. Available online: http://www.ars.usda.gov/ba/bhnrc/ndl (accessed on 10 July 2014).
15. Rimando, A.M.; Perkins-Veazie, P.M. Determination of citrulline in watermelon rind. *J. Chromatogr. A* **2005**, *1078*, 196–200. [CrossRef] [PubMed]
16. Ghavipour, M.; Saedisomeolia, A.; Djalali, M.; Sotoudeh, G.; Eshraghyan, M.R.; Moghadam, A.M.; Wood, L.G. Tomato juice consumption reduces systemic inflammation in overweight and obese females. *Br. J. Nutr.* **2013**, *109*, 2031–2035. [CrossRef] [PubMed]
17. Gann, P.H.; Ma, J.; Giovannucci, E.; Willett, W.; Sacks, F.M.; Hennekens, C.H.; Stampfer, M.J. Lower prostate cancer risk in men with elevated plasma lycopene levels: Results of a prospective analysis. *Cancer Res.* **1999**, *59*, 1225–1230. [PubMed]
18. Stahl, W.; Sies, H. Antioxidant activity of carotenoids. *Mol. Aspects Med.* **2003**, *24*, 345–351. [CrossRef]
19. Moran, N.E.; Cichon, M.J.; Riedl, K.M.; Grainger, E.M.; Schwartz, S.J.; Novotny, J.A.; Erdman, J.W., Jr.; Clinton, S.K. Compartmental and noncompartmental modeling of (1)(3)c-lycopene absorption, isomerization, and distribution kinetics in healthy adults. *Am. J. Clin. Nutr.* **2015**, *102*, 1436–1449. [CrossRef] [PubMed]
20. Tsitsimpikou, C.; Kioukia-Fougia, N.; Tsarouhas, K.; Stamatopoulos, P.; Rentoukas, E.; Koudounakos, A.; Papalexis, P.; Liesivuori, J.; Jamurtas, A. Administration of tomato juice ameliorates lactate dehydrogenase and creatinine kinase responses to anaerobic training. *Food Chem. Toxicol.* **2013**, *61*, 9–13. [CrossRef] [PubMed]
21. Harms-Ringdahl, M.; Jenssen, D.; Haghdoost, S. Tomato juice intake suppressed serum concentration of 8-oxodg after extensive physical activity. *Nutr. J.* **2012**, *11*, 29. [CrossRef] [PubMed]
22. Wu, G.; Morris, S.M., Jr. Arginine metabolism: Nitric oxide and beyond. *Biochem. J.* **1998**, *336*, 1–17. [CrossRef] [PubMed]
23. Sureda, A.; Cordova, A.; Ferrer, M.D.; Tauler, P.; Perez, G.; Tur, J.A.; Pons, A. Effects of l-citrulline oral supplementation on polymorphonuclear neutrophils oxidative burst and nitric oxide production after exercise. *Free Radic. Res.* **2009**, *43*, 828–835. [CrossRef] [PubMed]
24. Bradley, S.J.; Kingwell, B.A.; McConell, G.K. Nitric oxide synthase inhibition reduces leg glucose uptake but not blood flow during dynamic exercise in humans. *Diabetes* **1999**, *48*, 1815–1821. [CrossRef] [PubMed]
25. Mandel, H.; Levy, N.; Izkovitch, S.; Korman, S.H. Elevated plasma citrulline and arginine due to consumption of citrullus vulgaris (watermelon). *J. Inherit. Metab. Dis.* **2005**, *28*, 467–472. [CrossRef] [PubMed]
26. Collins, J.K.; Wu, G.; Perkins-Veazie, P.; Spears, K.; Claypool, P.L.; Baker, R.A.; Clevidence, B.A. Watermelon consumption increases plasma arginine concentrations in adults. *Nutrition* **2007**, *23*, 261–266. [CrossRef] [PubMed]
27. Root, M.M.; McGinn, M.C.; Nieman, D.C.; Henson, D.A.; Heinz, S.A.; Shanely, R.A.; Knab, A.M.; Jin, F. Combined fruit and vegetable intake is correlated with improved inflammatory and oxidant status from a cross-sectional study in a community setting. *Nutrients* **2012**, *4*, 29–41. [CrossRef] [PubMed]
28. Akashi, K.; Miyake, C.; Yokota, A. Citrulline, a novel compatible solute in drought-tolerant wild watermelon leaves, is an efficient hydroxyl radical scavenger. *FEBS Lett.* **2001**, *508*, 438–442. [CrossRef]

29. Müller, L.; Fröhlich, K.; Böhm, V. Comparative antioxidant activities of carotenoids measured by ferric reducing antioxidant power (FRAP), abts bleaching assay (αTEAC), DPPH assay and peroxyl radical scavenging assay. *Food Chem.* **2011**, *129*, 139–148. [CrossRef]

30. Benzie, I.F.; Strain, J.J. The ferric reducing ability of plasma (FRAP) as a measure of "antioxidant power": The frap assay. *Anal. Biochem.* **1996**, *239*, 70–76. [CrossRef] [PubMed]

31. Edwards, A.J.; Vinyard, B.T.; Wiley, E.R.; Brown, E.D.; Collins, J.K.; Perkins-Veazie, P.; Baker, R.A.; Clevidence, B.A. Consumption of watermelon juice increases plasma concentrations of lycopene and beta-carotene in humans. *J. Nutr.* **2003**, *133*, 1043–1050. [PubMed]

32. Tarazona-Diaz, M.P.; Alacid, F.; Carrasco, M.; Martinez, I.; Aguayo, E. Watermelon juice: Potential functional drink for sore muscle relief in athletes. *J. Agric. Food Chem.* **2013**, *61*, 7522–7528. [CrossRef] [PubMed]

33. Cutrufello, P.T.; Gadomski, S.J.; Zavorsky, G.S. The effect of L-citrulline and watermelon juice supplementation on anaerobic and aerobic exercise performance. *J. Sports Sci.* **2015**, *33*, 1459–1466. [CrossRef] [PubMed]

34. U.S. Department of Agriculture. USDA National Nutrient Database for Standard Reference, Release 27. 2015. Available online: http://www.ars.usda.gov/main/site_main.htm?modecode=80-40-05-25 (accessed on 17 July 2015).

35. Dill, D.B.; Costill, D.L. Calculation of percentage changes in volumes of blood, plasma, and red cells in dehydration. *J. Appl. Physiol.* **1974**, *37*, 247–248. [PubMed]

36. Knab, A.M.; Nieman, D.C.; Gillitt, N.D.; Shanely, R.A.; Cialdella-Kam, L.; Henson, D.; Sha, W.; Meaney, M.P. Effects of a freeze-dried juice blend powder on exercise-induced inflammation, oxidative stress, and immune function in cyclists. *Appl. Physiol. Nutr. Metab.* **2014**, *39*, 381–385. [CrossRef] [PubMed]

37. Meaney, M.P.; Nieman, D.C.; Henson, D.A.; Jiang, Q.; Wang, F.Z. Measuring granulocyte and monocyte phagocytosis and oxidative burst activity in human blood. *J. Vis. Exp.* **2016**, in press.

38. Shanely, R.A.; Knab, A.M.; Nieman, D.C.; Jin, F.; McAnulty, S.R.; Landram, M.J. Quercetin supplementation does not alter antioxidant status in humans. *Free Radic. Res.* **2010**, *44*, 224–231. [CrossRef] [PubMed]

39. Wu, G.; Meininger, C.J. Analysis of citrulline, arginine, and methylarginines using high-performance liquid chromatography. *Methods Enzymol.* **2008**, *440*, 177–189. [PubMed]

40. Nieman, D.C.; Nehlsen-Cannarella, S.L.; Fagoaga, O.R.; Henson, D.A.; Utter, A.; Davis, J.M.; Williams, F.; Butterworth, D.E. Influence of mode and carbohydrate on the cytokine response to heavy exertion. *Med. Sci. Sports Exerc.* **1998**, *30*, 671–678. [CrossRef] [PubMed]

41. Perkins-Veazie, P.; Collins, J.K.; Davis, A.R.; Roberts, W. Carotenoid content of 50 watermelon cultivars. *J. Agric. Food Chem.* **2006**, *54*, 2593–2597. [CrossRef] [PubMed]

42. Rodriguez, N.R.; Di Marco, N.M.; Langley, S. American College of Sports Medicine position stand: Nutrition and athletic performance. *Med. Sci. Sports Exerc.* **2009**, *41*, 709–731. [PubMed]

43. Fujisawa, T.; Mulligan, K.; Wada, L.; Schumacher, L.; Riby, J.; Kretchmer, N. The effect of exercise on fructose absorption. *Am. J. Clin. Nutr.* **1993**, *58*, 75–79. [PubMed]

44. Jeukendrup, A.E.; Jentjens, R. Oxidation of carbohydrate feedings during prolonged exercise: Current thoughts, guidelines and directions for future research. *Sports Med.* **2000**, *29*, 407–424. [CrossRef] [PubMed]

45. Sawka, M.N.; Burke, L.M.; Eichner, E.R.; Maughan, R.J.; Montain, S.J.; Stachenfeld, N.S. American College of Sports Medicine position stand. Exercise and fluid replacement. *Med. Sci. Sports Exerc.* **2007**, *39*, 377–390. [PubMed]

46. Cao, G.; Prior, R.L. Comparison of different analytical methods for assessing total antioxidant capacity of human serum. *Clin. Chem.* **1998**, *44*, 1309–1315. [PubMed]

47. Duthie, G.; Robertson, J.; Maughan, R.; Morrice, P. Blood antioxidant status and erythrocyte lipid peroxidation following distance running. *Arch. Biochem. Biophys.* **1990**, *282*, 78–83. [CrossRef]

48. Perheentupa, J.; Raivio, K. Fructose-induced hyperuricaemia. *Lancet* **1967**, *2*, 528–531. [CrossRef]

49. McAnulty, S.R.; Hosick, P.A.; McAnulty, L.S.; Quindry, J.C.; Still, L.; Hudson, M.B.; Dibarnardi, A.N.; Milne, G.L.; Morrow, J.D.; Austin, M.D. Effect of pharmacological lowering of plasma urate on exercise-induced oxidative stress. *Appl. Physiol. Nutr. Metab.* **2007**, *32*, 1148–1155. [CrossRef] [PubMed]

50. Quindry, J.C.; Kavazis, A.N.; Powers, S.K. Exercise-induced oxidative stress: Are supplemental antioxidants warranted? In *The Encyclopaedia of Sports Medicine*; John Wiley & Sons Ltd.: Chichester, UK, 2013; pp. 263–276.

51. Kruger, K.; Pilat, C.; Schild, M.; Lindner, N.; Frech, T.; Muders, K.; Mooren, F.C. Progenitor cell mobilization after exercise is related to systemic levels of G-CSF and muscle damage. *Scand. J. Med. Sci. Sports* **2015**, *25*, e283–e291. [CrossRef] [PubMed]

52. Mooren, F.C.; Volker, K.; Klocke, R.; Nikol, S.; Waltenberger, J.; Kruger, K. Exercise delays neutrophil apoptosis by a G-CSF-dependent mechanism. *J. Appl. Physiol.* **2012**, *113*, 1082–1090. [CrossRef] [PubMed]

53. Yamada, M.; Suzuki, K.; Kudo, S.; Totsuka, M.; Nakaji, S.; Sugawara, K. Raised plasma G-CSF and il-6 after exercise may play a role in neutrophil mobilization into the circulation. *J. Appl. Physiol.* **2002**, *92*, 1789–1794. [CrossRef] [PubMed]

54. Moinard, C.; Nicolis, I.; Neveux, N.; Darquy, S.; Benazeth, S.; Cynober, L. Dose-ranging effects of citrulline administration on plasma amino acids and hormonal patterns in healthy subjects: The citrudose pharmacokinetic study. *Br. J. Nutr.* **2008**, *99*, 855–862. [CrossRef] [PubMed]

55. Hickner, R.C.; Tanner, C.J.; Evans, C.A.; Clark, P.D.; Haddock, A.; Fortune, C.; Geddis, H.; Waugh, W.; McCammon, M. L-citrulline reduces time to exhaustion and insulin response to a graded exercise test. *Med. Sci. Sports Exerc.* **2006**, *38*, 660–666. [CrossRef] [PubMed]

56. Suzuki, T.; Morita, M.; Kobayashi, Y.; Kamimura, A. Oral L-citrulline supplementation enhances cycling time trial performance in healthy trained men: Double-blind randomized placebo-controlled 2-way crossover study. *J. Int. Soc. Sports Nutr.* **2016**, *13*, 6. [CrossRef] [PubMed]

57. Bailey, S.J.; Blackwell, J.R.; Lord, T.; Vanhatalo, A.; Winyard, P.G.; Jones, A.M. L-citrulline supplementation improves O_2 uptake kinetics and high-intensity exercise performance in humans. *J. Appl. Physiol.* **2015**, *119*, 385–395. [CrossRef] [PubMed]

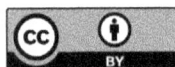

nutrients

MDPI

Article

Dietary Intakes and Supplement Use in Pre-Adolescent and Adolescent Canadian Athletes

Jill A. Parnell [1,*], Kristin P. Wiens [2] and Kelly A. Erdman [3]

[1] Department of Health and Physical Education, Mount Royal University, 4825 Mount Royal Gate SW, Calgary, AB T3E 6K6, Canada
[2] Department of Behavioral Health and Nutrition, University of Delaware, 026 North College Avenue, Newark, DE 19716, USA; kwiens@udel.edu
[3] Sport Medicine Centre, University of Calgary, 2500 University Dr NW, Calgary, AB T2N 1N4, Canada; kerdman@csicalgary.ca
*   Correspondence: jparnell@mtroyal.ca; Tel.: +1-403-440-8672

Received: 14 July 2016; Accepted: 16 August 2016; Published: 26 August 2016

Abstract: Young athletes experience numerous dietary challenges including growth, training/competition, unhealthy food environments, and travel. The objective was to determine nutrient intakes and supplement use in pre-adolescent and adolescent Canadian athletes. Athletes (n = 187) aged 11–18 years completed an on-line 24-h food recall and dietary supplement questionnaire. Median energy intake (interquartile range) varied from 2159 kcal/day (1717–2437) in 11–13 years old females to 2905 kcal/day (2291–3483) in 14–18 years old males. Carbohydrate and protein intakes were 8.1 (6.1–10.5); 2.4 (1.6–3.4) in males 11–13 years, 5.7 (4.5–7.9); 2.0 (1.4–2.6) in females 11–13 years, 5.3 (4.3–7.4); 2.0 (1.5–2.4) in males 14–18 y and 4.9 (4.4–6.2); 1.7 (1.3–2.0) in females 14–18 years g/kg of body weight respectively. Median vitamin D intakes were below the recommended dietary allowance (RDA) and potassium was below the adequate intake (AI) for all athlete groups. Females 14–18 years had intakes below the RDA for iron 91% (72–112), folate 89% (61–114) and calcium 84% (48–106). Multivitamin-multiminerals, vitamin C, vitamin D, vitamin-enriched water, protein powder, sport foods, fatty acids, probiotics, and plant extracts were popular supplements. Canadian pre-adolescent and adolescent athletes could improve their dietary intakes by focusing on food sources of calcium, vitamin D, potassium, iron, and folate. With the exceptions of vitamin D and carbohydrates during long exercise sessions, supplementation is generally unnecessary.

Keywords: diet analysis; youth athletes; nutrient intakes; dietary supplements; ergogenic aids

1. Introduction

Young athletes experience numerous nutritional challenges including: Meeting nutrient needs for growth, training/competition, the maintenance of health, concurrent sporting pursuits, challenging schedules (school, training, socializing, work, etc.), a lack of knowledge, a reliance on others for the purchase and preparation of foods, unhealthy eating environments in their locations of training and competition, and travel [1–4]. Additionally, the eating patterns and attitudes towards foods, set during adolescence, can impact an individual's lifelong relationship with food and nutrition [1]. Currently, targeted recommendations for youth are lacking, forcing the default use of adult recommendations.

Nutrient needs during adolescence are relatively high as compared to adulthood to support development [5] and these athletes require reliable guidance to ensure health and the prevention of injuries as they progress in their sporting endeavors. Dietary intakes in young athletes have been found to be superior to their non-athletic counterparts [6–8]. Conversely, the increased demands of intense physical activity imply that the consequences of a deficiency are greater in this demographic.

Furthermore, young athletes may have increased nutrient needs suggesting a direct comparison to intakes in non-athletes does not accurately represent the physiological impact of their dietary intakes. In young athletes, nutrients identified as of concern due to insufficient intakes include: Carbohydrates (especially during exercise), vitamin E, vitamin D, calcium, iron, magnesium, and zinc [5,9–11]. There is also a concern that the pressures associated with athletic performance can promote eating disorders with increased rates typically found in adult elite athletes as compared to non-athletes [12]. The role of sport in fostering eating disorders in youth is controversial with some finding a protective effect in young, female athletes as compared to non-athletes [13]. Additional investigation is required though it appears that the level of competition and sport type are critical with an increased risk in elite athletes as compared to recreational level athletes and those competing in sports that encourage leanness [13,14].

Few studies have evaluated the dietary patterns of young Canadian athletes, particularly those participating in sport at the community/provincial level. The primary aim of this study was to quantify dietary intakes in young Canadian athletes, from a wide variety of sports, competing primarily at the community or provincial level. A secondary aim was to evaluate dietary supplement use in the contexts of nutrient needs, health, and performance.

2. Materials and Methods

2.1. Participants

Male (n = 84) and female (n = 103) athletes aged 11 to 18 years were recruited from the province of Alberta through sporting communities and the public school system. The term "athlete" was defined as competing at the city level or higher and training ≥5 h per week. A sample size of 150 allowed the reporting of estimates to a margin of error of no more than 8% with a 95% confidence level [15].

2.2. Procedures

Athletes and/or their parents/guardians completed the Food Behaviour Questionnaire (FBQ). The FBQ is a web-based 24-h diet recall developed by Canadian researchers for diet analysis in youth [16]. Sport drinks were included in the questionnaire; however, other sport foods and supplements were not included, as they could not be linked to the Canadian Nutrient File for analysis. Questions regarding meal timing and training/competition were added to the FBQ. Basal metabolic rate (BMR) was calculated by the Schofield equation and participants with energy intake/BMR ≤0.89 were classified as low energy reporters [17] and removed from analyses.

A dietary supplement questionnaire [18] was incorporated into the FBQ and included sport foods, vitamin/mineral supplements, fatty acid supplements, plant extracts, probiotics, and ergogenic aids. All questionnaires were previously tested for reliability and validity [16,18]; however, the dietary supplement questionnaire was originally delivered in a face-to-face manner. Consequently, the electronic format was tested for reliability in a subset of 21 athletes who completed both a paper and electronic version. Weighted kappa coefficients [19] found questions had fair to moderate agreement with the exception of frequency of use for vitamin E, vitamin-enriched water, glutamine, sport drinks, recovery drinks, probiotics, sport gels/gummies, and caffeine pills.

2.3. Ethical Considerations

Individualized access information for the consent form and questionnaire was sent to the parent's/guardian's email account (except for those 18 years of age). Parental consent and athlete assent was provided electronically prior to commencing the questionnaire. The Mount Royal University Human Research Ethics Board (2013-19) and a school board (2013 1127 L) approved the study.

2.4. Statistical Analyses

Athletes were categorized based on Dietary Reference Intakes (DRIs): Male 11–13 years, female 11–13 years, male 14–18 years, and female 14–18 years. Estimated energy requirements (EER) were determined using the Institute of Medicine's EER equations and an "active" value for physical activity [20] (pp. 181–182). For macronutrient intakes, absolute values, intakes adjusted for body weight, and percent of total energy intake were calculated. Micronutrients are presented as absolute values and the percent of the Recommended Dietary Allowance (RDA) or Adequate Intake (AI). Percent RDA or AI was calculated by taking the intake for each athlete and dividing it by the established RDA or AI for that age and gender [21] and multiplying by 100. Supplement use was quantified as the percent of respondents who consumed the supplement Regularly, Occasionally ("Specific Times" or "I've Tried It"), and Never ("Never" or "Unfamiliar"). Data was checked for normality using the Shapiro-Wilk test. Differences for macronutrients in the percent of total calories and g/kg/body weight and micronutrient percent of Recommended Dietary Allowance (%RDA) or Adequate Intake (%AI) [21] were determined using a Kruskal–Wallis non-parametric test and difference between genders and age groups were assessed using Dunn's test for post-hoc pairwise comparisons. In cases where the data was normally distributed, a one-way ANOVA with a Bonferroni post-hoc comparison within age and gender was also calculated. Differences in percent of athletes meeting Canada's Food Guide [22] servings and dietary supplement/ergogenic aids use were determined using a Pearson's Chi-squared test and the effect size reported as V = Cramer's V. A p-value of < 0.05 was considered to be statistically significant. All analyses were performed using SPSS version 22 (IBM Corporation, Armonk, NY, USA) and Stata 14 (StataCorp, College Station, TX, USA).

3. Results

3.1. Participant Characteristics

The FBQ was completed by 187 participants, however, two females 11–13 years, two males 11–13 years, 12 females 14–18 years, and three males 14–18 years were identified as low-energy reporters and were removed from the analyses. Descriptive characteristics for the remaining 168 participants who completed the FBQ are presented in Table 1. Eight percent of young females, 15% of older females, 4% of young males, and 0% of older males reported trying to lose weight (p = 0.030; V = 0.204), whereas 3% of young females, 0% of older females, 15% of young males, and 42% of older males reported trying to gain weight (p < 0.001; V = 0.381). Energy intakes as a percent of EER were 98% (83–125) in 11–13 years old males, 91% (76–112) in 11–13 years old females, 85% (70–107) in 14–18 years old males, and 89% (73–104) in 14–18 years old females; there were no statistically significant differences between the groups.

3.2. Nutrient Intakes

Macronutrient intakes are presented in Table 2. Younger males had greater carbohydrate intakes based on body weight as compared to older males (p = 0.001) and older females (p < 0.001). Protein intakes based on body weight were highest in young males and greater as compared to older females (p < 0.001) and older males (p = 0.046), however the dietary assessment did not include protein supplements. The percent of calories coming from sugar and fats was consistent across all groups, however, based on body weight, young males had greater intakes of total fat as compared to older females (p < 0.001).

Micronutrient intakes are described in Table 3. Athletes' median intakes met or exceeded the RDA for all vitamins with the exception of vitamin D, folate (14–18 years females) and vitamin A (females 11–13 years and males 14–18 years). Females did not consume the RDA for calcium and older females did not meet the RDA for iron. Athletes did not meet the AI for potassium. Sodium intakes exceeded the upper limit in 89% of males 11–13 years, 65% of females 11–13 years, 83% of males 14–18 years, and 69% of females 14–18 years (p = 0.061; V = 0.209).

Servings according to Eating Well with Canada's Food Guide can be found in Table 4. Differences between the groups were noted in milk and alternatives where older females had the fewest percent of participants meeting the recommendation (p = 0.010; V = 0.259) and in the meat and alternatives where older males had a lower percent meeting the recommendations (p = 0.002; V = 0.294).

Table 1. Descriptive characteristics.

Descriptive Characteristics	All	Males 11–13 Years	Females 11–13 Years	Males 14–18 Years	Females 14–18 Years
Participants	168	26	37	53	52
Age years	14 (13–16)	12 (11–13)	13(12–13)	15 (15–16)	15 (14.5–17)
Weight kg	56 (12.9)	47 (9.9)	46 (8.7)	67 (12.2)	57 (7.2)
Height m	1.7 (1.6–1.8)	1.6 (1.5–1.6)	1.6 (1.5–1.6)	1.8 (1.8–1.9)	1.7 (1.6–1.7)
BMI kg/m^2	19.9 (18.3–21.7)	18.5 (16.9–19.9)	18.7 (17.7–20.6)	21.2 (19.6–22.2)	20.5 (19.0–21.9)
Level of Competition					
Club	55	7	14	21	13
Provincial	60	16	19	10	15
National	33	0	3	15	15
International	20	3	1	7	9
Sport Classification					
Endurance	42	5	9	13	15
Intermittent	69	7	16	26	20
Aesthetic	24	1	11	1	11
Power/Strength	33	13	1	13	6
Response Rate					
Total Assigned ID	327				
Food Recall	187 (57%)				
Low Energy Reporters	19 (10%)	2 (7%)	2 (5%)	3 (5%)	12 (19%)
Dietary Supplements	173 (53%)				

Descriptive characteristics are provided for all participants that reported adequate energy intakes on their Food Behaviour Questionnaire. Age, height, and BMI are median (interquartile range) and weight is mean (standard deviation). Values in "[]" under "Response Rate" refer to the percent of participants who completed the food recall and dietary supplement portions of the questionnaire, as well as those who were removed because they were low energy reporters [17].

Table 2. Reported energy and macronutrient intakes.

Nutrient	Male 11–13 (n = 26)	Female 11–13 (n = 37)	Male 14–18 (n = 53)	Female 14–18 (n = 52)	p
Energy kcal/day	2745 (2165–3555)	2159 (1717–2437)	2905 (2291–3483)	2177 (1764–2540)	
Carbohydrates g/day	386 (282–442)	264 (207–344)	353 (282–464)	281 (218–333)	0.435
Carbohydrates %kcal *	56 (45–61)	54 (49–59)	52 (42–56)	52 (47–59)	<0.001
Carbohydrates g/kg BW	8.1 (6.1–10.5)	5.7 (4.5–7.9) [a]	5.3 (4.3–7.4) [b]	4.9 (4.4–6.2) [c]	<0.001
Fibre g	25 (20–35)	19 (14–28)	25 (18–33)	23 (19–29)	
Sugar g	144 (115–191)	93 (71–146)	146 (109–183)	106 (81–145)	
Sugar % kcal *	24 (17–28)	20 (16–26)	20 (16–26)	22 (17–25)	0.741
Protein g/day	114 (82–162)	94 (67–112)	123 (104–159)	97 (76–113)	0.660
Protein %kcal	16 (13–20)	16 (15–19)	17 (15–21)	17 (14–20)	
Protein g/kg BW	2.4 (1.6–3.4)	2.0 (1.4–2.6)	2.0 (1.5–2.4) [b]	1.7 (1.3–2.0) [c]	<0.001
Fat g/day	92 (79–128)	72 (53–95)	108 (88–133)	79 (60–102)	
Fat %kcal *	33 (26–38)	31 (26–36)	33 (28–40)	33 (28–39)	0.700
Fat g/kg BW	2.2 (1.4–2.7)	1.7 (1.2–2.1)	1.7 (1.3–2.1)	1.4 (1.1–1.8) [c]	0.002
Saturated Fat g	33 (27–43)	23 (18–32)	38 (18–47)	24 (17–34)	
Saturated Fat %kcal *	11 (9–13)	10 (8–13)	11 (9–14)	11 (8–14)	0.723
MUFAs g	29 (23–42)	25 (16–33)	35 (29–42)	23 (18–30)	
PUFAs g	13 (9–23)	11 (7–18)	17 (13–24)	12 (9–18)	
Trans Fat g	0.5 (0.1–1.1)	0.2 (0.1–0.9)	0.5 (0.2–0.9)	0.1 (0–0.5)	
Cholesterol g	315 (174–484)	253 (105–388)	408 (271–629)	255 (176–393)	

Intakes are presented as median (interquartile range). BW, body weight; kcal, kilocalories; MUFAs, monounsaturated fatty acids; and PUFA, polyunsaturated fatty acids. Significant differences in %kcal and g/kg/BW were determined by a Kruskal-Wallis non-parametric test and [a] difference between age groups within gender; [b] difference between genders within age group; [c] difference between age group within gender; and [c] difference between genders within different age groups were assessed using Dunn's test for post-hoc pairwise comparisons. Variables with * are normally distributed thus an ANOVA was also performed and the differences remained non-significant.

Table 3. Micronutrient intakes from food sources.

Nutrient	Male 11–13 (n = 26)	Females 11–13 (n = 37)	Males 14–18 (n = 53)	Female 14–18 (n = 52)	p
Thiamin mg/day	1.9 (1.4–2.3)	1.4 (1.0–1.8)	2.1 (1.6–3.0)	1.6 (1.1–2.1)	0.073
%RDA	203 (140–240)	155 (112–204)	175 (137–246)	156 (113–213)	
Riboflavin mg/day	2.9 (2.2–3.9)	2.1 (1.6–3.0)	3.4 (2.6–4.1)	2.1 (1.4–2.7)	<0.001
%RDA	317 (248–434)	237 (182–336) [a]	258 (200–314) [b]	207 (143–271) [a,c]	
Niacin mg/day	40 (30–59)	33 (24–43)	45 (37–63)	37 (24–45)	0.024
%RDA	335 (250–494)	274 (200–359)	282 (230–393)	264 (173–325) [c]	
Vitamin B6 mg/day	2.1 (1.4–3.2)	1.3 (1.0–1.9)	2.4 (1.6–3.1)	1.6 (1.2–2.3)	0.002
%RDA	208 (142–315)	133 (104–193) [a]	185 (127–238)	132 (103–192) [a,c]	
Folate µg/day	412 (314–651)	309 (260–382)	486 (339–642)	357 (244–457)	<0.001
%RDA	138 (105–217)	103 (87–127) [a]	122 (85–161)	89 (61–114) [a,c]	
Vitamin B12 µg/day	5.5 (3.6–8.4)	4.0 (2.5–5.9)	7.5 (4.2–10.3)	3.5 (2.3–5.6)	<0.001
%RDA	303 (198–465)	223 (137–326)	313 (174–429)	147 (95–233) [a,b,c]	
Vitamin C mg/day	160 (65–262)	97 (54–141)	143 (81–279)	164 (105–240)	0.187
%RDA	356 (143–583)	216 (119–313)	191 (107–372)	252 (161–369)	
Vitamin D µg/day	8.4 (4.7–16.4)	4.3 (1.4–7.4)	9.2 (5.7–15.2)	3.1 (1.7–6.3)	<0.001
%RDA	56 (31–109)	29 (10–49) [a]	62 (38–101) [c]	21 (11–42) [a,c]	
Vitamin A RAE µg/day	933 (651–1191)	463 (287–842)	864 (702–1121)	697 (353–1065)	0.005
%RDA	156 (108–199)	77 (48–140) [a]	96 (78–125) [b]	100 (50–152) [c]	
Calcium mg/day	1419 (1113–2233)	1040 (715–1492)	1686 (1169–2251)	1090 (625–1377)	<0.001
%RDA	109 (86–172)	80 (55–115) [a]	130 (90–173) [c]	84 (48–106) [a,c]	
Iron mg/day	18 (12–20)	13 (10–17)	18 (15–22)	14 (11–17)	<0.001
%RDA	228 (150–250)	166 (130–211)	165 (137–195)	91 (72–112) [a,b,c]	
Zinc mg/day	14 (10–16)	10 (7–13)	15 (12–18)	9 (7–13)	<0.001
%RDA	177 (121–204)	121 (88–167) [a]	138 (107–166)	103 (79–140) [a,c]	
Potassium mg/day	3934 (3156–5150)	2534 (2125–3716)	4292 (3483–5012)	3240 (2274–3940)	<0.001
%AI	87 (70–114)	56 (47–83) [a]	91 (73–107) [c]	69 (48–84) [a,c]	
Sodium mg/day	3476 (2648–4573)	2701 (2089–3388)	3651 (2967–4676)	2928 (2144–3564)	<0.001
%AI	232 (177–305)	180 (139–226) [a]	243 (198–312) [c]	195 (143–238) [a]	

Intakes are median (interquartile range). Percent RDA or AI for each athlete was calculated by taking their intake and dividing it by the established RDA or AI for that age and gender [21] and multiplying by 100. Significant differences in percent RDA or AI were determined by a Kruskal–Wallis non-parametric test and [a] difference between genders within age group; [b] difference between age group within gender; and [c] difference between genders within different age groups were assessed using Dunn's test for post-hoc pairwise comparisons.

Table 4. Canada's Food Guide servings.

Nutrient	Male 11–13 (n = 26)	Female 11–13 (n = 37)	Male 14–18 (n = 53)	Female 14–18 (n = 52)	p
Vegetables and Fruits	6.5 (4.0–10.0)	4.0 (3.0–7.0)	7.0 (4.0–9.0)	7.0 (5.0–9.0)	
Met %	62 (n = 16)	35 (n = 13)	40 (n = 21)	54 (n = 28)	0.093
Grains	9.0 (6.0–11.0)	6.0 (4.0–9.0)	8.0 (6.0–11.0)	7.0 (5.0–8.0)	
Met %	81 (n = 21)	65 (n = 24)	68 (n = 36)	65 (n = 34)	0.516
Milk and Alt.	3.0 (3.0–6.0)	3.0 (2.0–4.0)	4.0 (3.0–6.0)	2.0 (1.0–3.5)	
Met %	77 (n = 20)	57 (n = 21)	76 (n = 40)	48 (n = 25)	**0.010**
Meat and Alt.	3.0 (1.0–3.0)	3.0 (2.0–3.0)	3.0 (2.0–5.0)	3.0 (2.0–3.0)	
Met %	89 (n = 23)	89 (n = 33)	59 (n = 31)	77 (n = 40)	**0.002**
Other	4.0 (2.0–6.0)	3.0 (2.0–6.0)	4.0 (3.0–6.0)	3.5 (2.0–6.5)	
Met %	N/A	N/A	N/A	N/A	

Eating Well with Canada's Food Guide [22] servings are presented as median (interquartile range). Percent met was calculated as the percent of athletes meeting the minimum recommended daily amounts. Significant differences in the percent of athletes in the groups meeting the minimum recommendations were determined by a Pearson's Chi-squared test.

3.3. Supplements

The use of dietary supplements and ergogenic aids is presented as those who consume the supplement regularly, occasionally, or never (Table 5). Given the broad definition of dietary supplements and the inclusion of occasional use over the past 3 months, 100% of athletes reported some usage. Multivitamin-multiminerals, vitamin C, vitamin D, sport bars, and protein powders were the most commonly consumed supplements on a regular basis. Supplements athletes frequently reported using occasionally included vitamin C, vitamin-enriched water, protein powders, sport bars and drinks, plant extracts, and gels/gummies. When supplement use was analyzed according to gender alone, differences were noted in fatty acid intakes with 17% of males reporting regular use, 5% occasional use and 78% never, whereas females reported regular use at 8%, occasional use at 15% and never at 77% ($p = 0.045$; V = 0.189). Furthermore, 18% of males used sport drinks regularly, 69% occasionally and 13% never as compared to females at 7% regularly, 70% occasionally, and 23% never ($p = 0.040$; V = 0.193). Analysis by age groups 11–13 years and 14–18 years found increased use of protein powder in the older age group with regular use 18%, occasional 45%, and never 37% vs. 10% regular, 23% occasional, and 68% never in 11–13 years ($p = 0.001$; V = 0.296). None of the athletes reported regular use of energy drinks, however, 14–18 years old had occasional use at 27% vs. 3% in 11–13 years ($p < 0.001$; V = 0.294). There were no other significant differences between gender or age groups in supplement use.

Table 5. Dietary supplements and ergogenic aids.

Supplement % Athletes	Males 11–13 (n = 26)			Females 11–13 (n = 36)			Males 14–18 (n = 52)			Females 14–18 (n = 59)			
	R	O	N	R	O	N	R	O	N	R	O	N	p
MVMM	46	15	39	36	19	44	40	19	40	22	27	51	0.346
B Vitamins	0	8	92	6	6	89	6	17	77	3	10	86	0.482
Vitamin C	15	23	62	19	31	50	27	23	50	19	27	54	0.862
Vitamin E	0	4	96	3	11	86	2	6	92	3	12	85	0.747
Vitamin D *	19	0	81	19	3	78	14	0	87	24	0	76	0.453
Vitamin Water	8	39	54	3	61	36	10	46	44	7	48	46	0.629
Iron	0	0	100	3	3	94	2	6	92	5	12	83	0.251
Calcium	0	0	100	6	8	86	8	10	83	3	7	90	0.471
Magnesium	0	4	96	3	3	94	2	6	92	0	2	98	0.735
Protein Powder	12	19	69	8	25	67	25	42	33	12	48	41	**0.004**
Beta Alanine	4	0	96	0	0	100	0	6	94	0	0	100	**0.047**
BCAA	4	0	96	3	0	97	2	6	92	3	2	95	0.598
Glutamine	4	0	96	0	0	100	0	4	96	0	2	98	0.230
Glucosamine	0	0	100	0	0	100	2	4	94	0	5	95	0.495
Fatty Acids	19	8	73	17	11	72	15	4	81	3	17	80	0.090
Sport Drink	15	65	19	8	69	22	19	71	10	7	70	24	0.264
Recovery Drink	15	8	77	0	14	86	4	23	73	5	17	78	0.109
Energy Drink	0	4	96	0	3	97	0	33	67	0	22	78	**0.001**
Sport Bar	15	46	39	14	69	17	33	50	17	25	51	24	0.110
Creatine	4	0	96	0	0	100	2	8	90	2	0	98	0.092
Caffeine	0	0	100	0	0	100	0	2	98	0	0	100	0.505
Gel/Gummy	8	46	46	0	47	53	2	29	69	0	37	63	0.079
Plant Extracts	4	31	65	3	39	58	2	31	67	3	37	59	0.968
Probiotics	4	19	77	3	19	78	0	14	87	0	20	80	0.559

Dietary supplement use is presented as percent of athletes who completed the dietary supplement portion of the questionnaire (n = 173). * Vitamin D was determined from responses to "Other Vitamins". MVMM, multivitamin-multimineral; BCAA, branched chain amino acids; R, regularly; O, occasionally; and N, never. Significant differences in the percent of athletes in the groups consuming the supplement were determined by a Pearson's Chi-squared test.

4. Discussion

This research is significant as it analyzes dietary intakes and supplement use across a broad range of sport types in a cohort of younger, understudied athletes. Studies focused on a single sport are extremely valuable to the cohort of athletes they represent, however, are less able to provide information regarding general nutrition concerns.

4.1. Overall Diet Quality and Energy Intakes

Adolescents typically adhere to a dietary pattern that is energy dense, however, low in nutrients [23]. Conversely, studies do report improved dietary intakes in adolescent athletic populations as compared to their sedentary peers [6–8]. Athletes have increased rates of disordered eating as compared to non-athletes, however, this concerns is more applicable to older athletes competing at higher levels than the majority of our sample [12]. Notably, the decline in diet quality in our female 14–18 years cohort, as compared to other groups, could be indicative of a trend towards increased rates of disordered eating; coaches and parents should carefully monitor this group. When athletes self-reported on the quality of their diet, 3% thought their diet was poor, 72% rated their diet as average, and 25% selected excellent.

Assessment of the athletes' Canada's Food Guide servings can provide an understanding of overall diet quality, however, Canada's Food Guide does not take into consideration high levels of physical activity. Consequently, it is possible that Table 4 underestimates the percentage of athletes consuming insufficient numbers of servings. It can reasonably be concluded that milk and alternatives is a food category of concern for young female athletes, a risk that increases with age. Furthermore, all athletes need to be encouraged to consume more vegetables and fruits. Another factor, potentially limiting performance in some athletes, may be inadequate intakes of whole grains, as grains are often good sources of carbohydrates, food folic acid, and iron. The relatively high contribution of sugars and saturated fats to total calories and servings from the "other" category, suggest young athletes need to focus on healthier choices and reducing processed and fast foods. A conclusion further supported by the high sodium intakes.

Energy intakes are slightly lower than the EER. An energy deficit is commonly reported in athletes [5,24,25], however, it is extremely difficult to accurately assess energy needs in young athletes [1] and self-reported dietary records are limited. Furthermore, BMI data indicates that underweight is not a prominent concern in this cohort of athletes.

4.2. Macronutrients

It is difficult to assess the adequacy of macronutrient intakes in young athletes due to a lack of recommendations and a default to adult values [26,27]. Carbohydrate recommendations based on body weight rather than percent of total calories are thought to best reflect athlete needs and range from 3 to 12 g/kg/BW depending on exercise load [28]. Carbohydrate intakes meet the minimum requirements in all our athlete groups. Importantly, when carbohydrate intakes were analyzed by sport type, endurance and intermittent athletes had median intakes of 5.5 g/kg/BW; whereas, aesthetic and power athletes had higher intakes at 6.2 g/kg/BW and 5.8 g/kg/BW respectively. Therefore, it may be advisable to emphasize carbohydrates for young endurance athletes. Inadequate carbohydrate intake in young athletes has been noted in other studies [5,11,26,27]. Dietary fibre intakes did not meet recommendations, suggesting that information on the quantity and quality of carbohydrates should be provided.

Protein recommendations have recently increased and range from 1.2 to 2.0 g/kg/BW depending on the type and amount of physical activity [29]. Furthermore, it has been estimated that protein intakes of 1.5 g/kg BW are required for nitrogen balance in young sprinters [30] and can, therefore, be assumed sufficient for most young athletes. Average protein intakes, from food alone, exceeded the upper recommendation for performance in all groups except 14–18 years old females, suggesting that this is not a nutrient of concern for young Canadian athletes; a finding supported by others [26,27]. Data in young, elite Canadian soccer players reports average protein intakes of 1.8 g/kg/BW [5]. Indeed, even elite, young female figure skaters reported an average protein intake of 1.2 g/kg/BW, despite total caloric intakes 44% less than their estimated needs [25]. It has been suggested that protein intakes are generally adequate or excessive because protein is overvalued among coaches and athletes [9,31].

Dietary fats ranged from 31% to 33% of total calories, which is at the high-end of the recommended 25%–35% [20]. Intakes of at least 30% have been consistently reported in adolescent athletes [1]. Young athletes may benefit from consuming fewer calories from fat and increasing calories from carbohydrates [11]. Conversely, if a young athlete were struggling to meet their caloric needs, healthy fats would be the most energy dense options.

4.3. Micronutrients

Athletes may have a greater need for select micronutrients, however, no widely accepted values are available [29]. Athletes met or exceeded the micronutrient recommendations in most cases. Notably, however, females between 14 and 18 years tended to have the lowest intakes relative to other groups, highlighting this group as higher risk. Importantly, when considering the micronutrient values as determined from 24-h recalls there is the possibility of underreporting. Underreporting was addressed in the methods by identifying low energy reporters, however could still be present to a lesser degree in the remaining sample, possibly inflating nutrient deficiencies.

Of particular apprehension in young athletes, especially females, is their ability to meet the recommendations for the bone-building nutrients such as vitamin D, calcium, and phosphorus [25]. Low bone mineral density has been reported in adolescent, female athletes, primarily those with amenorrhea [32]. Our results indicate vitamin D and calcium are of concern, with a high percentage of female athletes not meeting the RDA for these nutrients. Gibson et al. [5] also highlight vitamin D and calcium as nutrients of concern for young Canadian soccer players. The inadequate intakes of bone-related nutrients in our population may be associated with lower intakes of milk and alternatives.

Iron and folate (females 14–18 years) were also identified as nutrients where intakes often did not meet the RDA. Deficiencies in either of these nutrients can promote anemia, which can cause fatigue and suboptimal athletic performance [33]. Young female athletes are at a higher risk than their male counterparts for iron deficiencies due to losses from menses and lower energy intakes, and compared to their sedentary peers due to the increased requirements for intense training [29,33,34]. Diet assessments in other athletic populations also find inadequate intakes for iron and/or folate in young female athletes [5,10,11,25]. In Gibson et al. [5] although only 6% of athletes had iron intakes below the EAR, 89% had serum ferritin levels below 35 µg/L, a level thought to negatively impact performance.

Potassium was another nutrient where athletes did not meet the AI. Potassium has a role in muscle and nerve function and, consequently, is related to athletic performance. Although it is questionable whether intakes in the range noted here could negatively impact performance, it would still be prudent for athletes to increase their vegetable and fruit intakes to meet the Canada's Food Guide recommendations, as these foods are often good sources of potassium.

4.4. Supplements

Sport nutrition professionals agree that athletes should not use dietary supplements to compensate for a poor diet but rather consume whole foods to meet their nutrient needs. Only when this is not feasible should athletes rely on supplements [1,33].

Protein supplements were popular in our cohort; yet appear to be unnecessary given the high dietary intakes. Additionally, the need for a multivitamin-multimineral, vitamin C, and vitamin-enriched waters is questionable in the context of their nutrient intakes from food alone. Vitamin D supplementation is often recommended for athletes living at northern latitudes or training indoors and levels should be carefully monitored in young Canadian athletes to determine if supplementation is necessary [29]. Although calcium has been identified as a nutrient of concern in young female athletes, dietary changes rather than supplementation is recommended. Sport drinks, gummies, and gels could be justified during longer training sessions, as insufficient carbohydrate during exercise has been identified as a weakness in some young athletes [27]. Athletes should be cautious, however, to use these products only as needed and monitor calorie and sugar intakes [35].

Probiotics have the potential to reduce gastrointestinal symptoms and respiratory illnesses in athletes, however, additional research is needed to confirm these benefits and determine the types and effective dose [36].

Protein supplementation and energy drink consumption increased with age, a trend that we have previously reported [18]. Furthermore, others have found that dietary supplement use in youth increases with age [37]. Additional research is required to determine the reasons for these trends. However, it should be noted that the older athletes were also more likely to compete at a higher level; thus, the level of competition could be a factor, as these products are often viewed as performance-enhancing. Regardless, energy drink consumption is concerning in this demographic as they are contraindicated for those under the age of 18 years [35]. Male athletes were also more likely to use sport drinks. The reason for this is unclear, however, it may be linked to an overall concern regarding energy intake in females, as they were also more likely to be low energy reporters. Alternatively, we have previously demonstrated that young, Canadian male athletes are more likely than their female counterparts to use supplements for overall athletic performance [11] and others have found increased use in young males [37].

Our results are limited in that they are based on a single 24-h food recall and there is low reliability for a few dietary supplements, however, these limitations are somewhat offset by the large sample size. Additionally, we did not assess physical stages of maturation and it must be acknowledged that young athletes develop at different rates with considerable variation likely within the groups. The analysis was based on DRI recommendations; however, these are generalized and not specific to the individual or their athletic pursuits. Furthermore, multiple comparisons were made with a 5% level of significance, so it could be expected that up to 5% of results could be due to chance alone. Although caution should be taken when interpreting the findings, the reporting of all potentially important associations was deemed to outweigh the cost of a false positive in this case. Future research should be conducted to either refute or corroborate the findings.

5. Conclusions

Athlete support personnel should focus on food sources of vitamin D and calcium, iron, and folate (females). Supplementation is generally unnecessary, with the possible exceptions of vitamin D and iron, under physician supervision. Carbohydrate supplements should be emphasized to balance depletion versus overconsumption. Our research is novel in that, to our knowledge, it provides the first large scale, multi-sport assessment of dietary intakes in pre-adolescent and adolescent Canadian athletes. The information gained can be practically used to inform athlete support personnel regarding common trends and areas of nutritional concern in young athletes.

Acknowledgments: The Canadian Foundation of Dietetic Research funded the project. The authors would like to thank Jodi Siever for her assistance with the statistical analysis. Funds for covering the costs to publish in open access were provided by Mount Royal University.

Author Contributions: J.A.P., K.P.W., and K.A.E. conceived and designed the experiments; J.A.P. performed the experiments; J.A.P. and K.P.W. analyzed the data; J.A.P., K.P.W., and K.A.E. wrote the paper.

Conflicts of Interest: The authors declare no conflict of interest. The founding sponsors had no role in the design of the study; in the collection, analyses, or interpretation of data; in the writing of the manuscript, and in the decision to publish the results.

References

1. Desbrow, B.; McCormack, J.; Burke, L.M.; Cox, G.R.; Fallon, K.; Hislop, M.; Logan, R.; Marino, N.; Sawyer, S.M.; Shaw, G.; et al. Sports Dietitians Australia Position Statement: Sports nutrition for the adolescent athlete. *Int. J. Sport Nutr. Exerc. Metab.* **2014**, *24*, 570–584. [CrossRef] [PubMed]
2. Rosenbloom, C.A.; Loucks, A.B.; Ekblom, B. Special populations: The female player and the youth player. *J. Sports Sci.* **2006**, *24*, 783–793. [CrossRef] [PubMed]

3. Thomas, M.; Nelson, T.F.; Harwood, E.; Neumark-Sztainer, D. Exploring parent perceptions of the food environment in youth sport. *J. Nutr. Educ. Behav.* **2012**, *44*, 365–371. [CrossRef] [PubMed]
4. Walsh, M.; Cartwright, L.; Corish, C.; Sugrue, S.; Wood-Martin, R. The body composition, nutritional knowledge, attitudes, behaviors, and future education needs of senior schoolboy rugby players in Ireland. *Int. J. Sport Nutr. Exerc. Metab.* **2011**, *21*, 365–376. [CrossRef] [PubMed]
5. Gibson, J.C.; Stuart-Hill, L.; Martin, S.; Gaul, C. Nutrition status of junior elite Canadian female soccer athletes. *Int. J. Sport Nutr. Exerc. Metab.* **2011**, *21*, 507–514. [CrossRef] [PubMed]
6. Garcin, M.; Doussot, L.; Mille-Hamard, L.; Billat, V. Athletes' dietary intake was closer to French RDA's than those of young sedentary counterparts. *Nutr. Res.* **2009**, *29*, 736–742. [CrossRef] [PubMed]
7. Cavadini, C.; Decarli, B.; Grin, J.; Narring, F.; Michaud, P.-A. Food habits and sport activity during adolescence: Differences between athletic and non-athletic teenagers in Switzerland. *Eur. J. Clin. Nutr.* **2000**, *54*, S16–S20. [CrossRef] [PubMed]
8. Croll, J.K.; Neumark-Sztainer, D.; Story, M.; Wall, M.; Perry, C.; Harnack, L. Adolescents involved in weight-related and power team sports have better eating patterns and nutrient intakes than non-sport-involved adolescents. *J. Am. Diet. Assoc.* **2006**, *106*, 709–717. [CrossRef] [PubMed]
9. Juzwiak, C.R.; Amancio, O.M.S.; Vitalle, M.S.S.; Pinheiro, M.M.; Szejnfeld, V.L. Body composition and nutritional profile of male adolescent tennis players. *J. Sports Sci.* **2008**, *26*, 1209–1217. [CrossRef] [PubMed]
10. Koehler, K.; Braun, H.; Achtzehn, S.; Hildebrand, U.; Predel, H.-G.; Mester, J.; Schanzer, W. Iron status in elite young athletes: Gender-dependent influences of diet and exercise. *Eur. J. Appl. Physiol.* **2012**, *112*, 513–523. [CrossRef] [PubMed]
11. Papadopoulou, S.; Papadopoulou, S.; Gallos, G. Macro- and mico-nutrient intake of adolescent Greek female volleyball players. *Int. J. Sport Nutr. Exerc. Metab.* **2002**, *12*, 73–80. [CrossRef] [PubMed]
12. Joy, E.; Kussman, A.; Nattiv, A. 2016 update on eating disorders in athletes: A comprehensive narrative review with a focus on clinical assessment and management. *J. Sports Med.* **2016**, *50*, 154–162. [CrossRef] [PubMed]
13. Rosendahl, J.; Bormann, B.; Aschenbrenner, K.; Aschenbrenner, F.; Strauss, B. Dieting and disordered eating in German high school athletes and non-athletes. *Scand. J. Med. Sci. Sport* **2009**, *19*, 731–739. [CrossRef] [PubMed]
14. Kong, P.; Harris, L.M. The sporting body: Body image and eating disorder symptomatology among female athletes from leanness focused and nonleannes focused sports. *J. Psychol.* **2015**, *149*, 141–160. [CrossRef] [PubMed]
15. Russ Lenth's Power and Sample-Size Page. Available online: http://homepage.stat.uiowa.edu/~rlenth/Power/ (accessed on 29 July 2015).
16. Hanning, R.M.; Royall, D.; Toews, J.E.; Blashill, L.; Wegener, J.; Driezen, P. Web-Based Food Behaviour Questionnaire: Validation with grades six to eight students. *Can. J. Diet. Pract. Res.* **2009**, *70*, 172–178. [CrossRef] [PubMed]
17. Kontogianni, M.D.; Farmake, A.-E.; Vidra, N.; Sofrona, S.; Magkanari, F.; Yannakoulia, M. Associations between lifestyle patterns and body mass index in a sample of Greek children and adolescents. *J. Am. Diet. Assoc.* **2010**, *110*, 215–221. [CrossRef] [PubMed]
18. Wiens, K.; Erdman, K.A.; Stadnyk, M.; Parnell, J.A. Dietary supplement usage, motivation, and education in young Canadian athletes. *Int. J. Sport Nutr. Exerc. Metab.* **2014**, *24*, 613–622. [CrossRef] [PubMed]
19. Viera, A.J.; Garrett, J.M. Understanding interobserver agreement: The Kappa Statistic. *Fam. Med.* **2005**, *37*, 360–363. [PubMed]
20. Institute of Medicine. *Dietary Reference Intakes for Energy, Carbohydrate, Fiber, Fat, Fatty Acids, Cholesterol, Protein and Amino Acids*; National Academies Press: Washington, DC, USA, 2005; pp. 181–182.
21. Dietary Reference Intakes Tables and Application. Available online: http://iom.nationalacademies.org/Activities/Nutrition/SummaryDRIs/DRI-Tables.aspx (accessed on 25 November 2015).
22. Eating Well with Canada's Food Guide. Available online: http://www.hc-sc.gc.ca/fn-an/food-guide-aliment/index-eng.php (accessed on 25 November 2015).
23. Diethelm, K.; Jankovic, N.; Moreno, L.A.; Huybrechts, I.; De Henauw, S.; De Vriendt, T.; Gonzalez-Gross, M.; Leclercq, C.; Gottrand, F.; Gilbert, C.G.; et al. Food intake of European adolescents in the light of different food-based dietary guidelines: Results of the HELENA (Healthy Lifestyle in Europe by Nutrition in Adolescence) Study. *Public Health Nutr.* **2012**, *15*, 386–398. [CrossRef] [PubMed]

24. Aerenhouts, D.; Deriemaeker, P.; Hebbelinck, M.; Clarys, P. Energy and macronutrient intake in adolescent sprint athletes: A follow-up study. *J. Sports Sci.* **2011**, *29*, 73–82. [CrossRef] [PubMed]
25. Dwyer, J.; Eisenberg, A.; Prelack, K.; Song, W.O.; Sonneville, K.; Ziegler, P. Eating attitudes and food intakes of elite adolescent female figure skaters: A cross sectional study. *J. Int. Soc. Sports Nutr.* **2012**, *9*, 1–7. [CrossRef] [PubMed]
26. Nikic, M.; Jakovljevi, S.; Pediši, Ž.; Venus, D.; Šatali, Z. Adequacy of nutrient intakes in elite junior basketball players. *Int. J. Sport Nutr. Exerc. Metab.* **2014**, *24*, 516–523. [CrossRef] [PubMed]
27. Baker, L.B.; Heaton, L.E.; Nuccio, R.P.; Stein, K.W. Dietitian-observed macronutrient intakes of young skill and team-sport athletes: Adequacy of pre, during, and postexercise nutrition. *Int. J. Sport Nutr. Exerc. Metab.* **2014**, *24*, 166–176. [CrossRef] [PubMed]
28. Burke, L.M.; Hawley, J.A.; Wong, S.H.S.; Jeukendrup, A.E. Carbohydrates for training and competition. *J. Sports Sci.* **2011**, *29*, S17–S27. [CrossRef] [PubMed]
29. Thomas, D.T.; Erdman, K.A.; Burke, L.M. Position of the Academy of Nutrition and Dietetics, Dietitians of Canada, and the American College of Sports Medicine: Nutrition and Athletic Performance. *J. Acad. Nutr. Diet.* **2016**, *116*, 501–528. [CrossRef] [PubMed]
30. Aerenhouts, D.; Van Cauwenberg, J.; Poortmans, J.R.; Hauspie, R.; Clarys, P. Influence of growth rate on nitrogen balance in adolescent sprint athletes. *Int. J. Sport Nutr. Exerc. Metab.* **2013**, *23*, 409–417. [CrossRef] [PubMed]
31. Juzwiak, C.R.; Ancona-Lopez, F. Evaluation of nutrition knowledge and dietary recommendations by coaches of adolescent Brazilian athletes. *Int. J. Sport Nutr. Exerc. Metab.* **2004**, *14*, 222–235. [CrossRef] [PubMed]
32. Nichols, J.F.; Rauh, M.J.; Barrack, M.T.; Barkai, H.-S. Bone mineral density in female high school athletes: Interactions of menstrual function and type of mechanical loading. *Bone* **2007**, *41*, 371–377. [CrossRef] [PubMed]
33. American Dietetic Association; Dietitians of Canada; American College of Sports Medicine. Nutrition and athletic performance. *Med. Sci. Sports Exerc.* **2009**, *41*, 709–731.
34. Nielsen, P.; Nachtigall, D. Iron supplementation in athletes. Current recommendations. *Sport Med.* **1998**, *26*, 207–216. [CrossRef]
35. Committee on Nutrition and the Council on Sports Medicine and Fitness. Sports drinks and energy drinks for children and adolescents: Are they appropriate? *Pediatrics* **2011**, *127*, 1182–1189.
36. Pyne, D.B.; West, N.P.; Cox, A.J.; Cripps, A.W. Probiotics supplementation for athletes-clinical and physiological effects. *Eur. J. Sport Sci.* **2015**, *15*, 63–72. [CrossRef] [PubMed]
37. Evans, M.J.; Ndetan, H.; Perko, M.; Willimas, R.; Walker, C. Dietary supplement use by children and adolescents in the United States to enhance sport performance: Results of the National Health Interview Survey. *J. Prim. Prev.* **2012**, *33*, 3–12. [CrossRef] [PubMed]

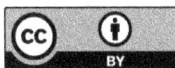

nutrients

MDPI

Article

Effects of a Short-Term High-Nitrate Diet on Exercise Performance

Simone Porcelli [1,*], Lorenzo Pugliese [1], Enrico Rejc [2], Gaspare Pavei [3], Matteo Bonato [4], Michela Montorsi [1,5], Antonio La Torre [4], Letizia Rasica [1,4] and Mauro Marzorati [1,6]

[1] Institute of Molecular Bioimaging and Physiology, National Research Council, Segrate 20090, Italy; lorenz.pugliese@gmail.com (L.P.); michela.montorsi@unisanraffaele.gov.it (M.Mo.); letizia.rasica@ibfm.cnr.it (L.R.); mauro.marzorati@ibfm.cnr.it (M.Ma.)
[2] Department of Neurological Surgery, Kentucky Spinal Cord Research Center, University of Louisville, Louisville, KY 40202, USA; enricorejc@kentuckyonehealth.org
[3] Department of Pathophysiology and Transplantation, Università degli Studi di Milano, Milano 20100, Italy; gaspare.pavei@unimi.it
[4] Department of Biomedical Sciences for Health, Università degli Studi di Milano, Milano 20100, Italy; matteo.bonato@unimi.it (M.B.); antonio.latorre@unimi.it (A.L.T.)
[5] Department of Human Sciences and Promotion of Quality of Life, Telematic University S. Raffaele, Roma 00166, Italy
[6] Department of Psychology, Exercise and Sport Science Degree Course, Catholic University of the Sacred Heart, Milan 20100, Italy
* Correspondence: simone.porcelli@ibfm.cnr.it; Tel.: +39-02-2171-7220

Received: 1 August 2016; Accepted: 24 August 2016; Published: 31 August 2016

Abstract: It has been reported that nitrate supplementation can improve exercise performance. Most of the studies have used either beetroot juice or sodium nitrate as a supplement; there is lack of data on the potential ergogenic benefits of an increased dietary nitrate intake from a diet based on fruits and vegetables. Our aim was to assess whether a high-nitrate diet increases nitric oxide bioavailability and to evaluate the effects of this nutritional intervention on exercise performance. Seven healthy male subjects participated in a randomized cross-over study. They were tested before and after 6 days of a high (HND) or control (CD) nitrate diet (~8.2 mmol·day^{-1} or ~2.9 mmol·day^{-1}, respectively). Plasma nitrate and nitrite concentrations were significantly higher in HND (127 ± 64 μM and 350 ± 120 nM, respectively) compared to CD (23 ± 10 μM and 240 ± 100 nM, respectively). In HND (vs. CD) were observed: (a) a significant reduction of oxygen consumption during moderate-intensity constant work-rate cycling exercise (1.178 ± 0.141 vs. 1.269 ± 0.136 L·min^{-1}); (b) a significantly higher total muscle work during fatiguing, intermittent sub-maximal isometric knee extension (357.3 ± 176.1 vs. 253.6 ± 149.0 Nm·s·kg^{-1}); (c) an improved performance in Repeated Sprint Ability test. These findings suggest that a high-nitrate diet could be a feasible and effective strategy to improve exercise performance.

Keywords: nitric oxide; oxygen cost of exercise; intermittent high-intensity exercise; diet

1. Introduction

Nitric oxide (NO) is a gaseous signaling molecule linked to a variety of physiological functions in mammalian cells, including the regulation of blood flow, mitochondrial biogenesis, excitation–contraction coupling, calcium handling, oxidative stress, and skeletal muscle repair [1]. NO is produced endogenously via the L-arginine-NO pathway by the nitric oxide synthase (NOS) enzymes in nervous tissue, the cardiovascular system (by the endothelium), and skeletal muscle [2,3]. However, an alternative source of NO has recently been described [4]. In fact, inorganic nitrate (NO_3^-), ingested from dietary sources (e.g., beetroot) or pharmacologic compounds (e.g., sodium/potassium nitrate), can be reduced in vivo to nitrite (NO_2^-) and subsequently converted to NO by numerous NO_2^- reductases [5].

A growing body of evidence demonstrates that acute (2–3 h) and short term (3–6 days) pharmacological (e.g., sodium/potassium nitrate) or dietary (e.g., beetroot juice) NO_3^- supplementation reduces whole body oxygen cost during moderate-intensity exercise, and improves exercise tolerance—at least in sedentary or moderately-trained subjects [6–12]. Given that the alternative NO_3^-–NO_2^-–NO pathway seems to increase NO bioavailability, especially in an acidic environment and in relatively hypoxic tissues [13], human studies have also been conducted in order to assess whether NO_3^- supplementation positively affects muscle contraction properties at higher exercise intensities, when muscle PO_2 and pH decline to a greater extent [14].

On the other side, it has been observed that maximal voluntary or involuntary (electrically evoked) isometric contraction, force–frequency relationship, and fatigability of quadriceps muscles are substantially unchanged following 4 days [15], 7 days [16], or 15 days [17] of NO_3^- supplementation. At the same time, nitrate supplementation has unclear effects on high-intensity intermittent activities. Although some studies have found an improvement of high-intensity intermittent performance following NO_3^- supplementation [18–21], others have failed to observe a positive effect [22,23]. The reasons for these controversial results may be attributed to differences in duration and dose of the supplementation scheme, in the exercise protocols employed [24], and in the individual aerobic fitness level of the participants.

So far, most of the studies that have investigated the ergogenic effects of dietary nitrate supplementation have used either beetroot juice or sodium nitrate. To our knowledge, only one study has evaluated the effects of a dietary intervention (acute whole baked beetroot assumption) on exercise performance [25]. Since recent studies have demonstrated that a high-nitrate vegetable diet can increase plasma NO_3^- and NO_2^- concentrations to similar level of beetroot or nitrate salt ingestion [26,27], this form of NO_3^- supplementation could represent an alternative dietary intervention able to positively affect exercise performance.

The aim of this study was to test the hypothesis that a diet containing NO_3^--rich vegetables increases plasma NO_3^- and NO_2^- concentrations and positively influences exercise performance. In particular, we expect that a diet high in NO_3^- can reduce the oxygen cost of exercise at moderate intensity and increase muscle performance during high-intensity intermittent activities.

2. Materials and Methods

2.1. Subjects

In this randomized crossover study, seven healthy males recreationally involved in basketball, badminton, and futsal (mean ± SD; age, 25 ± 2 years; body mass, 66.3 ± 6.0 kg; height, 1.74 ± 0.05 m) volunteered to participate in this study. Considering the standard deviations (SDs) of circulating nitrate levels based upon our previous findings [11], this *n* value allowed the detection of significant differences between groups (if present) with an alpha level of 0.05 and a beta level of 0.20 (Prism 6.0, GraphPad Software, La Jolla, CA, USA). Before the start of the study, participants underwent a complete medical screening (medical history, physical examination, and resting electrocardiogram) to ensure that there were no contraindications to study participation. An incremental cycle ergometer test up to exhaustion was also performed for the determination of peak oxygen consumptio ($\dot{V}O_2$ peak) and peak work rate (41.2 ± 4.7 mL·kg^{-1}·min^{-1}; 226 ± 49 W). All subjects gave their written informed consent to participate after the experimental procedures, associated risks, and potential benefits of participation had been explained. All procedures were in accordance with the recommendations found in the Declaration of Helsinki (2000) of the World Medical Association.

2.2. Study Design

Individual subjects' diet was recorded during a 7 day period, before the experimental phase. NO_3^- usual intake was estimated considering vegetable and fruit intake, according to reference tables [28]. Then, a nutritionist elaborated two diet schemes: a control diet (CD), with a NO_3^- intake similar to that usually ingested, and a diet with a high nitrate intake (HND). HND and CD diets were iso-energetic (about 2200 kcal) in accordance with subjects' habitual energy intake and matched to physical activity levels, and they contained a similar distribution of macronutrients (55% carbohydrates, 15% proteins, 30% fats), except for nitrate [29,30]. Fruits and vegetables ensured the different NO_3^- intake (Table 1).

Table 1. Dietary intake prescribed by the nutritionist for high-nitrate and control diet. The relative amounts of NO_3^- content for servings are also shown. CD: control diet; HND: high-nitrate diet.

CD		
Food	**Approximate Amount for Daily Servings**	**NO_3^- Content**
salad mix	180 g	2.4 mmol
broccoli	60 g	0.4 mmol
orange	150 g	0.0 mmol
cranberry juice	0.5 L	0.1 mmol
HND		
Food	**Approximate Amount for Daily Servings**	**NO_3^- Content**
raw spinach	40 g	4.8 mmol
cooked collard greens	80 g	3.2 mmol
banana	130 g	0.1 mmol
pomegranate juice	0.5 L	0.1 mmol

The intake of NO_3^- corresponded to ~8.2 mmol·day^{-1} and ~2.9 mmol·day^{-1} in HND and CD, respectively. Subjects were invited to follow the diet scheme for 6 days and were evaluated at days 5 and 6. A 20 day washout period separated the two interventions. Subjects were instructed to strictly respect the nutritionists' indications. Participants were not informed about the aims of the study and were led to believe that both interventions may be beneficial on exercise performance. Subjects were also required to abstain from using antibacterial mouthwash and chewing gum, as these are known to alter the oral bacteria responsible for the reduction of NO_3^- to NO_2^- [31].

2.3. Experimental Overview

All tests were performed at the same time of the day (± 1 h). Subjects were instructed to arrive at laboratory about 3 h postprandial and to avoid caffeine and alcohol intake and strenuous exercise in the 24 h preceding each testing session. Subjects visited the laboratory on two consecutive days at the end of both HND and CD.

On day one, subjects performed one repetition of a moderate-intensity constant work rate cycling exercise. Measures of maximal voluntary torque and total muscle work—estimated as the sum of impulses generated during fatiguing intermittent sub-maximal knee extensions—were also recorded (see below for further details). On day two, a second repetition of the moderate-intensity constant work rate cycling exercise was performed. After 30 min of rest, a cycling Repeated Sprint Ability test (RSA) was carried out (see below for further details). Prior to data collection, subjects were fully familiarized with exercise testing procedures.

2.4. Exercise Tests

Moderate intensity constant-work rate cycling exercise. An electromagnetically-braked cycle ergometer (Corival; Lode, Groningen, The Netherlands) was utilized. Subjects exercised at their freely chosen pedal frequency (80 ± 5 rpm). Each subject performed two repetitions of a 6-min constant work rate moderate-intensity exercise (CWR). Transitions from unloaded pedaling to the imposed work rate were attained in ~3 s. The work rate was chosen to correspond to 50% of peak work rate reached during the incremental test.

Isometric knee extensions. Subjects were seated on a special chair, secured by a safety belt tightened around the shoulders and abdomen, with the arms grasping handlebars and the legs hanging vertically down. A strap was tightened around the subject's dominant ankle, and was linked by a steel chain to a fixed frame. The chain length was regulated to obtain a knee angle of 110 degrees. The fixed frame was positioned behind the ankle to perform the isometric knee extensions. Subjects began the experimental session by performing a warm-up, which consisted of 20 sub-maximal isometric contractions at a self-selected intensity. After that, they performed two exercises in the same experimental session with the dominant lower limb only:

(A) Maximal voluntary contraction (MVC): subjects were asked to perform three MVCs of three-to-four seconds in duration each. To prevent fatigue, after each contraction subjects rested for two minutes. The highest force was multiplied by the moment arm in order to calculate maximal voluntary torque (MVT).

(B) Fatiguing intermittent submaximal knee extension: based on pilot studies, subjects performed intermittent isometric knee extensions of 3.5 s, with 10 s of rest between them. The target torque to reach and maintain during each contraction was set at 75% of the actual MVT (i.e., at the same relative intensity, in HND and CD). Two different auditory feedbacks were given to subjects: (1) a "ring", preceded by a countdown, determined the start and the end of each contraction; (2) a monotonic sound highlighted the reaching of the torque target level. Experimental sessions ended when subjects were not able to reach the target torque for two consecutive contractions.

Repeated Sprint Ability test (RSA). RSA consisted of five "all out" 6-second sprints on a cycle ergometer (894E, Monark Exercise AB, Vansbro, Sweden) separated by 24 s of inactive recovery [32]. Subjects pedaled in a seated position, and the mechanical resistance (F) was set at 0.74 N·kg^{-1} body mass.

2.5. Measurements

Physiological variables. Pulmonary ventilation ($\dot{V}E$), $\dot{V}O_2$, and carbon dioxide output ($\dot{V}CO_2$) were determined breath-by-breath by a computerized metabolic cart (Vmax29c; SensorMedics, Bilthoven, The Netherlands). Heart rate (HR) was determined from the electrocardiogram signal. Gain values (G)—the variable estimating the O_2 cost of cycling—were calculated as $\Delta \dot{V}O_2$ ($\dot{V}O_2$ at the end of CWR minus resting $\dot{V}O_2$) divided by work rate. Blood lactate concentration ([La]$_b$) was measured at rest and at several times during recovery on 20 µL of capillary blood obtained from a pre-heated earlobe by an enzymatic method (Biosen C-line; EKF Diagnostics GmbH, Barleben, Germany). The highest [La]$_b$ was taken as [La]$_b$ peak.

Force recording. A force sensor (TSD121C, BIOPAC Systems, Inc., Goleta, CA, USA) was connected in series to the chain, which connected the fixed frame of the special chair to the strap tightened around the subject's right ankle. Force analog output was sampled at a frequency of 1 kHz using a data acquisition system (MP100, BIOPAC Systems, Inc., Goleta, CA, USA) connected to a personal computer by means of an USB port.

Surface Electromyography (EMG) recording. EMG data were collected from the right (dominant) thigh: vastus lateralis (VL) was selected as the main knee extensor muscle. Pre-gelled surface EMG electrodes (circular contact area of 1 cm diameter, BIOPAC Systems, Inc., Goleta, CA, USA) were placed (inter-electrode distance equal to 20 mm) at two-thirds on the line from the anterior spina iliaca superior to the lateral side of the patella [33]. In order to ensure a good electrode–skin interface, prior to the application of the electrodes, the subject's skin was shaved, rubbed with an abrasive paste, and cleaned with a paper towel. EMG electrodes were placed at the beginning of the experimental session, and were not removed between the two exercises. The locations of the electrodes during the first experimental session were marked on the skin with a permanent ink pen. In order to place electrodes in the same positions prior to the second session, the subjects were asked to refresh these contours daily. To record the EMG data, the electromyography system (EMG100C, BIOPAC Systems, Inc., Goleta, CA, USA; Low Pass Filter: 500 Hz; High Pass Filter: 10 Hz; Noise Voltage (10–500 Hz): 0.2 µV (rms);

Zin: 2 M ohm; CMRR: 110 dB) was used. EMG data were sampled at a frequency of 1 kHz using a data acquisition system (MP100, BIOPAC Systems, Inc., Goleta, CA, USA), and processed using the program LabChart 7 Reader (ADInstruments Pty Ltd., Bella Vista, NSW, Australia).

Force and EMG analysis. As for MVC, a 500 ms window was centered at the maximal force exertion to calculate MVT (see above) and to analyze the surface electromyography (sEMG), its intensity being quantified by root mean square (RMS). During intermittent submaximal isometric contractions, no mechanical work is performed, so the torque-time integral (TTI) was used to estimate muscle work [34]. For each single knee extension, TTI and RMS of vastus lateralis (RMS-VL)—expressed as a percentage of maximal voluntary contraction (%MVC)—were calculated. In addition, the average value of RMS-VL calculated over the first three knee extensions was compared to the one obtained during the last three knee extensions, in order to investigate the fatigue effect on muscle activation (adapted from Mulder et al., 2007) [35].

Power recording. The power (P) values were calculated as $P = F \times d \times RPM$, where F is the resistance set ($0.74 \ N \cdot kg^{-1}$ body mass), d is the distance covered by the flywheel at each revolution, and RPM is the number of revolutions per minute. Instantaneous P values were sampled at 50 Hz and then averaged each second. Peak Power (PP) was considered the maximal value of power recorded over a second.

Blood sampling. Resting blood samples were collected to determine plasma levels of nitrate and nitrite before the experimental phase and on day 6 of both diet periods, at least 2.5 h after the last meal. Venous blood was drawn from the antecubital vein into a 5-mL EDTA Vacutainer tube (Vacutainer, Becton, Dickinson and Company, Franklin Lakes, NJ, USA). Plasma was immediately separated by centrifuge (5702R, Eppendorf, Hamburg, Germany) at $1000\times g$ for 10 min at 4 °C. Plasma samples were then ultrafiltered through a 10 kDa molecular weight cut-off filter (AmiconUltra; Millipore, EMD Millipore Corporation, Billerica, MA, USA) using an ultracentrifuge (4237R, ALC, Milan, Italy) at $14,000\times g$ for 60 min at 4 °C to reduce background absorbance due to the presence of hemoglobin. The ultrafiltered material was recovered and used to measure nitrite and nitrate concentration by the Griess method using a commercial kit (Cayman, BertinPharma, Montigny le Bretonneux, France). Samples were read by the addition of Griess reagents at 545 nm by a microplate reader spectrophotometer (Infinite M200, Tecan Group Ltd., Männedorf, Switzerland). A linear calibration curve was computed from pure nitrite and nitrate standard. All samples were determined in duplicate, and the inter-assay coefficient of variation was in the range indicated by the manufacturer.

2.6. Statistics

Data were expressed as mean ± SD. A paired *t*-test was performed on all tests data to compare HND and CD. A two-way ANOVA for repeated measures with Bonferroni correction was applied when multiple comparisons were made. The significance level was set at $p < 0.05$. Statistical analysis was performed by a software package (Prism 6.0; GraphPad Software, La Jolla, CA, USA).

3. Results

3.1. Nitrate and Nitrite Plasma Levels

Before the experimental phase, plasma NO_3^- and NO_2^- concentrations were 24 ± 8 μM and 118 ± 32 nM, respectively. Following CD, plasma NO_3^- and NO_2^- concentrations were 23 ± 10 μM and 240 ± 100 nM, respectively, and not statistically different. After HND, plasma NO_3^- and NO_2^- concentrations significantly increased to 127 ± 64 μM and 350 ± 120 nM, respectively.

3.2. Moderate-Intensity Constant Work Rate Cycling Exercise

Mean values of the main physiological variables determined during the last ~30 s of CWR (carried out at the same absolute work rate in the two conditions) are presented in Table 2.

Table 2. Mean ($\pm$SD) values of the main respiratory, cardiovascular, and metabolic variables determined at the end of the moderate-intensity constant work rate exercise after high (HND) and control nitrate diet (CD). $\dot{V}O_2$: oxygen uptake; $\dot{V}CO_2$: carbon dioxide output; R: gas exchange ratio; $\dot{V}E$: pulmonary ventilation; [La]$_b$: blood lactate concentration; HR: heart rate; * $p < 0.05$, significantly different between high and control diet.

	Work W	$\dot{V}O_2$ L·min^{-1}	$\dot{V}O_2$ mL·kg^{-1}·min^{-1}	$\dot{V}CO_2$ L·min^{-1}	R	$\dot{V}E$ L·min^{-1}	[La]$_b$ mM	HR b·min^{-1}
CD	74 ± 5	1.269 ± 0.136	18.9 ± 1.6	1.127 ± 0.118	0.89 ± 0.05	34.5 ± 3.6	5.15 ± 2.18	116 ± 17
HND	74 ± 5	1.178 ± 0.141 *	17.9 ± 2.8 *	1.049 ± 0.137 *	0.90 ± 0.05	33.0 ± 4.3	4.68 ± 1.84	112 ± 15

$\dot{V}O_2$ and $\dot{V}E$ values were significantly lower in HND vs.   CD. The values of G (estimating the O_2 cost of cycling) were significantly reduced by the high-nitrate diet (11.0 ± 1.2 vs. 13.3 ± 2.2 mL·min^{-1}·W^{-1}), even if they remained substantially closer to those usually observed in normal subjects (10 mL·min^{-1}·W^{-1}). Heart rate and blood lactate values were not different in the two conditions.

3.3. Isometric Knee Extension

MVT was not significantly different between HND (2.8 ± 0.5 Nm·kg^{-1}) and CD (2.9 ± 0.6 Nm·kg^{-1}). As for fatiguing intermittent submaximal exercise, after HND, the number of contractions performed was higher than after CD (47.1 ± 18.3 and 32.5 ± 12.4, respectively). The sum of TTI recorded was higher ($p < 0.05$) in HND (357.3 ± 176.1 Nm·s·kg^{-1}) than in CD (253.6 ± 149.0 Nm·s·kg^{-1}) (Figure 1A).

During the first three knee extensions (Begin), the average values of RMS-VL in both HND and CD (66.7 ± 7.6 %MVC and 67.8 ± 7.3 %MVC, respectively) were significantly lower compared to the average values of the last three contractions (End) (80.6 ± 12.7 %MVC and 80.0 ± 11.0 %MVC, respectively) (Figure 1B). No differences in RMS-VL values were detected between HND and CD.

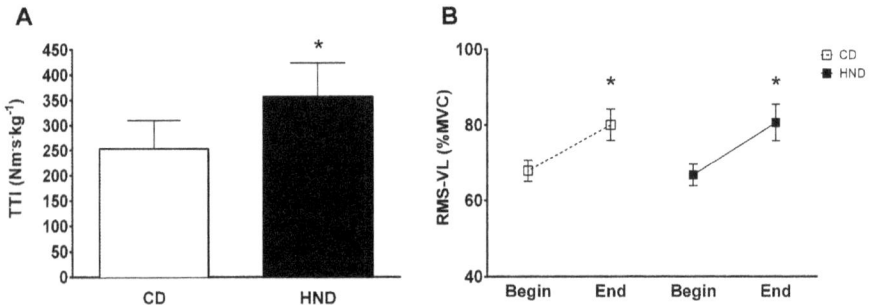

Figure 1. Knee extension fatiguing intermittent submaximal test. (**A**) Mean values (±SD) of total torque-time integral (TTI) and (**B**) root mean square of vastus lateralis (RMS-VL) recorded during the fatiguing intermittent submaximal test after control and high-nitrate diet. * $p < 0.05$.

3.4. Repeated Sprint Ability (RSA)

There was no difference in absolute PP output (Figure 2) of the first two sprints between HND (701.9 ± 80.8 W and 704.2 ± 80.0 W) and CD (669.6 ± 81.8 W, 675.9 ± 92.1 W).

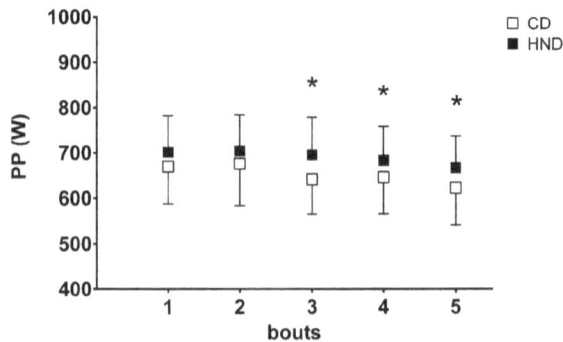

Figure 2. Repeated sprint ability test. Mean values (±SD) of peak power output (PP) obtained during the five bouts of the repeated sprint ability test (RSA) performed on a cycle ergometer after CD and HND. * $p < 0.05$.

In contrast, the PP output of the 3rd, 4th, and 5th sprints were significantly higher in HND (696.0 ± 83.1 W, 682.5 ± 76.2 W, 666.1 ± 70.7 W, respectively) than in CD (641.4 ± 76.2 W, 645.6 ± 80.2 W, 622.2 ± 81.4 W, respectively). No significant difference in $[La]_b$ during recovery was observed between the two conditions.

4. Discussion

In the present study, we examined the effects of a diet ensuring a high nitrate intake (by vegetables and fruits) on nitrate/nitrite plasma levels and exercise performance. Our results show that 6 days of a HND (~8.2 mmol·day^{-1}), compared to a CD (~2.9 mmol·day^{-1}), induced a significant rise of plasma nitrate and nitrite concentrations. These findings were associated with a reduced oxygen cost of aerobic exercise and an increased performance during high-intensity intermittent activities.

4.1. Plasma Nitrate/Nitrite Levels

Plasma nitrate concentration increased by ~500% and plasma nitrite concentration increased by ~50% after 6 days of HND, whereas no significant changes were observed after CD. The effects of HND in the present study are comparable to those reported in previous studies where supplementation with green leafy vegetables was pursued [26,36]. Moreover, the plasma nitrate and nitrite levels achieved are very close to those observed in studies that have used either beetroot juice [7] or sodium nitrate [11] as a supplement. Thus, our data indicate that a short-term diet containing nitrate rich vegetables significantly affects nitric oxide bioavailability. However, it should be noted that subjects were instructed to consume their meal about 3 h prior to exercise testing. Thus, this experimental design does not guarantee the exclusion of the combined chronic and acute effect of nitrate ingestion on plasma nitrate and nitrite concentrations [37].

4.2. Constant Work Rate Cycling Exercise

The increase of nitrate/nitrite plasma levels observed after high-nitrate diet was associated with a 7.2% reduction of oxygen consumption during a moderate intensity constant work rate exercise. This reduction was associated with lower pulmonary ventilation, whereas heart rate and blood lactate concentration were not influenced. In humans, Larsen et al. [4] first reported a lower oxygen cost during submaximal exercise following nitrate supplementation. Subsequently, this result has been confirmed by several randomized controlled trials in both healthy subjects (for a review, see [38]) and patients with chronic disease conditions that severely impair oxygen delivery and/or utilization, such as chronic obstructive pulmonary disease, heart failure, or peripheral arterial disease [39]. From these studies, it has been hypothesized that the underlying mechanisms of a reduced oxygen cost of exercise involve: (1) an enhanced mitochondrial oxidative phosphorylation efficiency, measured as the amount of oxygen consumed per ATP produced (P/O ratio) [3,6]; or (2) a reduced ATP cost of muscle force production due to a reduction in the ATP cost of cross-bridge cycling (actomyosin ATPase) and/or Ca^{2+} handling (Ca^{2+}-ATPase) [8]. Although we did not investigate the molecular effect of an increased NO bioavailability in this study, the results indicate that a diet containing nitrate-rich vegetables can influence the oxygen cost of moderate intensity exercise and could represent a useful ergogenic intervention to improve exercise tolerance similarly to either pharmacological (e.g., $NaNO_3^-$ and KNO_3^-) or dietary (e.g., beetroot juice) NO_3^- supplementations.

4.3. Intermittent High-Intensity Activities

In this study we observed similar values of maximal voluntary isometric force of the knee extensors after both high-nitrate and control diet. This result is consistent with the literature on the effects of nitrate supplementation (in the form of beetroot juice) on maximal voluntary force of young healthy physically active males [15–17]. At the same time, following HND, there was a significant improvement of muscle performance during both fatiguing submaximal knee extension exercise and Repeated Sprint Ability test. Indeed, HND resulted in an increased muscle work (higher number of muscle contractions and torque–time integral) during isometric knee extension and in an improved peak power output during the last bouts of the repeated sprint ability test. Although the present study did not evaluate specific muscular adaptations, the possible mechanisms underlying the induced enhancement in performance may involve several factors. A previous work in mice has shown an increase in myoplasmic free Ca^{2+} concentration, Ca^{2+} binding protein calsequestrin 1 and dihydropyridine receptors following several days of nitrate supplementation [40]. In humans, a reduced accumulation of intracellular phosphate ($[P_i]$) during contraction has been documented following nitrate supplementation [8]. Finally, Fulford et al. [17] reported that 15 days of dietary nitrate supplementation reduces the phosphocreatine cost of force production during repeated isometric maximal voluntary contractions of quadriceps muscle. Thus, it should be hypothesized that after HND, subjects were able to perform greater muscle work according to an increased Ca^{2+} sensitivity and sarcoplasmatic Ca^{2+} release. Additionally, a higher restoration of phosphocreatine (PCr) during the recovery phases between the contractions may have occurred. It is known that after beetroot juice supplementation, PCr degradation is reduced and lower inorganic phosphate and adenosine di-phosphate have been observed, reflecting an enhanced fatigue resistance from metabolite accumulation. In this study, the occurrence of an improved contraction efficiency (a reduced PCr depletion to force production) and/or an enhanced excitation–contraction coupling [16,17] without different levels of fatigue is supported by EMG data. Indeed, RMS value recorded from vastus lateralis was significantly higher at the end of the knee extensions fatiguing protocol compared to resting condition, but it was similar following HND and CD. Finally, it must be acknowledged that the increased bioavailability of nitric oxide has been also related to an enhanced mitochondrial oxidative phosphorylation efficiency and—especially in fast twitch fibers—to an improved muscle perfusion [38,40]. Thus, we cannot exclude that an increased production of ATP for the same oxygen consumption, as well as an increase in muscular blood flow and oxygenation after HND, could have contributed to a reduction in metabolic perturbation [20,41].

Another interesting finding of the present study is that the Repeated Sprint Ability test was significantly improved after HND. Although there was no difference in Peak Power output developed during the first two sprints, following HND, the Peak Power output of 3rd, 4th, and 5th sprint was significantly higher than that recorded after CD. These results are in accordance with Thompson et al. and Aucouturier et al., who found an improved repeated sprint performance after NO_3^- supplementation in team-sports players [20,21]. At the same time, these results are in contrast with other studies in which no effects on intermittent exercise performance after NO_3^- ingestion were observed [22,23]. The differences may be related to several factors. Christensen et al., for example, observed that nitrate supplementation did not change either peak or mean power for all six 20 s sprints [22]. However, the subjects recruited for this study were highly trained cyclists (~70 mL·kg^{-1}·min^{-1}), and it has been demonstrated that subjects with a high level of aerobic fitness may not benefit from NO_3^- supplementation [11,42]. Martin et al. did not find any beneficial effects on repeated sprint exercise after NO_3^- ingestion [23]. Nevertheless, they had found an elevated standard deviation in subjects' $\dot{V}O_2$max (49.6 ± 11.8 mL·kg^{-1}·min^{-1}), there was no information about plasma NO_3^- and NO_2^- concentrations after supplementation, and an active recovery was used between sprints. Finally, Buck et al. showed no effects on female athletes after acute NO_3^- ingestion [43]; it is likely that an acute nitrate supplementation can be less consistent than a short term one [38]. Moreover, the potential ergogenic effects of nitric oxide bioavailability in females have to be fully understood [44].

4.4. Study Limitations

In the present study, the dose of 8.2 mmol·day^{-1} of NO_3^- in HND was chosen according to the most effective pharmacological or dietary (beetroot juice) supplementation regimes adopted in previous studies [3,7–9,11]. Although this amount is significantly higher than the estimated average nitrate intake of 1–2 mmol·day^{-1} in the US and European populations, previous studies have utilized a similar nitrate intake as an effective intervention to reduce arterial hypertension [30,45]. This study shows that

Nutrients **2016**, *8*, 534

increasing daily dietary nitrate intake may also have important implications on exercise performance. We did not investigate possible adverse effects of our diet intervention, even if the subjects did not report any problem and the period of observation was quite short (6 days). However, these result need to be confirmed by further larger studies before reconsidering dietary recommendations. Furthermore, even if the two interventions differed from nitrate intake, we cannot exclude the possibility that other dietary compounds could be responsible for the performance changes.

5. Conclusions

In conclusion, this study has shown that the ingestion of nitrate-rich foods can increase plasma nitrate/nitrite concentrations and improve exercise performance. In particular, this nutritional intervention reduced energy demand during moderate-intensity exercise, enhanced muscle work during fatiguing intermittent submaximal contractions, and improved repeated sprint performance, whereas maximal isometric force or peak power output were not affected. These results suggest that a high-nitrate diet could be a feasible strategy for increasing plasma nitrate/nitrite levels and improving moderate intensity aerobic or high-intensity intermittent performance.

Acknowledgments: We thank the participants for their contributions and dedication to this research project. We also thank the following people for their valuable help: Simona Mrakic-Sposta, Giuseppe Bellistri, Sarah Moretti, and Alessandra Vezzoli.

Author Contributions: S.P., L.P., E.R., G.P., M.B. and A.L.T. conceived and designed the experiments; S.P., L.P., E.R., G.P. and M.B. performed the experiments; S.P., L.P., E.R., G.P., M.B. and L.R. analyzed the data; M.Mo. contributed reagents/materials/analysis tools; S.P., E.R. and M.Ma. wrote the paper.

Conflicts of Interest: The authors declare no conflict of interest.

References

1. Stamler, J.S.; Meissner, G. Physiology of nitric oxide in skeletal muscle. *Physiol. Rev.* **2001**, *81*, 209–237. [PubMed]
2. Lundberg, J.O.; Weitzberg, E.; Cole, J.A.; Benjamin, N. Nitrate, bacteria and human health. *Nat. Rev. Microbiol.* **2004**, *2*, 593–602. [CrossRef] [PubMed]
3. Larsen, F.J.; Weitzberg, E.; Lundberg, J.O.; Ekblom, B. Dietary nitrate reduces maximal oxygen consumption while maintaining work performance in maximal exercise. *Free Radic. Biol. Med.* **2010**, *48*, 342–347. [CrossRef] [PubMed]
4. Larsen, F.J.; Weitzberg, E.; Lundberg, J.O.; Ekblom, B. Effects of dietary nitrate on oxygen cost during exercise. *Acta Physiol.* **2007**, *191*, 59–66. [CrossRef] [PubMed]
5. Lundberg, J.O.; Weitzberg, E.; Gladwin, M.T. The nitrate-nitrite-nitric oxide pathway in physiology and therapeutics. *Nat. Rev. Drug. Discov.* **2008**, *7*, 156–167. [CrossRef] [PubMed]
6. Larsen, F.J.; Schiffer, T.A.; Borniquel, S.; Sahlin, K.; Ekblom, B. Dietary inorganic nitrate improves mitochondrial efficiency in humans. *Cell Metab.* **2011**, *13*, 149–159. [CrossRef] [PubMed]
7. Bailey, S.J.; Winyard, P.; Vanhatalo, A.; Blackwell, J.R.; Dimenna, F.J.; Wilkerson, D.P.; Tarr, J.; Benjamin, N.; Jones, A.M. Dietary nitrate supplementation reduces the O_2 cost of low-intensity exercise and enhances tolerance to high-intensity exercise in humans. *J. Appl. Physiol.* **2009**, *4*, 1144–1155. [CrossRef] [PubMed]
8. Bailey, S.J.; Fulford, J.; Vanhatalo, A.; Winyard, P.G.; Blackwell, J.R.; DiMenna, F.J.; Wilkerson, D.P.; Benjamin, N.; Jones, A.M. Dietary nitrate supplementation enhances muscle contractile efficiency during knee-extensor exercise in humans. *J. Appl. Physiol.* **2010**, *109*, 135–148. [CrossRef] [PubMed]
9. Vanhatalo, A.; Bailey, S.J.; Blackwell, J.R.; Dimenna, F.J.; Pavey, T.G.; Wilkerson, D.P.; Benjamin, N.; Winyard, P.G.; Jones, A.M. Acute and chronic effects of dietary nitrate supplementation on blood pressure and the physiological responses to moderate-intensity and incremental exercise. *Am. J. Physiol. Regul. Integr. Comp. Physiol.* **2010**, *299*, R1121–R1131. [CrossRef] [PubMed]
10. Lansley, K.E.; Winyard, P.G.; Bailey, S.J.; Vanhatalo, A.; Wilkerson, D.P.; Blackwell, J.R.; Gilchrist, M.; Benjamin, N.; Jones, A.M. Acute dietary nitrate supplementation improves cycling time trial performance. *Med. Sci. Sports Exerc.* **2011**, *43*, 1125–1131. [CrossRef] [PubMed]

11. Porcelli, S.; Ramaglia, M.; Bellistri, G.; Pavei, G.; Pugliese, L.; Montorsi, M.; Rasica, L.; Marzorati, M. Aerobic Fitness Affects the Exercise Performance Responses to Nitrate Supplementation. *Med. Sci. Sports Exerc.* **2015**, *47*, 1643–1651. [CrossRef] [PubMed]

12. Hoon, M.W.; Johnson, N.A.; Chapman, P.G.; Burke, L.M. The effect of nitrate supplementation on exercise performance in healthy individuals: A systematic review and meta-analysis. *Int. J. Sport. Nutr. Exerc. Metab.* **2013**, *23*, 522–532. [CrossRef] [PubMed]

13. Modin, A.; Bjorne, H.; Herulf, M.; Alving, K.; Weitzberg, E.; Lundberg, J.O. Nitrite-derived nitric oxide: A possible mediator of 'acidic-metabolic' vasodilation. *Acta Physiol. Scand.* **2001**, *171*, 9–16. [CrossRef] [PubMed]

14. Richardson, R.S.; Knight, D.R.; Poole, D.C.; Kurdak, S.S.; Hogan, M.C.; Grassi, B.; Wagner, P.D. Determinants of maximal exercise V'O2 during single leg knee-extensor exercise in humans. *Am. J. Physiol.* **1995**, *268*, H1453–H1461. [PubMed]

15. Hoon, M.W.; Fornusek, C.; Chapman, P.G.; Johnson, N.A. The effects of nitrate supplementation on muscle contraction in healthy adults. *Eur. J. Sport. Sci.* **2015**, *15*, 712–719. [CrossRef] [PubMed]

16. Haider, G.; Folland, J.P. Nitrate Supplementation Enhances the Contractile Properties of Human Skeletal Muscle. *Med. Sci. Sports Exerc.* **2014**, *46*, 2234–2243. [CrossRef] [PubMed]

17. Fulford, J.; Winyard, P.G.; Vanhatalo, A.; Bailey, S.J.; Blackwell, J.R.; Jones, A.M. Influence of dietary nitrate supplementation on human skeletal muscle metabolism and force production during maximum voluntary contractions. *Pflugers Arch.* **2013**, *465*, 517–528. [CrossRef] [PubMed]

18. Bond, H.; Morton, L.; Braakhuis, A.J. Dietary nitrate supplementation improves rowing performance in well-trained rowers. *Int. J. Sport Nutr. Exerc. Metab.* **2012**, *4*, 251–256. [CrossRef]

19. Wylie, L.J.; Mohr, M.; Krustrup, P.; Jackman, S.R.; Ermıdis, G.; Kelly, J.; Black, M.I.; Bailey, S.J.; Vanhatalo, A.; Jones, A.M. Dietary nitrate supplementation improves team sport-specific intense intermittent exercise performance. *Eur. J. Appl. Physiol.* **2013**, *113*, 1673–1684. [CrossRef] [PubMed]

20. Aucouturier, J.; Boissière, J.; Pawlak-Chaouch, M.; Cuvelier, G.; Gamelin, F.X. Effect of dietary nitrate supplementation on tolerance to supramaximal intensity intermittent exercise. *Nitric Oxide* **2015**, *49*, 16–25. [CrossRef] [PubMed]

21. Thompson, C.; Wylie, L.J.; Fulford, J.; Kelly, J.; Black, M.I.; McDonagh, S.T.; Jeukendrup, A.E.; Vanhatalo, A.; Jones, A.M. Dietary nitrate improves sprint performance and cognitive function during prolonged intermittent exercise. *Eur. J. Appl. Physiol.* **2015**, *115*, 1825–1834. [CrossRef] [PubMed]

22. Christensen, P.M.; Nyberg, M.; Bangsbo, J. Influence of nitrate supplementation on O_2 kinetics and endurance of elite cyclists. *Scand. J. Med. Sci. Sports* **2012**, *23*, e21–e31. [CrossRef] [PubMed]

23. Martin, K.; Smee, D.; Thompson, K.G.; Rattray, B. No improvement of repeated-sprint performance with dietary nitrate. *Int. J. Sports Physiol. Perform.* **2014**, *9*, 845–850. [CrossRef] [PubMed]

24. Wylie, L.J.; Bailey, S.J.; Kelly, J.; Blackwell, J.R.; Vanhatalo, A.; Jones, A.M. Influence of beetroot juice supplementation on intermittent exercise performance. *Eur. J. Appl. Physiol.* **2016**, *116*, 415–525. [CrossRef] [PubMed]

25. Murphy, M.; Eliot, K.; Heuertz, R.M.; Weiss, E. Whole Beetroot Consumption Acutely Improves Running Performance. *J. Acad. Nutr. Diet.* **2012**, *112*, 548–552. [CrossRef] [PubMed]

26. Bondonno, C.P.; Liu, A.H.; Croft, K.D.; Ward, N.C.; Yang, X.; Considine, M.J.; Puddey, I.B.; Woodman, R.J.; Hodgson, J.M. Short-term effects of nitrate-rich green leafy vegetables on blood pressure and arterial stiffness in individuals with high-normal blood pressure. *Free Radic. Biol. Med.* **2014**, *77*, 353–362. [CrossRef] [PubMed]

27. Ashworth, A.; Mitchell, K.; Blackwell, J.R.; Vanhatalo, A.; Jones, A.M. High-nitrate vegetable diet increases plasma nitrate and nitrite concentrations and reduces blood pressure in healthy women. *Public Health Nutr.* **2015**, *18*, 2669–2678. [CrossRef] [PubMed]

28. EFSA. Opinion of the Scientific Panel on Contaminants in the Food chain on a request from the European Commission to perform a scientific risk assessment on nitrate in vegetables. In *The EFSA Journal*; EFSA: Parma, Italy, 2008; pp. 1–79.

29. Appel, L.J.; Moore, T.J.; Obarzanek, E.; Vollmer, W.M.; Svetkey, L.P.; Sacks, F.M.; Bray, G.A.; Vogt, T.M.; Cutler, J.A.; Windhauser, M.M.; et al. A clinical trial of the effects of dietary patterns on blood pressure. *N. Engl. J. Med.* **1997**, *336*, 1117–1124. [CrossRef] [PubMed]

30. Hord, N.G.; Tang, Y.; Bryan, N.S. Food sources of nitrates and nitrites: The physiologic context for potential health benefits. *Am. J. Clin. Nutr.* **2009**, *90*, 1–10. [CrossRef] [PubMed]

31. Govoni, M.; Jansson, E.A.; Weitzberg, E.; Lundberg, J.O. The increase in plasma nitrite after a dietary nitrate load is markedly attenuated by an antibacterial mouthwash. *Nitric Oxide* **2008**, *19*, 333–337. [CrossRef] [PubMed]

32. Bishop, D.; Spencer, M.; Duffield, R.; Lawrence, S. The validity of a repeated sprint ability test. *J. Sci. Med. Sport* **2001**, *4*, 19–29. [CrossRef]

33. Hermens, H.J.; Freriks, B.; Disselhorst-Klug, C.; Rau, G. Development of recommendations for SEMG sensors and sensor placement procedures. *J. Electromyogr. Kinesiol.* **2000**, *10*, 361–374. [CrossRef]

34. Russ, D.W.; Elliott, M.A.; Vandenborne, K.; Walter, G.A.; Binder-Macleod, S.A. Metabolic costs of isometric force generation and maintenance of human skeletal muscle. *Am. J. Physiol. Endocrinol. Metab.* **2002**, *282*, E448–E457. [CrossRef] [PubMed]

35. Mulder, E.R.; Kuebler, W.M.; Gerrits, K.H.; Rittweger, J.; Felsenberg, D.; Stegeman, D.F.; de Haan, A. Knee extensor fatigability after bedrest for 8 weeks with and without countermeasure. *Muscle Nerve* **2007**, *36*, 798–806. [CrossRef] [PubMed]

36. Sobko, T.; Marcus, C.; Govoni, M.; Kamiya, S. Dietary nitrate in Japanese traditional foods lowers diastolic blood pressure in healthy volunteers. *Nitric Oxide* **2010**, *22*, 136–140. [CrossRef] [PubMed]

37. Wylie, L.J.; Ortiz de Zevallos, J.; Isidore, T.; Nyman, L.; Vanhatalo, A.; Bailey, S.J.; Jones, A.M. Dose-dependent effects of dietary nitrate on the oxygen cost of moderate-intensity exercise: Acute vs. chronic supplementation. *Nitric Oxide* **2016**, *57*, 30–39. [CrossRef] [PubMed]

38. Jones, A.M. Dietary nitrate supplementation and exercise performance. *Sports Med.* **2014**, *44*, S35–S45. [CrossRef] [PubMed]

39. Omar, S.A.; Webb, A.J.; Lundberg, J.O.; Weitzberg, E. Therapeutic effects of inorganic nitrate and nitrite in cardiovascular and metabolic diseases. *J. Intern. Med.* **2016**, *279*, 315–336. [CrossRef] [PubMed]

40. Hernàndez, A.; Schiffer, T.A.; Ivarsson, N.; Cheng, A.J.; Bruton, J.D.; Lundberg, J.O.; Weitzberg, E.; Westerblad, H. Dietary nitrate increases tetanic $[Ca^{2+}]i$ and contractile force in mouse fast-twitch muscle. *J. Physiol.* **2012**, *590*, 3575–3583. [CrossRef] [PubMed]

41. Ferguson, S.K.; Hirai, D.M.; Copp, S.W.; Holdsworth, C.T.; Allen, J.D.; Jones, A.M.; Musch, T.I.; Poole, D.C. Impact of dietary nitrate supplementation via beetroot juice on exercising muscle vascular control in rats. *J. Physiol.* **2013**, *591*, 547–557. [CrossRef] [PubMed]

42. Wilkerson, D.P.; Hayward, G.M.; Bailey, S.J.; Vanhatalo, A.; Blackwell, J.R.; Jones, A.M. Influence of acute dietary nitrate supplementation on 50 mile time trial performance in well-trained cyclists. *Eur. J. Appl. Physiol.* **2012**, *112*, 4127–4134. [CrossRef] [PubMed]

43. Buck, C.L.; Henry, T.; Guelfi, K.; Dawson, B.; McNaughton, L.R.; Wallman, K. Effects of sodium phosphate and beetroot juice supplementation on repeated-sprint ability in females. *Eur. J. Appl. Physiol.* **2015**, *115*, 2205–2213. [CrossRef] [PubMed]

44. Bescòs, R.; Surenda, A.; Tur, J.A.; Pons, A. The effect of nitric-oxide-related supplements on human performance. *Sports Med.* **2012**, *42*, 99–117. [CrossRef] [PubMed]

45. Kapil, V.; Webb, A.J.; Ahluwalia, A. Inorganic nitrate and the cardiovascular system. *Heart* **2010**, *96*, 1703–1709. [CrossRef] [PubMed]

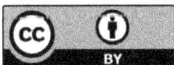

![nutrients logo] *nutrients*

MDPI

Article

Effect of a Nutritional Intervention in Athlete's Body Composition, Eating Behaviour and Nutritional Knowledge: A Comparison between Adults and Adolescents

Marcus Nascimento [1], Danielle Silva [1], Sandra Ribeiro [2], Marco Nunes [3], Marcos Almeida [4] and Raquel Mendes-Netto [2,*]

[1] Department of Nutrition, Federal University of Sergipe, São Cristóvão 49100-000, Brazil; marcusnascimentone@gmail.com (M.N.); daniellegoes@ufs.br (D.S.)
[2] School of Public Health, University of São Paulo, São Paulo 01246-904, Brazil; smlribeiro@usp.br
[3] Department of Medicine, Federal University of Sergipe, São Cristóvão 49100-000, Brazil; nunes.ma@ufs.br
[4] Department of Physical Education, Federal University of Sergipe, São Cristóvão 49100-000, Brazil; mb.almeida@gmail.com
*   Correspondence: raquelufs@gmail.com; Tel.: +55-79-2105-6662

Received: 24 June 2016; Accepted: 26 August 2016; Published: 7 September 2016

Abstract: The objective of the present study is to evaluate and compare the effect of a nutritional intervention between adolescent and adult. In a before and after quasi-experimental clinical study, 32 athletes (21 adults, age range 20–32 years; 11 adolescents, age range: 12–19 years) participated in a nutritional counselling consisting of four consultations separated by an interval of 45 to 60 days. The athlete's eating behaviour, body composition and nutrition knowledge were evaluated at the beginning and at the end of the protocol. Both groups increased lean body mass and nutritional knowledge. Adolescents increased their mid-arm muscle circumference and improved meal frequency, and daily water intake. Athletes of both groups improved their ingestion of vegetables and fruits and decreased the ingestion of sweets and oils. Adolescents showed a higher prevalence of individuals that remained within or approached to the recommendations of sweets. This is the first study to evaluate and compare the effect of a nutritional intervention between adolescent and adult athletes body composition, eating behaviour and nutritional knowledge. The nutritional counselling has been effective in promoting beneficial changes on the athlete's eating behaviour, nutritional knowledge and body composition, however, some healthy changes were only experienced by adolescents, especially in the frequency of meals and the intake of sweets.

Keywords: body composition; nutritional intervention; athletes; eating behaviour

1. Introduction

A balanced diet is important for an improved sports performance and for health. During exercise, athletes may suffer from the depletion of glycogen stores, dehydration and muscle damage. Thus, the ingestion of nutrient rich foods (lean meat/milk, fruits, vegetables and complex carbohydrates) and water may improve thermoregulation, enhance energy stores, maximize muscle protein synthesis and provide the supply of vitamins and minerals [1].

Although the importance of adequate nutrition has been well established [1], many athletes have shown several nutritional inadequacies [2–5]. Some authors have suggested that the dietary errors found in an athletic population may be due to low levels of nutritional knowledge and a lack of adequate nutritional counselling [6].

One strategy to improve the nutrition knowledge of athletes and coaches could be tailored nutrition programs. In the 1990s, some universities settled upon nutritional educational programs linked to their own sports department [7,8]. More recently, other nutritional interventions have also been developed [9,10]. However, these programs did not have their effectiveness evaluated, and they reflect a different reality from which most athletes are exposed, as they have extensive protocols and are dependent on a multi-disciplinary team.

There are few published studies involving nutritional interventions in athletes, and due to the different methodologies used, the results are inconsistent. Collison [11] did not find changes in the dietary intake of athletes, after participating in two nutritional workshops. In contrast, Carmo, Marins and Peluzio [12] observed a significant reduction in the dietary fat intake and the body fat percentage in Jiu-Jitsu athletes, after nine months of nutritional counselling.

Adolescent athletes are at a high nutritional risk because of the high energy cost of training. In addition, a number of nutrients are needed for the processes of growth and development. Proteins are needed to maximize muscle protein synthesis, calcium and vitamin D are important in the development and maintenance of skeleton, essential fatty acids may provide energy to support the growth and maturation, iron would prevent adverse athletic performance due to suboptimal iron stores, and so forth [1]. Nonetheless, few studies have studied nutritional interventions in this type of population, and most of them have only focused on improving the athlete's hydration practices [13,14] or their nutritional knowledge [15]. It is necessary to investigate this type of program in order to develop specific strategies to these individuals.

In this context, the objective of the present study is to evaluate and compare the effect of a nutritional intervention in athlete's body composition, eating behaviour and nutritional knowledge. Our secondary aim is to compare the effect of the nutritional intervention between adult and adolescent athletes.

2. Materials and Methods

This study was conducted according to the guidelines laid down in the declaration of Helsinki and all procedures involving human subjects were approved by the Research Ethics Committee of the University Hospital UFS (CAAE 08574213.4.0000.5546).

The work was conducted with athletes from a Brazilian program for athlete support, the "Bolsa Atleta", in the city of Aracaju, Brazil. This program provides financial aid to featured athletes who compete in the Olympic, Paralympic, and non-Olympic sports.

Data regarding the number of athletes of the program were provided by the SEJESP (Department of Youth and Sports in the city of Aracaju, Brazil). The program includes different athletes yearly, based on their sports results (state competitions). At the time of this study, 80 athletes were enrolled, from which five were in the gold category (international competitions), 25 in the silver category (national competitions), and 50 in the bronze category. After checking the inclusion and exclusion criteria, the eligible athletes were invited. These athletes were invited to take part of the study.

The inclusion criterion was based upon being a beneficiary of the program. There were no age or gender restrictions. The exclusion criteria were being in any concomitant nutritional counselling programs, or having any disease or health condition that required a specialized dietary planning.

2.1. Study Design

The work consisted of a quasi-experimental clinical trial with a pre and post design. The data collection took place from February 2012 to March 2014.

Written informed consent was obtained from all subjects. In the case of the adolescents, the consent form was sent to their respective responsible parents or guardians.

The program consisted of four visits with nutritional counselling and one lecture related to Brazilian Food Guide. [16,17]. During the intervention period, dietary and anthropometric measurements were performed. The data obtained before (first visit) and after the nutritional intervention (fourth visit) were compared. Figure 1 shows the experimental design of the study.

	Nutrition Counselling (45 to 60 days between consultations)			
	1st	2nd	3rd	4th
Anthropometry	X			X
Dietary Assesment	X	X	X	X
Nutrition Orientations	X	X	X	X
Healthy eating and Brazilian Food Guide lecture		X		

Figure 1. Experimental design of the study.

2.2. Anthropometric Evaluation

The anthropometric measures were performed following the techniques proposed by Lohman et al. [18]. Height was measured to the nearest 0.1 cm using a stadiometer (Altura Exata®, Altura Exata, Belo Horizonte, Brazil and body weight was measured to the nearest 0.1 kg using an electronic scale (P150M®, LÍDER, Araçatuba, Brazil). The mid-arm circumference was measured to the nearest 0.1 cm using a flexible and non-elastic tape (Sanny®, Sanny, São Bernardo do Campo, Brazil). All measurements were performed while the subjects wore no shoes and only light clothes.

Using a Lange Skinfold Calliper, the following skinfold thickness measurements were taken: triceps, subscapular, suprailiac, abdomen, thigh, axilla, and chest. These were measured to the nearest 0.1 mm, with the average of three measurements at each site being used for analysis. Evans et al. [19] equation was used for determining body fat percentages in both male and female adult athletes. In the adolescents, the percentage of body fat was estimated by Lohman's equation [20]. The triceps skinfold and the mid-arm muscle circumference were used to calculate the mid-arm muscle circumference (MAMC) in both groups [21].

2.3. Dietary Intake Assesment

The dietary intake was assessed by a sports nutritionist using a 24-h food recall. This method consisted of a written or verbal report about the food intake during the previous 24 h. The data on the food currently consumed, weight information, portion sizes, and food preparation techniques, were also collected.

A photo album was used as a resource to assist the respondents in remembering the food portions consumed, and thereby increasing the reliability of the information provided. This album consisted of utensils and food designs in three normal sizes (small, medium, and large) [22,23].

The energy content of each athlete's food intake was calculated using the Nutrition Data System for Research Software (NDSR) Version 2011 (NCC, Minneapolis, MN, USA) The daily water intake included water from food and beverages. The water consumption during training was based on the water from beverages used. Soft drinks, tea, or coffee, were not included in the water analysis.

The food servings were compared with the recommendations proposed by the Brazilian Food Pyramid [16,17]. As athletes might have different nutritional inadequacies, which may influence the nutrition advices given, we decided to analyse the nutrition intervention effects on food portions by grouping athletes according to their classification in adequate, low or high consumers of each food group [16,17]. The prevalence of the individuals who approached or remained within the recommendations of the protocol was also analysed.

The interval between meals was calculated from the mean interval between each meal. The characterisation of each meal was defined based on Burke et al. [4]. Breakfast was regarded as the first meal of the day between 05:00 and 10:00, the morning snack as the meal between 10:00 and 11:59, lunch as the meal between 12:00 and 14:59, the afternoon snack as the meal between 15:00 and 17:59, dinner as the meal between 18:00 and 20:59, and supper between 21:00 and 04:59.

Any food or energy containing drink consumed within a 30-min period was considered a "meal". The morning snack, the afternoon snack, and supper, were grouped into a single category called "snacks", while breakfast, lunch, and dinner, were considered to be "main meals". The prevalence of meal omission was also calculated. Furthermore, the time adequacy of pre and post-training meals were analysed according to the recommendations proposed by Aragon and Shoenfeld [24], where the interval between the pre-training and the post-training meals should be of three to four hours.

2.4. Nutritional Intervention

The nutritional intervention was divided into four face-to-face consultations, lasting for 45 to 60 min (Figure 1). The nutritional advice was given by only one sports nutritionist in order to minimize bias. Training routines, diet, anthropometric measurements, and personal data, were collected during the first meeting. From the initial analysis of eating habits and athlete's routine, specific dietary counselling was given and goals were set to improve diet quality. To increase the athlete's adherence, three days of the week were made available for consultations. At the end of the meetings, or by telephone, the athletes were scheduled for revaluations, and these occurred in the range of 45 to 60 days after the previous evaluation.

During the intervention, the athletes individually participated in a nutritional educational lecture about the Brazilian Food Guide [16,17] (2nd meeting). The participants were presented and clarified about the principles of healthy eating, focusing on the importance of each food group. The educational protocol aimed to improve the nutritional knowledge and to motivate the adoption of dietary practices that would promote health and athletic performance.

Adherence to guidelines was verified at each follow-up evaluation, as well as the dietary adjustments, in accordance with the current objectives of training and competition. At the end of each visit, the athletes received a list of specific nutritional advice. In addition, the aspects described in Figure 2 were reinforced during all meetings. To maintain the athlete's motivation, a group was created on a social network, whereby all participants received information about healthy eating tips and recipes. The information was posted monthly by the sports nutritionist and included advice about the preparation of pre and post-training meals, healthy hydration practices during training and competitions and other sport nutrition issues.

Theme	Orientation	Objective
Hydration	• Use of water bottles (500 mL) during training, school or other daily activities; • Drink at least one bottle in the morning, afternoon and every hour of training.	Improve water intake and availability
Meal Frequency	• Bring or buy snacks at work or school, to be consumed at least every two hours; • Feeding at least one hour before training; • Feeding at least one hour after training;	Improve meal frequency and food availability
Diet Quality	• Intake of vegetables associated with a raw vegetable oil everyday, at least at lunch; • Intake of different kinds of fruit as snacks and at breakfast • Reduction of the ingestion of sweets, salty, fried foods and soft drinks.	Improve fruits and vegetables intake and reduce the ingestion of convenience foods.

Figure 2. Issues addressed in the consultations.

2.5. Nutritional Knowledge

A nutritional knowledge test based on the studies of Gonçalves [25] and Zawila, Steib and Hoogenboom [26] was applied. The questionnaire had 14 questions divided into three sections. The first section contained three multi-choice questions about the basic aspects of nutrition. The second part consisted of a question related to the Brazilian Food Guide Pyramid, where the athletes had to fill in the pyramid with the correct food groups. The third section addressed the issue of sports nutrition and was comprised of a matter containing 10 statements to which the athletes should mark "yes" if they agreed with the statement, "no" if they disagreed with the statement, or "do not know" if they were unsure. The correct issues were worth a plus point and the wrong or "do not know" answers received no points. The average percentage of correct answers was calculated and they were compared between the groups before and after the intervention.

The questionnaire had its discriminative validity determined in a previous study by our research group [27]. The test was applied to 19 graduates of the 4th period of nutrition and to 16 adolescent athletes. To be considered valid, the questionnaire should be able to differentiate the participants at different levels of knowledge. After the application, the students had a significantly higher mean percentage of correct answers (97.4%) than did the athletes (57%).

2.6. Statistical Analysis

The statistical analysis was performed using SPSS Software Version 17.0 (SPSS Inc., Chicago, IL, USA). The data normality was verified by the Kolmorgorov–Smirnov test. Normally distributed data were presented as a mean and standard error (SE), while non-normally distributed variables were log-transformed before statistical analyses to avoid skewed data and are presented as geometric means and back-transformed 95% confidence intervals (95% CI) [28].

Student's *t*-tests and Pearson's chi-square test were used to access whether any demographic, anthropometric or dietary measures where different between groups at baseline. The significance of within-group changes in numeric variables (within-group analyses) was determined using paired *t*-tests. The categorical data was compared over time using McNemar's Test. Since there were baseline differences between groups with respect to anthropometric measures, number of meals, interval between meals, daily water intake and water intake during training, a general linear model univariate analysis (ANCOVA) was used to determine whether the change scores of these variables (post-pre) where different between adolescents and adults, after adjusting for pre-intervention values.

The internal consistency of the nutritional knowledge questionnaire was obtained by the Cronbach's alpha coefficient (α). This coefficient ranges between 0.00 (no reliability) to 1.00 (perfect reliability). The minimum value of 0.70 was recommended by Rowland, Arkkelin and Crisler [29]. Statistical analyses of the intervention effects on nutrition knowledge were carried out using a two factor (group and time) analysis of variance (ANOVA). For all analysis, a statistical significance was set at $p < 0.05$.

3. Results

After checking the inclusion and exclusion criteria, 67 athletes were eligible to participate in the research. Of these, only 32 athletes completed the four-consultation protocol. The reasons for attrition, as well as the description of the final sample are at Figure 3. The participants were 32 athletes of the following sports: fighting (boxing, taekwondo, karate, judo, jiu-jitsu, capoeira, and wrestling, $n = 16$), athletics ($n = 3$), cycling ($n = 1$), swimming ($n = 6$), tennis ($n = 2$), beach volleyball ($n = 1$), surfing ($n = 1$), rowing ($n = 1$) and sailing ($n = 1$). The sample consisted of 21 adolescents (65.6%, age range: 12–19 years) and 11 adults (34.4%, age range: 20–32 years), with a mean age of 15.4 years (SE: 0.35) and 23.7 years (SE: 0.53), respectively. All of the adults were male, while six adolescents (28.6%) were female and 15 were male (71.4%). There was no difference in the results when they were analysed without the female athletes; thus, they were included. The adolescents and the adults had an average of 12.8 (SE: 1) h and 16.2 (SE: 1.2) h of training per week, respectively.

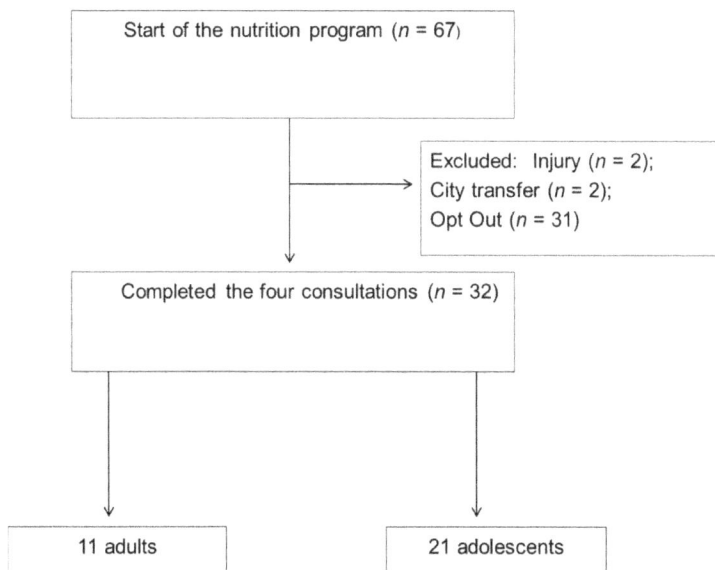

Figure 3. Study diagram.

Most of the athletes in both groups (95.2% of adolescents and 81.8% of adults) had a goal of maintaining or gaining lean mass. Only one adolescent (4.8%) and two adults (18.2%) had the intention of reducing body mass.

Table 1 shows the anthropometric and body composition values of the athletes before and after nutritional counselling. Both groups increased their body mass and lean body mass (kg), however, only the adolescents increased MAMC. There were no differences in the changes between the groups (ANCOVA, $p > 0.05$).

Table 1. Mean (SE) of athlete's anthropometry and body composition.

Variables	Group	Intervention ($n = 32$)		ANCOVA [1]
		Pre	Post	p-Value [1]
Body mass (kg)	Adults	69.2 (2.0)	71.4 (2.1) [3]	0.06
	Adolescents	56.1 (2.2)	57.6 (2.0) [3]	
BMI (kg/m^2)	Adults	24.8 (1.3)	25.1 (1.2)	0.056
	Adolescents	20 (1)	20.3 (0.8)	
MAMC	Adults	26.8 (11)	26.9 (12)	0.21
	Adolescents	22.4 (0.6)	23.8 (0.8) [3]	
ΣSKF [2]	Adults	80.4 (9)	93.1 (13)	0.57
	Adolescents	20.6 (2)	20.3 (1.4)	
Fat mass (%)	Adults	12.6 (1.4)	14.2 (1.5)	0.58
	Adolescents	14 (1.5)	13.7 (1.1)	
Lean mass (kg)	Adults	60 (1.7)	61.1 (1.6)	0.03
	Adolescents	48 (1.8)	49.2 (1.6)	
Fat (kg)	Adults	8.9 (1.1)	10.3 (1.3)	0.001
	Adolescents	8 (0.8)	8.4 (0.6)	

[1] p-values refer to differences between groups, using ANCOVA on the changes, adjusting for baseline values; [2] Adolescents: sum of two skinfold, adults: sum of seven skinfolds; [3] $p < 0.05$, pre versus post.

The analysis showed an increase in the number of meals for young athletes, as well as a significant reduction in the interval between the meals; however, there were no group effects on the changes in these variables (ANCOVA, $p > 0.05$) (Figure 4). The adolescents also showed a significant reduction of meal and snack omissions. Both groups increased the time adequacy of pre-training and post-training meals (Figure 4). As all of the adults were suited to the recommendations, it was not possible to apply within-group inferences.

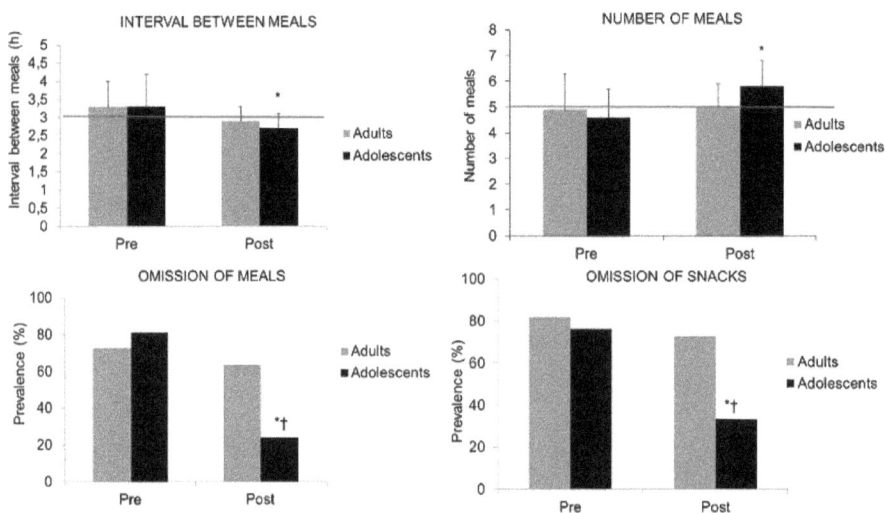

Figure 4. *Cont.*

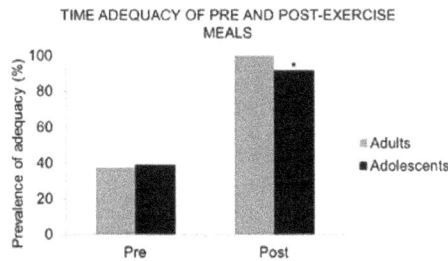

Figure 4. Number of meals, interval between meals, meal omission, snack omission, and time adequacy of pre and post-training meals, before and after nutritional counselling. The red lines indicate the recommendations of at least five meals a day (number of meals) and a maximum of three hours between meals. * $p < 0.05$, pre versus post. † $p < 0.05$, adults versus adolescents.

The within-group analysis showed that there was a statistically significant increase in daily water intake among the adolescents (Table 2). There were no differences in the change scores between the groups (ANCOVA, $p > 0.05$).

Table 2. Geometric mean (95% CI) of daily water intake and water ingestion during training.

Variables	Group	Intervention ($n = 32$)		ANCOVA
		Pre Mean (95% CI)	Post Mean (95% CI)	p-Value [1]
Daily Water (L)	Adults	4.8 (2.3–9)	5 (2.4–10)	0.30
	Adolescents	3.3 (2–5.6)	3.6 (2.1–6) [3]	
Water during training (mL/h) [2]	Adults	233 (5–1107)	576 (63–5268)	0.44
	Adolescents	192 (17–2101)	417 (175–993)	

[1] p-values refer to differences between groups, using ANCOVA on the changes, adjusting for baseline values; [2] $n = 21$; [3] $p < 0.05$, pre versus post.

Table 3 shows the athletes ingestion of food portions according to their baseline classification. Participants with low intake of legumes and vegetables increased their ingestion. Athletes that demonstrated high intakes of meat and eggs, sweets and oils decreased their ingestion after the intervention. We also found a high prevalence (more than 50%) of individuals that remained within or approached to the recommendations of cereals, fruits, vegetables, meat and eggs, and oils and fats. When these values were compared between groups, the adolescents showed a higher prevalence of individuals that remained within or approached to the recommendations of sweets (Adolescents: 71.4%, adults: 18%).

Table 3. Intake of food portions before and after the intervention.

Portions	Portion Intakes Classification	Age Group		Intervention [1] ($n = 32$)		Guidelines [2]
		Adult n (%)	Adolescents n (%)	Pre	Post	
Cereals	Adequate	7(50)	7(50)	9.8 (6.7–14)	6.1 (3.5–10) [3]	6–9
	Low	4(22.2)	14(77.8)	3(1.7–5.5)	3.8 (2.1–6.8)	
Fruits	Adequate	8 (34.8)	15(65.2)	6.6 (5–8.7)	4.8 (2.6–8.6) [3]	3–5
	Low	3(33.3)	6(66.7)	2.4 (1.2–5)	4.6 (1.6–12) [3]	
Vegetables	Adequate	2(34.6)	4(65.4)	6.3 (2.5–16)	2.5 (1.4–4.8) [3]	3–5
	Low	9 (34.6)	17 (66.7)	1.6 (1.6–3.1)	2.2 (0.8–7.8) [3]	
Meats and Eggs	Adequate	4 (25)	12 (75)	2.1 (1.6–3)	2.8 (1.8–4)	1–2
	High	7 (43.8)	9 (56.3)	4 (3–5)	2.8 (1.7–4) [3]	

Table 3. Cont.

| Portions | Portion Intakes Classification | Age Group | | Intervention [1] (n = 32) | | Guidelines [2] |
		Adult n (%)	Adolescents n (%)	Pre	Post	
Dairy	Adequate	3 (23.1)	10 (76.9)	5 (3.8–6.8)	3.3 (1.4–8)	3
	Low	8 (42.1)	11 (57.9)	1.8 (1.1–2.9)	2.5 (1.7–3.7) [3]	
Beans and nuts	High	8 (34.8)	15 (65.2)	4 (2.8–6)	2.6 (1.2–5.5) [3]	1
	Adequate	3 (33.3)	6 (66.7)	1.2 (0.8–1.8)	2.8 (0.2–6.4) [3]	
Fats and Oils	Adequate	4 (21.1)	15 (78.9)	2(1.6–2.6)	2.7(1.6–4.7) [3]	1–2
	High	7 (53.8)	6 (46.2)	4.8 (3.3–7)	2.5 (1.5–4) [3]	
Sweets	Adequate	9 (45)	11 (55)	2 (1.4–2.8)	3.4 (1.9–6) [3]	1–2
	High	2 (16.7)	10 (83.3)	8.4 (6–12)	2.9 (1.4–6) [3]	

[1] Data expressed as geometric means (95% CI); [2] Phillip (1999); [3] $p < 0.05$, pre versus post.

The nutrition knowledge questionnaire internal consistency value was obtained through Cronbach's coefficient. These values showed an acceptable reliability for the adults (0.84) and the adolescents (0.81). Both groups had an increment in total and food pyramidal nutritional knowledge (Table 4).

Table 4. Mean (SE) of athlete's nutritional knowledge before and after the intervention.

| Nutrition Knowledge Categories | Group | Intervention (n = 32) | | ANOVA (p-Value) | | |
		Before	After	Group	Time	Group × Time
Total	Adults	70 (9)	89 (10) [1]	0.75	<0.001	0.47
	Adolescents	73.6 (15)	84.6 (11) [1]			
Basic Nutrition	Adults	89.7 (23)	92 (18)	0.94	0.42	0.77
	Adolescents	92 (12)	97 (13)			
Food Pyramid	Adults	28.4 (26)	77 (14) [1]	0.85	0.001	0.56
	Adolescents	37 (28)	52 (25) [1]			
Sports Nutrition	Adults	84.5 (11)	87.2 (24)	0.84	0.15	0.97
	Adolescents	83.3 (18,7)	92 (17)			

[1] $p < 0.05$, pre versus post.

4. Discussion

To our knowledge, this is the first study to evaluate and compare the effect of a nutritional intervention between adolescent and adult athletes. The results have shown that both groups improved their body composition, their dietary intake and nutrition knowledge, however, the adolescent had a higher improvement on body composition, meal frequency and sweets intake than adults.

4.1. Body Composition

After about eight months of nutritional counselling, the adolescent athletes increased their MAMC, while and showed a trend towards significance to increase their lean mass ($p = 0.051$). Since the results were consistent with the objectives outlined in the consultations, the specific nutritional advice that was given may have contributed to the changes in their body composition (most of the athletes reported that lean mass gain or maintenance as a goal).

It should be noted that adults had a higher increase in fat than adolescents (ANCOVA, $p < 0.05$). An increase in body fat may occur during nutrition interventions focusing on body mass gain [30]. However, due to a more anabolic profile [31], the adolescent athletes may have had a greater capacity to gain muscle mass than the adults, without changes in fat mass.

Other nutritional intervention studies have shown significant changes in an athlete's body composition and also had their planning directed to their goal. Garthe et al. [30] supported a total of 21 athletes for at least eight weeks who aimed to gain body mass. The participants received nutritional counselling by two nutritionists and at the end of the study they showed an increase in their body mass and their lean body mass (approximately 1.7 kg). More recently, Carmo, Marins and Peluzio [12] found a significant reduction in body mass and body fat percentage in 20 Jiu-Jitsu athletes after participating in a specific nutritional intervention for reducing body mass.

These results are of great relevance, as athletes may have difficulty in achieving the desired body shape, and they tend to adopt inappropriate strategies which can be harmful to health and sports performance [11]. In these situations, nutritional counselling should be indicated as a strategy to promote changes with a greater efficiency and quality.

4.2. Meal Frequency

The division of the total caloric intake in frequent meals (with a three-hour interval) can be beneficial for athletes, since it reduces the risk of gastrointestinal distress and provides a greater flexibility in the amount and the variety of food to be ingested. These factors may help to improve diet quality and nutrient distribution throughout the day [3]. However, both age groups of athletes showed a high prevalence of meal omission, mainly of snacks, which contributed to the inadequacy in the number of meals and the interval between them.

The increasing availability of healthy foods is seen as a facilitator of eating behaviour changes, especially among adolescents, since they are exposed to foods of a low nutritional value and a high energy density, especially in school [32]. Thus, during these consultations, the athletes received instructions regarding the preparation of practical snacks with a high nutritional content, which should be consumed at home, work, or at school, in order to increase healthy food accessibility and meal frequency. These guidelines were also reinforced by their social network, where they received tips on examples of healthy meals.

After the nutritional intervention, the adolescents increased their number of meals, reduced the interval between them, as well as an omission of snacks. In addition, both of the groups increased their time adequacy of pre and post-training meals.

Despite the scarcity of studies about athletes that perceive barriers for healthy eating, the literature suggests that they may have difficulty in maintaining an adequate frequency of meals, due to the exhausting routine caused by a high work load of training and associated with other tasks (e.g., work and school) [33]. An anamnesis taken showed that all of the adolescents attended school lessons in the morning and sports training in the afternoon, or at night, while the adults, in addition to training and studying, had much of the day filled with working hours. Studies that have focused on the analysis of adults have perceived barriers to adopt a healthy eating habit, observed that the most cited reason is a lack of time for the preparation and the consumption of food [34]. Thus, our hypothesis is that by having a greater number of obligations than adolescents (family, education, and employment), the adults have found a greater difficulty in feeding, especially between "main meals", despite having the same hours of training.

4.3. Water Intake

Despite of the importance athlete's hydration behaviour, to our knowledge, only two studies have analysed the effect of nutritional interventions on athlete's hydration practices. Kavouras et al. [14] and Cleary et al. [13] have improved the hydration status in young athletes, by individual prescriptions, and have increased the accessibility of this nutrient, respectively.

In the present study, the participants were advised to drink water from 500 mL bottles at different times of the day. These strategies could facilitate quantification and the perception of water intake, as well as improving its availability. After nutritional counselling, the adolescents increased their daily water intake. For both groups, although their improvement in water intake during training was not statistically significant, the result was clinically relevant, since they doubled their ingestion.

4.4. Food Portions

There are several methods to evaluate dietary intake. The average intake of a nutrient, or the prevalence of individuals facing a guideline are the most used, however, some considerations need to be analysed when performing nutritional intervention studies. The literature suggests that small progressive changes in a diet are more effective and sustainable than big ones [35]. The time necessary for an eating behaviour change may vary depending on the social and environmental factors specific to each individual. Thus, one must expect an individual to pass from an intake category of "inadequate" to "adequate". This may be a conservative assessment (e.g., not eat any fruit portion and begin to consume four servings), preventing the detection of small changes. Some studies have used an average as the evaluation method. However, as athletes can have different types of food inadequacies within the same sample, the average intake of a nutrient may include athletes who have an inadequate intake and those who are adequate. This grouping can lead to a bias in the results interpretation, since those with an intake within the recommendations, were oriented to maintain it, contributing to the average intake unchanging after the intervention. Thus, to reduce this bias, athletes were grouped according to their baseline classification of food portions ingestion.

After the intervention, athletes classified as low consumers of fruits, vegetables, dairy and high consumers of sweets, meat and fats and oils approached to the recommendations of the Brazilian Food Pyramid, which could be considered a positive effect of the nutrition intervention. Data analysis also showed that athletes maintained their adequate intake of most of the food portions. However, participants appeared to have had more difficulties in maintaining the adequacy of sweets, fat and oils and vegetables. Considering that these food habits might take a longer time to change, dieticians should carefully monitor the ingestion of these food portions during nutrition interventions. As athletes are exposed to numerous barriers that preclude a balanced diet, and even for those guidelines that are being met, the strategies have been tightened at each visit. Thus, the maintenance of an adequate intake could also be considered a positive effect.

Both of the groups showed a high prevalence of individuals that approached to or remained adequate within the recommendations, however, when analysing the ingestion of sweets, this prevalence was higher among adolescents. The preference for a sweet taste has been identified in studies involving both adolescents and adults and has been considered a barrier to the ingestion of other food groups [36,37]. In this study, as all athletes were residential, it is possible that the presence of parents in the adolescent consultations may have aided the adherence to the nutritional advices. This would be especially evident with regard to food intake and frequency, as parents were responsible for the courses preparation and its organisation, and thus would provide a greater support for the athletes. Iglezias-Gutiérrez et al. [38] observed that food preferences might not influence an adolescent athletes dietary intake. This might be due to the influence of the family environment on the purchase and selection of meals, which may reduce the chances of ingesting foods that were considered "preferred".

4.5. Nutritional Knowledge

Both groups had an increase in their nutritional knowledge, especially with regard to the topics that related to the Brazilian Food Guide Pyramid. This finding is of a great importance, as athletes receive nutritional information from various sources, mainly from coaches and trainers, who have shown a lack of nutritional knowledge. In addition, unreliable information sources, such as the Internet, magazines, friends, relatives, and media, are widely used for information [6].

In addition to the dissemination of nutritional information topics, specific orientations to the needs and difficulties of each athlete were provided in the present study by a sports nutritionist, which has been considered the most qualified professional to give nutritional advices to athletes. This approach may have been responsible for the better results being found in relation to the researchers that have only used nutritional educational strategies, such as seminars and lectures [11].

Despite the fact that the nutritional intervention strategy has promoted beneficial changes in body composition, dietary intake, and athlete's nutritional knowledge, it is worth noting that the participants had a low adherence to the protocol adopted. Only 50% of the participants who started the protocol finished the four consultations. Due to the high number of bookings for each athlete, we hypothesized that they had difficulties in making time for the consultations during their daily routine. Future research should focus on the main barriers faced by athletes to adopt healthy eating, and factors such as boredom and tedious teachings may influence the adherence to different types of nutritional intervention. As family and coaches may possibly influence athlete's food habits, the research protocols should also include these particular populations.

4.6. Practical Applications

When consulting athletes it is important for nutritionists to take into account the time for meal preparation, as well as its possibility of storage time, especially in the case of snacks. A minimum of five meals/day is recommended, however, these meals should be gradually inserted to facilitate an athlete's adaptation, especially in the pre- and post-training period.

The development of practical strategies to increase water availability might be useful, especially in places where it is done through drinking fountains or sports that are practiced in open spaces such as beaches and fields. Even with the existence of general hydration recommendations (500 mL/h of training), it is important, to first of all, respect an athlete's tolerance to the prescribed amount of liquid. The prescription of high-water-content food (e.g., Fruits) may also enhance hydration during the day.

4.7. Limitations

Despite the relevance of the results of this study, some methodological limitations must be taken into consideration. The analysis of food intake using a single 24-h recall is a limiting factor on the basis of the intra-individual variability provided by the instrument. However, it was necessary the use of this method due to the operational difficulty in accessing the same participant more than one time, as the athletes trained in different places and had to move to the place of data collection. According to Magkos and Yannankolia [39], the use of a single 24-h recall might be an alternative when you cannot use the instrument more than one time. Other works also used this method [40,41].

5. Conclusions

The present study has shown that the nutritional intervention was effective in promoting beneficial changes in athletes' body composition, eating behaviour, and nutritional knowledge. However, some healthy changes were only experienced by adolescents, especially in the frequency of meals and the intake of sweets.

Acknowledgments: The authors wish to thank the SEJESP (Department of Youth and Sports in the city of Aracaju, Brazil) for their assistance with this project.

Author Contributions: Marcus Nascimento participated in the project design, acquisition, analysis and interpretation of data and drafting the article. Danielle Silva, Sandra Ribeiro, Marco Nunes and Marcos Almeida made substantial contributions to the design of the work, interpretation of data, and revised it critically for important intellectual content. Raquel Mendes-Netto is the coordinator of the project and has been involved with all stages of the article elaboration. All authors have given final approval of the version to be published.

Conflicts of Interest: The authors declare no conflict of interest.

References

1. Thomas, D.T.; Erdman, K.A.; Burke, L.M. Position of the academy of nutrition and dietetics, dietitians of Canada and the American college of sports medicine: Nutrition and athletic performance. *J. Acad. Nutr. Diet.* **2016**, *116*, 501–528. [CrossRef] [PubMed]

2. Dwyer, J.; Eisenberg, A.; Prelack, K.; Song, W.O.; Sonneville, K.; Ziegler, P. Eating attitudes and food intakes of elite adolescent female figure skaters: A cross sectional study. *J. Int. Soc. Sports. Nutr.* **2012**, *9*. [CrossRef] [PubMed]

3. Erdman, K.A.; Tunnicliffe, J.; Lun, V.M.; Reimer, R.A. Eating patterns and composition of meals and snacks in elite Canadian athletes. *Int. J. Sport Nutr. Exerc. Metable* **2013**, *23*, 210–219. [CrossRef]

4. Burke, L.M.; Slater, G.; Broad, E.M.; Haukka, J.; Modulon, S.; Hopkins, W.G. Eating patterns and meal frequency of elite Australian athletes. *Int. J. Sport. Nutr. Exerc. Metable* **2003**, *13*, 521–538. [CrossRef]

5. Nogueira, J.; da Costa, T. Nutrient intake and eating habits of triathletes on a Brazilian diet. *Int. J. Sport Nutr. Exerc. Metable.* **2004**, *14*, 684–697. [CrossRef]

6. Heaney, S.; O'Connor, H.; Michael, S.; Gifford, J.; Naughton, G. Nutrition knowledge in athletes: A systematic review. *Int. J. Sport Nutr. Exerc. Metable* **2011**, *21*, 248–261. [CrossRef]

7. Vinci, D.M. Effective nutrition support programs for college athletes. *Int. J. Sport Nutr.* **1998**, *8*, 308–320. [CrossRef] [PubMed]

8. Clark, K. Working with college athletes, coaches, and trainers at a major university. *Int. J. Sport Nutr.* **1994**, *4*, 135–141. [CrossRef] [PubMed]

9. Quatromoni, P.A. Clinical observations from nutrition services in college athletics. *J. Am. Diet. Assoc.* **2008**, *108*, 689–694. [CrossRef] [PubMed]

10. Karpinski, C. Exploring the feasibility of an academic course that provides nutrition education to collegiate student-athletes. *J. Nutr. Educ. Behav.* **2012**, *44*, 267–270. [CrossRef] [PubMed]

11. Collison, S.B. Impact of nutrition education on female athletes. *Am. J. Health Behav.* **1996**, *20*, 14–23.

12. Carmo, M.C.L.; Marins, J.C.B.; Peluzio, M.C.G. Intervenção nutricional em atletas de Jiu-jitsu. *Rev. Bras. Ciênc Mov.* **2014**, *22*, 97–110. (In Portuguese) [CrossRef]

13. Cleary, M.A.; Hetzler, R.K.; Wasson, D.; Wages, J.J.; Stickley, C.; Kimura, I.F. Hydration behaviors before and after an educational and prescribed hydration intervention in adolescent athletes. *J. Athl. Train.* **2012**, *47*, 273–281. [PubMed]

14. Kavouras, S.; Arnaoutis, G.; Makrillos, M.; Garagouni, C.; Nikolaou, E.; Chira, O.; Ellinikaki, E.; Sidossis, L.S. Educational intervention on water intake improves hydration status and enhances exercise performance in athletic youth. *Scand. J. Med. Sci. Sports.* **2012**, *22*, 684–689. [CrossRef] [PubMed]

15. Gonçalves, C.B.; Nogueira, J.A.D.; Costa, T.H.M. The food pyramid adapted to physically active adolescents as a nutrition education tool. *Rev. Bras. Ciênc Esporte.* **2014**, *36*, 29–44. (In Portuguese) [CrossRef]

16. Phillipi, S.T.; Latterza, A.R.; Cruz, A.T.R.; Ribeiro, L.C. Pirâmide Alimentar Adaptada: Guia para a escolha dos alimentos. *Rev. Nutr.* **1999**, *2*, 65–80. (In Portuguese) [CrossRef]

17. Phillipi, S.T. *Pirâmide dos Alimentos: Fundamentos Básicos Da Nutrição*, 2nd ed.; Editora Manole Ltda.: São Paulo, Brazil, 2014; p. 424. (In Portuguese)

18. Lohman, T.G.; Roche, A.F.; Martorell, R. *Anthropometric Standardization Reference Manual*; Human Kinetics Books: Champaign, IL, USA, 1988.

19. Evans, E.M.; Rowe, D.A.; Misic, M.M.; Prior, B.M.; Arngrímsson, S.A. Skinfold prediction equation for athletes developed using a four-component model. *Med. Sci. Sports Exerc.* **2005**, *37*, 2006–2011. [CrossRef] [PubMed]

20. Lohman, T. Applicability of body composition techniques and constants for children and youths. *Exerc. Sport Sci. Rev.* **1985**, *14*, 325–357. [CrossRef]

21. Martorell, R.; Yarbrough, C.; Lechtig, A.; Delgado, H.; Klein, R.E. Upper arm anthropometric indicators of nutritional status. *Am. J. Clin. Nutr.* **1976**, *29*, 46–53. [PubMed]

22. Galeazzi, M.; Meireles, A.; Viana, R.; Zabotto, C.; Domene, S.; Cunha, D. *Registro Fotográfico Para Inquéritos Dietéticos: Utensílios e Porções*; Unicamp: Goiânia, Brazil, 1996. (In Portuguese)

23. Lopez, R.P.S.; Botelho, R.A. *Álbum Fotográfico de Porções Alimentares*, 1st ed.; Sariava: São Paulo, Brazil, 2008. (In Portuguese)

24. Aragon, A.A.; Schoenfeld, B.J. Nutrient timing revisited: Is there a post-exercise anabolic window. *J. Int. Soc. Sports Nutr.* **2013**, *10*. [CrossRef] [PubMed]

25. Gonçalves, C.B. Consumo Alimentar e Entendimento da Pirâmide Alimentar Adaptada em Adolescentes Fisicamente Ativos do Distrito Federal. Master's Thesis, Universidade de Brasília, Brasília, Brazil, 2009. (In Portuguese)

26. Zawila, L.G.; Steib, C.S.M.; Hoogenboom, B. The female collegiate cross-country runner: Nutritional knowledge and attitudes. *J. Athl. Train.* **2003**, *38*, 67–74. [PubMed]

27. Leite, M.M.R.; Machado, A.C.S.B.; Silva, D.G.; Raposo, O.F.F.; Mendes-Netto, R.S. Conocimiento sobre alimentación Y nutricióndespues del desarrollo de actividades de educación alimentaria entre niños y adolescentes deportistas. *Pensar a Prática* **2016**, accepted.

28. Bland, J.M.; Altman, D.G. Transformations, means and confidence intervals. *BMJ* **1996**, *312*, 1079. [CrossRef] [PubMed]

29. Rowland, D.; Arkkelin, D.; Crisler, L. *Computer-Based Data Analysis: Using SPSSx iIn the Social and Behavioral Sciences*; Nelson-Hall: Chicago, IL, USA, 1991.

30. Garthe, I.; Raastad, T.; Refsnes, P.E.; Sundgot-Borgen, J. Effect of nutritional intervention on body composition and performance in elite athletes. *Eur. J. Sport Sci.* **2013**, *13*, 295–303. [CrossRef] [PubMed]

31. Meylan, C.; Cronin, J.B.; Oliver, J.; Hopkins, W.; Contretras, B. The effect of maturation on adaptations to strength training and detraining in 11–15 years olds. *Scand. J. Med. Sci. Sports* **2014**, *24*, 156–164. [CrossRef] [PubMed]

32. Nestle, M.; Wing, R.; Birch, L.; DiSogra, L.; Drewnowski, A.; Middleton, S.; Sigman-Grant, M.; Sobal, J.; Winston, M.; Economos, C. Behavioral and social influences on food choice. *Nutr. Rev.* **1998**, *56*, 50–64. [CrossRef]

33. Martínez Sanz, J.M.; Urdampilleta, A.; Micó, L.; Soriano, J.M. Aspectos psicológicos y sociológicos en la alimentación de los deportistas. *Cuad. Psicol. Dep.* **2012**, *12*, 39–48. (In Portuguese) [CrossRef]

34. Kearney, J.; Mcelhone, S. Perceived barriers in trying to eat healthier–results of a pan-EU consumer attitudinal survey. *Br. J. Nutr.* **1999**, *81*, S133–S137. [CrossRef] [PubMed]

35. Hill, J.O. Can a small-changes approach help address the obesity epidemic? A report of the Joint Task Force of the American Society for Nutrition, Institute of Food Technologists, and International Food Information Council. *Am. J. Clin. Nutr.* **2009**, *89*, 477–484. [CrossRef] [PubMed]

36. Macdiarmid, J.; Loe, J.; Kyle, J.; McNeill, G. "It was an education in portion size". Experience of eating a healthy diet and barriers to long term dietary change. *Appetite* **2013**, *71*, 411–419. [CrossRef] [PubMed]

37. Stevenson, C.; Doherty, G.; Barnett, J.; Muldoon, O.T.; Trew, K. Adolescents' views of food and eating: Identifying barriers to healthy eating. *J. Adolesc.* **2007**, *30*, 417–434. [CrossRef] [PubMed]

38. Iglesias-Gutiérrez, E.; García-Rovés, P.M.; García, Á.; Patterson, Á.M. Food preferences do not influence adolescent high-level athletes' dietary intake. *Appetite* **2008**, *50*, 536–543. [CrossRef] [PubMed]

39. Magkos, F.; Yannakoulia, M. Methodology of dietary assessment in athletes: Concepts and pitfalls. *Curr. Opin. Clin. Nutr. Metable* **2003**, *6*, 539–549. [CrossRef]

40. Goston, J.L.; Mendes, L.L. Perfil nutricional de praticantes de corrida de rua de um clube esportivo da cidade de Belo Horizonte, MG, Brasil. *Rev. Bras. Med. Esporte* **2011**, *17*, 13–17.

41. Ribeiro, S.M.L.; Freitas, A.M.P.; Pereira, B.; Vilalva, R.; Krinski, K.; Souza-Júnior, T.P. Dietary practices and anthropometric profile of professional male surfers. *J. Sports Sci.* **2015**, *3*, 79–88.

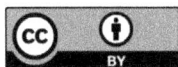

![nutrients logo] *nutrients*

MDPI

Article

The Diet Quality of Competitive Adolescent Male Rugby Union Players with Energy Balance Estimated Using Different Physical Activity Coefficients

Tracy Burrows [1,3], Simon K. Harries [2,3], Rebecca L. Williams [1,3], Cheryl Lum [1] and Robin Callister [2,3,*]

1   School of Health Sciences, Faculty of Health and Medicine, The University of Newcastle, Callaghan 2308, NSW, Australia; Tracy.Burrows@newcastle.edu.au (T.B.); Rebecca.Williams@newcastle.edu.au (R.L.W.); cheryllum1610@gmail.com (C.L.)
2   School of Biomedical Sciences and Pharmacy, Faculty of Health and Medicine, The University of Newcastle, Callaghan 2308, NSW, Australia; Simon.Harries@uon.edu.au
3   Priority Research Centre in Physical Activity and Nutrition, University of Newcastle, Callaghan 2308, NSW, Australia
*   Correspondence: Robin.Callister@newcastle.edu.au; Tel.: +61-024-921-5650; Fax: +61-024-921-7053

Received: 3 August 2016; Accepted: 31 August 2016; Published: 7 September 2016

Abstract: Objectives: The aims of the current study were to comprehensively assess the dietary intakes and diet quality of a sample of Australian competitive adolescent rugby union players and compare these intakes with National and Sports Dietitians Association (SDA) Recommendations for adolescent athletes. A secondary aim investigated applying different physical activity level (PAL) coefficients to determine total energy expenditure (TEE) in order to more effectively evaluate the adequacy of energy intakes. Design: Cross-sectional. Methods: Anthropometrics and dietary intakes were assessed in 25 competitive adolescent male rugby union players (14 to 18 years old). Diet was assessed using the validated Australian Eating Survey (AES) food frequency questionnaire and diet quality was assessed through the Australian Recommended Food Score. Results: The median dietary intakes of participants met national recommendations for percent energy (% E) from carbohydrate, protein and total fat, but not carbohydrate intake when evaluated as g/day as proposed in SDA guidelines. Median intakes of fibre and micronutrients including calcium and iron also met national recommendations. Overall diet quality was classified as 'good' with a median diet quality score of 34 (out of a possible 73); however, there was a lack of variety within key food groups including carbohydrates and proteins. Non-core food consumption exceeded recommended levels at 38% of the daily total energy intake, with substantial contributions from takeaway foods and sweetened beverages. A PAL coefficient of 1.2–1.4 was found to best balance the energy intakes of these players in their pre-season. Conclusions: Adolescent rugby players met the percent energy recommendations for macronutrients and attained an overall 'good' diet quality score. However, it was identified that when compared to specific recommendations for athletes, carbohydrate intakes were below recommendations and these players in their pre-season reported high consumption of non-core foods, particularly sugar sweetened drinks and low intakes of vegetables.

Keywords: nutrients; food frequency questionnaire; rugby; adolescents

---

1. Introduction

Adolescence is a life stage where dietary requirements for energy, protein, carbohydrates and other nutrients such as iron, zinc, and calcium are increased [1]. Meeting these dietary needs is important for adolescent growth, development and overall health, including protection against chronic disease [1]. This life stage is of interest from a dietary perspective as ambiguity often exists for calculating an adolescent's requirements, as this stage covers a diverse age range and requirements can be highly variable. Adolescents who participate in regular exercise training and sports competition may have additional nutrient needs to meet their increased energy expenditure, muscle development and maintenance, as well as performance and recovery requirements [2]. In recognition of these unique needs Sports Dietitians Australia (SDA) published a Position Statement, "Sports Nutrition for the Adolescent Athlete" [2], which provides nutrition recommendations for this population. These recommendations reinforce the importance of eating for long-term health, as well as meeting specific diet and hydration needs related to exercise. SDA guidelines specifically recommend adequate intakes of calcium and iron due to an elevated risk of deficiency of these nutrients, and that these nutrient needs should be met by food rather than supplement sources [2]. The SDA statement is directed at two groups of athletes: Active adolescent athletes and competitive adolescent athletes, but not elite athletes. The competitive group are those with demonstrated sports talent who are engaged in higher volumes of training and competition. The Australian Institute of Sport, which is the leading sports training facility in Australia, also provides dietary recommendations suggesting athletes should consume a regular spread of high quality protein foods to supply the body with appropriate quantities of essential amino acids, and high quality carbohydrate foods defined as those that are nutrient dense with consideration given to glycaemic index [3].

Rugby union is an intermittent field-based team sport, involving repeated short bursts of high intensity activity interspersed with longer periods of low intensity activity [4]. Rugby union players require high levels of strength and power to perform activities such as running, sprinting, tackling, and pushing or competing for the ball. Some positions, for example rugby forwards, require a larger body mass, with higher levels of muscle mass, but these players generally have a higher percentage of body fat. Elite rugby union players are taller, heavier and have lower body fat levels than their sub-elite counterparts [4].

The nutritional demands of rugby players vary across the game's seasons (pre-season, competitive, and off-season) [5] and likely differ depending on playing position [6]. In addition to the variations in energy needs of adolescents due to age, gender, growth and maturation, the varying levels of energy expenditure across a year make it challenging to estimate the physical activity levels (PAL) for use in estimating daily total energy expenditure (TEE) to determine the adequacy of dietary energy intake. Few studies have specifically investigated dietary intakes in adolescent rugby players. Existing studies do not comprehensively report dietary intakes; studies have examined short-term dietary intake such as single-meal consumption after training [7], reported on major or selective food groups or nutrients [8,9], and identified poor nutritional knowledge relating to sports performance [10]. Both the Australian Dietary Guidelines (ADG) and the SDA position statement recommend variety in the daily diet of adolescent athletes; however, to date no studies have investigated overall diet quality in this population group.

The aims of the current study were to comprehensively assess the dietary intakes and diet quality of a sample of Australian competitive adolescent rugby union players and compare these intakes with National and SDA recommendations for adolescent athletes. A secondary aim investigated applying different PAL coefficients to determine total energy expenditure (TEE) in order to more effectively evaluate the adequacy of energy intakes.

2. Participants and Methods

2.1. Participants

Competitive adolescent male rugby players (aged 14 to 18 years) were recruited from two sub-elite representative rugby union squads from the Hunter region, NSW, Australia. Sample size was based on the power to detect differences between groups for changes in box squat performance, which was the primary outcome measure of this study [11]. Data collection took place at the beginning of the pre-season period in February 2012. Ethics approval for this study was obtained from the University of Newcastle Human Research Ethics Committee and all participants provided written informed consent; parental consent was also provided. The study was registered with the Australia and New Zealand Clinical Trials registry (ACTRN12612000278831).

2.2. Anthropometric Assessments

These were conducted by trained research assistants between 9:00 a.m. and 10:30 a.m. during a morning assessment session at the University of Newcastle. Participants were advised with consistent information to eat a light breakfast and to perform no exercise training on the day before assessments. Height was recorded using a calibrated stadiometer (Harpenden portable stadiometer with high speed Veeder-Root counter, Holtain Ltd., Pembrokeshire, UK) and bodyweight determined using calibrated scales (CH-150kp, A&D Mercury Pty Ltd., Seven Hills, NSW, Australia). Repeat assessments were performed to ensure accuracy of measures. If there was a difference of 0.3 cm or 0.1 kg between the two measurements, a third measure was taken. Body Mass Index (BMI) was calculated using standardised equations and BMI z score calculated using Lambda, Mu, Sigma (LMS) methods [12]. Body composition was determined via bio-impedance analysis using the INBODY720 Body Comp analyser (InBody720, Biospace Co., Ltd., Seoul, Korea) with body fat (kg and %), fat free mass (FFM) (kg) and skeletal muscle mass (SMM) (kg) determined. The InBody720 has been shown to display a high level of agreement with dual energy X-ray absorption spectroscopy (DEXA), the gold standard for body composition analysis, in the measurement of body fat mass (ICC males = 0.93, $p < 0.001$ [13]), and compared to computed tomography when measuring visceral fat area ($r = 0.76$) [14].

2.3. Dietary Intakes

This was assessed using the Australian Eating Survey (AES), a 120-item semi-quantitative food frequency questionnaire (FFQ) validated for use in Australian children for energy and nutrient intakes, as well as fat profiles and fruit and vegetable intakes through a range of objective biomarkers [15–17]. This dietary assessment method was chosen over alternate methods as it has a longer reporting period and is more likely to capture usual/habitual dietary intakes. An individual response for each food is required, with consumption frequency options ranging from 'Never' to '4 or more times per day' and for some beverages up to '7 or more glasses per day', but varied depending on the item. The AES groups items according to their food group as follows: Core foods which include breads and cereals, fruit, vegetables (including potatoes), dairy, meat and meat alternatives (legumes, nuts, eggs, tofu), and non-core foods which include those foods characterised as high in sugar, salt or fat, such as sweetened drinks, packaged snacks, confectionary and takeaway foods. Fifteen supplementary questions assessed dietary behaviours including use of vitamin supplements (dosage and length of use) and frequency of take-out food.

2.4. Diet Quality

The quality of diet was assessed through the Australian Recommended Food Score (ARFS), which is a validated food-based diet quality index modelled on the Recommended Food Score by Kant and Thompson [18,19] and the Australian Child and Adolescent Recommended Food Score (ACARFS) [20,21]. The ARFS focuses on dietary quality and variety within food groups recommended in the Australian Dietary Guidelines (ADG) [1]. It is calculated by using a subset of 70 AES FFQ questions. The ARFS has sub-scales of food groups including fruits, vegetables, grains, protein sources, vegetarian protein sources, dairy and condiments. Most foods are awarded one point for a consumption frequency of ≥once per week, but varies based on national dietary guidelines [1,22] with bonus points for grained varieties of breads and cereals and low fat dairy. The ARFS score was calculated by summing the points for each item, the total score ranges from zero to 73.

Nutrient intakes were computed using the Australian AusNut 1999 database (All Foods) Revision 17 primarily, and AusFoods (Brands) Revision 5 (Australian Government Publishing Service, Canberra,

Australia). The estimated mean individual daily intakes for macro- and micro-nutrients were calculated using FoodWorks (version 3.02.581, Xyris Software, Highgate Hill, Queensland, Australia). The computed data was then compared to standardized national data [23]. To standardise the assessment of fibre intakes for participants with differing energy intakes, grams of fibre/1000 kJ were calculated. Servings of fruits and vegetables were calculated by summing the weight or energy of food items in the AES coded as fruits or vegetables and dividing by the serve size dictated in the Australian Guide to Healthy Eating (AGHE) (fruits, 150 g and vegetables, 75 g, grains, meat/alternatives and dairy 500–600 kJ/serve). All other foods were quantified using multiples of standard child portions from the 1995 Australian National Nutrition Survey of children and adolescents, which are suitable for use in this population group.

2.5. Physical Activity Level (PAL) Calculations

In order to determine whether energy intakes met energy needs, equations were used to predict exercise and total energy expenditure (TEE) and from this calculate energy availability. The Schofield equation using both height and weight values is the preferred equation for estimating resting energy expenditure (REE) in children and adolescents [24]. To better estimate TEE, a PAL coefficient can be applied to account for exercise related increases in EE. PAL recommendations are available for adult athletes however there is a lack of consensus of PAL levels to use in adolescent athletes [25–27]. For the purpose of this study, a range of coefficient values were applied to calculated REE to reflect a range of activity levels. These included: No PAL, and PAL 1.2, 1.4, 1.6 and 1.8.

2.6. Data Analysis

Participant demographics and data from the food frequency questionnaires were analyzed using SPSS. Data were not normally distributed so non-parametric tests were used and data are presented as median and interquartile range. Wilcoxon rank tests were used to compare differences between estimated energy needs and reported energy intake. Bland Altman plots were produced according to standardised methods [28] to assess levels of agreement between reported and estimated energy requirements. Statistical significance was set at the 5% level ($p < 0.05$).

3. Results

3.1. Participant Characteristics

Participant characteristics are reported in Table 1. The median (IQR) age of players was 16 (2) years with a BMI of 23.6 (5.5) kg/m^2 Body composition analysis showed body fat was 11.7 (6.2) kg, fat free mass was 66.1 (13.7) kg and skeletal muscle mass was 37.9 (9.9) kg. Participants reported that, on average, they were currently doing one hour or less per day of exercise.

3.2. Energy Needs and Energy Intakes

The median (IQR) BMR of the rugby players was 8379 (1254) kJ and total estimated energy requirements ranged from 10,055 (1505) kJ to 15,083 (2258) kJ when using a PAL of 1.2 up to 1.8, respectively. Reported dietary intakes as per the AES FFQ are summarised in Tables 2 and 3. The median (IQR) reported energy intake was 10,372 (4974) kJ.

Applying a PAL coefficient of 1.2 or 1.4 produced the closest TEE for energy balance between the reported intakes and calculated expenditures. Using a PAL of 1.2 or 1.4, the mean differences between TEE and reported energy intakes were −614 kJ ($p = 0.480$) and +1129 kJ ($p = 0.209$) respectively. Applying no PAL or the larger coefficients of 1.6 and 1.8, reflecting more extensive exercise, provided larger discrepancies with differences of 2872 kJ ($p = 0.004$) and 4516 kJ ($p < 0.000$) for PAL 1.6 and 1.8, respectively.

Table 1. Participant characteristics of adolescent rugby players.

Characteristic	Median (IQR)
Age (year)	16 (2)
Weight (kg)	76.5 (10.0)
Height (cm)	179.6 (6.5)
Body fat (kg)	11.7 (6.2)
Body fat (%)	14.0 (6.6)
Fat free mass (kg)	66.1 (13.7)
Skeletal Muscle Mass (kg)	37.9 (9.9)
Basal Metabolic Rate (/day)	
kJ	8379 (1254)
kCal	1995 (299)
Estimated Energy Requirement (kJ)	
PAL 1.2	10,055 (1505)
PAL 1.4	11,731 (1756)
PAL 1.6	13,407 (2007)
PAL 1.8	15,083 (2258)
Estimated Exercise Expenditure (kJ)	
PAL 1.2	1676 (251)
PAL 1.4	3352 (502)
PAL 1.6	5028 (753)
PAL 1.8	6704 (1003)

3.3. Macronutrients: Fats, Protein and Carbohydrates

The median intake of all participants met the recommended percentage of daily total energy intake for Australians (% TE) from macronutrients for energy derived from carbohydrate (45%–65% TE), total fat (20%–35% TE) and protein intakes (15%–25% TE) (Table 2). Reported intakes of saturated fats (15% E) exceeded the national recommended intake of <10% TE, with the median intake of 15% TE with 4% of total energy intake from poly-unsaturated fat and 12% from monounsaturated.

Protein intakes in this study were found to be similar when compared to the Australian Health Survey (AHS) data of 14- to 18-year-old males in the general population and were within 4% of each other [24]. When intakes for this study were compared directly to SDA recommendations, protein requirements in g/kg were also met with the median intake of 1.5 g/kg/day.

Carbohydrate intakes in this study were within 7% of those averages found for adolescent males in the AHS [23]. When expressed as g/kg, as recommended by the SDA for carbohydrates, the median intake of this population was below that suggested with a median intake of 3.6 g/kg compared to the recommended 5–7 g/kg/day for those following a moderate exercise program [2,3].

3.4. Micronutrients

Intakes of iron and calcium met both National Dietary Recommendations (Table 2) and SDA recommendations. Intakes of calcium and iron were higher in rugby players in this study than in adolescent males of the same age in the general Australian population (AHS data) [23] with a calcium intake approximately 200 mg higher (approximately 0.8 serve/day) and iron intake 2 mg higher. The fibre intake met recommendations assessed both as grams per day (RDI 28 g/day) and when adjusted for energy intake as g/1000 kJ. The fibre intake of these males was on average 5 g/day higher than that of the general population who had an intake of 23 g/day [29].

Table 2. Energy and nutrient intakes of adolescent male rugby players and comparison with National Dietary Recommendations and SDA recommendations.

Nutrient	Median (IQR)	% Total Daily Energy	Health Recommendations [1]	SDA Recommendations [2]
Energy (kJ)	10,372 (4974)	X	X	
Protein (total g)	108.1 (75.9)	19 (5)	15%–25% of energy	
g/kg/day	1.53 (0.86)	X	0.8 g/kg	1.3–1.8 g/kg
Fat (g)	88.5 (54.9)	34 (8)	20%–35% energy	
Saturated fat (g)	39.8 (21.5)	15 (4)	8%–10% of energy	
Polyunsaturated fats (g)	9.4 (6.6)	4(1)		
Monounsaturated fats (g)	29.9 (16.4)	12 (3)		
Carbohydrates (g)	317 (153)	48 (12)	45%–65% of energy	
g/kg/day	3.59 (2.40)	X	X	5–7 g/kg
Sugars (g)	149.4 (117.4)	X	X	
Fibre (g)	33.4 (15.1)	X	28 g/day	
Fibre/1000 kJ	2.6 (0.6)	X	X	
Calcium (mg)	1124 (713)	X	1050 mg/day	
Iron (mg)	15.9 (7.9)	X	8 mg/day	

EAR—Estimated average requirements, ARFS—Australian Recommended Food Score: A measure of diet quality, X no specific recommendations/NA.

3.5. Fluid Intake

Only 23% of adolescents reported consuming >seven glasses of water/day. Consumption of sugar-sweetened beverages was deemed high with soft drinks (not diet), fruit juice-based drinks and cordial (make up) consumed at intakes >two glasses/day by 26%, 44% and 23% of participants, respectively. Fruit juice-based drinks were the most commonly consumed sweetened drink in these players. Vitamin supplements were reported as being consumed by only 8% (*n* = 2) of the participants, at a dose of three to five vitamin tablets per week.

3.6. Food Groups and Diet Quality

Table 3 presents the dietary intakes from major food groups and food subgroups as well as the total diet quality score for both rugby players in this study and males of the same age in the general population. The median % TE derived from core foods for males in this study (breads and cereals, vegetables, fruits, meat and meat alternatives, milk and dairy) was 62% (IQR 19) and for males in the general population it was 59%. The reported number of servings of fruit (which excludes juice) was 4.7 servings/day for males in this study, which exceeded the AGHE recommendation of two servings/day. Only 46% of male children and adolescents in the general population consume the recommended two servings/day, consuming a mean of 1.5 servings and median 1.1 servings [30]. Intakes of vegetables in these adolescent rugby players were well below recommendations at 1.1 servings/day compared to the recommendation of five servings/day. Males of the same age in the general population also had suboptimal intakes of vegetables consuming a mean of 2.2 (median 2.1) servings/day. Intakes of grains were 3.7 servings/day in this study and a mean of 5.7 (5.5 median) servings/day in males in the general population, with both well short of the recommended seven servings/day. Meat/alternatives in the rugby players at 3.4 servings/day was higher than in the general population (1.7 servings/day). Neither the males in this study nor in the general population met the 3.5 servings/day recommendation for dairy intake, consuming 2.1 and 1.6 servings/day, respectively.

The median % TE derived from non-core foods in this study was 38% (IQR 19) and that of males in the general population was 40.7%, both of which exceed the recommendation of 5%–10% of the total energy intake. The main sources of non-core food energy in these rugby players were 4.4% TE from sweetened drinks (soft drinks/cordials/sports drinks/juice), 5.4% TE from packaged snacks (muesli/snack bars), 3.8% TE from confectionary (chocolates/candy), and 8.1% TE from takeout meals, which includes hamburgers, fries, pies and sausage rolls.

3.7. Diet Quality Scores

The median ARFS score was 34 out of a possible 73 points, which is classified as 'good' (range 32 or above) diet quality [28]. A breakdown into the ARFS subgroups identified a lack of variety within subgroups, with median scores for vegetables at 12 out of a possible score of 21, fruit at six out of 12, dairy at 4.5 out of 11, meat at three out of seven and meat/alternatives at two out of six.

Table 3. Food group intakes of adolescent male rugby players.

Food Sub Groups	Population				Health Recommendations (Servings/Day) [1]
	14–18 Years Old Rugby Players		14–18 Years Old Males—AHS		
	Median (IQR) (Servings/Day)	% Total Daily Energy	Mean (Servings/Day)	% Total Daily Energy	
Fruit	4.7 (5.0)	X	1.5	X	2
Vegetables	1.1 (0.5)	X	2.2	X	5 1/2
Grains	3.7 (2.8)	X	5.7	X	7
Meat/alternatives	3.4 (2.5)	X	1.7	X	2 1/2
Dairy	2.1 (2.1)	X	1.6	X	3 1/2
Discretionary foods	7.5 (3.7)	38.4	X	40.7	0–5 *
Energy (kJ): sweetened drinks	508 (616)	4.4 (8.2)			X
Energy (kJ): packaged snacks	549 (780)	5.4 (7.8)			X
Energy (kJ): confectionary	376 (516)	3.8 (4.8)			X
Energy (kJ): takeaway	913 (521)	8.1 (4.8)			X

Diet Quality	Score		
	14–18 Years Old Rugby Players	Adults (18+ Years)	
Total ARFS (out of 73)	34 (13)	X	36 (10.5) [21]	X

AHS—Australian Health survey; % TE—percentage of total energy; * Approximate number of additional servings from the five food groups or unsaturated spreads and oils or discretionary choices.

4. Discussion

This study investigated the dietary intakes and diet quality of competitive adolescent male rugby players using a validated FFQ. These players had adequate macronutrient profiles for carbohydrate, total fat and protein intakes but exceeded national recommendations for saturated fat. Micronutrient intakes, including calcium and iron, were also adequate. Excess energy was derived from non-core foods, particularly fruit juices and other sweetened drinks, and there was inadequate vegetable consumption when compared to national recommendations. Overall diet quality was classified as 'good', although the results indicate a substantial scope to improve diet variety, particularly within the fruit, vegetable and dairy food groups.

The energy requirements of the adolescent athletes were met by their dietary intakes when a PAL coefficient of 1.2 or 1.4 was used. It is important to recognise that these players were assessed immediately prior to the commencement of pre-season training. The period over which they reported their diet was the off-season. Players reported less than one hour of physical activity a day during this period. This suggests that they may need to increase their energy intake once training and then playing commence, and that the PAL required to calculate energy needs would likely approach 1.6 for this period of the year.

Macronutrients: Protein intakes were found to be meeting and/or exceeding SDA recommendations in competitive adolescent rugby players, for both percentage of total energy intake and g/kg. For carbohydrate intakes, this population group was found to have adequate intakes compared to national dietary recommendations for percentage of total energy intake. However, when compared to SDA recommendations for carbohydrate intake expressed as g/kg, their intakes were found to be inadequate for those undertaking moderate exercise training. Given these players were just commencing their pre-season, their physical activity levels were likely lower than they would become during pre-season training and the competition season where their estimated requirements for carbohydrate could increase to as much 6–10 g/kg [3]. Total fat intakes were found to be within recommended ranges for this age group; however, saturated fats exceeded recommendations. This is likely to have been largely derived from non-core foods which also exceeded recommendations.

Micronutrients: Recommended intakes were met for calcium and iron, which were a focus in this study as they are specifically mentioned in the SDA position statement as important to adolescent health. Although the players did not meet the recommended servings of dairy foods per day, which are recognised as excellent sources of calcium, these players still met their calcium requirements, indicating they are likely deriving calcium from alternate food sources including nuts and beans. These athletes did not rely on vitamin supplements to meet these nutrient needs, with few participants reporting regular intake. Dietary intakes of fibre were met, which provides some indication of the quality of the carbohydrate intake of these rugby players. In this study, fibre intake was adjusted for energy intake and reported per 1000 kJ so it is not simply reflective of higher energy intake. Fibre intake is likely to be derived from carbohydrate-based sources from whole grains including breakfast cereals often containing moderate amounts of fibre which are more nutrient dense than refined flour sources. Servings of fruit were adequate but not vegetable intakes. Increased intakes of vegetables are associated increased intakes of nutrients. It is recommended that intakes of vegetables be increased in these adolescent athletes to ensure intakes of other vitamins and minerals such as magnesium for muscle function [31] and antioxidants for inflammation [32].

The consumption of non-core foods was higher than desirable, with energy from takeout and sugar-sweetened beverages being the major contributors. Participants consumed low quantities of water compared with fluid intakes from other sources. Sweetened drinks including soft drinks and cordial but particularly fruit juice-based drinks were commonly consumed; sports drinks were not directly assessed in this study. This finding may be reflective of the broader food environment where current food trends such as smoothies and juice bars increase the availability and perception that these drinks are healthy [33]. It is acknowledged that increased consumption of high-energy-density items such as sweetened drinks may help in achieving the energy needs of adolescent athletes; however, this may also have implications for excess energy intake and oral health [34]. Energy-dense items may also be considered convenient for adolescents and might characterise adolescent diets, which are increasingly influenced by peers and the media, as they start to assert independence and control of their food intakes and preferences [35,36]. This is consistent with other research where adolescents consume intakes of energy-dense nutrient-poor foods well above the national recommendation of 5% of energy. In this study, non-core foods were found to contribute approximately 38% of daily energy, which is consistent with national dietary surveys where reported intakes constitute up to 41% of daily energy [37]. Elite rugby athletes are required to have speed, agility, strength and power; this high consumption of non-core foods may compromise the players' body composition, fitness, and performance [38].

Both the Australian Dietary Guidelines (ADG) and the SDA position statement recommend variety in daily diet. The SDA recommendations particularly emphasise the quality of carbohydrate and protein foods for adolescent athletes [2]. This is consistent with the broader ADG, which recommend variety in daily diet in addition to variety within food groups, as this is more likely to produce a diet with a more comprehensive and complete range of nutrients. Quality carbohydrate foods generally include those that are not highly processed and are made from whole grains with adequate quantities of fibre. The quality of foods in this study was assessed through the ARFS, which values both food quality and variety among food groups and within groups; for example, the meat and alternatives group includes a range of foods such as meat, eggs, and fish, all of which differ in their nutrient profiles. Although the overall ARFS score for the players' diets was considered good, the scores of important food subgroups such as fruit, vegetables, dairy and protein foods were less than 50% of the available points, which reflects a lack of variety within these food groups [28]. Improvements in consumption of these foods could be targeted in future interventions.

Studies suggest adolescents consume supplements for health benefits, energy and enhancement of sports performance [39–41]. Common supplements used by athletes include sports drinks, protein powders and creatine; however, there was very little use of supplements in this study. Less than 10% of players reported consuming vitamin supplements, which was less than expected [39]. Recent studies which used a four-day food diary to assess dietary intake reported that 74% of 14- to 19-year-old rugby players consumed dietary supplements [9]. Details on the assessment of supplements used by participants in this study were limited to consumption patterns and frequency of intake; the types of supplements (i.e., protein or antioxidants) and reasons for use were not assessed. These should be investigated more thoroughly in future studies.

Nutrition education has been identified as an area of need for adolescent athletes previously in the literature [10], especially for adolescent rugby players. While previous studies did not describe areas for nutrition education, the results from this study provide a starting point for areas which require improvement to improve overall health and performance. These include education on food groups, particularly non-core foods (sweetened drinks, takeaways), as a strategy to decrease overall saturated fat and optimise fat profiles, and the importance of overall diet quality and diet variety within food groups to ensure adequacy of diet.

The AES FFQ used in this study has been validated against a number of objective dietary standards including double-labelled water, plasma carotenoids and red blood cell membrane fatty acids; however, it is acknowledged that FFQs, like most dietary assessment tools, are prone to bias, being a self-report measure [42]. The FFQ used assesses the usual dietary intake with a reporting period of the previous six months; there is no assessment of the timing of intake. Studies in athletes [40] demonstrate that timing of dietary intake is an important factor to maximise performance and should be assessed in future studies through use of a diet history, a food and training diary or direct observations. Timing of meals and snacks may be particularly important for nutrients such as protein and should be investigated in future studies, as an amount of approximately 20 g of protein throughout or immediately following strength training enhances acute protein synthetic responses to the training stimulus [43]. Body composition in this study was measured using an INBODY720 Body Composition Analyzer and not the recognised gold standard DEXA method for assessing body composition. Other limitations to the study include the small sample size, estimation of energy expenditure through a standardised equation rather than measurement of resting energy expenditure, and that the population studied was from one country and two squads from the same region; while all participants were advised to have light breakfast before assessments, there may have been some variation in intake prior to assessments. Future studies investigating dietary habits in competitive adolescents should consider a multi-centre trial and assessing diet during different stages of the training and competitive seasons.

5. Conclusions

This study examined the nutrient profiles and diet quality of competitive adolescent rugby players. The key findings were that these players met the percent energy recommendations for macronutrients and attained an overall 'good' diet quality score. However, it was identified that when compared to specific recommendations for athletes, carbohydrate intakes were below recommendations and these players in their pre-season reported high consumption of non-core foods, particularly sugar-sweetened drinks, and low intakes of vegetables, highlighting particular areas for dietary education. During the off-season, a PAL of 1.2 or 1.4 appears appropriate for determining energy balance; however, further research should investigate the use of PALs at different training loads.

Acknowledgments: The authors of this study would like to thank Australian Rugby Union Ltd. and Hunter Junior Rugby Union Inc. No external funding was used for this project.

Author Contributions: S.H. and R.C. designed the study and collected data. T.B. led the write up and analysis of this manuscript with R.W. and C.L. also major contributors. All authors contributed and approved the final manuscript.

Conflicts of Interest: The authors have no competing interests relating to the content of this manuscript. There were no other contributors to this manuscript.

References

1. NHMRC. Australian Dietary Guidelines (2013). Available online: https://www.nhmrc.gov.au/guidelines-publications/n55? (accessed on 20 August 2013).

2. Desbrow, B.; McCormack, J.; Burke, L.M.; Cox, G.R.; Fallon, K.; Hislop, M.; Logan, R.; Marino, N.; Sawyer, S.M.; Shaw, G.; et al. Sports dietitians Australia position statement: Sports nutrition for the adolescent athlete. *Int. J. Sport Nutr. Exerc. Metab.* **2014**, *24*, 570–584. [CrossRef] [PubMed]

3. AIS. Australian Institute of Sport-Nutrition Fact Sheets. Available online: http://www.ausport.gov.au/ais/nutrition/factsheets (accessed on 3 September 2016).

4. Duthie, G.; Pyne, D.; Hooper, S. Applied physiology and game analysis of rugby union. *Sports Med.* **2003**, *33*, 973–991. [CrossRef] [PubMed]

5. Holway, F.E.; Spriet, L.L. Sport-specific nutrition: Practical strategies for team sports. *J. Sports Sci.* **2011**, *29*, S115–S125. [CrossRef] [PubMed]

6. Potgeiter, S.; Visser, J.; Croukamp, I.; Markides, M.; Nascimento, J.; Scott, K. Body composition and habitual and match-day dietary intake of the FNB maties varsity cup rugby players. *S. Afr. J. Sports Med.* **2014**, *26*, 35–43. [CrossRef]

7. Thivel, D.; Maso, F.; Aouiche, S.; Coigent, B.; Doré, E.; Duché, P. Nutritional responses to acute training sessions in young elite players. *Appetite* **2015**, *84*, 316–321. [CrossRef] [PubMed]

8. Imamura, H.; Iide, K.; Yoshimura, Y.; Kumagai, K.; Oshikata, R.; Miyahara, K.; Oda, K.; Miyamoto, N.; Nakazawa, A. Nutrient intake, serum lipids and iron status of colligate rugby players. *J. Int. Soc. Sports Nutr.* **2013**, *10*. [CrossRef] [PubMed]

9. Smith, D.R.; Jones, B.; Sutton, L.; King, R.F.; Duckworth, L.C. Dietary intakes of elite 14–19 year old English academy rugby players during a pre-season training period. *Int. J. Sport Nutr. Exerc. Metab.* **2016**. [CrossRef] [PubMed]

10. Walsh, M.; Cartwright, L.; Corish, C.; Sugrue, S.; Wood-Martin, R. The body composition, nutritional knowledge, attitudes, behaviors, and future education needs of senior schoolboy rugby players in Ireland. *Int. J. Sport Nutr. Exerc. Metab.* **2011**, *21*, 365–376. [CrossRef] [PubMed]

11. Harries, S.; Lubans, D.; Callister, R. Comparison of resistance training progression models on maximal strength in sub-elite adolescent rugby union players. *J. Sci. Med. Sport* **2016**, *19*, 163–169. [CrossRef] [PubMed]

12. Cole, T.; Pan, H. *Lms Growth Computer Program, 2.12*; Medical Research Council: Cambridge, UK, 2002.

13. Ling, C.H.; de Craen, A.J.; Slagboom, P.E.; Gunn, D.A.; Stokkel, M.P.; Westendorp, R.G.; Maier, A.B. Accuracy of direct segmental multi-frequency bioimpedance analysis in the assessment of total body and segmental body composition in middle-aged adult population. *Clin. Nutr.* **2011**, *30*, 610–615. [CrossRef] [PubMed]

14. Ogawa, H.; Fujitani, K.; Tsujinaka, T.; Imanishi, K.; Shirakata, H.; Kantani, A.; Hirao, M.; Kurokawa, Y.; Utsumi, S. Inbody 720 as a new method of evaluating visceral obesity. *Hepato-Gastroenterology* **2011**, *58*, 42–44. [PubMed]

15. Burrows, T.; Berthton, B.; Garg, M.; Collins, C. Validation of food frequency questionnaire using red blood cell membrane fatty acids. *Eur. J. Clin. Nutr.* **2012**, *66*, 825–829. [CrossRef] [PubMed]

16. Burrows, T.L.; Warren, J.M.; Colyvas, K.; Garg, M.L.; Collins, C.E. Validation of overweight childrens fruit and vegetable intake using plasma carotenoids. *Obesity* **2009**, *17*, 162–168. [CrossRef] [PubMed]

17. Collins, C.; Watson, J.; Guest, M.; Boggess, M.; Duncanson, K.; Pezdirc, K.; Rollo, M.; Hutchesson, M.; Burrows, T. Reproducibility and comparative validity of a food frequency questionnaire for adults. *Clin. Nutr.* **2014**, *33*, 906–914. [CrossRef] [PubMed]

18. Kant, A.; Thompson, F. Measures of overall diet quality from a food frequency questionnaire: National health interview survey 1992. *Nutr. Rev.* **1997**, *17*, 1443–1456. [CrossRef]

19. Marshall, S.; Burrows, T.; Collins, C. Systematic review of diet quality indices and their associations with health-related outcomes in children and adolescents. *J. Hum. Nutr. Diet.* **2014**, *27*, 577–598. [CrossRef] [PubMed]

20. Marshall, S.; Watson, J.; Burrows, T.; Guest, M.; Collins, C.E. The development and evaluation of the Australian child and adolescent recommended food score: A cross-sectional study. *Nutr. J.* **2012**, *11*, 96. [CrossRef] [PubMed]
21. Collins, C.E.; Burrows, T.L.; Rollo, M.E.; Boggess, M.M.; Watson, J.F.; Guest, M.; Duncanson, K.; Pezdirc, K.; Hutchesson, M.J. The comparative validity and reproducibility of a diet quality index for adults: The Australian recommended food score. *Nutrients* **2015**, *7*, 785–798. [CrossRef] [PubMed]
22. Smith, A.; Kellet, E.; Schmerlaib, Y. *The Australian Guide to Healthy Eating*; Commonwealth Department of Health and Family Services under the National Food and Nutrition Policy Program: Canberra, Australia, 1998.
23. ABS. Australian Bureau of Statistics Australian Health Survey: Usual Nutrient Intakes, 2011–2012. Available online: http://www.abs.gov.au/ausstats/abs@.nsf/Lookup/4364.0.55.008main+features12011-12 (accessed on 3 September 2016).
24. Rodriguez, G.; Moreno, L.; Sarri, A.; Fleta, J.; Bueno, M. Resting energy expenditure in children and adolescents: Agreement between calorimetry and prediction equations. *Clin. Nutr.* **2000**, *21*, 255–260. [CrossRef]
25. Carlsohn, A.; Scharhag-Rosenberger, F.; Cassel, M.; Weber, J.; Guzman, A.; Mayer, F. Physical activity levels to estimate the energy requirement of adolescent athletes. *Pediatr. Exerc. Sci.* **2011**, *23*, 261–269. [CrossRef] [PubMed]
26. Shetty, P.S. Human energy requirements. Scientific back-ground papers from the joint FAO/WHO/UNU expert consultation. *Public Health Nutr.* **2005**, *8*, 929–1228.
27. Torun, B.; Davies, P.; Livingstone, M.; Paolisso, M.; Sackett, R.; Spurr, G. Energy requirements and dietary energy recommendations for children and adolescents 1 to 18 years old. *Eur. J. Clin. Nutr.* **1996**, *50*, S37–S81. [PubMed]
28. Altman, D.G.; Bland, J.M. Measurement in medicine: The analysis of method comparison studies. *J. R. Stat. Soc.* **1983**, *32*, 307–317. [CrossRef]
29. ABS. Australian Bureau of Statistics. Australian Health Survey: First Results 2014–2015. Available online: http://www.abs.gov.au/AUSSTATS/abs@.nsf/DetailsPage/4364.0.55.0012014-15?OpenDocument (accessed on 3 September 2016).
30. ABS. Australian Health Survey: Consumption of Food Groups from the Australian Dietary Guidelines, 2011–2012. Available online: http://www.Abs.Gov.Au/ausstats/abs@.Nsf/mf/4364.0.55.012 (accessed on 15 July 2016).
31. Volpe, S. Magnesium and the athlete. *Curr. Sports Med. Rep.* **2015**, *14*, 279–283. [CrossRef] [PubMed]
32. Watson, T.; Callister, R.; Taylor, R.; Sibbritt, D.; MacDonald-Wicks, L.; Garg, M.L. Antioxidant restriction and oxidative stress in short-duration exhaustive exercise. *Med. Sci. Sports Exerc.* **2005**, *37*, 63–71. [CrossRef] [PubMed]
33. Bucher, T.; Siegrist, M. Children's and parents' health perception of different soft drinks. *Br. J. Nutr.* **2015**, *113*, 526–535. [CrossRef] [PubMed]
34. Mishra, M.; Mishra, S. Sugar sweetenend beverages: General and oral health hazards in children and adolescents. *Int. J. Clin. Pediatr. Den.* **2011**, *4*, 119–123. [CrossRef]
35. Savige, G.S.; Ball, K.; Worsley, A.; Crawford, D. Food intake patterns among Australian adolescents. *Asia Pac. J. Clin. Nutr.* **2007**, *16*, 738–747. [PubMed]
36. Truswell, A.S.; Darton-Hill, I. Food habits of adolescents. *Nutr. Rev.* **2009**, *39*, 73–88. [CrossRef]
37. Rangan, A.M.; Randall, D.; Hector, D.J.; Gill, T.P.; Webb, K.L. Consumption of 'extra' foods by Australian children: Types, quantities and contribution to energy and nutrient intakes. *Eur. J. Clin. Nutr.* **2008**, *62*, 356–364. [CrossRef] [PubMed]
38. Duthie, G.M.; Pyne, D.B.; Hopkins, W.G.; Livingstone, S.; Hooper, S.L. Anthropometry profiles of elite rugby players: Quantifying changes in lean mass. *Br. J. Sport Med.* **2006**, *40*, 202–207. [CrossRef] [PubMed]
39. O'Dea, J.A. Consumption of nutritional supplements among adolescents: Usage and perceived benefits. *Health Educ. Res.* **2003**, *18*, 98–107. [CrossRef] [PubMed]
40. Calfee, R.; Fadale, P. Popular ergogenic drugs and supplements in young athletes. *Pediatrics* **2006**, *117*, 577–589. [CrossRef] [PubMed]
41. Schwenk, T.L.; Costley, C.D. When food becomes a drug: Nonanabolic nutritional supplement use in athletes. *Am. J. Sports Med.* **2002**, *30*, 907–916. [PubMed]

Nutrients **2016**, *8*, 548

42. Burrows, T.; Martin, R.; Collins, C. A systematic review of the validity of dietary assessment methods in children when compared with the method of doubly labelled water. *J. Am. Diet Assoc.* **2010**, *110*, 1501–1510. [CrossRef] [PubMed]

43. Phillips, S.; VanLoom, L. Dietary protein for athletes: From requirements to optimum adaptation. *J. Sport Sci.* **2011**, *29*, S29–S38. [CrossRef] [PubMed]

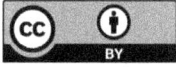

nutrients [MDPI]

Article

Supplemental Protein during Heavy Cycling Training and Recovery Impacts Skeletal Muscle and Heart Rate Responses but Not Performance

Andrew C. D'Lugos, Nicholas D. Luden, Justin M. Faller, Jeremy D. Akers, Alec I. McKenzie and Michael J. Saunders *

Department of Kinesiology, James Madison University, 261 Bluestone Drive MSC 2302, Harrisonburg, VA 22807, USA; dlugosac@dukes.jmu.edu (A.C.D.); ludennd@jmu.edu (N.D.L.); fallerjm@dukes.jmu.edu (J.M.F.); akersjd@jmu.edu (J.D.A.); mckenzai@dukes.jmu.edu (A.I.M.)
* Correspondence: saundemj@jmu.edu; Tel.: +1-540-568-8121

Received: 11 July 2016; Accepted: 29 August 2016; Published: 7 September 2016

Abstract: The effects of protein supplementation on cycling performance, skeletal muscle function, and heart rate responses to exercise were examined following intensified (ICT) and reduced-volume training (RVT). Seven cyclists performed consecutive periods of normal training (NT), ICT (10 days; average training duration 220% of NT), and RVT (10 days; training duration 66% of NT). In a crossover design, subjects consumed supplemental carbohydrate (CHO) or an equal amount of carbohydrate with added protein (CP) during and following each exercise session (CP = +0.94 g/kg/day protein during ICT; +0.39 g/kg/day during RVT). A 30-kilometer time trial performance (following 120 min at 50% W_{max}) was modestly impaired following ICT (+2.4 ± 6.4% versus NT) and returned to baseline levels following RVT (−0.7 ± 4.5% versus NT), with similar responses between CHO and CP. Skeletal muscle torque at 120 deg/s benefited from CP, compared to CHO, following ICT. However, this effect was no longer present at RVT. Following ICT, muscle fiber cross-sectional area was increased with CP, while there were no clear changes with CHO. Reductions in constant-load heart rates (at 50% W_{max}) following RVT were *likely* greater with CP than CHO (−9 ± 9 bpm). Overall it appears that CP supplementation impacted skeletal muscle and heart rate responses during a period of heavy training and recovery, but this did not result in meaningful changes in time trial performance.

Keywords: carbohydrate; protein; chocolate milk; muscle repair; sports nutrition

---

1. Introduction

Athletes perform condensed periods of overload training to elicit compensatory adaptations and performance gains. These planned periods of heavy training often lead to transient decrements in physiological function and performance capacity [1–3]. Numerous reports suggest that co-ingestion of carbohydrate and protein (CP) proximal to a single session of heavy exercise can enhance subsequent performance compared to carbohydrate (CHO) treatments matched for carbohydrate content [4], or total calories [5–8]. CP supplementation may therefore be a feasible strategy to promote recovery, minimize performance decrements, and maximize compensatory adaptations during periods of heavy training and recovery. However, comparatively few studies have assessed the efficacy of CP supplementation over multiple days of training, and although there are some reports that CP can enhance subsequent performance under these conditions [9–11], the effects of CP on functional recovery across multiple days of training remains unclear [12–14].

An important feature shared by the aforementioned multi-day studies is that performance levels were sustained over multiple days of heavy training, even in the CHO control conditions. Very little is known about the value of CP supplementation during an extended period of rigorous training that leads to impaired physical function and performance. One related study examined the effects of a protein-enriched diet (3.0 vs. 1.5 g/kg/day) during seven days of intensified training followed by seven days of reduced-volume training [15]. Higher protein intake resulted in 'possible attenuation' of performance decrements following the intensified training period, as well as a 'possible benefit' on performance restoration after the reduced-training period. By contrast, a recent study supplemented CP during exercise throughout six days of strenuous training that elicited decrements in performance, and reported no differences in performance versus an isocaloric CHO supplement (with CP provided post-exercise in both conditions) [16]. However, neither of these studies specifically examined the impact of CP when provided immediately post-exercise, which is potentially significant because relatively modest increases in protein intake provided post-exercise (i.e., 0.4 g/kg/h) have been shown to positively impact next-day exercise performance versus CHO [8]. Therefore, a primary purpose of the present investigation was to investigate the effects of CP provided during and post-exercise on exercise performance following multiple days of strenuous cycling training, and a subsequent period of recovery.

The ostensible benefit of CP supplementation during heavy periods of endurance training could be mediated through the effects of protein on skeletal muscle. There is evidence that skeletal muscle undergoes a markedly different global transcriptional response to endurance exercise when protein is added to a supplement containing carbohydrate and fat [17]. Among other pathways, gene expression related to immune and inflammatory processes and extracellular matrix and cytoskeletal remodeling appeared to be favorably influenced by the presence of exogenous protein. In support of these molecular alterations, CP supplementation close to acute heavy endurance exercise can better preserve subsequent whole muscle function and reduce indices of post-exercise muscle damage (i.e., muscle soreness and biomarkers of sarcolemma permeability) compared to CHO alone [18,19]. Several reports also indicate that CP can continue to attenuate markers of muscle damage across multiple days of exercise [9,12,20,21]. However, very little is known about how this may impact whole muscle function and performance during periods of heavy training and subsequent recovery. Thus, the present study was also designed to examine the effects of CP supplementation on changes in muscle fiber cross-sectional area (CSA), muscle function, and markers of muscle damage during consecutive periods of strenuous cycling training and recovery.

CP intake may also impact endurance performance via changes in cardiovascular responses during exercise. For instance, cycling performance was enhanced during the latter stages of an 8-day stage race in those consuming CP versus CHO alone [22]. The CP group also had attenuated changes in body temperature during exercise, and tended to have lower exercise heart rates, suggesting performance benefits were related to altered cardiovascular responses with CP. This view is strengthened by observations in untrained individuals that CP ingestion was associated with increased plasma albumin content and plasma volume expansion [23–25], resulting in increased stroke volume and decreased heart rate during exercise versus placebo [24,25]. So, there is emerging evidence that CP may influence cardiovascular responses during repeated days of heavy cycling, but these effects have not yet been systematically investigated in endurance athletes. Therefore, the present study also examined the effects of CP supplementation on heart rate responses during constant-load cycling following consecutive periods of strenuous cycling training and recovery.

2. Materials and Methods

2.1. Subjects

Ten endurance-trained cyclists from James Madison University and the Harrisonburg area volunteered for this study. All subjects were experienced cyclists who reported ≥ 7 h·week^{-1} of cycling training for ≥ 2 months prior to the investigation (including at least one ride ≥ 3 h every 14 days), and demonstrated VO$_{2\text{peak}}$ values ≥ 50 mL·kg^{-1}·min^{-1}. One subject failed to complete the study due to time demands and another was unable to adhere to dietary and training controls. An additional subject completed all trials, but exhibited substantial variations in exercise performance between baseline trials conducted at the onset of each experimental condition (i.e., variability in time trial performance >3 SD larger than those from all other subjects). Thus, performance data for this subject was removed, and data are reported for 7 subjects (5 males, 2 females; age, 25 ± 8 year; height, 173 ± 12 cm; weight, 71 ± 12 kg; VO_{2peak}, 63 ± 9 mL·kg^{-1}·min^{-1}). Subjects gave consent to participate after receiving written and oral information regarding experimental procedures and potential risks. All procedures were approved by James Madison University's Institutional Review Board (Protocol #12-0487).

2.2. Preliminary Testing

An incremental-load cycling test was conducted on a computerized ergometer (Velotron, Racermate Inc., Seattle, WA, USA) to determine VO_{2peak}, as described previously [26]. Oxygen uptake was assessed throughout the test using indirect calorimetry via an automated Moxus Modular Metabolic System (AEI Technologies, Bostrop, TX, USA). VO_{2peak} was recorded as the highest 30-s mean VO_2 value, and was used to determine if subjects met the inclusion criteria. Power output at VO_{2peak} (W_{max}) was used to prescribe workloads for subsequent testing.

2.3. Experimental Design

The general study design is illustrated in Figure 1. Briefly, following a baseline period of normal training (NT), subjects completed two 20-day training blocks separated by a washout period (WO). Each training block was divided into 10 days of intensified cycling training (ICT) followed by 10 days of reduced volume training (RVT). Nutritional supplementation (CHO or CP) was provided throughout the ICT and RVT periods. A double-blind crossover design was utilized such that each subject received both nutrition interventions, with order of nutritional treatments randomly counterbalanced. Due to uneven subject retention, two subjects completed the CP trial first, and five subjects completed the CHO trial first. Details regarding training and nutritional interventions are provided below.

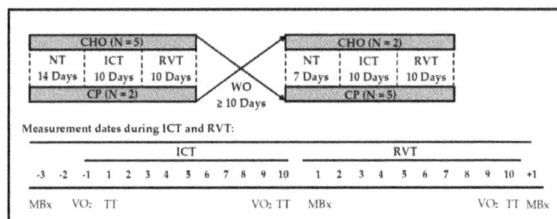

Figure 1. General Study Design. NT = normal training; ICT = intensified cycle training (daily training duration = ~220% NT); RVT = reduced volume training (~65% of NT); WO = washout; CHO = carbohydrate supplementation; CP = carbohydrate + protein supplementation; MBx = Muscle function and biopsy; VO_2 = VO_{2peak}; TT = Cycling time trial, constant-load exercise, and blood biomarkers.

2.3.1. Normal Training

The first 7 days of NT were used to quantify normal training volumes to prescribe training volumes and intensities for the remainder of the study. The second 7 days were used to conduct familiarization trials and preliminary testing for exercise protocols while maintaining total training duration and intensity at normal training levels. Subjects utilized bicycle wheels equipped with a PowerTap system (Saris Cycling Group Inc., Madison, WI, USA) to quantify power output, heart rate, cycling duration and distance during all training sessions conducted outside the laboratory. Power output and heart rate during cycling were used as indices of training intensity, whereas training duration (min) was used to quantify training volume.

2.3.2. Intensified Cycling Training

ICT consisted of 10 days in which average daily training duration was increased to ~220% of NT levels. This overload was comparable to previous training protocols that resulted in impaired performance following ICT [2,27]. Preloaded time trials (120 min at 50% W_{max} + 30-km maximal effort, described below) and VO_{2peak} tests were completed on the days shown in Figure 1 (additional preloaded time trials were conducted on days 4 and 7 to contribute to total training loads). Additional training was conducted outside of the laboratory; subjects followed individualized training guidelines to achieve 220% of NT training duration. Training was quantified with a PowerTap system, as described above. During the second treatment phase, subjects were provided with specific durations and intensities to match the training stimulus with the first treatment phase.

2.3.3. Reduced Volume Training

Average daily training duration was reduced to ~65% of NT levels during RVT, with the intent of restoring or improving cycling performance following ICT [15,28]. Preloaded 30-kilometer time trials and VO_{2peak} tests were completed on the days shown in Figure 1. Otherwise, all training during RVT was completed outside the laboratory, quantified as described above to verify compliance with the training guidelines. During the second treatment phase, subjects were provided with specific durations and intensities to match the training stimulus with the first treatment phase.

2.3.4. Washout (WO) Period

WO consisted of individualized periods of recovery to accommodate schedules, with the intent of restoring NT loads prior to the second phase of the study. A minimum of 10 days of WO was provided, resulting in ≥27 days between the two periods of ICT (i.e., 10 days RVT + 10 days WO + 7 days NT). In female subjects, the washout period was timed to ensure that each treatment phase (CHO or CP) began on the same day of the menstrual cycle, to offset any potential influences of menstrual phase on study outcomes.

2.4. Treatment Beverages

Treatment beverages were administered during (750 mL·h^{-1}) and immediately following (11.8 mL·kg·BW^{-1}) all training sessions throughout ICT and RVT. Recovery beverages were consumed within 30 min of terminating exercise. Participants avoided any other beverage or food intake for 2 h following each exercise session, with the exception of ad libitum water consumption.

The treatment beverages consumed during exercise were either a commercially available carbohydrate-electrolyte beverage (CHO), providing 45 g·h^{-1} carbohydrate (sucrose/dextrose), 423 mg·h^{-1} sodium, and 97 mg·h^{-1} potassium (Gatorade®, PepsiCo, Inc., Purchase, NY, USA); or an identical beverage plus 17.7 g·h^{-1} of hydrolyzed whey protein isolate powder (American Casein Company, AMCO, Burlington, NJ, USA), providing 15 g Pro·h^{-1} (CP). The post-exercise treatment beverages were either a chocolate-flavored carbohydrate beverage (CHO), containing 1.2 g CHO kg·BW^{-1} (maltodextrin/sucrose), 0.09 g fat kg·BW^{-1}, 3.3 mg·kg·BW^{-1} sodium, and 4.4 mg·kg·BW^{-1} potassium (Clif Shots, Clif Bar and Co., Emeryville, CA, USA); or commercially-available low-fat chocolate milk (TruMoo®, Dean Foods, El Paso, TX, USA), containing 1.2 g CHO·kg·BW^{-1} (lactose/sucrose), 0.4 g protein·kg·BW^{-1}, 0.11 g fat·kg·BW^{-1}, 9.0 mg·kg·BW^{-1} sodium, and 21.0 mg·kg·BW^{-1} potassium (CP).

2.5. Dietary Controls

Participants were provided detailed instructions on dietary procedures and recording techniques by a Registered Dietician Nutritionist (RD/RDN). All subjects were provided with a digital food scale for food measurement, and completed a food intake record (FIR) during NT (4 days) and ICT (10 days for each treatment) and RVT (10 days for each treatment). The FIR were analyzed using the Nutrition Data System for Research (University of Minnesota, Minneapolis, MN, USA) and evaluated by the RD/RDN for quality assurance. FIR from NT were analyzed to ensure that baseline carbohydrate intake was >6.5 g/kg/day (all subjects exceeded this level). The FIR obtained from the first treatment phase (ICT and RVT) were used to develop replicable menus for the second treatment phase, which included three alternative choices for each food item that matched calories and macronutrients. Participants were instructed to use these menus to replicate their dietary habits during the second phase of the crossover design. During this second treatment phase participants submitted their FIR each day by 4:00 p.m. and researchers analyzed dietary intakes immediately upon receipt. Researchers responded to participants via text message or e-mail with specific dietary prescriptions for the remainder of the day to ensure that daily calories and macronutrient intakes remained consistent with the previous treatment period.

During all exercise trials conducted in the laboratory, subjects received 250 mL of beverage every 20 min until exercise completion. For all rides performed outside the laboratory, participants received bottles of treatment beverage measured to achieve 750 mL/h of fluid ingestion for the duration of each training ride. Subjects returned empty bottles to the investigators (including any remaining solution, to ensure compliance) following each ride. Following each exercise session, participants received recovery beverages and were instructed to finish the beverage within 30 min of terminating exercise. Participants avoided any other beverage/food intake for 2 h following each exercise session, with the exception of ad libitum water consumption. During the time period between the onset of each training session and two hours following each training session, participants received no nutrients other than the CHO or CP treatment beverages. All laboratory testing was performed after an 8–10 h overnight fast (ad libitum water consumption). In addition, participants were provided with standardized boxed-lunches on all days they reported to the laboratory (8/20 days per treatment period), which standardized dietary intake for approximately 6 h after each exercise session.

2.6. Dependent Measurements

2.6.1. Cycling Performance and Responses to Constant-Load Exercise

Cycling tests were conducted on a computerized cycle ergometer (VeloTron, Racermate Inc., Seattle, WA, USA) at the completion of NT, ICT and RVT (see Figure 1). Trials began with 120 min of cycling at 50% W_{max} (from VO_{2peak} test during NT of the first treatment phase). This provided a period of constant-load exercise in which physiological measurements (described below) could be compared between training periods and treatments at the same absolute intensity. It also provided a prolonged, metabolically demanding duration of exercise prior to the second portion of the trial; a self-paced, simulated 30-kilometer time trial (TT), which was used to quantify cycling performance. Measurements obtained during the cycling tests are described below:

Cardiorespiratory Responses to Constant-Load Exercise

Oxygen uptake (VO_2) and respiratory exchange ratio (RER) were assessed using a Moxus Modular Metabolic System (AEI Technologies, Pittsburgh, PA, USA) at 25–30 min of constant-load cycling at 50% W_{max}. Values were averaged over the final three min of data collection, following two minutes of breathing equilibration.

Heart rate (Suunto, Vaanta, Finland) and ratings of perceived exertion (RPE; 6–20 Borg Scale) were recorded at 30 min of cycling at 50% W_{max}. Finger-stick blood samples (~0.5 mL) were obtained at the same time; glucose and lactate levels were determined immediately from whole blood using automated instrumentation (YSI 2300 STAT glucose/lactate analyzer, Yellow Springs, OH, USA).

Cycling Performance

The 30-kilometer TT finishing times and average power output were used as measures of cycling performance. Subjects were encouraged to treat the TT portion of each trial as a competitive event and provide a maximal effort. Subjects received no performance feedback during the TT other than elapsed distance, and no verbal encouragement was provided. A pedestal fan was placed ~2 m from the handlebars and utilized on high speed setting for consistency across trials. This protocol has been utilized previously in our laboratory with good reproducibility (coefficient of variation between repeated trials of 3.6%).

2.6.2. VO_{2peak} and Body Weight

Subjects completed graded exercise tests to obtain VO_{2peak} values following NT, ICT and RVT (see Figure 1), using protocols described above. Body weight was measured prior to the onset of these trials, following an overnight fast and voiding of the bladder, and while wearing only cycling shorts (all subjects) and sports bra (females).

2.6.3. Peak Isokinetic Torque

Torque of the knee extensors from a single, randomly selected leg was assessed using an isokinetic dynamometer (Biodex Medical System Inc., Shirley, NY, USA) following NT, ICT and RVT (Figure 1). Following 5 min of standardized warm-up on a cycle ergometer, peak isokinetic torque was assessed at 240 deg·s^{-1} and 120 deg·s^{-1}. Four maximal trials were completed at each velocity, with the highest value recorded as the peak value. Trials were separated by 30 s of rest. Furthermore, opposite legs were used for peak torque assessments between CHO and CP training phases.

2.6.4. Muscle Soreness

Subjects rated their perceived muscle soreness using a 100 mm visual analog scale, with 0 indicating no muscle soreness and 100 indicating extreme soreness, as described previously [13]. Scores were obtained at the end of each training period (Figure 1).

2.6.5. Muscle Fiber Cross-Sectional Area

Muscle biopsies were obtained from the *vastus lateralis* (VL) following each training phase (Figure 1). Biopsy samples were processed, stored, and mounted onto microscope slides as previously described [29]. Briefly, slides were incubated in primary antibodies directed against laminin, myosin heavy chain (MHC) I and IIa (Developmental Studies Hybridoma Bank, Iowa City, IA, USA). Following a series of washes, slides were then incubated in appropriate fluorescently labeled secondary antibodies (Invitrogen, Molecular Probes, Carlsbad, CA, USA) and visualized on an upright fluorescent microscope (Nikon Eclipse TE2000-E, Tokyo, Japan). Fiber CSA was measured using ImageJ software (National Institutes of Health, Bethesda, MD, USA). Due to insufficient tissue yields for two subjects during RVT (with CP supplementation), this time point was excluded from statistical analysis.

2.6.6. Biomarkers

Fasting venous blood samples were obtained from an antecubital vein following 10 min of supine rest following NT, ICT and RVT (prior to each TT). After 30 min of coagulation, samples were centrifuged at 3000 rpm for 10 min at 4 °C. Serum was separated and stored at −80 °C for later analysis.

Serum albumin was assessed via the bromocresol green method using spectrophotometry at an optical density of 620 nm, according to standardized procedures provided by the manufacturer (KA1612, Abnova, Walnut, CA, USA). Serum creatine kinase was analyzed by an enzymatic kinetic assay (Pointe Scientific, Canton, MI, USA) on an automated biochemical analyzer (ChemWell-T 4600, Awareness Technology Inc., Palm City, FL, USA). Serum cortisol concentrations were measured using a Quantikine® high sensitivity enzyme-linked immunoassay (KGE008, R&D Systems, Minneapolis, MN, USA). The minimal detectable concentrations were 0.01 g·dL^{-1} for albumin, 1.0 U/L for creatine kinase, and 0.156 ng·mL^{-1} for cortisol.

2.6.7. Statistical Analyses

For each measurement variable, magnitude-based inferences about the data were derived using methods described by Hopkins [30]. All data was log transformed to diminish the effects of non-uniformity. The threshold for the smallest meaningful treatment effect was quantified as 0.2*SD (obtained from NT in the CHO condition) for all variables other than cycling performance (see below). A published spreadsheet was used to determine the likelihoods of the true treatment effect (of the population) reaching the meaningful change threshold [31]. Likelihoods were classified as: <1% *almost certainly no chance*, 1%–5% = *very unlikely*, 5%–25% = *unlikely*, 25%–75% = *possible*, 75%–95% = *likely*, 95%–99% = *very likely*, and >99% = *most likely*. If the likelihood of the effect reaching the threshold was <25% and the effect was clear, it was classified as a 'trivial' effect. If 90% confidence intervals included values that exceeded the threshold for both a positive and negative effect, effects were classified as unclear.

As recommended by Paton and Hopkins [32], the smallest worthwhile change in performance was defined as $0.3 \times$ the within-subject variation of competitive cyclists across repeated trials (CV = 1.3% for time and estimated 3.25% for power), which translated to an effect of 0.22 min or 2.0 watts in the current study. Clinical inference criteria were used from published spreadsheets to classify the effects of treatment on performance time [31]. The statistical power of our research design was calculated using a publicly available spreadsheet created for studies using magnitude-based inferences [33]. Based on a minimum sample size of seven subjects (and estimating within-subject variability based on prior studies in our laboratory using the same measurement protocol), the present design and statistical approach possessed the statistical power to detect changes in time trial performance of 3% (1.7 min) with a power of 0.9; effects on time trial performance of 2% (1.1 min) could be detected with an estimated power of 0.54.

For ease of interpretation, data are displayed as raw means $\pm$ SD and/or mean difference between treatments $\pm$ CL (90% confidence limit). Effects of treatment order were examined using the same statistical approach described above. No meaningful effects of treatment order were observed for any variables (i.e., order effects *unclear* or *trivial*), other than VO_{2peak} (*likely*) and skeletal muscle function measurements (Peak Torque 120 (NT vs. RVT) = *very likely*; Peak Torque 240 (ICT and NT vs. RVT) = *very likely*). Therefore, order-adjusted outcomes are reported where appropriate in addition to raw values.

3. Results

3.1. Training Loads and Nutrient Intake

Training duration, power output, and heart rate during NT, ICT, and RVT are reported in Table 1. These data were used to quantify compliance with the prescribed training program, and assess the consistency of training completed between the CHO and CP treatment phases. Average daily training duration during ICT was increased to 222% of NT levels (*most likely* increased versus NT in both CHO and CP). Duration during RVT was 66% of NT levels (*most likely* decreased versus NT in both CHO and CP). Average training intensity decreased slightly but consistently during ICT. Specifically, average power output and heart rates during ICT training were lower versus NT and RVT in both CHO and CP (all semantic inferences = *likely/very likely/most likely*). Thus, training during ICT represented a substantial increase in average daily training duration, at a slightly lower average exercise intensity. The RVT training represented a substantial decrease in training duration, at the same average intensity as NT. As intended, overall training demands between CHO and CP were very similar within each training period.

Macronutrient intake during ICT and RVT are reported in Table 2. Differences in macronutrient intake between CHO and CP are shown independent of treatment beverages (Dietary Macronutrients) and including the treatments (Total Macronutrient Intake). During ICT, dietary macronutrients were virtually identical between CHO and CP phases, and the increased protein/calories from the CP treatment beverages resulted in higher total protein/calories in CP. During RVT, subjects tended to consume slightly less dietary carbohydrate and fat (and thus calories) in CP. Due to the higher protein/calories from the CP treatment beverages, this resulted in similar total caloric intake between CHO and CP.

Table 1. Training Loads (Mean ± SD) during Normal, Intensified, and Reduced-Volume Training.

Variable	NT			ICT			RVT		
	CHO	CP	CP-CHO Effects	CHO	CP	CP-CHO Effects	CHO	CP	CP-CHO Effects
Duration (min/day)	61.5 ± 8.3	63.0 ± 6.0	1.5 ± 4.1	137.1 ± 14.8	139.9 ± 16.9	2.7 ± 3.9	41.2 ± 4.9	42.2 ± 5.2	1.1 ± 1.8
			52/39/10			20/79/1			40/58/2
			Unclear			Likely trivial			Possible
Power output (W)	189 ± 31	182 ± 30	−8 ± 13	165 ± 32	167 ± 26	2 ± 6	193 ± 37	193 ± 36	0 ± 5
			7/21/72			30/66/3			4/93/3
			Unclear			Possible			Likely trivial
Heart Rate (bt·min^{-1})	150 ± 16	146 ± 14	−4 ± 5	139 ± 13	137 ± 13	−2 ± 6	150 ± 13	146 ± 11	−4 ± 5
			2/32/65			5/60/35			1/28/72
			Possible			Unclear			Possible

Effects are mean ± 90% CI, % likelihoods of positive/trivial/negative effects, and semantic inference. NT = normal training; ICT = intensified cycle training; RVT = reduced volume training; CHO = carbohydrate supplementation; CP = carbohydrate + protein supplementation.

Table 2. Macronutrient Intake (Mean ± SD) during Intensified Training and Reduced-Volume Training.

	Dietary Macronutrients (Day)			During-Exercise		Post-Exercise		Total Macronutrient Intake (Day)		
	CHO	CP	CP-CHO Effects	CHO	CP	CHO	CP	CHO	CP	CP-CHO Effects
ICT Period										
Carbohydrate (g)	337 ± 100	331 ± 114	−6 ± 15 1/88/11 Likely trivial	112 ± 11	112 ± 11	86 ± 14	86 ± 14	535 ± 110	529 ± 122	−6 ± 15 1/92/7 Likely trivial
Protein (g)	120 ± 38	118 ± 38	−3 ± 11 9/46/45 Unclear	0 ± 0	38 ± 4	0 ± 0	29 ± 5	120 ± 38	184 ± 44	64 ± 12 100/0/0 Most likely
Fat (g)	118 ± 29	118 ± 34	0 ± 7 1/97/2 V.L. trivial	0 ± 0	2 ± 0	7 ± 1	8 ± 1	124 ± 30	127 ± 35	3 ± 7 13/84/3 Likely trivial
Calories (kcal)	2948 ± 779	2899 ± 878	−49 ± 122 1/79/20 Likely trivial	447 ± 46	612 ± 61	404 ± 65	532 ± 85	3799 ± 841	4043 ± 951	244 ± 122 91/9/0 Likely
RVT Period										
Carbohydrate (g)	317 ± 89	292 ± 104	−25 ± 31 3/27/70 Possible	33 ± 4	33 ± 4	50 ± 9	50 ± 9	400 ± 94	376 ± 106	−25 ± 31 3/27/70 Possible
Protein (g)	112 ± 22	110 ± 21	−2 ± 10 18/48/35 Unclear	0 ± 0	11 ± 1	0 ± 0	17 ± 3	112 ± 22	138 ± 24	26 ± 11 100/0/0 Most likely
Fat (g)	105 ± 20	97 ± 13	−8 ± 8 0/68/31 Possible	0 ± 0	1 ± 0	4 ± 1	5 ± 1	108 ± 21	102 ± 14	−6 ± 8 2/30/69 Possible
Calories (kcal)	2706 ± 569	2527 ± 543	−178 ± 198 2/26/72 Possible	132 ± 15	180 ± 20	236 ± 43	310 ± 56	3074 ± 608	3018 ± 577	56 ± 188 6/68/25 Unclear

Effects are mean ± 90% CI, % likelihoods of positive/trivial/negative effects, and semantic inference. CHO = carbohydrate supplementation; CP = carbohydrate + protein supplementation.

3.2. Dependent Measurements

3.2.1. Cycling Time Trial (TT) Performance

Pre-loaded 30-km TT times are shown in Figure 2, and tended to get slower from NT (CHO: 56.0 ± 5.3 min; CP: 55.6 ± 6.2 min) to ICT (CHO: 57.3 ± 8.3 min; CP: 57.2 ± 7.8 min) and return to baseline levels following RVT (CHO: 55.3 ± 5.3; CP: 55.7 ± 7.8 min), with no between-treatment effects. Similarly, all treatment differences in power output between CHO (NT: 191 ± 48; ICT: 188 ± 53; RVT: 198 ± 41 W) and CP (NT: 201 ± 54; ICT: 187 ± 47; RVT: 201 ± 61 W) were unclear.

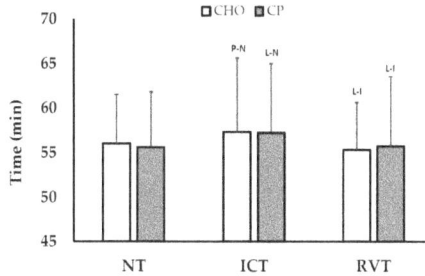

Figure 2. Cycling Performance (Mean $\pm$ SD) during Normal, Intensified, and Reduced-Volume Training. Within-treatment effects: P-N = *Possibly* different than NT; L-N = *Likely* different than NT; L-I = *Likely* different than ICT. No between-treatment effects were observed. NT = normal training; ICT = intensified cycle training; RVT = reduced volume training; CHO = carbohydrate supplementation; CP = carbohydrate + protein supplementation.

3.2.2. Responses during Constant-Load Exercise

Physiological responses during constant-load cycling were examined at 50% W_{max}, corresponding to 57%–62% VO_{2peak}. Heart rate responses are shown in Figure 3. Briefly, heart rate was possibly decreased following ICT with CP, but not altered in CHO. Following RVT, heart rates possibly increased in the CHO condition (versus ICT and NT), while heart rate remained attenuated with CP (versus NT). As a result of these combined effects, reductions in heart rate between NT-RVT with CP were *likely* greater than CHO.

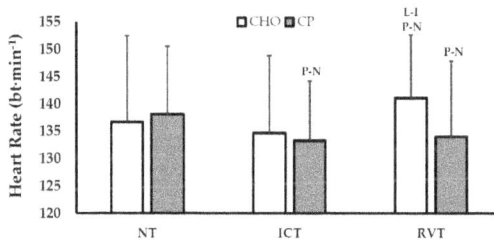

Figure 3. Heart Rate Responses (Mean $\pm$ SD) during Constant-Load Cycling (50% Wmax). Within-treatment effects: P-N = *Possibly* different than NT; L-I = *Likely* different than ICT. Between-treatment effects: NT-ICT = *Unclear* (% chance of larger/trivial/smaller attenuation in heart rate with CP, compared to CHO = 51/39/10), ICT-RVT = *Possible* (74/24/2), NT-RVT = *Likely* (85/12/2). NT = normal training; ICT = intensified cycle training; RVT = reduced volume training; CHO = carbohydrate supplementation; CP = carbohydrate + protein supplementation.

Constant-load exercise data for VO_2, RER, glucose, lactate, and RPE are reported in Table 3. Treatment differences between training periods for most variables were unclear. However, RER responses exhibited differences between treatments. In general, RER tended to decrease from NT-ICT with CP, and return to baseline levels following RVT. By contrast, RER values trended upwards throughout the course of the study in the CHO condition.

3.2.3. VO_{2peak} and Body Weight

VO_{2peak} possibly increased in the CHO condition from NT-ICT and from NT-RVT (NT: 4457 ± 833 mL/min; ICT: 4592 ± 736 mL/min; RVT: 4675 ± 887 mL/min) but not CP (NT: 4337 ± 973 mL/min; ICT: 4335 ± 1032 mL/min; RVT: 4433 ± 1107 mL/min). As a result, changes in VO_{2peak} from NT-ICT and NT-RVT were possibly greater with CHO versus CP (an order-adjusted analysis to account for effects of treatment order provided the same semantic inference). All treatment differences in body weight between CHO (NT: 70.7 ± 11.7; ICT: 70.1 ± 11.3; RVT: 70.6 ± 11.3 kg) and CP (NT: 70.9 ± 11.7; ICT: 71.0 ± 11.4; RVT: 70.9 ± 11.6 kg) were *most likely* trivial.

3.2.4. Muscle Function, Size and Soreness

Peak torque values for each training period and nutritional treatment are shown in Figure 4. In general, declines in peak torque from NT to ICT tended to be greater with CHO than with CP. However, treatment differences did not persist following RVT (this interpretation is consistent with order-adjusted analyses to account for effects of treatment order from NT-RVT, as all treatment effects at that time point were unclear).

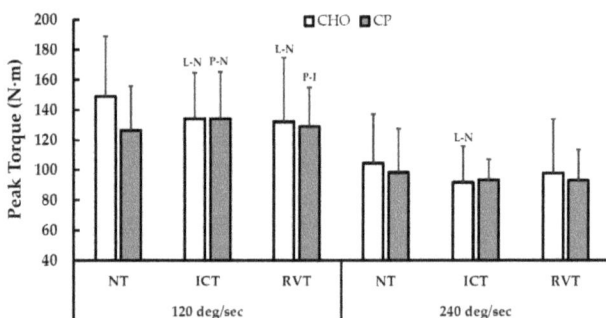

Figure 4. Effects of Training Periods and Nutritional Supplementation on Peak Knee Extensor Torque. Within-treatment effects: P-N = *Possibly* different than NT; L-N = *Likely* different than NT; P-I = *Possibly* different than ICT. Between-treatment effects at 120 deg/s: NT-ICT = *Likely* (% chance of smaller/trivial/larger decrease in torque with CP, compared to CHO = 95/5/1), ICT-RVT = *Unclear* (32/35/33), NT-RVT = *Unclear* (59/31/10). Between-treatment effects at 240 deg/s: NT-ICT = *Unclear* (64/25/11), ICT-RVT = *Likely* (2/14/84), NT-RVT = *Unclear* (16/29/55). NT = normal training; ICT = intensified cycle training; RVT = reduced volume training; CHO = carbohydrate supplementation; CP = carbohydrate + protein supplementation.

Changes in muscle fiber cross-sectional area are shown in Table 4. There were no clear changes amongst fiber CSA throughout the CHO treatment. However, with CP supplementation, MHC I CSA *very likely* increased ($13.6\% \pm 8.0\%$) and MHC IIa *likely* increased ($16.4\% \pm 19.4\%$) from NT to ICT. This resulted in a *likely* treatment difference in MHC I fiber CSA response from NT to ICT (comparisons to the RVT time point are not available due to insufficient tissue yields for 2 subjects in CP). Muscle soreness values for each training period are shown in Figure 5. Soreness *very likely* increased from NT to ICT (with both CHO and CP) and *very likely* decreased to baseline levels following RVT, with no clear treatment differences.

Table 3. Physiological Responses (Mean ± SD) during Constant-Load Cycling (50% W_{max}).

Variable	NT		ICT		RVT		Treatment Differences		
	CHO	CP	CHO	CP	CHO	CP	NT-ICT	ICT-RVT	NT-RVT
VO_2 (mL·min⁻¹)	2767 ± 368	2704 ± 496	2679 ± 404 [P-N]	2563 ± 418 [L-N]	2671 ± 389	2587 ± 501 [L-N]	−53 ± 190	32 ± 204	−20 ± 275
							13/47/40	33/46/21	27/36/37
							Unclear	Unclear	Unclear
Heart Rate (bt·min⁻¹)	137 ± 16	138 ± 13	135 ± 12	133 ± 14 [P-N]	141 ± 15 [P-N]	134 ± 13 [P-N]	−3 ± 9	−6 ± 6	−9 ± 9
							10/39/51	2/24/74	2/12/85
							Unclear	Possible	Likely
RER	0.81 ± 0.04	0.83 ± 0.02	0.84 ± 0.11	0.80 ± 0.04 [L-N]	0.87 ± 0.02 [ML-N]	0.84 ± 0.03 [L-I]	−0.05 ± 0.05	0.01 ± 0.08	−0.04 ± 0.03
							4/3/93	49/12/39	2/2/96
							Likely	Unclear	Very likely
Glucose (mg·dL⁻¹)	87 ± 8	80 ± 6	93 ± 7 [L-N]	83 ± 11	91 ± 5	86 ± 7 [L-N]	−3 ± 16	5 ± 16	2 ± 9
							30/13/57	66/11/23	56/23/21
							Unclear	Unclear	Unclear
Lactate (mmol·L⁻¹)	1.1 ± 0.5	1.0 ± 0.5	0.9 ± 0.1	1.0 ± 0.4	1.1 ± 0.6	0.9 ± 0.2	0.1 ± 0.8	−0.3 ± 0.7	−0.2 ± 0.8
							46/20/35	18/24/58	31/20/50
							Unclear	Unclear	Unclear
RPE (6–20)	12.0 ± 1.0	11.7 ± 2.3	12.3 ± 1.9	12.0 ± 2.2 [P-N]	11.4 ± 2.2 [L-N]	11.6 ± 2.2 [P-I]	0.0 ± 1.1	0.4 ± 0.6	0.4 ± 1.3
							44/28/28	73/24/3	66/18/16
							Unclear	Possible	Unclear

Treatment effects are mean ± 90% CI, % likelihoods positive/trivial/negative effects, and semantic inference. [P-N] = *possibly different than NT*, [L-N] = *likely different than NT*, [VL-N] = *very likely different than NT*, [ML-N] = *most likely different than NT*, [P-I] = *possibly different than ICT*, [L-I] = *likely different than ICT*. NT = normal training; ICT = intensified cycle training; RVT = reduced volume training; CHO = carbohydrate supplementation; CP = carbohydrate + protein supplementation; VO_2 = oxygen uptake; RER = respiratory exchange ratio; RPE = rating of perceived exertion.

Table 4. Muscle Fiber Size (Mean ± SD) following Normal, Intensified, and Reduced-Volume Training.

Variable	NT		ICT		RVT		Treatment Differences		
	CHO	CP	CHO	CP	CHO	CP	NT-ICT	ICT-RVT	NT-RVT
Peak Torque at 120 deg/s (N·m)	110 ± 29	93 ± 22	99 ± 23 [L-N]	99 ± 23 [P-N]	98 ± 31 [L-N]	95 ± 19	17 ± 12 95/5/1 Likely	−2 ± 23 32/35/33 Unclear	14 ± 18 84/12/4 Likely positive ADJ = 6 ± 16 59/31/10 Unclear
Peak Torque at 240 deg/s (N·m)	77 ± 24	72 ± 22	68 ± 18 [L-N]	69 ± 10	72 ± 27	69 ± 15	6 ± 16 64/25/11 Unclear	−5 ± 12 10/42/48 Unclear ADJ = −11 ± 11 2/14/84 Likely	1 ± 18 47/29/24 Unclear ADJ = −6 ± 16 16/29/55 Unclear
MHC I CSA (μm²)	5273 ± 1355	4823 ± 1319	5356 ± 897	5401 ± 1119 [VL-N]	5925 ± 1680	N/A	496 ± 856 80/16/4 Likely	N/A	N/A
MHC II CSA (μm²)	5605 ± 1512	5105 ± 2004	5685 ± 1457	5840 ± 1822 [L-N]	6131 ± 1852	N/A	655 ± 1276 76/17/7 Unclear	N/A	N/A
Muscle Soreness (mm, 0–100)	39 ± 20	35 ± 24	65 ± 12 [VL-N]	55 ± 26 [VL-N]	38 ± 20 [VL-I]	34 ± 22 [VL-I]	−6 ± 21 52/26/22 Unclear	5 ± 20 54/19/27 Unclear	0 ± 17 61/13/26 Unclear

Treatment effects are mean ± 90% CI, % likelihoods of positive/trivial/negative effects, and semantic inference. [P-N] = *possibly different than NT*, [L-N] = *likely different than NT*, [VL-N] = *very likely different than NT*, [VL-I] = *very likely different than ICT*. ADJ = values adjusted for *very likely* effects of treatment order. NT = normal training; ICT = intensified cycle training; RVT = reduced volume training; CHO = carbohydrate supplementation; CP = carbohydrate + protein supplementation.

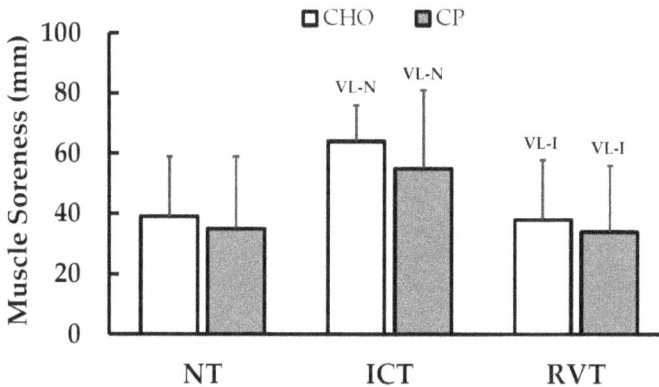

Figure 5. Effects of Training Periods and Nutritional Supplementation on Muscle Soreness (Mean ± SD). Within-treatment effects: VL-N = *Very likely* different than NT; VL-I = *Very likely* different than ICT; No between-treatment effects were observed. NT = normal training; ICT = intensified cycle training; RVT = reduced volume training; CHO = carbohydrate supplementation; CP = carbohydrate + protein supplementation.

3.2.5. Serum Biomarkers: Albumin, Creatine Kinase, and Cortisol

Serum albumin levels tended to increase from NT to ICT to a similar extent between CHO (*likely*, 0.5 ± 0.5 g·dL^{-1}) and CP (*unclear*, 0.4 ± 0.6 g·dL^{-1}). There were no clear treatment effects on albumin levels. Serum albumin levels were as follows for CHO (NT: 5.73 ± 1.07; ICT: 6.23 ± 0.67; RVT: 6.05 ± 1.03 g·dL^{-1}) and CP (NT: 5.48 ± 0.76; ICT: 5.91 ± 0.54; RVT: 6.03 ± 0.64 g·dL^{-1}). Reported values are from 6 subjects, as one subject was unable to provide serum samples for all time points.

Creatine kinase levels possibly decreased from NT to ICT (-25 ± 28 U/L) with CHO but not PRO (1 ± 20 U/L; *unclear*), leading to *likely* treatment differences at these time points. All other treatment comparisons in creatine kinase between CHO (NT: 157 ± 82; ICT: 135 ± 61; RVT: 94 ± 42 U/L) and CP (NT: 127 ± 47; ICT: 128 ± 34; RVT: 137 ± 79 U/L) were unclear.

There were no clear differences in serum cortisol levels between any time points, and no treatment effects. Serum cortisol levels were: CHO = NT: 103 ± 37; ICT: 97 ± 32; RVT: 94 ± 42 ng/mL and CP = NT: 125 ± 47; ICT: 114 ± 26; RVT: 107 ± 33 ng/mL.

4. Discussion

The central objective of this study was to assess the effects of CP supplementation on time trial performance, skeletal muscle function and morphology, and heart rate responses following a prolonged period of heavy training and recovery. Cycling performance was modestly impaired following ICT (2.4% slower versus NT) and restored with RVT, with no apparent performance differences between CP and CHO. Peak isokinetic torque of the knee extensors was diminished following ICT in the CHO condition, but was better preserved with CP. Similarly, both MHC I and MHC IIa cross-sectional areas were unchanged following ICT with CHO, but were increased with CP. In addition, reductions in constant-load heart rate between NT-RVT tended to be greater with CP than CHO. Altogether it appears that CP supplementation impacted select physiological parameters during heavy training and recovery, but not on a magnitude that influenced time trial performance.

The current result that repeated days of CP supplementation had no effect on performance versus CHO is supported by previous data from our laboratory [12,13]. However, the distance runners studied by Luden et al. [12] tapered their training volumes slightly during a six-day intervention period, and the subjects of Gilson and colleagues [13] completed a 4-day period of soccer training with only minimal increases in training volume (+12% versus normal training). Consequently, we designed the current study to deliver a rigorous training stimulus in an attempt to maximize the potential value of CP supplementation. Along with elevated muscle soreness, and impaired skeletal muscle function, the 10-day ICT intervention impaired cycling time trial performance by 2.4%. This was comparable to a recent study which reported that power output during a 5-min time trial was reduced by 3.8% following a rigorous 6-day training camp in cyclists [16]. Similar to the present study, these investigators reported that supplemental protein during intensified training did not affect changes in performance versus supplemental CHO alone. By contrast, Witard and associates [15] reported that increased dietary protein intake (3.0 vs. 1.5 g/kg/day) modestly attenuated performance declines following a week of intensified training that elicited large declines in performance in the control condition (>10%). However, it should be noted that the protocols for protein supplementation during heavy training also varied considerably between these studies. Witard and colleagues [15] provided a relatively large amount of additional protein (+104 g/day) throughout the day, whereas Hansen [16] provided ~65 g of supplemental protein only during exercise, and the present study supplemented ~67 g of protein during/following exercise. Thus, based on the limited studies in this area, it could be speculated that CP supplementation may elicit performance benefits when larger amounts of protein are provided during heavy training that results in sizeable decreases in performance, while smaller amounts of supplemental protein do not appear to impact performance during heavy training that elicits only modest impairments in performance.

Discrepancies between prior studies regarding the influence of CP on performance following periods of heavy training may also be affected by dietary protein intake and the resulting protein balance. For instance, Rowlands and colleagues noted that positive effects on performance were observed when CP supplementation was compared to a relatively low-protein control diet (0.92 g/kg/day; [9]), or versus a moderate-protein diet which elicited a mildly negative protein balance (1.6 g/kg/day; [10]). Yet when CP supplementation was compared to a moderate-protein control diet which produced positive daily nitrogen balance, no effects of CP on performance were observed (1.5 g/kg/day; [14]). Protein balance status could also possibly explain the differences between our findings and the aforementioned results from Witard and colleagues [15]. It is possible that the protein intake in the control diet (described above) resulted in negative protein balance during heavy training. By contrast, the slightly higher dietary protein intake in the control condition of the present study (1.7 g/kg during ICT, 1.6 g/kg during RVT) could have been sufficient to elicit positive protein balance, minimizing the potential effects of CP on performance. This is consistent with aforesaid findings from Hansen and associates [16], who reported no effects of protein supplementation versus CHO when protein intake was controlled between groups at 1.7 g/kg/day. However, another study from this group reported that orienteers who received protein supplementation before and after exercise improved 4-kilometers run performance at the end of a one-week training camp, versus those who received a control diet containing 1.8 g/kg/day of protein [11]. However, nitrogen balance was not assessed in any of these studies, and numerous methodological differences make it difficult to directly compare results between studies (i.e., Hansen's study of orienteers utilized a between-subject design, weight-bearing exercise mode, and two training sessions per day).

Though cycling performance was not influenced by treatment, both skeletal muscle function and morphology were favorably influenced by CP. Muscle function was *likely* affected by treatment at a contractile velocity of 120 deg·s^{-1}. Following ICT, peak knee extensor torque was *possibly* enhanced with CP, but *likely* impaired with CHO. Interestingly, the treatment effect was *unclear* at 240 deg·s^{-1}, despite peak torque *likely* being lower after ICT with CHO but not CP. The more apparent benefit of CP on whole muscle function at 120 deg·s^{-1} suggests that the slower contractile velocity (and higher torque output) is a more sensitive measure of peak muscle function. This notion is supported by the findings of Coutts et al. who observed clear effects of heavy training on peak isokinetic torque at 60 deg·s^{-1}, but not at 300 deg·s^{-1} [34]. Regardless, this is the first evidence that peak skeletal muscle force is better preserved with CP supplementation during an extended period of heavy training.

The practical advantage of this outcome is questionable though, as the treatment effect on muscle function neither persisted through RVT nor did it translate to better cycling performance. The latter may be attributable to the fact that the angular velocity during cycling exercise is much closer to 240- than 120 deg·s^{-1} [35]. The apparent benefit of CP throughout ICT on muscle function may in part be due to increased muscle fiber CSA observed with CP but not CHO. Contrary to earlier reports that fiber CSA decreases following heavy training [36–38], MHC I (*very likely*) and MHC IIa CSA (*likely*) increased following ICT with CP, but not CHO. The mechanisms mediating this response are beyond the scope of the current investigation, but CP may have increased muscle fiber size by augmenting protein synthesis rates in the early hours following exercise [39–41], resulting in a potentially greater net protein balance compared to CHO [39,40]. Because our CP treatment provided additional protein and calories, we cannot conclude definitively that the effects of CP on muscle function and morphology were the result of protein per se. However, augmented protein synthesis rates have been reported with CP versus isocaloric CHO treatments in prior studies [39]. Further research is needed to delineate how potential effects of protein intake on peak muscle function and fiber size translate to cycling specific performance.

CK levels and perceived muscle soreness together offer insight into the possible effects of muscle damage on changes in muscle function with training and nutrition. Muscle soreness increased as a result of ICT and decreased following RVT, as expected [3]. However, CP had no apparent influence on muscle soreness responses, which differs from a number of prior studies that have reported attenuated post-exercise soreness with CP ingestion [12,18,20,21]. CHO was associated with *possibly* reduced CK levels following ICT compared to CP, which is contrary to earlier findings showing CP-attenuated CK levels after heavy training [9,12,21]. However, the magnitude of all changes in CK in the present study (i.e., across time points and between treatments) were very small, suggesting that the effects of training and diet on CK were negligible.

Another purpose of this investigation was to assess the effects of CP supplementation on submaximal heart rate responses. During CP, constant-load heart rates *possibly* decreased following ICT, and remained *possibly* suppressed following RVT. By contrast, constant-load heart rates during CHO did not change to a meaningful degree following ICT, and *possibly* increased from ICT-RVT. As a result, reductions in heart rate during constant-load cycling were *likely* greater with CP than CHO between NT-RVT (-9 ± 9 bpm). This apparent effect of CP on heart rate is also supported by data obtained from the training sessions (Table 1). Despite exercising at an identical average power output (between treatments) during RVT, average heart rates during training were *possibly* lower in CP versus CHO (-4 ± 5 bpm). These observations are generally consistent with findings from Goto and colleagues, who reported that protein supplementation magnified training-induced reductions in heart rate following 5 days of aerobic training in previously untrained subjects [25]. Attenuated heart rate responses during exercise could be viewed as a positive adaptation to CP ingestion as they may reflect protein-mediated increases in plasma volume and stroke volume, suggesting possible reductions in cardiovascular and heat strain during exercise [23–25]. However, this interpretation should be made cautiously since plasma volume and stroke volume were not measured in the present study. Additionally, prior studies reported that increased plasma and/or stroke volume were related to increased plasma albumin levels with protein supplementation [23–25] and though plasma albumin levels tended to increase from NT-ICT, no differences were observed between CHO and CP. The extended training periods in the study precluded a careful examination of the time course of albumin changes, and the predicted influences of CP on plasma volume potentially confounds measurements of albumin concentration in the existing model, so it is unclear whether total albumin levels were affected by CP. Meaningful increases in plasma and/or stroke volume would also be expected to increase VO$_{2\text{peak}}$ values, even in previously trained athletes [42]. However, there was no evidence that CP improved VO$_{2\text{peak}}$ values versus CHO (conversely, there were *possible* increases in VO$_{2\text{peak}}$ with CHO, but not CP). Lastly, we cannot exclude the possibility that the decreased exercise heart rates with CP were associated with overtraining-induced central nervous system dysfunction [43], rather than a positive adaptation to training. Therefore, despite potentially reduced heart rate responses during constant-load cycling, the overall effects of CP ingestion on cardiovascular adaptations following ICT/RVT training were equivocal.

5. Conclusions

The present study extends prior findings regarding the effects of carbohydrate and protein (CP) supplementation during periods of intensified training and recovery. We observed novel findings that CP (provided during and immediately post-exercise) was associated with: (1) favorable influences on skeletal muscle function and morphology following intensified cycling training; and (2) differences in constant-load heart rates versus supplemental carbohydrate (CHO), after intensified training and recovery. Despite these potentially beneficial outcomes, CP supplementation did not attenuate the modest decreases in time trial performance observed following intensified training. Future investigators are encouraged to examine the effects of differing doses and timing of CP administration during intensified training on performance outcomes. Multi-site collaborative studies assessing the effects of CP on performance should also be considered. This approach would allow the recruitment of large sample sizes, increasing the potential to detect small but athletically relevant effects on performance.

Acknowledgments: This project was funded by a grant from the Dairy Research Institute (M.J.S. and N.D.L.). The authors thank the research participants for their particular dedication and effort in this demanding protocol. They also wish to recognize the important contributions of numerous research assistants who contributed to data collection for the project.

Author Contributions: M.J.S. and N.D.L. conceived and designed the experiments; A.C.D., N.D.L., J.M.F., J.D.A., A.I.M. and M.J.S. performed the experiments; A.C.D., N.D.L., J.M.F., J.D.A., A.I.M. and M.J.S. analyzed the data; A.C.D., N.D.L. and M.J.S. wrote the paper, J.M.F., J.D.A. and A.I.M. edited the manuscript.

Conflicts of Interest: M.J.S. has served as a member of advisory committees for the National Dairy Council, and the National Fluid Milk Processor Promotion Board, and has received fees and travel reimbursement for work related to this role. Otherwise, no conflicts of interest, financial or otherwise, are declared by the authors. The funding sponsors had no role in the design of the study; in the collection, analyses, or interpretation of data; in the writing of the manuscript, and in the decision to publish the results.

References

1. Jeukendrup, A.E.; Hesselink, M.K.; Snyder, A.C.; Kuipers, H.; Keizer, H.A. Physiological changes in male competitive cyclists after two weeks of intensified training. *Int. J. Sports Med.* **1992**, *13*, 534–541. [CrossRef] [PubMed]
2. Halson, S.L.; Bridge, M.W.; Meeusen, R.; Busschaert, B.; Gleeson, M.; Jones, D.A.; Jeukendrup, A.E. Time course of performance changes and fatigue markers during intensified training in trained cyclists. *J. Appl. Physiol.* **2002**, *93*, 947–956. [CrossRef] [PubMed]
3. Achten, J.; Halson, S.L.; Moseley, L.; Rayson, M.P.; Casey, A.; Jeukendrup, A.E. Higher dietary carbohydrate content during intensified running training results in better maintenance of performance and mood state. *J. Appl. Physiol.* **2004**, *96*, 1331–1340. [CrossRef] [PubMed]
4. Saunders, M.J.; Kane, M.D.; Todd, M.K. Effects of a carbohydrate-protein beverage on cycling endurance and muscle damage. *Med. Sci. Sports Exerc.* **2004**, *36*, 1233–1238. [CrossRef] [PubMed]
5. Berardi, J.M.; Noreen, E.E.; Lemon, P.W. Recovery from a cycling time trial is enhanced with carbohydrate-protein supplementation vs. Isoenergetic carbohydrate supplementation. *J. Int. Soc. Sports Nutr.* **2008**, *5*, 24. [CrossRef] [PubMed]
6. Ferguson-Stegall, L.; McCleave, E.L.; Ding, Z.; Doerner, P.G., 3rd; Wang, B.; Liao, Y.H.; Kammer, L.; Liu, Y.; Hwang, J.; Dessard, B.M.; et al. Postexercise carbohydrate-protein supplementation improves subsequent exercise performance and intracellular signaling for protein synthesis. *J. Strength Cond. Res.* **2011**, *25*, 1210–1224. [CrossRef] [PubMed]
7. Lunn, W.R.; Pasiakos, S.M.; Colletto, M.R.; Karfonta, K.E.; Carbone, J.W.; Anderson, J.M.; Rodrigues, N.R. Chcolate milk and endurance exercise recovery: Protein balance, glycogen, and performance. *Med. Sci. Sports Exerc.* **2012**, *44*, 682–691. [CrossRef] [PubMed]

8. Rustad, P.I.; Sailer, M.; Cumming, K.T.; Jeppesen, P.B.; Kolnes, K.J.; Sollie, O.; Franch, J.; Ivy, J.L.; Daniel, H.; Jensen, J. Intake of protein plus carbohydrate during the first two hours after exhaustive cycling improves performance the following day. *PLoS ONE* **2016**, *11*, e0153229. [CrossRef] [PubMed]

9. Rowlands, D.S.; Rossler, K.; Thorp, R.M.; Graham, D.F.; Timmons, B.W.; Stannard, S.R.; Tarnopolsky, M.A. Effect of dietary protein content during recovery from high-intensity cycling on subsequent performance and markers of stress, inflammation, and muscle damage in well-trained men. *Appl. Physiol. Nutr. Metab.* **2008**, *33*, 39–51. [CrossRef] [PubMed]

10. Thomson, J.S.; Ali, A.; Rowlands, D.S. Leucine-protein supplemented recovery feeding enhances subsequent cycling performance in well-trained men. *Appl. Physiol. Nutr. Metab.* **2011**, *36*, 242–253. [CrossRef] [PubMed]

11. Hansen, M.; Bangsbo, J.; Jensen, J.; Bibby, B.M.; Madsen, K. Effect of whey protein hydrolysate on performance and recovery of top-class orienteering runners. *Int. J. Sport Nutr. Exerc. Metab.* **2015**, *25*, 97–109. [CrossRef] [PubMed]

12. Luden, N.D.; Saunders, M.J.; Todd, M.K. Postexercise carbohydrate-protein- antioxidant ingestion decreases plasma creatine kinase and muscle soreness. *Int. J. Sport Nutr. Exerc. Metab.* **2007**, *17*, 109–123. [CrossRef] [PubMed]

13. Gilson, S.F.; Saunders, M.J.; Moran, C.W.; Moore, R.W.; Womack, C.J.; Todd, M.K. Effects of chocolate milk consumption on markers of muscle recovery following soccer training: A randomized cross-over study. *J. Int. Soc. Sports Nutr.* **2010**, *7*, 19. [CrossRef] [PubMed]

14. Nelson, A.R.; Phillips, S.M.; Stellingwerff, T.; Rezzi, S.; Bruce, S.J.; Breton, I.; Thorimbert, A.; Guy, P.A.; Clarke, J.; Broadbent, S.; et al. A protein-leucine supplement increases branched-chain amino acid and nitrogen turnover but not performance. *Med. Sci. Sports Exerc.* **2012**, *44*, 57–68. [CrossRef] [PubMed]

15. Witard, O.C.; Jackman, S.R.; Kies, A.K.; Jeukendrup, A.E.; Tipton, K.D. Effect of increased dietary protein on tolerance to intensified training. *Med. Sci. Sports Exerc.* **2011**, *43*, 598–607. [CrossRef] [PubMed]

16. Hansen, M.; Bangsbo, J.; Jensen, J.; Krause-Jensen, M.; Bibby, B.M.; Sollie, O.; Hall, U.A.; Madsen, K. Protein intake during training sessions has no effect on performance and recovery during a strenuous training camp for elite cyclists. *J. Int. Soc. Sports Nutr.* **2016**, *13*, 9. [CrossRef] [PubMed]

17. Rowlands, D.S.; Thomson, J.S.; Timmons, B.W.; Raymond, F.; Fuerholz, A.; Mansourian, R.; Zwahlen, M.C.; Metairon, S.; Glover, E.; Stellingwerff, T.; et al. Transcriptome and translational signaling following endurance exercise in trained skeletal muscle: Impact of dietary protein. *Physiol. Genom.* **2011**, *43*, 1004–1020. [CrossRef] [PubMed]

18. Greer, B.K.; Woodard, J.L.; White, J.P.; Arguello, E.M.; Haymes, E.M. Branched-chain amino acid supplementation and indicators of muscle damage after endurance exercise. *Int. J. Sport Nutr. Exerc. Metab.* **2007**, *17*, 595–607. [CrossRef] [PubMed]

19. Valentine, R.J.; Saunders, M.J.; Todd, M.K.; St Laurent, T.G. Influence of carbohydrate-protein beverage on cycling endurance and indices of muscle disruption. *Int. J. Sport Nutr. Exerc. Metab.* **2008**, *18*, 363–378. [CrossRef] [PubMed]

20. Flakoll, P.J.; Judy, T.; Flinn, K.; Carr, C.; Flinn, S. Postexercise protein supplementation improves health and muscle soreness during basic military training in marine recruits. *J. Appl. Physiol.* **2004**, *96*, 951–956. [CrossRef] [PubMed]

21. Skillen, R.A.; Testa, M.; Applegate, E.A.; Heiden, E.A.; Fascetti, A.J.; Casazza, G.A. Effects of an amino acid carbohydrate drink on exercise performance after consecutive-day exercise bouts. *Int. J. Sport Nutr. Exerc. Metab.* **2008**, *18*, 473–492. [CrossRef] [PubMed]

22. Cathcart, A.J.; Murgatroyd, S.R.; McNab, A.; Whyte, L.J.; Easton, C. Combined carbohydrate-protein supplementation improves competitive endurance exercise performance in the heat. *Eur. J. Appl. Physiol.* **2011**, *111*, 2051–2061. [CrossRef] [PubMed]

23. Okazaki, K.; Hayase, H.; Ichinose, T.; Mitono, H.; Doi, T.; Nose, H. Protein and carbohydrate supplementation after exercise increases plasma volume and albumin content in older and young men. *J. Appl. Physiol.* **2009**, *107*, 770–779. [CrossRef] [PubMed]

24. Okazaki, K.; Ichinose, T.; Mitono, H.; Chen, M.; Masuki, S.; Endoh, H.; Hayase, H.; Doi, T.; Nose, H. Impact of protein and carbohydrate supplementation on plasma volume expansion and thermoregulatory adaptation by aerobic training in older men. *J. Appl. Physiol.* **2009**, *107*, 725–733. [CrossRef] [PubMed]

25. Goto, M.; Okazaki, K.; Kamijo, Y.; Ikegawa, S.; Masuki, S.; Miyagawa, K.; Nose, H. Protein and carbohydrate supplementation during 5-day aerobic training enhanced plasma volume expansion and thermoregulatory adaptation in young men. *J. Appl. Physiol.* **2010**, *109*, 1247–1255. [CrossRef] [PubMed]

26. Baur, D.A.; Schroer, A.B.; Luden, N.D.; Womack, C.J.; Smyth, S.A.; Saunders, M.J. Glucose-fructose enhances performance versus isocaloric, but not moderate, glucose. *Med. Sci. Sports Exerc.* **2014**, *46*, 1778–1786. [CrossRef] [PubMed]

27. Costill, D.L.; Flynn, M.G.; Kirwan, J.P.; Houmard, J.A.; Mitchell, J.B.; Thomas, R.; Park, S.H. Effects of repeated days of intensified training on muscle glycogen and swimming performance. *Med. Sci. Sports Exerc.* **1988**, *20*, 249–254. [CrossRef] [PubMed]

28. Halson, S.L.; Lancaster, G.I.; Achten, J.; Gleeson, M.; Jeukendrup, A.E. Effects of carbohydrate supplementation on performance and carbohydrate oxidation after intensified cycling training. *J. Appl. Physiol.* **2004**, *97*, 1245–1253. [CrossRef] [PubMed]

29. Babcock, L.; Escano, M.; D'Lugos, A.; Todd, K.; Murach, K.; Luden, N. Concurrent aerobic exercise interferes with the satellite cell response to acute resistance exercise. *Am. J. Physiol. Regul. Integr. Comp. Physiol.* **2012**, *302*, R1458–R1465. [CrossRef] [PubMed]

30. Hopkins, W.G.; Marshall, S.W.; Batterham, A.M.; Hanin, J. Progressive statistics for studies in sports medicine and exercise science. *Med. Sci. Sports Exerc.* **2009**, *41*, 3–13. [CrossRef] [PubMed]

31. Hopkins, W. A spreadsheet for deriving a confidence interval, mechanistic inference and clinical inference from a p value. *Sportscience* **2007**, *1*, 16–20.

32. Paton, C.D.; Hopkins, W.G. Variation in performance of elite cyclists from race to race. *Eur. J. Sport Sci.* **2006**, *6*, 25–31. [CrossRef]

33. Atkinson, G. Estimating sample size for magnitude-based inferences. *Sportscience* **2006**, *10*, 63–70.

34. Coutts, A.; Reaburn, P.; Piva, T.J.; Murphy, A. Changes in selected biochemical, muscular strength, power, and endurance measures during deliberate overreaching and tapering in rugby league players. *Int. J. Sports Med.* **2007**, *28*, 116–124. [CrossRef] [PubMed]

35. Rosler, K.; Conley, K.E.; Howald, H.; Gerber, C.; Hoppeler, H. Specificity of leg power changes to velocities used in bicycle endurance training. *J. Appl. Physiol.* **1986**, *61*, 30–36. [PubMed]

36. Harber, M.P.; Gallagher, P.M.; Creer, A.R.; Minchev, K.M.; Trappe, S.W. Single muscle fiber contractile properties during a competitive season in male runners. *Am. J. Physiol. Regul. Integr. Comp. Physiol.* **2004**, *287*, R1124–R1131. [CrossRef] [PubMed]

37. Fitts, R.H.; Costill, D.L.; Gardetto, P.R. Effect of swim exercise training on human muscle fiber function. *J. Appl. Physiol.* **1989**, *66*, 465–475. [PubMed]

38. Kohn, T.A.; Essen-Gustavsson, B.; Myburgh, K.H. Specific muscle adaptations in type ii fibers after high-intensity interval training of well-trained runners. *Scand. J. Med. Sci. Sports* **2011**, *21*, 765–772. [CrossRef] [PubMed]

39. Howarth, K.R.; Moreau, N.A.; Phillips, S.M.; Gibala, M.J. Coingestion of protein with carbohydrate during recovery from endurance exercise stimulates skeletal muscle protein synthesis in humans. *J. Appl. Physiol.* **2009**, *106*, 1394–1402. [CrossRef] [PubMed]

40. Levenhagen, D.K.; Carr, C.; Carlson, M.G.; Maron, D.J.; Borel, M.J.; Flakoll, P.J. Postexercise protein intake enhances whole-body and leg protein accretion in humans. *Med. Sci. Sports Exerc.* **2002**, *34*, 828–837. [CrossRef] [PubMed]

41. Rowlands, D.S.; Nelson, A.R.; Phillips, S.M.; Faulkner, J.A.; Clarke, J.; Burd, N.A.; Moore, D.; Stellingwerff, T. Protein-leucine fed dose effects on muscle protein synthesis after endurance exercise. *Med. Sci. Sports Exerc.* **2015**, *47*, 547–555. [CrossRef] [PubMed]

42. Lorenzo, S.; Halliwill, J.R.; Sawka, M.N.; Minson, C.T. Heat acclimation improves exercise performance. *J. Appl. Physiol.* **2010**, *109*, 1140–1147. [CrossRef] [PubMed]

43. Lehmann, M.; Schnee, W. Decreased nocturnal catecholamine excretion parameter for an overtraining syndrom in athletes. *Int. J. Sports Med.* **1992**, *13*, 236–242. [CrossRef] [PubMed]

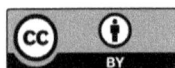

nutrients

MDPI

Review

A Systematic Review of Athletes' and Coaches' Nutrition Knowledge and Reflections on the Quality of Current Nutrition Knowledge Measures

Gina L. Trakman [1,*], Adrienne Forsyth [1], Brooke L. Devlin [2] and Regina Belski [1]

[1] School of Allied Health, La Trobe University, Melbourne 3086, Australia; A.forsyth@latrobe.edu.au (A.F.);
R.Belski@latrobe.edu.au (R.B.)

[2] Mary MacKillop Institute for Health Research, Australian Catholic University, Melbourne 3000, Australia;
Brooke.Devlin@acu.edu.au

* Correspondence: g.trakman@latrobe.edu.au; Tel.: +61-3-9479-5655

Received: 17 June 2016; Accepted: 7 September 2016; Published: 16 September 2016

Abstract: Context: Nutrition knowledge can influence dietary choices and impact on athletic performance. Valid and reliable measures are needed to assess the nutrition knowledge of athletes and coaches. Objectives: (1) To systematically review the published literature on nutrition knowledge of adult athletes and coaches and (2) to assess the quality of measures used to assess nutrition knowledge. Data Sources: MEDLINE, CINAHL, SPORTDiscuss, Web of Science, and SCOPUS. Study Selection: 36 studies that provided a quantitative measure of nutrition knowledge and described the measurement tool that was used were included. Data extraction: Participant description, questionnaire description, results (mean correct and responses to individual items), study quality, and questionnaire quality. Data synthesis: All studies were of neutral quality. Tools used to measure knowledge did not consider health literacy, were outdated with regards to consensus recommendations, and lacked appropriate and adequate validation. The current status of nutrition knowledge in athletes and coaches is difficult to ascertain. Gaps in knowledge also remain unclear, but it is likely that energy density, the need for supplementation, and the role of protein are frequently misunderstood. Conclusions: Previous reports of nutrition knowledge need to be interpreted with caution. A new, universal, up-to-date, validated measure of general and sports nutrition knowledge is required to allow for assessment of nutrition knowledge.

Keywords: nutritional knowledge; dietary knowledge; athlete; coach; sport; questionnaire; survey; measure; valid; sports nutrition

1. Introduction

A carefully planned nutrition program has significant positive effects on athletic performance [1–3]. There has recently been an increase in internationally endorsed dietary guidelines for athletes, reflected by the publication of several consensus statements on optimal intake and timing of food, fluid, and supplements [4,5]. Despite this, research indicates that many athletes have sub-optimal dietary intakes [6,7], which may be due to lack of time, finances, cooking skills, and access to cooking equipment when attempting to select and prepare appropriate meals and snacks [8]. Food choices may also be driven by factors such as cultural background, taste preferences, appetite, attitude towards nutrition, and nutrition knowledge [8–10].

Nutrition knowledge is one of the few modifiable determinants of dietary behaviors. Sports dietitians often center their dietary interventions on nutrition education to improve awareness of and compliance with expert dietary guidelines [10,11]. Nutrition education programs are rarely evaluated. There are a number of cross-sectional studies reporting on the nutrition knowledge of both athletes and coaches [12–14]. In a 2011 systematic review of the nutrition knowledge of recreational and elite athletes, scores across various nutrition knowledge questionnaires assessing general and sports specific nutrition were mediocre, with mean scores of approximately 45%–65% [7]. There appeared to be a weak, positive correlation between nutrition knowledge and good quality dietary intake. The review concluded that in order to confirm the nutrition knowledge of athletes, and the relationship between nutrition knowledge and dietary intake, further high-quality research was required [7]. A 2014 review on the relationship between nutrition knowledge and dietary intake in adults also suggested that while the relationship between nutrition knowledge and dietary behavior appears to be moderate at best, results may be affected by the quality of measures used to assess knowledge [6]. Several studies assessing nutrition knowledge in athletes, not included in either of the aforementioned reviews, have been published in recent years [12,15–23].

Despite researchers having raised concerns regarding the validity of current nutrition knowledge measures [6,7,22], a detailed review of their limitations has not been undertaken to date. It is important to consider the comprehensiveness of the tools used. That is, the extent to which they have assessed all the relevant topics of nutrition knowledge, such as knowledge of macronutrients, micronutrients, supplementation, and hydration. In nutrition knowledge measures, questions on each of these topics are often grouped together and referred to as nutrition "sub-sections". Previous reviews have identified concerns with drawing comparison between studies due to the heterogeneity of measures used; however, analysis of related nutrition sub-sections and responses to congruent questions across studies has not been performed. Several reports [9,11] and cross-sectional studies in elite Australian athletes and American College athletes have established that coaches are often a key source of nutrition information for athletes [16,24,25] but there has not been a systematic review of their nutrition knowledge.

Considering the importance of nutrition knowledge as a modifiable determinant of dietary behavior, the aims of the present review are to determine whether:

1. Athletes (aged 17 years and over) and coaches of adult athletes are aware of expert nutrition recommendations
2. There are gaps in particular topics (nutrition sub-sections) of nutrition knowledge
3. The quality (validity, reliability, and comprehensiveness) of measures that have been used to assess nutrition knowledge is acceptable.

2. Methods

2.1. Protocol and Registration

Methods for the review were in accordance with PRISMA guidelines and were registered with PROSEPERO [26].

2.2. Search Terms

A systematic search using the strategy nutrition knowledge or diet knowledge and athlete or sports people or sportsman and questionnaire or tool or measure or survey and valid or reliable, was conducted by one researcher (GT) from the earliest record until November 2015. A second search using the terms nutrition knowledge or diet knowledge and coach or questionnaire or tool or measure or survey was also conducted. Searched databases included MEDLINE, CINAHL, SPORTDiscuss, Web of Science, and SCOPUS. To ensure all related texts were captured, the reference lists of included articles were hand-searched.

2.3. Eligibility Criteria

Original research (cross-sectional, observational, randomized controlled trials) conducted in adult athletes (17 years and older) or coaches/athletic trainers of adult athletes, and published in peer-reviewed journals were included for review. Abstracts, conference posters, reviews, and unpublished theses were excluded. Athletes were defined as individuals involved in training and playing competitive sport. All 'levels' of athletic competition, for example, recreational, college, national, and international were accepted. Only English language studies were included. Studies needed to report an aspect of nutrition knowledge (general, overall sports, or specific sports nutrition e.g., hydration) using a measure that produced a numerical score. Studies that provided qualitative data only, or stated how many participants answered questions correctly/incorrectly, but failed to report overall quantitative results were excluded. The questionnaires could be in any format including self-administered, researcher-administered, online, or handwritten. To be included, studies also needed to provide a description of the tool used to assess knowledge including number of items, content, and question response categories (Table 1).

Table 1. Eligibility criteria.

	Included		Excluded
1.	Original research (cross-sectional, observational, randomized controlled trials)	1.	Abstracts, conference posters, reviews, and unpublished theses
2.	Athletes (aged 17 years and older) and coaches of adult athletes (recreational, elite)	2.	Adolescent athletes, all non-athletes other than coaches
3.	English language studies	3.	Non-English language studies
4.	Studies reporting a quantitative measures of nutrition knowledge that could be converted into a single 'score' (% total correct)	4.	Studies on nutrition attitudes, behavior, habits, or intake; studies where a mean nutrition knowledge score could not be determined
5.	Studies that described the tool used to assess knowledge including number of items, content and question response-categories	5.	Studies where it was unclear what (and how) the tool used actually measured nutrition knowledge

2.4. Selection Process

Duplicate and irrelevant articles were excluded on the basis of abstract and title by two authors (GT and AF). Articles deemed eligible for full-text review were retrieved and screened against the inclusion criteria by two authors (GT and AF) (Figure 1).

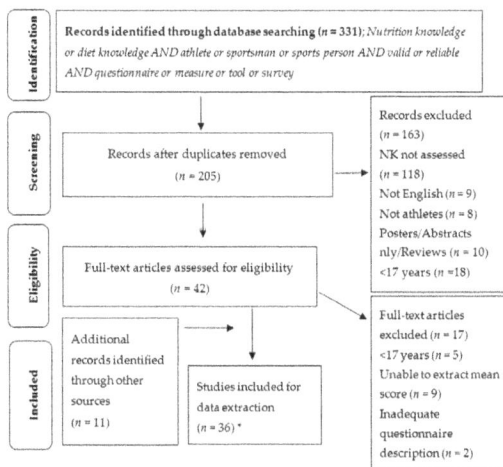

Figure 1. Flowchart of review process. * Secondary search using the term coach did not yield any additional relevant articles. NK = nutrition knowledge.

2.5. Data Extraction and Tool Quality

Data from eligible studies were extracted by one author (GT). Information retrieved included: country of study, participant description (age, gender, sport played/coached, athletic level), questionnaire description (item generation, number of questions, question-response format), and results (mean nutrition knowledge scores, as well as nutrition sub-sections where participants scored above and below the study's overall mean). All scores were converted into percentage correct for consistency. Athletic level was based on descriptions provided in the paper; if athletic level was not adequately described, judgments on athletic level were based on other available information such as participant recruitment. Where reported, responses to individual items were also extracted then collated and summarized based on congruent themes. If questionnaires were not available, authors were contacted and permission to review a copy of the tool that was used was requested.

Detailed data on the quality of the measures reported in the studies reviewed were recorded and used to calculate two separate quality scores: one for validity and reliability and another for questionnaire comprehensiveness. The validity and reliability score was based on a set of guidelines developed by Parmenter and Wardle [27]. Their recommendations are based upon psychometric validation techniques within the classical test theory (CTT) framework and are in line with leaders in the field of scale development, such as Kline [28] and Nunnally [29]. They outline several methods for the development and evaluation of questionnaires, including: item analysis (item difficulty/item discrimination); homogeneity/"internal consistency" assessed using Cronbach's alpha; face validity assessed using a cohort similar to the target audience; content validity assessed using a panel of experts; construct validity assessed using known-group comparisons; and test–retest reliability using Pearson's correlation. In accordance with these guidelines, a validity score out of six was given. The decision was made to assess face validity, as, although it is similar to content validity, it utilizes different focus groups (target audience, not experts) and has different aims (ensuring readability/tool assesses what it intends to, not ensuring the entire content of the domain is covered). Scales developed under CTT apply only to the group of people who took the test; therefore, it is necessary to re-run internal consistency calculations for new samples [30]. Accordingly, in instances where an existing measure or modified version of an existing tool was used, a point was not awarded for internal consistency unless Cronbach's alpha was reassessed. If this test had been performed in the original sample, a partial point was given (denoted by P). If a tool had been modified from a previous tool, or was a composite of various previous questionnaires, validation points were not awarded unless the new version had undergone psychometric testing.

For the comprehensiveness score, a point was awarded for each of the following nutrition sub-sections covered: general nutrition knowledge, carbohydrates, proteins, fats, micronutrients, hydration, pre-exercise nutrition, nutrition during competition, recovery nutrition, supplementation, and alcohol. A maximum of 11 points could be awarded. Decisions on whether a questionnaire included adequate coverage on each topic to be included as a nutrition sub-section were made by one author (GT), based on a combination of review of the actual tool (when available) and the description of the measure provided in the article.

2.6. Study Quality

The methodological quality of studies was assessed by two reviewers (GT and AF), using the "Academy of Nutrition and Dietetics" "Quality Criteria Checklist for Primary Research" [31]. Disagreements were resolved by a third reviewer (BD). The checklist rates studies as positive, neutral, or negative (poor) on 10 criteria. The criteria addressing study group comparisons (3), methods for handling withdrawals (4), use of blinding (5), and description of interventions/comparisons/description of intervening factors (6) could not be logically applied to cross-sectional or observational studies. All studies awarded positive quality ratings needed to adequately address selection bias, make appropriate study group comparisons, clearly describe any interventions, and use valid and reliable measurements. To receive a "Yes" for criterion (7),

"Were outcomes clearly defined and the measurements valid and reliable?", the questionnaire needed to undergo a least three different types of expected psychometric validation, outlined by Parmenter and Wardle [27], as above. Meta-analysis was not possible due to heterogeneity in measures used to assess nutrition knowledge.

3. Results

3.1. Study Selection

The original search yielded 331 results. After removal of duplicate and irrelevant records, 42 studies were retained for full-text review. An additional 11 records were identified through hand searching reference lists. Thus, a total of 53 full-text articles were screened for inclusion in the final review. Thirty-six of these met the inclusion criteria. The reasons for excluding the other articles included: the age of the participants being less than 17 years old ($n = 5$), inability to extract a mean score ($n = 9$), lack of adequate questionnaire description ($n = 2$), or failure to assess nutrition knowledge ($n = 1$) (Figure 1). A secondary search using the term 'coach' did not yield any additional relevant articles.

3.2. Study Characteristics

The majority of the studies ($n = 34$) employed a cross-sectional design, with the remaining two [32,33] using a questionnaire to assess the effectiveness of an education program at two time points. Of the 36 included studies, 15 assessed nutrition knowledge in American college athletes [13,23–25,32–42]; two of these also collected data on coaches and athletic trainers, stratifying the results [23,24]. There were an additional four studies [38,43–45] that assessed the knowledge of coaches alone. Six studies assessed college athletes outside of the USA (three in Iran [15,20,46]; one each in India [17], Malaysia [21], and Nigeria [18]). Five studies [12,14,16,22,47] were conducted with elite athletes and three studies [48–50] assessed knowledge in recreational athletes. Five studies [15,24,33,34,45] did not report what sport the athletes played. Across the remaining studies, the other sports that were represented included: Australian football (AFL) [16], basketball [13,20,23,35,37–40,42,44], baseball [23,25,37,38,42], cross-country [13,35,41,42,44], cycling [50], football [13,20,23,35,37,38,44], golf [13,23,35,37,40], gymnastics [13,35,40,49], hockey [35,40,47], lacrosse [23,35,39], soccer [13,23,32,38,42], softball [13,19,35,37,40,42,44], running and/or track and field [14,23,25,35,37,42,44,48], rugby [12,22,47,51], swimming [13,18,32,35,37,52], tennis [35,37,38,42,43], and triathlon [50]. Participant numbers ranged from five [17] to 595 [46]. Most studies were mixed-gender ($n = 19$) [13–15,18,20–24,35–37,39,44,46,47,50,53]. There were a total of 5231 participants: 2307 males, 2170 females, and 754 where gender was not reported. The mean age ranges of coaches and athletes were 33.0 to 43.2 years and 19.0 to 35.2 years, respectively. No studies reported the nutrition knowledge of older athletes (master's level) (Table 2).

3.3. Nutrition Knowledge Results

3.3.1. Demographic Factors Related to Nutrition Knowledge Scores

Seven out of 11 studies that reported on prior nutrition knowledge found that higher levels of (general) education, previously undertaking a nutrition course, or currently majoring in nutrition studies correlated with higher nutrition knowledge scores [14,20,40,41,46,48,50]. Fifteen studies reported on male versus female scores, and 10 of these studies reported no significant difference [14,15, 21,35,36,39,42,44,49,53]. All studies that assessed for differences between athletes from varying sports reported no significant differences in nutrition knowledge scores based on sport played [21,25,39,40]. Where reported, there was no significant difference in nutrition knowledge scores across National College Athletic Association (NCAA) divisions I, II, and III (ranked according to level of support and participation) [41,52].

Table 2. Nutrition knowledge of athletes and coaches.

References Author, Year, Country	Participant Characteristics Athletic Level	Sport Played	N (Gender)	Mean Age (Years) ± SD	Questionnaire Used/Item Generation and Number of Questions	Type of Questions	Mean Correct Nutrition Knowledge Score (%) ± SD	Questionnaire Nutrition Sub-Sections with Scores above Average Compared to the Total Mean Score within the Same Study (% ± SD Where Available)	Nutrition Sub-Sections with Scores below Average Compared to the Total Mean Score within the Same Study (% ± SD Where Available)	Quality Rating
Abood et al. [32], 2004, USA	College	Soccer, Swimming	n = 30 (F)	19.5 (SD NR)	Self-developed; n = 42	True/False	68.5	NR	NR	Neutral
Alaunyte et al. [12], 2015, UK	Elite	Rugby	n = 21 (M)	25 ± 5	Existing Questionnaire (A–C of GNKQ); n = 28	Multi-Choice, Open-Ended, Less/More/Not Sure/Same	72.82 ± 6.11	Recommendations made by experts (85.7 ± 13.0)	Food groups (71.2 ± 7.2) and Making healthier Food Choices (69.5 ± 14.0)	Neutral
Azizi and Hosseini [15], 2012, Iran	College/-Non-College	NR	n = 250 (130 M, 120 F); 121 College, 129 Non-College	College M: 24.71 ± 2.3, College F: 23.61 ± 2.10, Non-College M: 23.42 ± 1.8, Non-College F: 21.49 ± 2.8	Modified Questionnaire (Zawila et al. 2003); n = 40	True/False	54.0	Vitamins (61.2), Calcium and Iron (56.48), Weight Lose (57.95)	Macronutrients (50.7), Fiber (52.3), Sports Nutrition (49.74), General Nutrition (49.97)	Neutral
Azizi et al. [46], 2010, Iran	College	Sport Olympiad (range of sports)	n = 595 (298 M, 297 F)	M: 22.8 ± 1.9, F: 21.8 ± 1.8	Self-developed; n = 15	Strongly agree/agree/neutral/ disagree/strongly disagree	* 58.9 (M: 52.36 ± 6.2; F: 54.3 ± 6.3)	NR	NR	Neutral
Barbarne–Tudor et al. [43], 2011, Croatia	Coaches	Tennis	n = 58 (50 M, 8 F)	33 ± 10.8	Self-developed; n = 40	True/False	68.9 (SD not reported)	NR	NR	Neutral
Barr [48], 1987, USA	Recreational	Marathon runners	n = 104 (F) And n = 105 fitness class participants (F)	NR: 1.0% <20, 40.8% 20–29, 43.7% 30–39, 14.6% >40 years	Self-developed; n = 87	True/False/Don't Know	Athletes: 50.1 *; Fitness class participant: 42.6 * (SD not reported)	Knowledge about general nutrition (50.9)	Knowledge about sports nutrition (48.3)	Neutral
Botsis and Holden [44], 2015, USA	Coaches	Volleyball, Softball, Cross-Country, Track and Field, Football, and Basketball	n = 21 (16 M, 5 F)	NR	Existing Questionnaire (Zinn et al. 2006); n = 88	Agree/Disagree/Unsure, Multi-Choice	35 (SD not reported)	NR	NR	Neutral
Collison et al. [34], 1996, USA	College	NR	n = 51 (F) And n = 49 (F) comparison group	19.4 ± 1.2	Modified Questionnaire (Werblow et al., 1978); n = 35	Agree/Disagree	Athletes: 68.3 Comparison group: 77.1	NR	NR	Neutral
Condon et al. [35], 2007, USA	College	Ice hockey, Lacrosse, Basketball, Track and Field, Softball and Tennis	n = 165 (63 M, 102 F)	20 ± 1.3; M: 20.3 ± 1.5, F: 19.7 ± 1.1	Self-developed; n = 8	True/False, Open-ended, Multi-choice	50.0	NA	NA	Neutral
Corley et al. [53, 52], USA	College Coaches	Track and Field, Cross-Country, Swimming, Tennis, Basketball, Gymnastics, and Golf, and Men's Football, and Men's Wrestling	n = 105 (75 M, 30 F)	35	Self-developed; n = 15	True/False/Not Sure	* 60.09	NR	NR	Neutral
Danaher and Curley [45], 2014, Canada	College Coaches	NR	n = 5 (NR)	NR	Modified existing Questionnaire (Zinn et al., 2005); n = 95	Agree/Disagree/Unsure, Multi-Choice	56.3	Training diet (58.1), Pre-competition diet (58.1), weight loss and weight gain (57.5)	Fluid (49.5), Recovery diet (50.6), Dietary Supplements (53.8) * not statistically analyzed	Neutral

Table 2. Cont.

References	Participant Characteristics				Questionnaire					Quality Rating
Author, Year, Country	Athletic Level	Sport Played	N (Gender)	Mean Age (Years) ± SD	Questionnaire Used/Item Generation and Number of Questions	Type of Questions	Mean Correct Nutrition Knowledge Score (%) ± SD	Nutrition Sub-Sections with Scores above Average Compared to the Total Mean Score within the Same Study (% ± SD Where Available)	Nutrition Sub-Sections with Scores below Average Compared to the Total Mean Score within the Same Study (% ± SD Where Available)	
Davar [17], 2012, India	College	Hockey	n = 30 (F)	19.9 ± 2.7	Modified existing Questionnaire (Zawila et al 2003); n = 61	True/False, Open-Ended	38.8 (SD not reported)	Protein (41.1), Fats (53.5), Vitamins (39.3), Minerals (43.8), Hydration (51.6)	Energy (25.9), Carbohydrates (37.7), Weight management (32.3), Sports nutrition (36.5), Fiber (21.4)	Neutral
Devlin and Belski [16], 2015, Australia	Elite	Australian Football (AFL)	n = 46 (M)	23.5 ± 2.8	Modified Existing questionnaire (GNKQ + Shifflet); n = 123	Multi-Choice, Open-Ended, Less/More/Not Sure/Same	60.5 (SD for % score not reported)	Sources of nutrients (60.9), Sports Nutrition Knowledge (61.7)	Dietary recommendations (60.0), Sources of nutrients (57.0)	Neutral
Dunn et al. [13], 2007, USA	College	Basketball, Golf, Gymnastics, Softball, Swimming, Soccer, Tennis, Cross-country, Volleyball, Football	n = 190 (92 M, 98 F)	19.0	Existing Questionnaire (GNKQ); n = 124	Multi-Choice, Open-Ended, Less/More/Not Sure/Same	51.5 ± 13.57	Dietary recommendations (59.3), Food groups (54.4)	Dietary recommendations (60.0), Sources of nutrients (57.0)	Neutral
Folasire et al. [18], 2015, Nigeria	College	Ball-games' Racquet, 'Combat sports', Swimming	n = 110 (63 M, 47 F)	22.06 ± 2.39	Self-developed (used items from Zawila et al. 2003 and Supriya et al. 2013); n = 14	Yes/No/Not Sure	64.3 (SD not reported)	NR	NR	Neutral
Grete R et al. [19], USA	College	Softball	n = 185 (F)	NR	Self-developed; n = 80	Likert Scale	* 57.1	NR	NR	Neutral
Hamilton et al. [14], 1994, New Zealand	Elite	Distance Runners	n = 53 (41 M, 12 F)	24 ± 6	Self-developed; n = 48	Multi-choice	64.0: General M: 70 ± 14, General F: 78 ± 14, Sports M: 50 ± 16; Sports F: 58 ± 11	Vitamin C, energy and fiber (83.0–100), iron deficiency (98.0), recommended methods for weight loss (99.0), coronary heart disease (94.0–96.0). Protein as a fuel source, high carbohydrate foods and energy sources for vigorous exercise (74.0–98.0)	Foods high in saturated fat (42.0) and unsaturated fat (25.0), and changes in energy requirements with age (47.0). Carbohydrate loading, recommended ratio of dietary energy sources and ergogenic aids (6.0–17.0)	Neutral
Harrison et al. [47], 1991, New Zealand	Elite/non-elite*	Field Hockey, Basketball, Powerlifting, Netball (F only), Rugby Union (M only)	n = 122 (69 M, 53 F); 69 elite, 53 non-elite	23.75	Self-developed; n = 28	True/False/Not Sure, Open-Ended	Elite: 67.0 ± 12; non-elite: 56.0 ± 12	Energy sources (77.0 for elite)	Vitamins (9.0–50.0)	Neutral
Hoogenboom et al. [52], 2009, USA	College	Swimmers	n = 85 (F)	19 ± 1.6	Existing Questionnaire (Zawila et al., 2003); n = 76	Strongly agree/agree/neutral/disagree/strongly disagree	* 72.0 (SD not reported)	NR	NR	Neutral
Jessri et al. [20], 2010, Iran	College	Basketball, Football	n = 207 (109 M, 98 F)	21.8 ± 1.3	Modified existing Questionnaire (Zinn et al., 2006); n = 88	Agree/Disagree/Unsure, Multi-Choice	33.2 ± 12.3	Nutrient type (36.75), Weight Control (33.35)	Fluid (33.05), Supplements (30.35)	Neutral
Kunkel et al. [33], 2001, USA	College	NR	n = 32 (F)	NR	Existing Questionnaire (Werblow et al., 1978); n = 31	Multi-choice, Agree/Disagree/Not Sure	66.7 ± 8.3	Sports Knowledge questions (66.3)	General Knowledge questions (54.5)	Neutral

Table 2. Cont.

References	Participant Characteristics				Questionnaire Used/Item Generation and Number of Questions	Type of Questions	Mean Correct Nutrition Knowledge Score (%) ± SD	Questionnaire		Quality Rating
Author, Year, Country	Athletic Level	Sport Played	N (Gender)	Mean Age (Years) ± SD				Nutrition Sub-Sections with Scores above Average Compared to the Total Mean Score within the Same Study (% ± SD Where Available)	Nutrition Sub-Sections with Scores below Average Compared to the Total Mean Score within the Same Study (% ± SD Where Available)	
Nichols et al. [42], 2005, USA	College	Soccer, Basketball, Tennis, Cross-country, Track, Baseball, Softball, and Volleyball	$n = 139$ (62 M; 77 F)	19.8 ± 1.5; M: 20.1 ± 1.6, F: 19.6 ± 1.4	Self-developed; $n = 17$	True/false	81.8	N/A	N/A	Neutral
Rash et al. [36], 2007, USA	College	Track and Field	$n = 113$ (61 M; 53 F)	M:19.3 ± 1.2, F: 19.1 ± 1.1	Existing Questionnaire (Zawila et al., 2003); $n = 76$	Strongly agree/agree/neutral/disagree/strongly disagree	58.3 ± 13	Carbohydrates (75.4), Vitamins and Minerals (62.7)	Protein (54.7), Vitamin E (45.0), Vitamin C (38.4)	Neutral
Raymond-Barker et al. [49], 2007, England	Recreational	Endurance athletes (runners, cyclists, triathlon), and gymnasts	$n = 59$ (F)	33.88 ± 9.74	Modified existing Questionnaire (GNKQ); $n = 110$	Multi-Choice, Open-Ended, Yes/No/Not Sure, Agree/Disagree/Not Sure	74.2	NR	NR	Positive
Rosenbloom et al. [37], 2002, USA	College	Football, Track and Field, Baseball, Swimming, Basketball, Tennis, Golf, Softball, Volleyball	$n = 328$ (237 M; 91 F)	M: 19.0 ± 2.7, F: 19.0 ± 1.3	Self-developed; $n = 11$	Agree/Disagree/Don't Know	52.7 (SD not reported)	NR	NR	Neutral
Sedek and Yih [21], 2014, Malaysia	College	Futsal, Cricket, Pencak Silat, Volleyball, Silat Cekap, Taekwondo	$n = 100$ (50 M; 50 F), And $n = 100$ non-athletes (50 M; 50 F)	20.8 ± 1.8	Modified existing Questionnaire (Paugh et al., 2005); $n = 29$	Strongly agree/agree/neutral/disagree/strongly disagree	* Athletes: 83.7 ± 6.84 Non-athletes: 83.5 ± 6.23	NR	NR	Neutral
Shifflett et al. [24], 2002, USA	College Athletes and	NR	Athletes: $n = 65$ (12 M: 53 F); Coaches: $n = 68$ (39 M; 29 F)	Athletes: M. 20.0 ± 2.00; F: 20.0 ± 2.00; Coaches: M: 43.10 ± 9.7; F: 37.6 ± 9.4	Self-developed; $n = 19$	Multi-Choice, Open-Ended	Athletes: 55.0; Coaches: 60.8	NR	NR	Neutral
Shoaf et al. [25], 1986, USA	College	Baseball, Football, Track	$n = 75$ (M)		Self-developed; $n = 25$	Multi-Choice	43.8 (SD not reported as %)	NR	NR	Neutral
Smith-Rockwell et al. [38], 2001, USA	College Coaches	Baseball, Basketball, Cheerleading, Football, Cross-Country, Lacrosse, Rowing, Soccer, Swimming, Tennis, Track and field Volleyball, Wrestling	$n = 53$ (Gender NR)	34.2 ± 9.7	Self-Developed; $n = 19$	True / False / Multi-Choice	67.0	Weight control (71), Nutrition supplements (90), Other topics: fluids, amenorrhea, sources of nutrition information (92)	Macronutrients (51), Micronutrients (53)	Neutral
Spendlove et al. [22], 2012, Australia	Elite	Surf lifesaving, Rugby League	$n = 175$ (76 M; 99 F) And $n = 116$ community members And $n = 53$ dietitians	18.9 ± 4.9	Existing Questionnaire (GNKQ) and Modified existing questionnaire (R-GNKQ); R-GNKQ: $n = 90$	Multi-Choice, Open-Ended, Less/More/Not Sure/Same	Athletes: R-GNKQ—65.3 (95% CI 8.3, 8.8); Community: 65.4 (95% CI 8.2, 8.9) Dietitians: 77.7 (95% CI 9.5, 10.8)	GNKQ: Dietary recommendations (65.4), Sources of Nutrients/Food groups (60.9), Choosing Everyday foods (60.0); R-GNKQ: Dietary recommendations (73.4, Choosing everyday foods 68.0)	GNKQ: Diet-disease relationship (57.6) GNKQ: Sources of nutrients/food groups (62.1), Diet-disease relationship (48.9)	Neutral

Table 2. Cont.

References	Participant Characteristics				Questionnaire					Quality Rating
Author, Year, Country	Athletic Level	Sport Played	N (Gender)	Mean Age (Years) ± SD	Questionnaire Used/Item Generation and Number of Questions	Type of Questions	Mean Correct Nutrition Knowledge Score (%) ± SD	Nutrition Sub-Sections with Scores above Average Compared to the Total Mean Score within the Same Study (% ± SD Where Available)	Nutrition Sub-Sections with Scores below Average Compared to the Total Mean Score within the Same Study (% ± SD Where Available)	
Torres-McGehee et al. [23], 2012, USA	College Athletes and College Coaches	Baseball, Basketball, Cheerleading, dance, Equestrian, Football, Golf, Ice-Hockey, Lacrosse, Soccer, Swimming & Diving, Tennis, Track and Field, Volleyball, and Wrestling	Athletes: n = 185 (Gender NR); Coaches: n = 131 (Gender NR); Athletic trainers: n = 91; Strength and Conditioning coaches: n = 71	NR	Self-developed; n = 20	Multi-Choice	Athletes: 54.9 ± 13.5 Coaches: 65.9 ± 14.3 Athletic trainers: 77.8 ± 10.3 Strength and Conditioning Coaches: 81.6 ± 10.3	Supplements and performance (66.3 ± 19.9)	Micronutrients and Macronutrients (51.8 ± 20.3), Weight management and Eating disorders (47.0 ± * 21.9), Hydration (54.7 ± 24.2)	Neutral
Weeden et al. [39], 2014, USA	College	Male Basketball, Football, Tennis, Track and Field, and Female, Basketball, Golf, Soccer, Tennis, Track and Field and Volleyball	n = 174 (86 M, 88 F)	20.0 ± 1.4	Self-developed; n = 24	Yes/No/Not Sure	56.4 ± 13.4	Hydration (80.0)	Weight management (32.0), dietary supplements (36.0)	Neutral
Werblow et al. [40], 1978, USA	College	Softball, Track and Field, Gymnastics, Basketball, Field Hockey, Tennis, Swimming, Diving, Volleyball, Golf	n = 94 (F)	NR	Self-developed; n = 31	Strongly agree/agree/neutral/disagree/strongly disagree	* 67.74 (SD not reported)	NR	NR	Neutral
Worme et al. [50], 1990, USA	Recreational	Triathlon	n = 71 (50 M, 21 F) And n = 28 non-athletes (21 M, 17 F)	35.3	Self-developed; n = 20	True/False	Athletes: 54.2 ± 2.0, Non-athletes: 56.5 ± 2.3	NR	NR	Neutral
Zawila et al. [41], 2003, USA	College	Cross-country runners	n = 60 (F)	19.8 ± 1.04	Self-developed; n = 76	Strongly agree/agree/neutral/disagree/strongly disagree	57.2 (SD nor reported)	NR	NR	Neutral
Zinn et al. [51], 2006, New Zealand	Elite Coaches	Rugby	n = 364 (M)	NR	Existing Questionnaire; n = 88	Agree/Disagree/Unsure, Multi-Choice	55.6 (SD for total score not reported)	Supplements and performance (79.9 ± 18.9)	Micronutrients and Macronutrients (58.0 ± 19.4), Weight management and Eating disorders (63.8 ± 20.9), Hydration (61.9 ± 22.4)	Neutral

F = female; M = male; * = more than 1 point awarded for correct answers; NR = not reported; GNQK = general nutrition knowledge questionnaire; Bold = percent score calculated by researchers as either (a) scores presented as figure out of total (b) nutrition sub-section means but not total score reported; NA = not applicable; "Quality ratings were decided using the Academy of Nutrition and Dietetics" "Quality Criteria Checklist for Primary Research".

3.3.2. Nutrition Knowledge Scores of Athletes versus Comparison Group (within Studies)

Five studies included a non-athlete comparison group [21,22,34,48,50]. A study of American college athletes found that athletes had lower nutrition knowledge scores than a non-athlete comparison group consisting of 28% nutrition majors [34]; however, a study of college athletes in Malaysia found athletes had similar levels of knowledge when compared to non-athlete controls whose prior exposure to nutrition education was not reported [21]. Recreational athletes scored better than matched fitness class participants [48] and a matched community sample [50]. In contrast, a sample of elite athletes scored lower than both a matched community sample and a cohort of dietitians [22] (Table 2).

Four studies also included athletes of various levels and/or both athletes and coaches [15,23,24,47]. University athletes in Iran were found to score better than non-university athletes [15] and elite athletes in New Zealand achieved higher scores than non-elite athletes [47]. Coaches scored better than athletes in the two studies that included both groups [23,24]. However, in all of these studies except the one comparing Iranian athletes [15], it was unclear whether the participants in various groups were comparable in terms of factors such as age, gender, and education (Table 2).

3.3.3. Comparison across Questionnaires (between Studies)

While a comparison of nutrition knowledge scores cannot be made across all studies due to the heterogeneity in measures and participants, some of the studies did use either the same tools or modified versions of such tools. The tool that Werblow et al. [40] developed for use in American college athletes was later modified and used in two other studies assessing similar groups [33,34]. Results in these studies were reasonably consistent at 68%, 68%, and 67%, respectively. The sports questionnaire developed by Zinn et al. [54], was used in three of the studies that assessed knowledge of coaches [44,45,51]. Scores observed in these studies were very similar, at 55%, 56%, and 56% respectively. The questionnaire developed by Zawila et al. [41] (for use in college runners) was based on a composite of two previous measures [40,48]. It was utilized by two other researchers assessing knowledge in American college athletes [36,52]. Three of the studies in non-USA college athletes [15,17,18] also used the tool by Zawila et al. [41] or one of the two original tools it was based upon. The results reported in the studies using these tools in American college athletes were 57%, 58%, and 72% and in Non-American college athletes were 54%, 39%, and 64%, respectively. Three of the five studies in elite athletes used a version of the "general nutrition knowledge questionnaire" [12,16,22]; scores in these studies were moderately disparate at 60.5%, 72.8%, and 65.3% respectively (Table 2).

3.4. Responses to Specific Nutrition Sub-Sections and Nutrition Questions

Given that there is a large degree of discrepancy in the question type and format across measures, scores reported as percentages provide little information regarding the actual knowledge (and gaps in knowledge) of participants. Therefore, in addition to reporting on the scores (% total correct) obtained in specific nutrition sub-sections (Table 2), we have provided a summary of nutrition sub-sections that were tested in each questionnaire (Table 3) and included a summary of responses to individual questions (Sections 3.4.1–3.4.10).

3.4.1. General versus Sports Nutrition Knowledge

The majority of studies assessed both general and sports nutrition knowledge. Four studies directly compared these nutrition sub-sections; scores were better in the sports nutrition knowledge compared to general nutrition knowledge section in two studies [16,33]; however, the opposite was true for the other two [47,48] (Table 2).

3.4.2. Weight Management and Energy Balance

Eight studies reported on weight management and energy balance nutrition sub-section scores [14,17,20,23,38,39,45,51] (Table 2). Several authors also described responses to specific questions related to this topic. In many of the studies, athletes had a sound understanding of safe weight loss practices based on current recommendations. For example, in a study of recreational athletes, 92% of participants [48] disagreed that fasting is a good way to decrease fat and increase muscle. Similarly, 100% of swimmers in the study by Hoogenboom et al. [52] felt that skipping meals was not an acceptable way to lose weight. About 75% of college athletes in the study by Rosenbloom et al. [37] knew that eating carbohydrate would not "make them fat". Nevertheless, misconceptions were evident; for example, 84% of female college athletes in the study by Collison et al. [34] and 92% of male and female college athletes in the study by Weeden et al. [39] agreed that "acidic foods such a grapefruit could assist with weight loss". Likewise, Harrison et al. [47] found that 84% of elite and 63% of non-elite athletes disagreed with the statement "you can lose weight by decreasing your food intake".

3.4.3. Macronutrients

All studies but one assessed knowledge of carbohydrates [46]. Protein was not assessed in five studies [18,35,46,48,50]. Fat was not assessed in seven studies [18,33,35,40,42,46,48] (Table 3). Across these studies, there was no discernible pattern regarding related nutrition sub-section scores (% total correct) being above or below the overall mean nutrition score (% total correct) (Table 2). Several studies also reported on responses to individual items related to the energy density, role, sources, and requirements of macronutrients.

Energy density: Devlin and Belski [16] found that only 22% of elite Australian Rules Football players were aware that fat is the most energy-dense macronutrient. Likewise, only 22% of U.S. college swimmers surveyed by Hoogenboom et al. [52], 28% of American college athletes surveyed by Collison et al. [34], and 18% of American college coaches in the study by Corley et al. [53] knew that carbohydrates and protein have the same amount of energy per gram.

Role: Sixty-nine per cent of Nigerian athletes in the study by Folasire et al. [18], 98% of elite athletes surveyed by Hamilton et al. [14], and 64% of college athletes in the study by Rosenbloom et al. [37] agreed with a statement indicating that that foods rich in carbohydrate should be the main source of energy. Rosenbloom et al. [37] and Rash et al. [36] also reported that about 46% and 40% of College American college athletes thought that protein was a source of fuel for muscles or believed protein was a good source of "immediate" energy. However, none of the coaches surveyed by Corley et al. [53] subscribed to similar beliefs.

Sources: Only 42% of elite athletes surveyed by Hamilton et al. [14] correctly answered questions on sources of saturated and unsaturated fat. Similarly, less than one-quarter of elite Australian Rules Football players in the study by Devlin and Belski [16] selected dairy as a source of saturated fat and less than one-fifth were aware of the saturated fat content of margarine and red meat. On the other hand, many of the elite Australian Rules Football players were able to identify foods that were low in both protein and carbohydrates [16], and 100% of coaches surveyed by Corley et al. [53] knew that sources of dietary carbohydrates include breads, crackers, and pastas.

Requirements: In the studies by Shifflett et al. [24] and Hoogenboom et al. [52] only 21% and 25% of college athletes, respectively, knew what proportion of energy should come from fat; slightly more, 41%, knew the proportion of energy that should come from protein [24,52]. Similarly, in the study by Weeden et al. [39], when asked what carbohydrate range was endorsed by experts, 53% of college athletes selected a value below the current recommendations.

Quality: Only 50% of elite and 26% of non-elite athletes surveyed by Harrison et al. [47] disagreed that "athletes who are vegetarians perform as well as non-vegetarian athletes". This belief was also reported by Rash et al. [36], where 82% of American college athletes believed that vegetarian athletes needed protein supplementation. Devlin and Belski [16] and Hamilton et al. [14] found that 80% of elite Australian Rules Football players [16] and 55% of elite athletes in New Zealand, respectively were aware that most of the fats in our diet should be unsaturated. In relation, all college coaches surveyed by Corley et al. [53] agreed that plant oils are healthier than animal fats.

3.4.4. Micronutrients

All studies except five [33,35,37,40,42] assessed knowledge of micronutrients (Table 3) and eight studies reported on micronutrient sub-section scores [14,15,17,23,36,38,47,51] (Table 2). Arazi and Hosseini [15] reported that the mean scores for the sections covering knowledge of "Vitamins" and "Calcium and Iron" were 61% and 56%, respectively. These scores were higher than the overall mean of 54%. These results were echoed in the study by Zawila et al. [41], where questions on iron were answered correctly by more than 70% of runners, and in the study by Hamilton et al. [14], where most swimmers answered questions on vitamin C (85%–100%) and iron deficiency (98%) correctly. In contrast, Rash et al. [36] reported that college athletes' scores on both vitamin C and vitamin E questions were below the overall mean scores. Information on responses to specific questions on the role, sources, and requirements of micronutrients was also included in some studies.

Role: Only 17% of college athletes surveyed by Weeden et al. [39] could identify the differences between fat and water soluble vitamins. Sixty-seven percent of college males [37] and 72% of college females [34] surveyed knew that vitamins do not provide extra energy, but 56% of a different sample of college athletes [36] and 56% of a sample of Nigerian college athletes [18] thought this statement was true. Just 19% of elite and 9% of non-elite athletes surveyed by Harrison et al. [47] selected "false" to the statement, "vitamin B-complex helps you to recover faster".

Sources: Ninety-six percent of recreational runners in the study by Barr [48] knew that bananas and avocados are good sources of potassium, 89% knew that bread is not a good source of calcium, and 56% knew "apples are a good source of vitamin C". On the contrary, many male college athletes in the study by Shoaf et al. [25] thought that milk was high in iron, and many triathletes in the study by Worme et al. [50] believed that iron was the main nutrient found in spinach.

Requirements: In the study by Zawila et al. [41], 60% of female athletes thought that calcium needs could be met by having just two glasses of milk. On the other hand, all female recreational marathon runners surveyed by Barr [48] knew that women need more iron than men and 69% of coaches surveyed by Corley et al. [53] correctly selected "false" for the statement "female athletes need more B vitamins than any other athlete".

3.4.5. Supplementation

Twenty-one studies included questions on supplementation [14,16,17,20,21,23–25,34,36–39,41,43–45, 47,51–53] (Table 3). Five studies reported on supplementation sub-section scores [14,20,23,38,45]; correct responses to this section were high in some studies, but low in others (Table 2). Many authors also provided information on how individual items pertaining to ergogenic aids, vitamins, and minerals, as well as protein supplementation, were answered.

Ergogenic aids: Shoaf et al. [25] found that supplement questions were answered correctly by 87% of male college athletes; items on creatine were answered correctly more than 70% of the time. Eighty-two percent of elite athletes surveyed by Hamilton et al. [14] knew that steroids are not safe, but only 26% were aware that caffeine can help extend performance.

Vitamins and Minerals: In the paper by Hamilton et al. [14] only 29% of elite athletes thought vitamin C supplements help fight colds. However, in other studies misconceptions were common: 72% of college coaches surveyed by Corley et al. [53] thought all vegetarian athletes required zinc supplementation; 50% of elite athletes surveyed by Hamilton et al. [14] believed multivitamins would increase energy levels and 45% though they were 'vital for topping up performance'. In relation, 76% of college athletes surveyed by Rash et al. [36] felt a general vitamin and mineral supplement was needed daily, 53% believed that they needed vitamin C supplements to boost immune function, and 56% believed that vitamin E supplementation was needed to protect red blood cells (RBC) from oxidative damage and to promote oxygen transport to RBC. In contrast, 89% of coaches in the study by Corley et al. [53] disagreed with the statement that vitamin pills could be taken in unlimited amounts and 72% knew that vitamin pills are not needed if a well-balanced diet is consumed.

Protein: Jessri et al. [20] reported that 43% of female and 47% male Iranian college athletes believed all athletes needed protein supplementation; and, while only 34% of elite athletes in the study by Hamilton [14] disagreed that "protein supplements build larger muscles and make you stronger", 79% of college coaches surveyed by Corley et al. [53] selected "false" for a similar statement. One-third of coaches surveyed by Zinn et al. [51] felt that protein powder was essential for weight loss.

3.4.6. Fluids

Twenty-three studies asked questions about fluids [14,16–21,23,24,36,37,39,41–45,47,48,51,53] (Table 3). Six studies reported on fluid (or hydration) sub-section scores [17,20,23,38,39,51]. In some studies, the scores (% total correct) in this section were above the overall mean; however, in others they were below the overall mean (Table 2). Several studies also reported on the frequency with which individual items related to the need for fluid, fluid timing, and fluid type were answered correctly.

Need for fluid: Weeden et al. [39] found that 92% of USA college respondents were able to identify the importance of water in body temperature regulation, and 97% knew the best sources of electrolytes. Rosenbloom et al. [37] found that 93% of college athletes agreed that dehydration decreases performance. Similarly, Corley et al. [53] found that 89% of coaches were aware that fluids are required to prepare for sweat losses.

Timing of fluid ingestion: Harrison et al. [47] reported that 79% of elite and 68% of non-elite athletes knew that you should drink during exercise lasting over one hour, and that 65% of elite 45% of non-elite athletes knew you should drink before exercise. Likewise, about 95% of college athletes in the study by Rosenbloom et al. [37] and 94% of college coaches in the study by Corley et al. [53] agreed ingestion of water was important before, during, and after exercise.

Type of fluid: Jessri et al. [20] stated that only 1.3% of female and 0.6% of male Iranian college athletes could identify the amount of carbohydrate a sports drink should contain. While Folasire et al. [18] reported that 59% of Nigerian university athletes knew that sports drinks were best to replace fluids, only 22% of American college athletes in the study by Rosenbloom et al. [37] agreed that they are better than water.

3.4.7. Pre-Competition Meal

Seventeen studies included questions on the pre-competition meal [14,16,18–21,23,25,35,37,43–45, 47,48,51,53] (Table 3). Only one author [45] reported on a pre-competition sub-score, indicating that scores in this section were above the overall mean scores (Table 2). Two studies [34,37] also reported on responses to individual items relevant to pre-competition nutrition. In the study by Collison et al. [34], 72% of athletes selected "false" for "carbohydrate loading will enhance performance in all events of 1 h or less", 95% agreed that "high carbohydrate meals require 2 to 3 h to be emptied from the stomach", and 66% agreed that "high-fat meals should not be eaten 2–3 h before competition". Conversely, Rosenbloom et al. [37] found that 63% of male and 71% of female college athletes thought sugar eaten before an event will adversely affect performance.

3.4.8. Nutrition during Competition

Only one paper included questions on nutrition during competition [48] (Table 3). There was no specific information on how these questions were answered.

3.4.9. Recovery Meal

Seven studies included questions on the recovery meal [16,20,24,44,45,48,51] (Table 3). No studies provided a summary of specific questions on recovery. However, both Danaher and Curley [45] and Zinn et al. [51] reported on recovery as a nutrition sub-section. Coaches performed poorly in the former study, but well in the latter (Table 2).

3.4.10. Alcohol

Only one paper assessed knowledge of alcohol [16] (Table 3). While 89% of elite Australian Rules Football players in this study were able to identify safe alcohol consumption guidelines, only 33% selected the correct alcoholic beverage when asked which was an example of a "standard drink", and just 38% correctly answered a question regarding grams of ethanol in a "standard drink" [16].

3.5. Quality Assessment of Included Articles/Risk of Bias

Quality analysis was performed for all studies that met inclusion criteria, and results of quality analysis did not alter decisions about inclusion. Only one of the studies received a positive ("Yes") rating [49]. All of the other included studies received a neutral rating indicating moderate study quality. Ratings were mostly affected by the lack of inclusion of a comparison group, and use of tools that had not undergone adequate validation. In many cases, participant characteristics were not well described.

3.6. Quality Assessment of Tools Used

The comprehensiveness scores ranged from one to 10 (Table 3). None of the studies used a questionnaire that covered all 11 nutrition sub-sections that were deemed relevant. Three studies received scores of less than or equal to two; however two of these [35,42] only aimed to test a single nutrition sub-section of nutrition knowledge—carbohydrates and hydration respectively. The third [15] received the very low score because it was unclear what was and was not tested. Thirteen studies [14,16,20,21,23,24,39,41,44,45,47,51,52] covered eight or more (that is, more than 75%) of the relevant nutrition sub-sections.

The validation scores ranged from zero to six out of six (Table 4). Four studies made no mention of validation [21,35,37,44], scoring zero. Two authors [16,41] used a combination of two previously validated questionnaires but did not perform any assessment of the composite tool, also scoring zero. Eight studies used questionnaires that underwent just one type of psychometric analysis [23,36, 41,42,47,48,50,53]. Two authors [36,52] used the questionnaire by Zawila et al. [41] with minor modification, assessing the tool for face and content validity, scoring two. Three studies [13,15,49] used questionnaires that had undergone five out of the six possible validation procedures. Just one study [22] scored 6, the maximum amount of available points. All of the studies that scored five to six for the validation score utilized the "general nutrition knowledge questionnaire" [55].

Table 3. Comprehensiveness rating (score either 0 or 1 for each category).

Author	Items	General	CHO	Protein	Fat	Micro	Pre	During	Recovery	Fluid	Supplement&TOH		Score
Abood et al. [32]	42	1	1	1	1	1	0	0	0	0	0	0	5
Alaunyte et al. [12]	28	1	1	1	1	1	0	0	0	0	0	0	4
Arazi and Hosseini [15]	40	1	1	1	1	1	U	U	U	U	U	U	4
Azizi et al. [46]	15	1	U	U	U	1	U	U	U	U	U	U	1
Barbaros-Tudor et al. [43]	87	1	1	1	1	1	1	1	0	1	1	0	7
Barr [48]	40	0	1	U	U	1	1	1	0	1	0	0	6
Botsis and Holden [44]	88	1	1	1	1	1	1	0	1	1	1	0	9
Collison et al. [34]	35	1	1	1	1	1	0	0	0	1	1	0	7
Condon et al. [35]	7	0	1	0	0	0	1	0	0	0	0	0	2
Corley et al. [53]	15	0	1	1	1	1	1	0	0	1	1	0	7
Danaher and Curley, 2014 [45]	88	1	1	1	1	1	1	0	1	1	1	0	9
Davar [17]	61	1	1	1	1	1	0	0	0	1	1	0	7
Devlin and Belski [16]	123	1	1	1	1	1	1	0	1	1	1	1	10
Dunn et al. [13]	124	1	1	1	1	1	0	0	0	1	0	0	5
Folasire et al. [18]	14	1	1	0	0	1	1	0	0	1	0	1	6
Grete R et al. [19]	20	1	U	1	1	1	1	0	0	1	0	0	7
Hamilton et al. [14]	48	1	1	1	1	1	1	0	0	1	1	0	8
Harrison et al. [47]	18	1	1	1	1	1	1	0	0	1	1	0	8
Hoogenboom et al. [52]	76	1	1	1	1	1	U	0	1	1	1	1	8
Jessri et al. [20]	88	1	1	1	1	1	1	U	1	1	1	1	9
Kunkel et al. [33]	31	1	1	1	U	U	U	U	U	U	U	U	3
Nichols et al. [42]	17	0	0	0	0	0	0	0	0	0	0	0	1
Rash et al. [36]	76	1	1	1	1	1	U	U	U	1	1	0	7
Raymond-Barker et al. [49]	110	0	1	1	1	1	0	0	0	0	0	0	5
Rosenbloom et al. [37]	11	0	1	1	1	0	1	0	0	1	1	0	6
Sedek and Yih [21]	29	1	1	1	1	1	1	0	0	1	1	1	9
Shifflett et al. [24]	20	1	1	1	1	1	0	0	1	1	0	0	8
Shoaf et al. [25]	25	1	1	1	1	1	1	0	0	0	1	0	7
Smith-Rockwell et al. [38]		1	1	1	1	1	0	0	0	1	1	0	7
Spendlove et al. [22]	113/90	1	1	1	1	1	0	0	0	0	0	0	5
Torres-McGehee et al. [23]	20	1	1	1	1	1	1	0	0	1	0	0	8
Weeden et al. [39]	24	1	1	1	1	1	0	0	0	0	1	1	8
Werblow et al. [40]	31	1	1	1	0	0	0	0	0	0	1	0	3
Worme et al. [50]	20	1	0	0	1	1	U	U	U	1	0	0	5
Zawila et al. [41]	76	1	1	1	1	1	U	U	U	1	1	1	8
Zinn et al. [51]	88	1	1	1	1	1	1	0	U	1	1	0	9

1 = adequate coverage of nutrition sub-section; 0 = inadequate coverage of nutrition sub-section; U = unclear (scored as 0). Decisions on whether a questionnaire included adequate coverage on each topic were made based on a combination of review of the actual tool (when available) and the description of the measure provided in the article.

Table 4. Validity and reliability rating score (either 0 or 1 for each category).

Author	Pre-Tested/Piloted	Face Validity	Content Validity	Item Discrimination	Internal Reliability	Construct Validity (Known Group Comparisons)	External Reliability	Total Score
Abood et al. [32]	Y; n = 6	0	1	0	0	0	1 (r = 0.86)	2
Alaunyte et al. [12]	N	1	1	1*	P (r = 0.7–0.97)	1*	1*	5
Arazi and Hosseini [15]	N	1	1	0	0	0	0	2 +
Azizi et al. [46]	Y; n = 30	0	1	0	1 (α = 0.85)	0	0	2
Barbaros-Tudor et al. [43]	Y; n = 34 for construct; n = 10 for face	1	1	0	1 (r =0.82)	1 (dietitians > undergrads)	0	4
Barr, [48]	N	0	1	0	0	0	0	1
Botsis and Holden [44]	N	0	1	0	0	1 (dietitians > other groups)	1 (r = 0.74–0.93)	2
Collison et al. [34]	Y; n = 19	0	1	0	0	0	1	2
Condon et al. [35]	N	0	0	0	0	0	0	0
Corley et al. [53]	Y; n = 22	U	0	0	1(α = 0.56)	0	0	1
Danaher and Curley [45]	Y; n = NR	1	1	0	0	1 (dietitians > other groups)	1 (r = 0.74–0.93)	4
Davar [17]	Y; n = 5	1	1	0	0	0	0	2 +
Devlin and Belski [16]	N	0	0	0	0	0	0	0
Dunn et al. [13]	N	1	1	1	P (r = 0.7–0.97)	1 (nutrition > business)	1 (r = 0.7)	5
Folasire et al. [18]	Y	U	1	0	1 (α = 0.75)	0	0	2
Grete R et al. [19]	Y; n = NR	1	1	0	0	0	0	2 +
Hamilton et al. [14]	Y; n = NR	1	1	0	0	0	0	
Harrison et al. [47]	Y; n =10	1	0	0	0	0	0	1
Hoogenboom et al. [52]	N	0	0	0	0	0	0	0
Jessri et al. [20]	N	1	1	0	0	0	0	2 +
Kunkel et al. [33]	N	1	1	0	P (r = 0.82)	1	0	3
Nichols et al. [42]	N	0	1	0	0	0	0	1
Rash et al. [36]	Y; n = 20	0	0	0	1 (α = 0.94–0.96)	0	0	1
Raymond-Barker et al. [49]	Y; n = 47	1	1	0	0	0	0	2 +
Rosenbloom et al. [37]	Y; n = 6	1	1	1	P (r = 0.7–0.97)	P (nutrition > business)	1 (r = 0.7)	5
Sedek and Yih [21]	N	0	0	0	0	0	0	0
Shifflett et al. [24]	N	0	0	0	P (α = 0.645)	0	0	0
Shoaf et al. [25]	Y; n = 123	0	1	1	1 (not stated)	0	0	3
Smith-Rockwell et al. [38]	Y; n = 56	0	1	0	1 (α = 0.72)	0	1 (r = 0.82)	3

242

Table 4. *Cont.*

Author	Pre-Tested/Piloted	Face Validity	Content Validity	Item Discrimination	Internal Reliability	Construct Validity (Known Group Comparisons)	External Reliability	Total Score
Spendlove et al. [22]	Y; n = 53	1	1	1*	1 (α = 0.34–0.93 for GNKQ and 0.4–0.95 for R-GNKQ)	1 (nutrition > business)	1 (r = 0.37–0.92 in GNKQ)	6
Torres-McGehee et al. [23]	Y; n = 12	0	1	0	0	0	0	2
Weeden et al. [39]	Y; n = 21	1	1	0	0	0	0	2 +
Werblow et al. [40]	Y; n = 14	1	1	0	0	0	0	2 +
Worme et al. [50]	Y; n = NR	0	1	0	0	0	0	1
Zawila et al. [41]	N	0	0	1	0	0	0	1
Zinn et al. [51]	N	0	0	0	0	0	0	0
Abood et al. [32]	Y; n = 100	0	1	0	0	1*	1* (r = 0.74–0.93)	3

Y = yes; N = no; n = number of participants; NR = 0 = psychometric validation not performed; 1 = psychometric validation performed; U = unclear; P = partial (internal consistency performed on original sample but not repeated), scored as 0; + = score of two, with both types of validation being qualitative (face and content validity but no quantitative statistical test performed); * = performed in original validation study but not-repeated in present study sample; r = Pearson's or Spearman's correlation coefficient as reported in paper (range represents scores across different nutrition sub-sections); α = Cronbach alpha value as reported in paper; NR = not reported.

4. Discussion

4.1. Study Selection and Study Characteristics

The aim of this review was to summarize current levels of knowledge in athletes (aged 17 years and older) and coaches, and to provide a detailed assessment of the quality of the tools used to assess nutrition knowledge. Our search yielded 36 studies that met the inclusion criteria; 10 [15–19,21,22,32,39,56] of the studies on athletes were published after 2010, when a previous complementary review on athletes was conducted [7]; there were also an additional seven [35,42–45,51,53] relevant studies that had been not included in the aforementioned review due to differing inclusion criteria. Males and females tended to be equally represented. The majority of research has been conducted with American college athletes [13,19,23,24,32–37,40–42,52], presumably because they are easy to recruit. Our search did not retrieve a single paper on the knowledge of elite athletes in North America; this is surprising considering the scope of elite athlete leagues in this region. Likewise, while a broad range of sports are covered across the literature, there was only one study in netball players [47], and athletes from many other popular Commonwealth sports, such as cricket, were underrepresented. There is a need for research that is representative of various types of athletes. A better understanding of specific athletes who may have poor knowledge will allow professionals working with these populations to advocate for increased education and support.

4.2. Quality Assessment of Included Articles and Quality Assessment of Tools Used

Akin to previous complimentary reviews [7,56], a key finding of this review was that there were issues with quality of the included studies, and the questionnaires used to assess nutrition knowledge were inadequately validated. Despite recommendations made in a 2011 review by Heaney et al. [7] that studies assessing nutrition knowledge should collect and report demographic data, include comparison groups, and use validated tools, the quality ratings of newer studies (i.e., those published since 2010) do not appear to be higher than the ratings of older studies. In relation, even though the validity of tools used to assess nutrition knowledge have been questioned in previous reviews [7,56], no new tool has been developed and validated. This is likely because the time and resources required for tool development can be prohibitive [27]. Most studies that did receive a high validation score (for the measurement instrument) used the "general nutrition knowledge questionnaire" [55], and since this does not assess sports nutrition knowledge, these studies received low scores on the comprehensiveness rating. There were a number of issues related to the content included in the tools. Only one of the questionnaires asked questions on alcohol, which is an important topic given the drinking culture among sports people [57,58]. There are also several important considerations in regards to the relevance/accuracy of some of the items. All of the questions on carbohydrate recommendations state requirements as percent total macronutrient contribution, however more recent consensus statements provide recommendations in grams per kilogram of body weight per day [2]. Furthermore, experts may no longer agree with the "correct" answers to some questions, for instance, Collison et al. [34] indicated that tea, cola, and coffee were NOT the best pre-athletic event beverages but it could be argued that these may be beneficial due to their caffeine content, which is a known ergogenic aid for some athletes [59]. Several other examples of outdated questions exist. Many of these are in relation to hydration, specifically with regards to thirst as an indicator for fluid needs [60]. It is axiomatic that the strong consensus regarding dietary strategies for optimal athletic performance should be reflected in questionnaires designed to assess nutrition knowledge [7]. Researchers developing tools to assess the nutritional knowledge of sports people should ensure they address the aforementioned limitations.

Another important factor to consider is whether tools are validated for the population they are being used with [7,61]. The questionnaire developed by Zinn, et al. [54] was used in two other studies in coaches [20,44], with just a 1.5% difference in scores between them [54,55], indicating it may have good validity in this cohort. On the other hand, the range of scores on the "general nutrition knowledge questionnaire" [12,13,16,22,49] was quite large (51.5%–74.2%), even when comparing across similar athletic levels (e.g., scores across studies in elite athletes using this tool ranged from 60.5% to 72.8%). This tool was developed for a British audience and has been modified for several other population groups including the Australian population. Interestingly, the highest scores on the "general nutrition knowledge" tool were achieved in British cohorts of elite and recreational athletes [12,49], middle scores in an Australian sample of elite athletes [22] and the lowest scores in a sample of college athletes in the USA [13]. While it is certainly possible that this variation was due to factors such as athletic level or age [7,22] it is worth considering that this tool was not culturally appropriate for North American athletes.

4.3. Nutrition Knowledge Results

Given that all studies received a neutral quality rating and that many of the measurement tools used were inadequately validated, it is difficult to definitively comment on the both the current status of nutrition knowledge of athletes and coaches, and the factors that may influence nutrition knowledge. One consistent finding was that education impacts nutrition knowledge; it is therefore important that questionnaires cater to various literacy levels (e.g., by including pictures) so that scores are reflective of actual nutrition knowledge, rather than literacy in general. It appears nutritional knowledge may also be affected by athletic level, and that coaches' knowledge is better than athletes'. Theoretically, it is plausible that elite athletes have greater access to resources and therefore higher levels of knowledge; likewise, it is likely that American college athletes have more support and funding than non-USA college athletes. In contrast to previous findings [7], our review did not suggest that gender or the type of sport played affects nutrition knowledge. Likewise, findings comparing athletes to non-athlete comprising groups were inconsistent. More quality research is needed to ascertain whether these associations are confounded by demographic factors, study quality, and questionnaire quality.

4.4. Responses to Specific Nutrition Sub-Sections

Scores reported as a percentage are fairly arbitrary unless they are being used to compare different groups within the same study, or changes to the same group over time. While several authors have suggested various "cutoff" points that signify adequate levels of knowledge (e.g., Torres-McGehee et al. [23] stated that >75% was indicative of adequate knowledge), these values add little meaning. It cannot be assumed that a questionnaire with 11 items covering a few relevant nutrition sub-sections is equivalent to a 76-item questionnaire that addresses multiple topics of general and sports nutrition knowledge. Therefore, we synthesized responses to nutrition sub-sections and individual questions. It is clear that there is considerable discrepancy between studies. In many cases, participants scored poorly in a section in one study, and well in the same section in another study. The lack of consistency makes drawing conclusions about gaps in knowledge difficult. Overall, however, it appears that understanding of the following topics was poor: energy density, the need for vitamin and mineral supplementation amongst athletes, the role of protein in muscle synthesis, sources of fat, and the need for protein supplementation among athletes trying to lose weight and athletes who follow a vegetarian diet. Awareness of areas of knowledge that require improvement is an important consideration when designing interventions (one-on-one) and education programs aimed at improving nutrition knowledge of athletes. Specific gaps in knowledge cannot be ascertained from nutrition knowledge results that are reported as percentage total correct responses. Researchers should consider the ways in which knowledge results are reported. It should be clear what topics (nutrition sub-sections) of knowledge were tested and whether the tool used was able to identify particular nutrition concepts that were not well understood.

5. Limitations

A major limitation of this review is that meta-analysis of scores across studies was not possible. This was due to the relatively small amount of included studies, the under-representation of various sporting disciplines and levels, the lack of representativeness within studies, the heterogeneity of participants across studies, and the heterogeneity of the measures used to assess nutrition knowledge.

There are also limitations related to how the tools have been rated (Table 4). It was often unclear how information collected during "pre-testing" was actually used to modify the questionnaire being piloted. Firstly, judgements were hindered by the vague description provided of the type and extent of validation that has been performed. For example, Sedek and Yih [21] stated that they used a questionnaire that has been validated by Paugh [62]. In fact, this was an unpublished thesis that only assessed Cronbach's alpha (α = 0.56). Secondly, validation scores were based on the steps outlined by Parmenter and Wardle [27], but their protocol does not describe factor analysis or Rasch analysis. Factor analysis assesses a scale's dimensionality, and therefore can be used to decide whether Cronbach's alpha is appropriate [30,63]. Rasch analysis is an Item Response Theory (IRT) technique, which allows for shorter scales, with multiple response formats to be developed [64]. Finally, although a point was awarded if a topic was deemed to be covered in adequate detail (Table 4), there was still a large variety in the depth and detail in which nutrition sub-sections were covered. For instance, while the questionnaires used by Collison et al. [34] and Zinn et al. [54] both covered supplements, the former only included two questions on the use of diuretics and multivitamins and the latter tested knowledge of creatine, hydroxy-beta-methlybutyrate (HBM), micronutrient supplementation, and appetite suppressants. The quality of individual items was not taken into account when designing the comprehensiveness score. The issues with individual items are beyond the scope of this review. They include, but are not limited to, ambiguous wording and reference to outdated recommendations as described in Section 4.2.

6. Conclusions

The quality and heterogeneous nature of the included studies and of current measures used to assess nutrition knowledge make assessment of general and sports nutrition knowledge in athletes and coaches difficult to ascertain. Specific gaps in knowledge also remain largely unclear, although analysis of individual items indicates that it is likely that energy density, supplementation, and the role of protein are commonly misunderstood topics. It is possible that there is a relationship between gender, athletic level (e.g., elite) and nutrition knowledge; however, more high-quality research is needed to confirm these assertions.

Nutrition knowledge is a modifiable determinant of dietary behavior, and therefore has the potential to have a significant impact on athletic performance. Accordingly, there is a need for additional high-quality research on this topic. However, the low quality of current measures of nutrition knowledge means that none of the currently available tools can confidently be endorsed for use in future studies. It is therefore the recommendation of the authors that a new, universal, up-to-date, validated measure of general and sports nutrition knowledge be developed. Such a tool should consider health literacy, cultural appropriation, and current consensus recommendations regarding nutrition for optimal athletic performance, and should undergo rigorous validation that includes techniques from within an item response theory framework. Moreover, the questionnaire should have the capacity to report a knowledge "profile", outlining gaps in knowledge and areas where knowledge is well understood. A quality tool would allow more robust assessment of knowledge of both athletes and coaches, having utility in clinical practice, the development and evaluation of education programs, and research in the field. Over time this new tool would allow more robust comparisons across various groups to be made.

Acknowledgments: Gina Trakman is currently undertaking her PhD studies and receives a La Trobe University scholarship. Open access fee was funded by author's research funds.

Author Contributions: All authors contributed to writing and revising the paper for intellectual content. Gina Louise Trakman (G.L.T.) and Adrienne Forsyth (A.F.) developed the search strategy, determined inclusion and exclusion criteria, screened articles for inclusion, and completed a quality analysis checklist. G.L.T. performed the search and extracted data. Brooke Lea Devlin (B.L.D.) completed quality analysis to resolve any disagreements between G.L.T. and A.F.

Conflicts of Interest: The authors declare no conflict of interest.

References

1. Rodriguez, N.R.; DiMarco, N.M.; Langley, S. Nutrition and athletic performance. *Med. Sci. Sports Exerc.* **2009**, *41*, 709–731. [PubMed]
2. Potgieter, S. Sport nutrition: A review of the latest guidelines for exercise and sport nutrition from the American College of Sport Nutrition, the International Olympic Committee and the International Society for Sports Nutrition. *S. Afr. J. Clin. Nutr.* **2013**, *26*, 6–16. [CrossRef]
3. Broad, E.M.; Cox, G.R. What is the optimal composition of an athlete's diet? *Eur. J. Sport Sci.* **2008**, *8*, 57–65. [CrossRef]
4. Jonnalagadda, S.S.; Ziegler, P.J.; Nelson, J.A. Food preferences, dieting behaviors, and body image perceptions of elite figure skaters. *Int. J. Sport Nutr. Exerc. Metab.* **2004**, *14*, 594–606. [CrossRef] [PubMed]
5. Sawka, M.N.; Burke, L.M.; Eichner, E.R.; Maughan, R.J.; Montain, S.J.; Stachenfeld, N.S. American College of Sports Medicine position stand. Exercise and fluid replacement. *Med. Sci. Sports Exerc.* **2007**, *39*, 377–390. [PubMed]
6. Spronk, I.; Kullen, C.; Burdon, C.; O'Connor, H. Relationship between nutrition knowledge and dietary intake. *Br. J. Nutr.* **2014**, *111*, 1713–1726. [CrossRef] [PubMed]
7. Heaney, S.; O'Connor, H.; Michael, S.; Gifford, J.; Naughton, G. Nutrition knowledge in athletes: A systematic review. *Int. J. Sport Nutr. Exerc. Metab.* **2011**, *21*, 248–261. [CrossRef] [PubMed]
8. Heaney, S.; O'Connor, H.; Naughton, G.; Gifford, J. Towards an understanding of the barriers to good nutrition for elite athletes. *Int. J. Sports Sci. Coach.* **2008**, *3*, 391–401. [CrossRef]
9. Ono, M.; Kennedy, E.; Reeves, S.; Cronin, L. Nutrition and culture in professional football. A mixed method approach. *Appetite* **2012**, *58*, 98–104. [CrossRef] [PubMed]
10. Birkenhead, K.L.; Slater, G. A review of factors influencing athletes' food choices. *Sports Med.* **2015**, *45*, 1511–1522. [CrossRef] [PubMed]
11. Clark, K.S. Sports nutrition counseling: Documentation of performance. *Top. Clin. Nutr.* **1999**, *14*, 34–40. [CrossRef]
12. Alaunyte, I.; Perry, J.L.; Aubrey, T. Nutritional knowledge and eating habits of professional rugby league players: Does knowledge translate into practice? *J. Int. Soc. Sports Nutr.* **2015**, *12*, 18. [CrossRef] [PubMed]
13. Dunn, D.; Turner, L.W.; Denny, G. Nutrition knowledge and attitudes of college athletes. *Sport J.* **2007**, *10*, 45.
14. Hamilton, G.; Thomson, C.; Hopkins, W. Nutrition knowledge of elite distance runners. *N. Z. J. Sports Med.* **1994**, *22*, 26–26.
15. Arazi, H.; Hosseini, R. A comparison of nutritional knowledge and food habits of collegiate and non-collegiate athletes. *SportLogia* **2012**, *8*, 100–107. [CrossRef]
16. Devlin, B.L.; Belski, R. Exploring general and sports nutrition and food knowledge in elite male Australian athletes. *Int. J. Sport Nutr. Exerc. Metab.* **2015**, *25*, 225–232. [CrossRef] [PubMed]
17. Davai, V. Nutritional knowledge and attitudes towards healthy eating of college-going women hockey players. *J. Hum. Ecol.* **2012**, *37*, 119–124.
18. Folasire, O.F.; Akomolafe, A.A.; Sanusi, R.A. Does nutrition knowledge and practice of athletes translate to enhanced athletic performance? Cross-sectional study amongst nigerian undergraduate athletes. *Glob. J. Health Sci.* **2015**, *7*, 215–225. [CrossRef] [PubMed]
19. Grete, R.H.; Carol, A.F.; Jane, E.E.; Kimberli, P. Nutrition knowledge, practices, attitudes, and information sources of mid-American conference college softball players. *Food Nutr. Sci.* **2011**, *2*, 109–117.
20. Jessri, M.; Jessri, M.; RashidKhani, B.; Zinn, C. Evaluation of Iranian college athletes' sport nutrition knowledge. *Int. J. Sport Nutr. Exerc. Metab.* **2010**, *20*, 257–263. [CrossRef] [PubMed]
21. Sedek, R.; Yih, T.Y. Dietary habits and nutrition knowledge among athletes and non-athletes in National University of Malaysia (UKM). *Pak. J. Nutr.* **2014**, *13*, 752–759. [CrossRef]

22. Spendlove, J.K.; Heaney, S.E.; Gifford, J.A.; Prvan, T.; Denyer, G.S.; O'Connor, H.T. Evaluation of general nutrition knowledge in elite Australian athletes. *Br. J. Nutr.* **2012**, *107*, 1871–1880. [CrossRef] [PubMed]
23. Torres-McGehee, T.M.; Pritchett, K.L.; Zippel, D.; Minton, D.M.; Cellamare, A.; Sibilia, M. Sports nutrition knowledge among collegiate athletes, coaches, athletic trainers, and strength and conditioning specialists. *J. Athl. Train.* **2012**, *47*, 205–211. [PubMed]
24. Shifflett, B.; Timm, C.; Kahanov, L. Understanding of athletes' nutritional needs among athletes, coaches, and athletic trainers. *Res. Q. Exerc. Sport* **2002**, *73*, 357–362. [CrossRef] [PubMed]
25. Shoaf, L.R.; McClellan, P.D.; Birskovich, K.A. Nutrition knowledge, interests, and information sources of male athletes. *J. Nutr. Educ.* **1986**, *18*, 243–245. [CrossRef]
26. International Prospective Register of Systematic Reviews. Available online: http://www.crd.york.ac.uk/PROSPERO/ (accessed on 18 March 2016).
27. Parmenter, K.; Wardle, J. Evaluation and design of nutrition knowledge measures. *J. Nutr. Educ.* **2000**, *32*, 269–277. [CrossRef]
28. Kline, P. *Handbook of Psychological Testing*; Routledge: Abingdon, UK, 2013.
29. Nunnally, J. *Psychometric Methods*; McGraw-Hill: New York, NY, USA, 1978.
30. Streiner, D.L. Starting at the beginning: An introduction to coefficient alpha and internal consistency. *J. Personal. Assess.* **2003**, *80*, 99–103. [CrossRef] [PubMed]
31. American Dietetic Association. Evidence Analysis Manual: Steps in the Ada Evidence Analysis. Available online: https://www.adaevidencelibrary.com/vault/editor/File/Evidence_Analysis_Manual_January_2008.pdf (accessed on 14 September 2016).
32. Abood, D.A.; Black, D.R.; Birnbaum, R.D. Nutrition education intervention for college female athletes. *J. Nutr. Educ. Behav.* **2004**, *36*, 135–137. [CrossRef]
33. Kunkel, M.E.; Bell, L.B.; Luccia, B.H.D. Peer nutrition education program to improve nutrition knowledge of female collegiate athletes. *J. Nutr. Educ.* **2001**, *33*, 114–115. [CrossRef]
34. Collison, S.B.; Kuczmarski, M.F.; Vickery, C.E. Impact of nutrition education on female athletes. *Am. J. Health Behav.* **1996**, *20*, 14–23.
35. Condon, E.M.; Dube, K.A.; Herbold, N.H. The influence of the low-carbohydrate trend on collegiate athletes' knowledge, attitudes, and dietary intake of carbohydrates. *Top. Clin. Nutr.* **2007**, *22*, 175–184. [CrossRef]
36. Rash, C.L.; Malinauskas, B.M.; Duffrin, M.W.; Barber-Heidal, K.; Overton, R.F. Nutrition-related knowledge, attitude, and dietary intake of college track athletes. *Sport J.* **2008**, *11*, 1–8.
37. Rosenbloom, C.A.; Jonnalagadda, S.S.; Skinner, R. Nutrition knowledge of collegiate athletes in a Division I National Collegiate Athletic Association institution. *J. Am. Diet. Assoc.* **2002**, *102*, 418–420. [CrossRef]
38. Smith-Rockwell, M.; Nickols-Richardson, S.M.; Thye, F.W. Nutrition knowledge, opinions, and practices of coaches and athletic trainers at a division 1 university. *Int. J. Sport Nutr. Exerc. Metab.* **2001**, *11*, 174–185. [CrossRef] [PubMed]
39. Weeden, A.; Olsen, J.; Batacan, J.; Peterson, T. Differences in collegiate athlete nutrition knowledge as determined by athlete characteristics. *Sport J.* **2014**, *17*, 1–13.
40. Werblow, J.A.; Fox, H.M.; Henneman, A. Nutritional knowledge, attitudes, and food patterns of women athletes. *J. Am. Diet. Assoc.* **1978**, *73*, 242–245. [PubMed]
41. Zawila, L.G.; Steib, C.M.; Hoogenboom, B. The female collegiate cross-country runner: Nutritional knowledge and attitudes. *J. Athl. Train.* **2003**, *38*, 67–74. [PubMed]
42. Nichols, P.E.; Jonnalagadda, S.S.; Rosenbloom, C.A.; Trinkaus, M. Knowledge, attitudes, and behaviors regarding hydration and fluid replacement of collegiate athletes. *Int. J. Sport Nutr. Exerc. Metab.* **2005**, *15*, 515. [CrossRef] [PubMed]
43. Barbaros-Tudor, P.; Radman, I.; Jankovic, G. Nutritional knowledge and dietary habits of croatian tennis coaches. In Proceedings of the 6th International Scientific Conference on Kinesiology: Integrative Power of Kinesiology, Zagreb, Croatia, 8–11 September 2011; pp. 102–105.
44. Botsis, A.E.; Holden, S.L. Nutritional knowledge of college coaches. *Sport Sci. Rev.* **2015**, *24*, 193–200. [CrossRef]
45. Danaher, K.; Curley, T. Nutrition knowledge and practices of varsity coaches at a Canadian university. *Can. J. Diet. Pract. Res.* **2014**, *75*, 210–213. [CrossRef] [PubMed]
46. Azizi, M.; Rahmani-Nia, F.; Malaee, M.; Malaee, M.; Khosravi, N. A study of nutritional knowledge and attitudes of elite college athletes in Iran. *Braz. J. Biomot.* **2010**, *4*, 105–112.

47. Harrison, J.; Hopkins, W.; MacFarlane, D.; Worsley, A. Nutrition knowledge and dietary habits of elite and non-elite athletes. *Aust. J. Nutr. Diet.* **1991**, *48*, 124–127.
48. Barr, S. Nutrition knowledge of female varsity athletes and university students. *J. Am. Diet. Assoc.* **1987**, *87*, 1660–1664. [PubMed]
49. Raymond-Barker, P.; Petroczi, A.; Quested, E. Assessment of nutritional knowledge in female athletes susceptible to the Female Athlete Triad syndrome. *J. Occup. Med. Toxicol.* **2007**, *2*, 10. [CrossRef] [PubMed]
50. Worme, J.D.; Doubt, T.J.; Singh, A.; Ryan, C.J.; Moses, F.M.; Deuster, P.A. Dietary patterns, gastrointestinal complaints, and nutrition knowledge of recreational triathletes. *Am. J. Clin. Nutr.* **1990**, *51*, 690–697. [PubMed]
51. Zinn, C.; Schofield, G.; Wall, C. Evaluation of sports nutrition knowledge of New Zealand premier club rugby coaches. *Int. J. Sport Nutr. Exerc. Metab.* **2006**, *16*, 214–225. [CrossRef] [PubMed]
52. Hoogenboom, B.J.; Morris, J.; Morris, C.; Schaefer, K. Nutritional knowledge and eating behaviors of female, collegiate swimmers. *N. Am. J. Sports Phys. Ther.* **2009**, *4*, 139–148. [PubMed]
53. Corley, G.; Demarest-Litchford, M.; Bazzarre, T.L. Nutrition knowledge and dietary practices of college coaches. *J. Am. Diet. Assoc.* **1990**, *90*, 705–709. [PubMed]
54. Zinn, C.; Schofield, G.; Wall, C. Development of a psychometrically valid and reliable sports nutrition knowledge questionnaire. *J. Sci. Med. Sport* **2005**, *8*, 346–351. [CrossRef]
55. Parmenter, K.; Wardle, J. Development of a general nutrition knowledge questionnaire for adults. *Eur. J. Clin. Nutr.* **1999**, *53*, 298–308. [CrossRef] [PubMed]
56. Spronk, I.; Heaney, S.E.; Prvan, T.; O'Connor, H.T. Relationship between general nutrition knowledge and dietary quality in elite athletes. *Int. J. Sport Nutr. Exerc. Metab.* **2015**, *25*, 243–251. [CrossRef] [PubMed]
57. O'Brien, K.S.; Kypri, K. Alcohol industry sponsorship and hazardous drinking among sportspeople. *Addiction* **2008**, *103*, 1961–1966. [CrossRef] [PubMed]
58. Martens, M.P.; Dams-O'Connor, K.; Beck, N.C. A systematic review of college student-athlete drinking: Prevalence rates, sport-related factors, and interventions. *J. Subst. Abuse Treat.* **2006**, *31*, 305–316. [CrossRef] [PubMed]
59. Maughan, R.; Greenhaff, P.; Hespel, P. Dietary supplements for athletes: Emerging trends and recurring themes. *J. Sports Sci.* **2011**, *29*, S57–S66. [CrossRef] [PubMed]
60. Goulet, E.D. Effect of exercise-induced dehydration on time-trial exercise performance: A meta-analysis. *Br. J. Sports Med.* **2011**, *45*, 1149–1156. [CrossRef] [PubMed]
61. Beaton, D.E.; Bombardier, C.; Guillemin, F.; Ferraz, M.B. Guidelines for the process of cross-cultural adaptation of self-report measures. *Spine* **2000**, *25*, 3186–3191. [CrossRef] [PubMed]
62. Paugh, S.L. Dietary Habits And Nutritional Knowledge of College Athletes. Available online: http://libweb.calu.edu/thesis/umi-cup-1011.pdf (accessed on 14 September 2016).
63. Thompson, B. *Exploratory and Confirmatory Factor Analysis: Understanding Concepts and Applications*; American Psychological Association: Columbia, MO, USA, 2004.
64. Tennant, A.; Conaghan, P.G. The Rasch measurement model in rheumatology: What is it and why use it? When should it be applied, and what should one look for in a Rasch paper? *Arthritis Care Res.* **2007**, *57*, 1358–1362. [CrossRef] [PubMed]

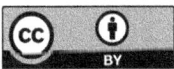

nutrients

MDPI

Article

Carbohydrate Mouth Rinsing Enhances High Intensity Time Trial Performance Following Prolonged Cycling

Nicholas D. Luden *, Michael J. Saunders, Andrew C. D'Lugos, Mark W. Pataky, Daniel A. Baur, Caitlin B. Vining and Adam B. Schroer

Human Performance Lab, Department of Kinesiology, James Madison University, Harrisonburg, VA 22807, USA; saundemj@jmu.edu (M.J.S.); dlugosac@jmu.edu (A.C.D.); patakymw@jmu.edu (M.W.P.); dab13b@my.fsu.edu (D.A.B.); viningcb@gmail.com (C.B.V.); abschroer@mix.wvu.edu (A.B.S.)
* Correspondence: ludennd@jmu.edu; Tel.: +1-540-568-4069

Received: 1 September 2016; Accepted: 14 September 2016; Published: 20 September 2016

Abstract: There is good evidence that mouth rinsing with carbohydrate (CHO) solutions can enhance endurance performance ($\geq$30 min). The impact of a CHO mouth rinse on sprint performance has been less consistent, suggesting that CHO may confer benefits in conditions of 'metabolic strain'. To test this hypothesis, the current study examined the impact of late-exercise mouth rinsing on sprint performance. Secondly, we investigated the effects of a protein mouth rinse (PRO) on performance. Eight trained male cyclists participated in three trials consisting of 120 min of constant-load cycling (55% W_{max}) followed by a 30 km computer-simulated time trial, during which only water was provided. Following 15 min of muscle function assessment, 10 min of constant-load cycling (3 min at 35% W_{max}, 7 min at 55% W_{max}) was performed. This was immediately followed by a 2 km time trial. Subjects rinsed with 25 mL of CHO, PRO, or placebo (PLA) at min 5:00 and 14:30 of the 15 min muscle function phase, and min 8:00 of the 10-min constant-load cycling. Magnitude-based inferential statistics were used to analyze the effects of the mouth rinse on 2-km time trial performance and the following physiological parameters: Maximum Voluntary Contract (MVC), Rating of Perceived Exertion (RPE), Heart Rate (HR), and blood glucose levels. The primary finding was that CHO 'likely' enhanced performance vs. PLA (3.8%), whereas differences between PRO and PLA were unclear (0.4%). These data demonstrate that late-race performance is enhanced by a CHO rinse, but not PRO, under challenging metabolic conditions. More data should be acquired before this strategy is recommended for the later stages of cycling competition under more practical conditions, such as when carbohydrates are supplemented throughout the preceding minutes/hours of exercise.

Keywords: cycling; endurance performance; maltodextrin; mouth wash; oralpharyngeal receptor; whey protein

1. Introduction

Carbohydrate (CHO) ingestion during exercise has been widely reported to enhance exercise performance, particularly during prolonged exercise when endogenous carbohydrates are limited. A large share of the CHO-induced performance gains during prolonged exercise are thought to be due to elevated carbohydrate oxidation rates late in exercise [1–4] and/or muscle/liver glycogen sparing [3,5,6]. Additionally, there is some evidence that CHO ingestion can also better shorter-duration (<1 h or intensity >75% VO_{2max}) exercise performance [4,7–9]; this is despite the lack of a clear metabolic advantage during these shorter exercise trials. An explanation for how CHO supplementation can improve high-intensity performance was provided by Carter and colleagues whereby CHO mouth rinsing (MR) (without swallowing) enhanced a time trial performance lasting ~1 h [10]. The authors speculated that the CHO MR affected the central nervous system by activating oropharangeal receptors. This was confirmed by subsequent work demonstrating that CHO mouth rinsing activates areas of the brain associated with reward and motor control, consequently accentuating excitatory/motor output and muscular performance [11].

The ergogenic value of CHO rinsing has now been examined in a variety of conditions and there is good evidence that CHO MR can enhance physical performance in certain scenarios. Interestingly, most data has indicated that the performance value of CHO MR is less prominent [12,13], and in many cases non-existent, when exercise is performed in a post-prandial/carbohydrate-fed state [12,14–17]. However, CHO MR has repeatedly been shown to elicit higher power output and faster race times in events lasting between 30 and 75 min when performed in a post-absorptive/fasted state [10–12,18–20], with three exceptions [16,21,22]. Though only examined on a few occasions, CHO MR does not typically benefit high-intensity/sprint performance [20,23,24]. The only deviation from this has been when repeated sprints were performed in a glycogen-depleted state [25], suggesting that high-intensity performance may be improved when CHO MR is delivered under conditions of fatigue or metabolic strain. Nothing is known about the potential for CHO MR to enhance short-duration trial performance at the end of prolonged exercise, analogous to a typical 'final surge' to the finish line late in the endurance competition. Therefore, we designed this project to test the hypotheses that mouth rinsing with CHO can enhance 2 km time trial performance when preceded by ~3 h of cycling.

We were also interested in providing initial insight into the effects of a mouth rinse comprised of protein on late-exercise sprint performance. Though controversial, there is some evidence that adding protein to a carbohydrate supplement confers greater performance gains than carbohydrate alone [26–30], but the underlying physiology responsible for this observation has not been determined. Although we are not aware of general protein receptors in the oropharangeal cavity, whey protein possesses a bitter taste, and mouth rinsing with a bitter solution (quinine) can lead to higher power outputs than a placebo rinse [31]. It has also been speculated that oropharangeal receptors may be sensitive to caloric content, as 'sweetness' is not what confers performance gains [11]. Thus, it is conceivable that a protein mouth rinse can alter performance but this possibility has not yet been investigated.

2. Materials and Methods

2.1. Subjects

Eight male endurance-trained cyclists (24 ± 6 years; height, 176 ± 5 cm; weight, 74 ± 7 kg; VO_{2max}, 63.8 ± 5.7 mL·kg^{-1}·min^{-1}) participated in this project. All subjects performed ≥3 days of cycling per week for ≥2 months prior to study enrollment. All participants were informed about study procedures and potential risks prior to consent. All procedures were approved by the James Madison University Institutional Review Board (IRB #14-0119).

2.2. Cardiorespiratory Fitness

Subjects performed an incremental exercise test to exhaustion on a bicycle ergometer (Velotron; Racermate, Seattle, WA, USA) to determine maximum oxygen uptake (VO_{2max}) and power output at VO_{2max} (W_{max}). Subjects began the protocol at a self-selected power output that would be "a manageable workload during a 60 min ride". Power was then increased by 25 watts (W) every 2 min until volitional exhaustion. Breath samples were continuously monitored with a calibrated Moxus Modular Metabolic System (AEI Technologies, Pittsburgh, PA, USA) and data were aggregated in 30 s increments. Peak power (W_{max}) in the final completed stage was used to prescribe exercise intensity for subsequent exercise trials.

2.3. Experimental Design

The study was carried out in a counterbalanced, double-blinded fashion, with trials separated by seven to 10 days each. Following cardiorespiratory fitness testing, subjects completed 1 familiarization trial and three experimental trials on the aforementioned cycle ergometer. Each trial consisted of: 120 min of constant-load cycling at 55% W_{max}, a simulated 30 km time trial (TT) (~57 min), 15 min of rest that included peak isometric force testing, 10 min of constant-load cycling (3 min at 35% W_{max} and 7 min at 55% W_{max}), and a computer simulated 2 km time trial (~4 min) (Figure 1). The inclusion of a variable and self-selected intensity 30 km time trial prior to the mouth rinse intervention instead of continuing constant-load cycling allowed us to assess 30 km TT reliability under placebo (water) conditions, as we have reported elsewhere [32]. This decision may have introduced additional variability for subsequent measures, though data gathered during the 30 km TT and finishing times indicate that subjects experienced similar physiological stimuli prior to each of the three MR treatments.

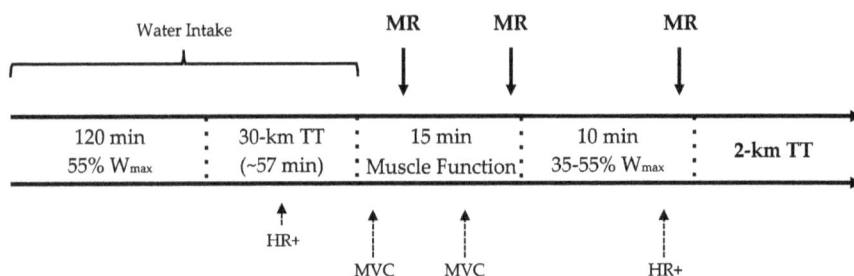

Figure 1. Experimental trial design with dependent measures. Water intake bracket indicates when only water was provided; HR+ with short arrow indicates heart rate (HR), rating of perceived exertion (RPE), and glucose measurements taken midway through the 30 km time trial (TT) prior to the mouth rinse (MR) intervention; HR+ with tall arrow indicates HR, RPE, and glucose measurements taken to determine the effects of the MR intervention; MVC, maximum voluntary.

Subjects were provided with 600 mL of water immediately prior to each trial, after which 150 mL of water was provided every 15 min during the 120 min steady-state ride and at three points during the 30 km TT (7.5 km, 15 km, and 22.5 km). Subjects were asked to void their bladders prior to all trials. A fan was placed ~2 m from the handlebars on high speed setting for uniform cooling during each trial and trials were conducted under thermoneutral conditions. All trials were performed in the morning, with no more than one hour separating start times for a given subject, two hours after consumption of a standardized breakfast (Section 2.6).

2.4. Mouth Rinse Solutions

The MR treatments contained 100 mL of deionized water (PLA) with the addition of either 6.4 g of maltodextrin (NOW Foods, Bloomingdale, IL, USA) or 6.4 g of hydrolyzed whey protein isolate (AMCO, Burlington, NJ, USA). Commercially available stevia was used to minimize differences in taste and smell.

During the three experimental trials (T1, T2, T3), subjects received 25 mL of each respective mouth rinse. Rinses were administered at three time points during the exercise trial: minutes 5:00 and 14:30 of the rest phase and at minute 8:00 of the 10 min constant-load segment (see Figure 1). Subjects swirled each rinse in their mouth for 5 s after which it was expectorated.

2.5. Dependent Measures

2.5.1. Cycling Performance

Finishing time from each 2 km cycling time trial was used as the performance measure.

2.5.2. Skeletal Muscle Function

Isometric peak torque (Maximum Voluntary Contraction, MVC) of the knee extensors was assessed at minutes 1:00 and 10:00 of the 15-min rest phase prior to the 2 km TT, as previously described [33]. Subjects performed three maximal attempts per test, each lasting 3 s, with one minute of rest between attempts. Peak force (N) was determined by the highest value from the three attempts, without visual feedback. While the 15 min rest period detracts from the ecological validity of the experimental design, it was necessary to facilitate muscle function testing before and after the MR intervention.

2.5.3. Heart Rate (HR), Rating of Perceived Exertion (RPE), and Blood Glucose

Heart rate was monitored throughout the duration of each exercise session using a chest-worn heart rate monitor (Suunto, Vantaa, Finland). Finger-stick blood samples were obtained at minute 8 of the 10 min constant-load phase. Glucose levels were determined immediately from whole blood using an automated analyzer (YSI 2300 STAT glucose, Yellow Springs, OH, USA). Subjective ratings of exertion using the Borg RPE scale were obtained simultaneously with blood sampling. Heart rate, RPE, and glucose were also assessed midway through the 30-km TT prior to the MR intervention.

2.6. Dietary and Physical Activity Controls

Subjects were instructed to maintain normal dietary habits throughout the study and were also provided with a standardized breakfast that was consumed 2 h prior to each trial (500 kcal; 90–100 g carbohydrate; 8–12 g protein, and 4–8 g of fat). Subjects completed a diet record for 24 h preceding the first experimental trial. Using a copy of the initial diet record, subjects were instructed to replicate their diet for the 24 h prior to each subsequent experimental trial. Subjects were instructed to refrain from heavy exercise for 48 h preceding each treatment trial, and were instructed to maintain consistent exercise habits between each of these trials. Subjects were also instructed to abstain from alcohol and caffeine for 24 and 12 h prior to each trial, respectively.

2.7. Statistical Analysis

All data were log transformed to diminish the effects of non-uniformity. Magnitude-based inferences about the data were derived using methods described by Hopkins and colleagues [34]. For performance, a previously established "smallest worthwhile change" in performance was used as the threshold value for a substantial treatment effect (CHO and PRO vs. PLA) [35]. The smallest worthwhile change in performance was defined as 0.3% of the within-subject variability of select groups of elite cyclists across repeated time trials (Coefficient of Variation = 1.3% for time), which translates to 0.8 s for the current project [36]. Published spreadsheets [37] were then used to determine the likelihood of the true treatment effect (of the population) reaching the substantial change threshold (0.8 s); these percent likelihoods were classified as <1% almost certainly no chance, 1%–5% = very unlikely, 5%–25% = unlikely, 25%–75% = possible, 75%–95% = likely, 95%–99% = very likely, and >99% = almost certain. Clinical inference criteria were used to classify the effects of treatment on performance. Specifically, if the percent chance of the effect reaching the substantial change threshold was <25% and the effect was clear, it was classified as "trivial." If the percent chance of the effect reaching the substantial change threshold for benefit exceeded 25% but the chance for harm was >0.5% the effect was classified as unclear. An exception to the 0.5% chance of harm criterion was made if the benefit/harm odds ratio was >66, in which case the effect was interpreted as clear and an inference was assigned.

For all other variables, the classification system detailed above was applied. However, the "smallest worthwhile change" was determined for each variable by multiplying the within-subject standard deviation under PLA conditions by 0.2. Further, mechanistic criteria were used such that if 90% confidence intervals included values that exceeded the substantial change threshold for both a positive and negative effect, effects were classified as unclear (>5% chance of reaching the substantial threshold for both a positive and negative effect), with no exceptions. For ease of interpretation, *p*-values derived from simple contrasts between treatments are included alongside the magnitude-based inferential outcomes.

3. Results

3.1. Cycling Pre-Load

As previously described, prior to MR intervention, subjects performed 120 min of constant-load cycling at 55% W_{max} (190 ± 22 Watts) followed by a 30 km TT. Data obtained midway (15 km) through the 30 km TT and finishing times are displayed in Table 1.

Table 1. The 30 km time trial prior to mouth rinse intervention.

Condition	Heart Rate (bpm)	RPE	Blood Glucose (mg/dL)	Finishing Time (min)
Placebo	150 ± 14	16 ± 1	68 ± 80	57.02 ± 5.21
Carbohydrate	148 ± 14	16 ± 1	68 ± 70	57.04 ± 2.75
Protein	144 ± 15	16 ± 1	66 ± 10	57.89 ± 7.38

Values are expressed as means ± SD. Data were obtained midway (15 km) through the 30 km TT. RPE = rating of perceived exertion. Data demonstrates that similar workloads were performed prior to the mouth rinse intervention.

3.2. Mouth Rinse Effects

3.2.1. Performance

CHO MR 'likely' enhanced the 2 km TT performance by 3.8% ± 4.7% (*p* = 0.11) compared to PLA, whereas the comparison between PRO vs. PLA was 'unclear' (0.4% ± 5.6%; *p* = 0.91). The 2 km TT data are displayed in Table 2 and Figure 2.

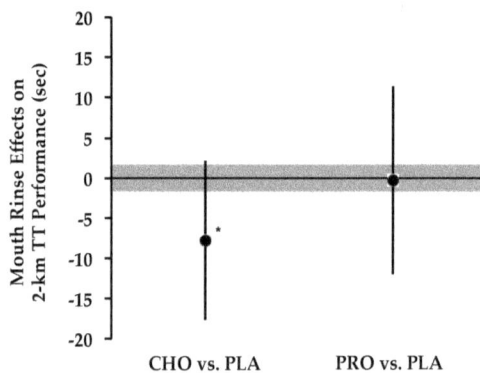

Figure 2. Effect of CHO and PRO mouth rinses on 2 km time trial (TT) Performance. Circles represent mean treatment difference compared to placebo. Bars depict 90% confidence interval. Shaded area notates threshold value for smallest meaningful effect. * 'Likely' faster than PLA.

Table 2. The 2 km performance, peak strength, and heart rate, rating of perceived exertion, and glucose.

Condition	Δ MVC (N)	Constant-Load—55% W_{max}			2 km TT Finishing Time (s)
		Heart Rate (bpm)	RPE	Blood Glucose (mg/dL)	
PLA	34 ± 40	150 ± 13	14 ± 20	59 ± 8	200.1 ± 10.8
CHO	25 ± 25	156 ± 10 *	14 ± 20	63 ± 7 **	192.4 ± 8.2 ††
PRO	10 ± 26 ‡	152 ± 60	14 ± 3	56 ± 10 †	199.9 ± 18.4

Values are expressed as means ± SD. Δ MVC, change in MVC from beginning to end of 15 min muscle function phase. RPE = rating of perceived exertion, MVC = maximum voluntary contraction. Statistics were used to separately compare PLA to CHO and PRO. Magnitude-based inferences for treatment comparisons are notated as follows: ‡ PRO vs. PLA, Possible (57%); * CHO vs. PLA, Likely (77%); ** CHO vs. PLA, Likely (92%); † PRO vs. PLA, Likely (77%); †† CHO vs. PLA, Likely (89%).

3.2.2. Skeletal Muscle Function

The MVC 'likely' increased from 456 ± 108 N to 490 ± 106 N during the 15 min muscle function period with PLA (7.9% ± 5.8%; $p = 0.03$), 'possibly' increased from 445 ± 61 N to 470 ± 70 N with CHO (5.3% ± 3.8%; $p = 0.03$), but had only a 'likely trivial' increase from 466 ± 84 N to 475 ± 75 N with PRO (2.5% ± 4.2%; $p = 0.78$). There was a 'possibly trivial' (68% likelihood; $p = 0.49$) difference between the change in MVC with PLA compared to CHO, whereas PRO had a 'possibly' smaller increase in MVC compared to PLA (57% likelihood; $p = 0.09$). Changes in MVC during the 15 min period are displayed in Table 2.

3.2.3. Heart Rate, RPE, and Blood Glucose

Heart rate during the 10 min constant-load phase was 'likely' higher with CHO compared to PLA (3.8% ± 5.3%; $p = 0.19$). The comparison between PRO and PLA was 'unclear' ($p = 0.73$). Differences in RPE between MR treatments were 'unclear'. Blood glucose levels during the 10 min constant-load phase were 'likely' higher with CHO relative to PLA (5.8% ± 4.1%; $p = 0.02$), and likely lower with PRO (−5.3% ± 7.0%; $p = 0.20$) compared to PLA. Mean HR, RPE, and blood glucose levels are displayed in Table 2.

4. Discussion

This project was primarily designed to examine the potential for a carbohydrate (CHO) mouth rinse to enhance high-intensity performance towards the end of prolonged exercise. We also included a separate experimental trial to investigate the possible benefit of mouth rinsing with a protein solution (PRO). The CHO mouth rinse 'likely' improved the 2 km TT performance (vs. PLA), whereas there were no systematic differences in the TT performance between PRO and PLA. This is the first evidence that late-exercise cycling TT performance can be improved by a CHO rinse, suggesting that endurance cyclists should consider CHO mouth rinsing to optimize performance during the late stages of competition, particularly when CHO supplementation is limited throughout exercise. The PRO MR data infers that previously reported benefits of adding PRO to a CHO supplement during prolonged exercise were not facilitated by detection of PRO in the mouth [26–30]. The ineffectiveness of the PRO rinse also indicates that physical gains from the CHO MR are specific to the presence of CHO.

The unique observation in this study is that the CHO MR enhanced short-duration TT performance lasting only ~3 min. Most previous work has demonstrated that CHO MR has little impact on short-duration, high-intensity 'performance' [20,23,24]. The only exception to this is the recent report that a repeated run-sprint performance was moderately enhanced by CHO MR, on the morning after a glycogen-depleting protocol [25]. Collectively, it now appears that MR can be effective for high-intensity exercise performance under difficult glycometabolic conditions. This is generally consistent with what is known about the efficacy of CHO rinsing during performances lasting longer than 30 min. The most pronounced improvements with CHO MR have been observed when exercise is commenced in a fasted state and when carbohydrate supplementation is withheld throughout exercise [12,13,38]. Further, the evidence supporting the performance advantages of CHO rinsing is much more consistent when the exercise is performed in a fasted state [10–12,18–20], in contrast to the null findings typically observed when the exercise is conducted in a fed state [12,14–17]. This indicates that the degree to which the presence of the carbohydrate in the mouth activates the reward/pleasure centers of the central nervous system (CNS) is related to carbohydrate availability or feeding latency time; specifically, that the CNS response to the presence of carbohydrate in the mouth is magnified under conditions of substantial energetic stress and/or when more time has elapsed since the most recent carbohydrate feeding. The current data would seem to support this hypothesis, though we did not directly examine CNS activity.

As mentioned earlier, CHO MR is believed to enhance physical performance by activating areas of the brain associated with reward/pleasure, thereby increasing excitatory/motor output and muscular performance. One criterion measure of this response is peak muscle strength, and though not unanimous [39], mouth rinsing with CHO can partially restore peak strength following fatiguing contractions [40], following 60 min of cycling [41], as well as attenuate force diminution during sustained muscle contractions [42]. We evaluated peak torque during a maximum voluntary contraction before and after the MR treatment, following the prolonged cycling stimulus. In contrast to our hypothesis, the CHO MR (+25 N) did not increase knee extensor torque more so than PLA (+34 N). The discrepancy between this and previous reports may be due to treatment dosing, specifically that the mouth rinse dose that separated pre- and post-strength measurements here may not have been enough to elicit a treatment effect. Strength measurements obtained in the current project were assessed before and after a single dose swirled in the mouth for 5 s, which is much shorter than the 10 s [40] and 60 s [42] rinses provided in the studies documenting strength improvements. This explanation is strengthened by a previous report that endurance performance is enhanced to a greater extent following 10 s compared to 5 s rinses [43]. Additionally, the decline in skeletal muscle force following 60 min of cycling was attenuated with a 5 s CHO MR, but the rinse was delivered seven times throughout the exercise session [41]. Therefore, additional mouth rinses or longer swill time may have been required to elicit strength gains. The obvious disconnect in the current dataset is that despite the absence of a CHO treatment effect on MVC, the CHO rinse did improve the 2 km TT performance. However, while the strength measurements were obtained after a single mouth rinse, two subsequent doses were administered prior to the 2 km TT.

Somewhat unexpectedly, the CHO MR was also associated with slightly elevated blood glucose levels and heart rate during constant-load cycling prior to the 2 km TT. Blood glucose following a CHO MR has been assessed during variable intensity exercise on a number of occasions and it has consistently been unaffected [12,38,44]. Though this possibly suggests that the rise in blood glucose resulted from the digestion of the MR constituents, we are inclined to believe that it was a centrally mediated response to the MR. The primary ingredient in the CHO MR, maltodextrin, cannot be digested into glucose residues in the oral cavity [45]. Further, investigators were present to administer the MR treatments and to ensure that the rinse was expectorated and not swallowed. In addition, while we did not measure the volume of the expectorate, any small amount of solution that may have been ingested was likely insufficient to significantly raise blood glucose levels. In support of a centrally mediated MR effect on blood glucose, the only other paper that measured blood glucose during constant-load exercise also noted elevated blood glucose levels [17]. The authors speculated that the increase in blood glucose following the CHO MR might have been due to an increase in hepatic glucose output facilitated by activation of hepatic and/or pancreatic sympathetic nerve activity [46]. Regardless of the mechanisms, much like the previous authors, we doubt the physiological relevance of the small differences in blood glucose levels (~3 mg/dL). There is good evidence that even larger discrepancies in blood glucose do not necessarily translate to a faster cycling performance [10,47,48]. Furthermore, the difference in blood glucose levels between PRO and PLA MR trials in the current study was also ~3 mg/dL, and the TT performances were virtually identical. Like blood glucose, heart rate was also slightly elevated during constant-load exercise following the CHO MR. There is no precedent for this response but it could also be related to an increase in sympathetic nerve activation mentioned earlier. It is also possible that the CHO MR led to an increase in cycling cadence, which has been shown to increase heart rate even when power output is clamped [49]. Unfortunately we do not have cadence data to test this hypothesis.

5. Conclusions

Here we present the first evidence that cyclists may want to consider mouth rinsing with a CHO solution prior to the closing kilometers of a competitive event. The practical relevance of this finding should be further established, as the mouth rinse solution was administered after approximately three hours of cycling without carbohydrate supplementation.

Acknowledgments: We thank all participants for their participation. This project was supported by James Madison University's College of Health and Behavioral Studies Faculty Research Grant (to NDL and MJS).

Author Contributions: Nicholas D. Luden, Michael J. Saunders, Andrew C. D'Lugos, and Caitlin W. Vining conceived and designed the experiments; Andrew C. D'Lugos, Mark W. Pataky, Daniel A. Baur, Caitlin B. Vining and Adam B. Schroer performed the experiments; Nicholas D. Luden analyzed the data; Nicholas D. Luden and Michael J. Saunders contributed reagents/materials/analysis tools; Nicholas D. Luden wrote the paper; and Michael J. Saunders, Andrew C. D'Lugos, Mark W. Pataky, Daniel A. Baur, Caitlin B. Vining, and Adam B. Schroer contributed major edits; Nicholas D. Luden, Michael J. Saunders, Andrew C. D'Lugos, Mark W. Pataky, Daniel A. Baur, Caitlin B. Vining, and Adam B. Schroer gave final approval of version to be published.

Conflicts of Interest: The authors declare no conflict of interest.

References

1. Coggan, A.R.; Coyle, E.F. Reversal of fatigue during prolonged exercise by carbohydrate infusion or ingestion. *J. Appl. Physiol.* **1987**, *63*, 2388–2395. [PubMed]
2. Coyle, E.F.; Hagberg, J.M.; Hurley, B.F.; Martin, W.H.; Ehsani, A.A.; Holloszy, J.O. Carbohydrate feeding during prolonged strenuous exercise can delay fatigue. *J. Appl. Physiol.* **1983**, *55*, 230–235. [PubMed]
3. Jeukendrup, A.E.; Wagenmakers, A.J.M.; Stegen, J.; Gijsen, A.P.; Brouns, F.; Saris, W.H.M. Carbohydrate ingestion can completely suppress endogenous glucose production during exercise. *Am. J. Physiol. Metab.* **1999**, *276*, E672–E683.
4. Neufer, P.D.; Costill, D.L.; Flynn, M.G.; Kirwan, J.P.; Mitchell, J.B.; Houmard, J. Improvements in exercise performance: Effects of carbohydrate feedings and diet. *J. Appl. Physiol.* **1987**, *62*, 983–988. [PubMed]
5. Stellingwerff, T.; Boon, H.; Gijsen, A.P.; Stegen, J.H.C.H.; Kuipers, H.; Van Loon, L.J.C. Carbohydrate supplementation during prolonged cycling exercise spares muscle glycogen but does not affect intramyocellular lipid use. *Pflugers Arch. Eur. J. Physiol.* **2007**, *454*, 635–647. [CrossRef] [PubMed]
6. De Bock, K.; Derave, W.; Ramaekers, M.; Richter, E.A.; Hespel, P. Fiber type-specific muscle glycogen sparing due to carbohydrate intake before and during exercise. *J. Appl. Physiol.* **2007**, *102*, 183–188. [CrossRef] [PubMed]
7. Anantaraman, R.; Carmines, A.A.; Gaesser, G.A.; Weltman, A. Effects of carbohydrate supplementation on performance during 1 hour of high-intensity exercise. *Int. J. Sports Med.* **1995**, *16*, 461–465. [CrossRef] [PubMed]
8. Below, P.R.; Mora-Rodríguez, R.; González-Alonso, J.; Coyle, E.F. Fluid and carbohydrate ingestion independently improve performance during 1 h of intense exercise. *Med. Sci. Sports Exerc.* **1995**, *27*, 200–210. [CrossRef] [PubMed]
9. Jeukendrup, A.; Brouns, F.; Wagenmakers, A.J.M.; Saris, W.H.M. Carbohydrate-electrolyte feedings improve 1 h time trial cycling performance. *Int. J. Sports Med.* **1997**, *18*, 125–129. [CrossRef] [PubMed]
10. Carter, J.M.; Jeukendrup, A.E.; Jones, D.A. The effect of carbohydrate mouth rinse on 1-h cycle time trial performance. *Med. Sci. Sports Exerc.* **2004**, *36*, 2107–2111. [CrossRef] [PubMed]
11. Chambers, E.S.; Bridge, M.W.; Jones, D. A Carbohydrate sensing in the human mouth: Effects on exercise performance and brain activity. *J. Physiol.* **2009**, *587*, 1779–1794. [CrossRef] [PubMed]

12. Lane, S.C.; Bird, S.R.; Burke, L.M.; Hawley, J. A Effect of a carbohydrate mouth rinse on simulated cycling time-trial performance commenced in a fed or fasted state. *Appl. Physiol. Nutr. Metab.* **2013**, *38*, 134–139. [CrossRef] [PubMed]

13. Fares, E.J.M.; Kayser, B. Carbohydrate mouth rinse effects on exercise capacity in pre- and postprandial states. *J. Nutr. Metab.* **2011**, *2011*. [CrossRef] [PubMed]

14. Beelen, M.; Berghuis, J.; Bonaparte, B.; Ballak, S.B.; Jeukendrup, A.E.; Van Loon, L.J.C. Carbohydrate mouth rinsing in the fed state: Lack of enhancement of time-trial performance. *Int. J. Sport Nutr. Exerc. Metab.* **2009**, *19*, 400–409. [CrossRef] [PubMed]

15. Ispoglou, T.; O'Kelly, D.; Angelopoulou, A.; Bargh, M.; O'Hara, J.P.; Duckworth, L.C. Mouth-rinsing with carbohydrate solutions at the postprandial state fail to improve performance during simulated cycling time trials. *J. Strength Cond. Res.* **2015**, *29*, 2316–2325. [CrossRef] [PubMed]

16. Trommelen, J.; Beelen, M.; Mullers, M.; Gibala, M.J.; Van Loon, L.J.C.; Cermak, N.M. A sucrose mouth rinse does not improve 1-Hr cycle time trial performance when performed in the fasted or fed state. *Int. J. Sport Nutr. Exerc. Metab.* **2015**, *25*, 576–583. [CrossRef] [PubMed]

17. Ataide-Silva, T.; Ghiarone, T.; Bertuzzi, R.; Stathis, C.G.; Leandro, C.G.; Lima-Silva, A.E. CHO mouth rinse ameliorates neuromuscular response with lower endogenous CHO stores. *Med. Sci. Sport Exerc.* **2016**, *48*, 1810–1820. [CrossRef] [PubMed]

18. Rollo, I.; Williams, C.; Gant, N.; Nute, M. The influence of carbohydrate mouth rinse on self-selected speeds during a 30-min treadmill run. *Int. J. Sport Nutr. Exerc. Metab.* **2008**, *18*, 585–600. [CrossRef] [PubMed]

19. Rollo, I.; Cole, M.; Miller, R.; Williams, C. The influence of mouth-rinsing a carbohydrate solution on 1 h running performance. *Med. Sci. Sports Exerc.* **2009**, *42*, 798–804. [CrossRef] [PubMed]

20. Bastos-Silva, V.J.; de Albuquerque Melo, A.; Lima-Silva, A.E.; Moura, F.A.; Bertuzzi, R.; de Araujo, G.G. Carbohydrate mouth rinse maintains muscle electromyographic activity and increases time to exhaustion during moderate but not high-intensity cycling exercise. *Nutrients* **2016**, *8*, 49. [CrossRef] [PubMed]

21. Kulaksız, T.N.; Koşar, Ş.N.; Bulut, S.; Güzel, Y.; Willems, M.E.T.; Hazir, T.; Turnagöl, H.H. Mouth rinsing with maltodextrin solutions fails to improve time trial endurance cycling performance in recreational athletes. *Nutrients* **2016**, *8*, 269. [CrossRef] [PubMed]

22. Ali, A.; Yoo, M.J.Y.; Moss, C.; Breier, B.H. Carbohydrate mouth rinsing has no effect on power output during cycling in a glycogen-reduced state. *J. Int. Soc. Sports Nutr.* **2016**, *13*, 19. [CrossRef] [PubMed]

23. Chong, E.; Guelfi, K.J.; Fournier, P.A. Effect of a carbohydrate mouth rinse on maximal sprint performance in competitive male cyclists. *J. Sci. Med. Sport* **2011**, *14*, 162–167. [CrossRef] [PubMed]

24. Přibyslavská, V.; Scudamore, E.M.; Johnson, S.L.; Green, J.M.; Stevenson Wilcoxson, M.C.; Lowe, J.B.; O'Neal, E.K. Influence of carbohydrate mouth rinsing on running and jumping performance during early morning soccer scrimmaging. *Eur. J. Sport Sci.* **2016**, *16*, 441–447. [CrossRef] [PubMed]

25. Kasper, A.M.; Cocking, S.; Cockayne, M.; Barnard, M.; Tench, J.; Parker, L.; McAndrew, J.; Langan-Evans, C.; Close, G.L.; Morton, J.P. Carbohydrate mouth rinse and caffeine improves high-intensity interval running capacity when carbohydrate restricted. *Eur. J. Sport Sci.* **2016**, *16*, 560–568. [CrossRef] [PubMed]

26. Ivy, J.; Res, P.; Sprague, R.; Widzer, M. Effect of a carbohydrate-protein supplement on endurance performance during exercise of varying intensity. *Int. J. Sport Nutr. Exerc. Metab.* **2003**, *13*, 382–395. [CrossRef] [PubMed]

27. Ferguson-Stegall, L.; McCleave, E.L.; Ding, Z.; Kammer, L.M.; Wang, B.; Doerner, P.G.; Liu, Y.; Ivy, J.L. The effect of a low carbohydrate beverage with added protein on cycling endurance performance in trained athletes. *J. Strength Cond. Res.* **2010**, *24*, 2577–2586. [CrossRef] [PubMed]

28. Saunders, M.J.; Moore, R.W.; Kies, A.K.; Luden, N.D.; Pratt, C.A. Carbohydrate and protein hydrolysate coingestions improvement of late-exercise time-trial performance. *Int. J. Sport Nutr. Exerc. Metab.* **2009**, *19*, 136–149. [CrossRef] [PubMed]

29. Saunders, M.; Luden, N.; Herrick, J. Consumption of an oral carbohydrate-protein gel improves cycling endurance and prevents postexercise muscle damage. *J. Strength Cond. Res.* **2007**, *21*, 678–684. [CrossRef] [PubMed]

30. Saunders, M.J.; Kane, M.D.; Todd, M.K.; Kent Todd, M. Effects of a carbohydrate-protein beverage on cycling endurance and muscle damage. *Med. Sci. Sports Exerc.* **2004**, *36*, 1233–1238. [CrossRef] [PubMed]

31. Gam, S.; Guelfi, K.J.; Fournier, P.A. Opposition of carbohydrate in a mouth-rinse solution to the detrimental effect of mouth rinsing during cycling time trials. *Int. J. Sport Nutr. Exerc. Metab.* **2013**, *23*, 48–56. [CrossRef] [PubMed]

32. Baur, D.A.; Schroer, A.B.; Luden, N.D.; Womack, C.J.; Smyth, S.A.; Saunders, M.J. Glucose-fructose enhances performance versus isocaloric, but not moderate, glucose. *Med. Sci. Sports Exerc.* **2014**, *46*, 1778–1786. [CrossRef] [PubMed]

33. Gilson, S.F.; Saunders, M.J.; Moran, C.W.; Moore, R.W.; Womack, C.J.; Todd, M.K. Effects of chocolate milk consumption on markers of muscle recovery following soccer training: A randomized cross-over study. *J. Int. Soc. Sports Nutr.* **2010**, *7*, 19. [CrossRef] [PubMed]

34. Hopkins, W.G.; Marshall, S.W.; Batterham, A.M.; Hanin, J. Progressive statistics for studies in sports medicine and exercise science. *Med. Sci. Sports Exerc.* **2009**, *41*, 3–13. [CrossRef] [PubMed]

35. Hopkins, W.G. How to Interpret Changes in an Athletic Performance Test. Available online: http://www.sportsci.org/jour/04/wghtests.htm (accessed on 5 September 2015).

36. Paton, C.C.D.; Hopkins, W.G.W. Variation in performance of elite cyclists from race to race. *Eur. J. Sport Sci.* **2006**, *6*, 25–31. [CrossRef]

37. Hopkins, W.G.W.G. A spreadsheet for deriving a confidence interval, mechanistic inference, and clinical inference from a *p* value. *Sport Sci.* **2007**, *11*, 16–19.

38. Pottier, A.; Bouckaert, J.; Gilis, W.; Roels, T.; Derave, W. Mouth rinse but not ingestion of a carbohydrate solution improves 1-h cycle time trial performance. *Scand. J. Med. Sci. Sport.* **2010**, *20*, 105–111. [CrossRef] [PubMed]

39. Painelli, V.S.; Roschel, H.; Gualano, B.; Del-Favero, S.; Benatti, F.B.; Ugrinowitsch, C.; Tricoli, V.; Lancha, A.H. The Effect of carbohydrate mouth rinse on maximal strength and strength endurance. *Eur. J. Appl. Physiol.* **2011**, *111*, 2381–2386. [CrossRef] [PubMed]

40. Jensen, M.; Stellingwerff, T.; Klimstra, M. Carbohydrate mouth rinse counters fatigue related strength reduction. *Int. J. Sport Nutr. Exerc. Metab.* **2015**, *25*, 252–261. [CrossRef] [PubMed]

41. Jeffers, R.; Shave, R.; Ross, E.; Stevenson, E.J.; Goodall, S. The effect of a carbohydrate mouth-rinse on neuromuscular fatigue following cycling exercise. *Appl. Physiol. Nutr. Metab.* **2015**, *40*, 557–564. [CrossRef] [PubMed]

42. Gant, N.; Stinear, C.M.; Byblow, W.D. Carbohydrate in the mouth immediately facilitates motor output. *Brain Res.* **2010**, *1350*, 151–158. [CrossRef] [PubMed]

43. Sinclair, J.; Bottoms, L.; Flynn, C.; Bradley, E.; Alexander, G.; McCullagh, S.; Finn, T.; Hurst, H.T. The effect of different durations of carbohydrate mouth rinse on cycling performance. *Eur. J. Sport Sci.* **2014**, *14*, 259–264. [CrossRef] [PubMed]

44. Watson, P.; Nichols, D.; Cordery, P. Mouth rinsing with a carbohydrate solution does not influence cycle time trial performance in the heat. *Appl. Physiol. Nutr. Metab.* **2014**, *39*, 1064–1069. [CrossRef] [PubMed]

45. Hofman, D.L.; Van Buul, V.J.; Brouns, F.J.P.H. Nutrition, health, and regulatory aspects of digestible maltodextrins. *Crit. Rev. Food Sci. Nutr.* **2016**, *56*, 2091–2100. [CrossRef] [PubMed]

46. Oppenheimer, S.M.; Gelb, A.; Girvin, J.P.; Hachinski, V.C. Cardiovascular effects of human insular cortex stimulation. *Neurology* **1992**, *42*, 1727–1732. [CrossRef] [PubMed]

47. Felig, P.; Cherif, A.; Minagawa, A.; Wahren, J. Hypoglycemia during prolonged exercise in normal men. *N. Engl. J. Med.* **1982**, *306*, 895–900. [CrossRef] [PubMed]

48. Flynn, M.G.; Costill, D.L.; Hawley, J.A.; Fink, W.J.; Neufer, P.D.; Fielding, R.A.; Sleeper, M.D. Influence of selected carbohydrate drinks on cycling performance and glycogen use. *Med. Sci. Sports Exerc.* **1987**, *19*, 37–40. [CrossRef] [PubMed]

49. Stebbins, C.L.; Moore, J.L.; Casazza, G.A. Effects of cadence on aerobic capacity following a prolonged, varied intensity cycling trial. *J. Sport. Sci. Med.* **2014**, *13*, 114–119.

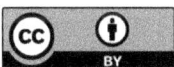

nutrients

MDPI

Review

Exercise, Appetite and Weight Control: Are There Differences between Men and Women?

Alice E. Thackray [1], **Kevin Deighton** [2], **James A. King** [1] **and David J. Stensel** [1,*]

[1] School of Sport, Exercise and Health Sciences, Loughborough University, Leicestershire LE11 3TU, UK; A.E.Thackray@lboro.ac.uk (A.E.T.); J.A.King@lboro.ac.uk (J.A.K.)

[2] Institute for Sport, Physical Activity and Leisure, Leeds Beckett University, Leeds LS6 3QS, UK; K.Deighton@leedsbeckett.ac.uk

* Correspondence: D.J.Stensel@lboro.ac.uk; Tel.: +44-1509-226-344

Received: 25 August 2016; Accepted: 18 September 2016; Published: 21 September 2016

Abstract: Recent years have witnessed significant research interest surrounding the interaction among exercise, appetite and energy balance, which has important implications for health. The majority of exercise and appetite regulation studies have been conducted in males. Consequently, opportunities to examine sex-based differences have been limited, but represent an interesting avenue of inquiry considering postulations that men experience greater weight loss after exercise interventions than women. This article reviews the scientific literature relating to the acute and chronic effects of exercise on appetite control in men and women. The consensus of evidence demonstrates that appetite, appetite-regulatory hormone and energy intake responses to acute exercise do not differ between the sexes, and there is little evidence indicating compensatory changes occur after acute exercise in either sex. Limited evidence suggests women respond to the initiation of exercise training with more robust compensatory alterations in appetite-regulatory hormones than men, but whether this translates to long-term differences is unknown. Current exercise training investigations do not support sex-based differences in appetite or objectively assessed energy intake, and increasing exercise energy expenditure elicits at most a partial energy intake compensation in both sexes. Future well-controlled acute and chronic exercise studies directly comparing men and women are required to expand this evidence base.

Keywords: appetite; appetite-regulatory hormones; compensation; energy balance; energy intake; exercise; sex-based differences; weight control

1. Introduction

Obesity is a major risk factor for several chronic diseases, including type 2 diabetes mellitus and cardiovascular disease, and remains a significant global burden from a public health and economic standpoint [1,2]. Weight loss as little as 3% of initial body mass is sufficient to promote favourable changes in several chronic disease risk markers and can be accomplished by increasing energy expenditure through exercise and/or reducing energy intake to achieve a sustained negative energy balance [3]. Recent years have witnessed significant research interest surrounding the interaction between exercise, appetite and energy balance, which has direct implications for the implementation of exercise as a weight management strategy [4].

Similar to many scientific fields, the majority of exercise and appetite regulation studies have traditionally focused research efforts on men. Consequently, much less is known about the interaction between exercise and appetite in women, and the opportunity to examine potential sex-based differences has been limited. A handful of exercise training studies have demonstrated that men experience greater reductions in body mass and body fat than women [5–7], although this is not a universal finding [8,9]. Authors supporting the concept of divergent weight loss outcomes have suggested that women demonstrate greater compensatory responses to exercise by more accurately balancing energy intake and expenditure in order to defend body fat stores and preserve reproductive function [10–12].

Exercise-induced changes in hormones implicated in appetite control and energy balance (e.g., acylated ghrelin, peptide YY (PYY), glucagon-like peptide-1 (GLP-1), insulin, and leptin) may contribute to sex-based differences in body fat loss after exercise [13]. Although based on a limited number of studies, a previous review concluded that women exhibit compensatory changes in appetite ratings and hormones conducive to appetite stimulation; a response that is not seen in men [11]. However, this conclusion has not been supported by more recent experimental studies, which have documented similar appetite, appetite-regulatory hormone and energy intake responses to acute and chronic exercise-induced energy deficits in men and women [8,14,15].

The purpose of this article is to review recent developments regarding appetite, appetite-regulatory hormone and energy intake responses to single bouts of exercise (acute responses) and exercise training (chronic responses) in men and women. Furthermore, this review will consider the potential implications of these findings for health and highlight important areas for future research.

2. Appetite-Regulatory Hormones

Appetite and energy intake are regulated at the physiological level by the neuroendocrine system, which involves complex interactions between central and peripheral mediated pathways [16,17]. Appetite-regulatory hormones include episodic gut signals that are sensitive to short-term fluctuations in feeding behaviour and control hunger and satiety on a meal-to-meal basis (e.g., acylated ghrelin, PYY, and GLP-1), and tonic hormonal signals that regulate long-term changes in energy balance and body fat (e.g., insulin, and leptin). A brief introduction to these hormones is presented here, but the interested reader is directed to a number of comprehensive reviews documenting the precise role of these hormones in the homeostatic regulation of appetite and energy balance [16–19].

Of the short-acting appetite regulatory signals, ghrelin is unique as the only known gut peptide that is orexigenic, and is predominantly secreted into the circulation by the oxyntic glands of the stomach. Ghrelin exists in the circulation in two forms (acylated and unacylated) and, although only 10%–20% of circulating ghrelin is acylated ghrelin, this form is believed to be solely responsible for appetite stimulation [20]. Circulating ghrelin concentrations increase preprandially and are rapidly suppressed postprandially on a meal-to-meal basis. This temporal pattern of fluctuation is indicative of an important role in coordinating meal initiation [21].

Working in opposition to ghrelin, on a meal-to-meal basis, several appetite-inhibiting hormones serve to promote post-meal satiation and satiety (e.g., PYY, GLP-1, cholecystokinin, pancreatic polypeptide, and amylin). Of primary relevance to this review, PYY is predominantly synthesised and secreted from the intestinal L-cells and is present peripherally in two forms (PYY_{1-36} and PYY_{3-36}), with PYY_{3-36} representing the most abundant and biologically active form. Concentrations of PYY are low in the fasted state and increase rapidly after meal intake, which highlights a potential role in meal termination and sensations of fullness between meals. Glucagon-like peptide-1 is also secreted from the intestinal L-cells in response to nutrient intake and similarly contributes to meal termination and satiety. It exists as an active (GLP_{7-36}) and inactive (GLP_{9-37}) form, with the active form rapidly degraded to its inactive form upon secretion into the circulation. The appetite-inhibiting effect of these hormones is further supported by studies demonstrating that peripheral administration of PYY_{3-36} [22] and GLP-1 [23] stimulates satiety and reduces ad libitum food intake in lean and obese individuals.

Leptin, secreted primarily from adipocytes, and insulin, released by the beta cells of the pancreas, are important regulators of energy balance, which are implicated in the long-term control of food intake and energy expenditure. Leptin and insulin are secreted in concentrations proportional to body fat mass, and act directly on the hypothalamus and other brain regions to exert anorexigenic effects. Circulating leptin and insulin concentrations are elevated in obese individuals, suggesting that a degree of resistance to the anorexigenic effects of these hormones may occur with obesity. This is further supported by evidence that the accumulation of adipose tissue weakens the inhibitory effect of fat mass on energy intake [24,25].

3. Exercise and Weight Loss

Exercise is an important component of weight management [3], and promotes a myriad of health benefits independent of weight loss [26]. It is well documented that exercise typically results in modest weight loss that can be enhanced when exercise is combined with dietary modifications [27,28]. However, the efficacy of exercise as a successful strategy for weight management varies markedly between individuals [29]. Interestingly, it has been suggested that sex may be a primary factor that affects the ability of structured exercise to promote weight loss and/or facilitate weight management [30].

The strongest evidence of a sex-based difference in the weight loss response to exercise was provided in the Midwest Exercise Trial by Donnelly and colleagues [6]. This study involved a 16-month supervised exercise training program at a set intensity and duration (five days per week, 20–45 min per session at 55%–70% peak oxygen uptake ($\dot{V}O_{2peak}$)) with ad libitum diet in previously sedentary men and women. After the exercise intervention, men lost an average of 5.2 kg in body weight and 4.9 kg in fat mass, whereas women maintained body weight and fat mass. Other studies have also demonstrated that men experience greater weight loss than women in response to a supervised program of exercise when exercise is prescribed at a similar duration and relative exercise intensity across the sexes [5,31,32].

However, in many of these studies, the exercise-induced energy expenditure was substantially greater in men than women. This has been suggested as a potential reason for the reported sex-based differences in exercise-induced weight loss [33], in accordance with evidence that the energy expenditure of exercise is the strongest predictor of fat loss during an exercise program [34,35]. Exercise training studies prescribing exercise based on energy expenditure have reported comparable body composition changes in response to the training stimulus in men and women [8,9,36]. Specifically, Donnelly and colleagues [9] have published findings from a subsequent randomised controlled trial as a follow-up to the Midwest Exercise Trial in which the exercise-induced energy expenditure was matched between men and women over a 10-month supervised aerobic exercise training intervention. In contrast to their earlier study [6], when the energy expenditure was equivalent between the sexes, similar reductions in body weight and body fat were seen between men and women [9].

A common finding in the literature is the degree of individual variation in the weight loss response to exercise training in both sexes [8,9,29,35,37,38]. It has been suggested that individual differences in compensatory behaviours that negate the exercise-induced energy deficit may be responsible for this variability [29]. Specifically, evidence of increased hunger and energy intake have been reported in individuals who experience a lower than expected weight loss after a period of exercise training [29,37,38]. Consequently, studies investigating the effect of exercise on appetite regulation (appetite perceptions, appetite-regulatory hormones, energy intake) in men and women are important and will be discussed in the following sections of this review.

4. Acute Effects of Exercise on Appetite, Appetite-Regulatory Hormones and Energy Intake

A plethora of studies have been conducted examining the appetite, appetite-regulatory hormone and energy intake responses to acute exercise in men, and to a much lesser extent, women. This research has been reviewed in detail elsewhere [4,39–43], but a brief synopsis of the most pertinent studies is presented in this article to frame the research literature which has examined sex-based differences.

4.1. Appetite and Appetite-Regulatory Hormones

The consensus of evidence in healthy, normal weight men suggests that acylated ghrelin concentrations are transiently suppressed, and satiety hormones, most notably PYY and GLP-1, are elevated during and immediately after an acute bout of exercise. Such hormonal changes often coincide with a transient reduction in subjective appetite responses, which has been described as "exercise-induced anorexia" [44]. These responses become apparent when acute exercise is performed $\geq$60% of $\dot{V}O_{2peak}$ typically [45–49], and have been replicated during a variety of exercise modes including running [45,46,48], cycling [47,50–53], swimming [54], resistance exercise [46,55] and high-intensity interval exercise [52,53,56]. Circulating appetite-regulatory hormones and appetite ratings typically return to control values within 30 to 60 min of exercise completion [39,46,48]; however, compensatory increases in appetite have been reported in some studies [52,54,57]. Furthermore, current evidence suggests that acute exercise elicits similar appetite and appetite-regulatory hormone responses in lean and overweight men [47], and does not stimulate compensatory changes in those who are overweight or obese [47,58].

Despite postulations that sex-based differences in appetite regulation may exist to enable women to preserve energy balance and reproductive function [10–12], several acute studies conducted in women suggest that they respond similarly to men. Specifically, transient alterations in appetite and appetite-regulatory hormone concentrations (acylated ghrelin, PYY_{3-36}, and GLP-1) have been reported in a direction expected to suppress appetite in healthy, recreationally active [15], endurance-trained [59] and overweight and obese [60] women. Furthermore, the majority of studies report no evidence of compensatory increases in appetite perceptions and appetite-regulatory hormones up to 7.5 h after a single bout of exercise in women [15,59–62].

However, exceptions have been observed in the literature with some studies demonstrating that women do not exhibit an acute exercise-induced suppression of appetite [62–64] or changes in appetite-regulatory hormones [61,62]. Furthermore, in contrast to the aforementioned studies in men and women, Larson-Meyer and colleagues [64] reported an increase in acylated ghrelin concentrations during the 2 h period after 60 min running at 70% $\dot{V}O_{2peak}$. Such discrepancies are likely related to differences in the exercise intensity, training status of participants, completion of exercise in the fasted or postprandial state, timing of meal intake and analytical methods used to quantify hormone concentrations.

Sex-based differences in the regulation of appetite in response to acute exercise have been examined directly in four studies [14,15,65,66]. The first acute exercise and appetite study that compared men and women was published by Kawano and colleagues [65]. The authors reported that 20 min of rope skipping exercise increased ratings of subjective hunger 30 min after exercise in women but not men; however, the absence of a control condition in this study and the somewhat unusual mode of exercise make this finding difficult to interpret. Furthermore, this study did not control for the potential confounding effects of the menstrual cycle, which represents an important consideration for acute exercise studies comparing men and women. In this regard, recent evidence suggests that compared with untailored programs, synchronising diet and exercise training interventions around the hormonal changes that occur during the menstrual cycle elicits greater weight loss [67] and improvements in muscle strength [68]. In addition, cyclical fluctuations in sex hormones (estrogen and progesterone) have been shown to alter appetite-regulatory hormone concentrations and energy intake in women across the menstrual cycle [69,70]. However, whether appetite responses to exercise in women are influenced by the menstrual cycle phase is not known and represents a research avenue to consider in the future.

Subsequent studies directly comparing men and women have also incorporated measures of appetite-regulatory hormones and energy intake (discussed below) alongside subjective appetite perceptions to provide a more comprehensive picture of potential sex-based differences in appetite regulation. In this regard, Hagobian and colleagues [14] examined the appetite and hormonal responses to a single bout of cycling performed at 70% $\dot{V}O_{2peak}$ until 30% of total daily energy expenditure was expended in healthy men and women matched for age and cardiorespiratory fitness. Importantly, the female participants were all studied during the early follicular phase of the menstrual cycle. The authors reported that appetite perceptions and appetite-regulatory hormone concentrations (acylated ghrelin and PYY$_{3-36}$) were not different during the 40 min after exercise in either sex. Similarly, in another acute study, breaking up prolonged sitting with light- or moderate-intensity walking did not alter appetite or concentrations of acylated ghrelin and total PYY over the 5 h observation period in either sex [66]. The walking interventions adopted in this study comprised a total of 28 min walking performed in 2 min bouts every 20 min. This intermittent pattern of exercise contrasts with the vast majority of acute exercise and appetite studies, which have reported transient perturbations in appetite and appetite-regulatory hormones in response to continuous, moderate- to high-intensity exercise protocols. Indeed, the authors recognise that the exercise stimulus may have been insufficient (in intensity and duration) to provoke transient changes in appetite and appetite-regulatory hormones.

Recently, Alajmi and colleagues [15] examined the effect of 60 min treadmill running at 70% $\dot{V}O_{2peak}$ on appetite and acylated ghrelin concentrations over 7 h in healthy men and women (studied during the follicular phase of the menstrual cycle). Despite the greater net energy expenditure during exercise in the men (3971 vs. 2536 kJ in men and women, respectively), both men and women exhibited an equivalent suppression in appetite and acylated ghrelin concentrations in response to acute exercise (Figure 1), with no evidence of compensatory responses to exercise in the 7 h observation period in either sex. Interestingly, the female participants in this study exhibited significantly greater acylated ghrelin concentrations compared with men. However, the relevance of this difference is unclear given subjective appetite ratings were greater in men than women. Furthermore, despite the greater appetite and lower acylated ghrelin concentrations in men than women, the appetite and acylated ghrelin responses to exercise were similar between the sexes.

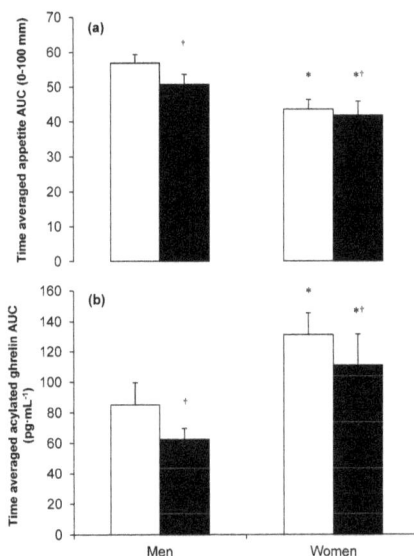

Figure 1. Time averaged total area under the curve (AUC) for appetite ratings (**a**); and plasma acylated ghrelin concentrations (**b**) in the control (□) and exercise (■) conditions. Each condition was 7 h and a single bout of exercise was performed between 0 to 1 h in the exercise condition (60 min running at 70% peak oxygen uptake). [†] Significant difference between exercise and control $p \leq 0.05$; [*] Significant difference between women and men $p \leq 0.05$. Values are mean (SEM), appetite ratings: $n = 10$ men, $n = 10$ women; acylated ghrelin: $n = 8$ men, $n = 8$ women. Data reproduced from reference [15]. © Wolters Kluwer Health, Inc. Reproduced with permission.

4.2. Energy Intake

Many of the studies highlighted above included an ad libitum meal in the post-exercise period to assess potential changes in energy intake after a single exercise stimulus. The majority of studies in men report no change in absolute energy intake after acute exercise when a single or multiple ad libitum meals are provided 30 min to 7.5 h after the cessation of exercise [48,49,52,53,55,71–73]; however, some studies have reported increases [50,74] or decreases [47,58,75] in energy intake after acute exercise. Nevertheless, two studies have demonstrated that 24 h energy intake is unchanged after acute exercise in healthy men quantified from laboratory-based ad libitum meals and overnight food bags [48,52].

Similarly, evidence suggests that ad libitum energy intake remains unchanged in response to acute exercise in healthy women [64,76–78] and overweight and obese women [61,62,76]. As an exception, Larson-Meyer and colleagues [64] reported that absolute energy intake (ad libitum meal provided 120 min after exercise) was unchanged after 60 min running at 70% $\dot{V}O_{2peak}$, but was increased after 60 min walking performed at the same relative intensity in a different group of women. The strength of this evidence is limited however by the between-measures design and the stark differences in body composition and cardiorespiratory fitness between the two groups. In another study, Pomerleau and colleagues [79] reported that ad libitum energy intake was increased 1 h after brisk walking at 70% $\dot{V}O_{2peak}$ in healthy, young women. However, this change did not translate to altered energy intake over the remainder of the day after the provision of an ad libitum meal 6.5 h after exercise and an overnight snack bag. This highlights the importance of monitoring feeding behaviour over longer time periods.

Regardless of whether absolute energy intake remained unchanged, increased or decreased in response to acute exercise in the studies cited thus far, relative energy intake (total energy intake minus net energy expenditure of exercise) is invariably lower after exercise compared with control in men and women. Whilst this suggests that the exercise-induced energy deficit is maintained after exercise, which may have significant implications for weight management, it should be noted that the short-term follow up in these studies prevents us from drawing conclusions about behavioural and physiological responses over a greater period of time.

Studies directly comparing men and women have demonstrated that total energy intake is greater in men compared with women [14,15], but this difference disappears after adjustment for lean body mass [15]. These findings coupled with the higher appetite ratings reported in men in the study conducted by Alajmi and colleagues [15] lend support to the theory that lean body mass, as the largest contributor to resting metabolic rate, is a primary determinant of appetite control and energy intake [24,25].

In addition to the appetite and hormone responses discussed in the previous section, Hagobian and colleagues [14] reported that absolute energy intake was unchanged in response to a single bout of cycling inducing a similar energy expenditure (30% of total daily energy expenditure) in men and women (energy expenditure: men, 975 kcal; women, 713 kcal) (Figure 2). The authors observed large variability in the energy intake responses (note large SDs on Figure 2 especially for men) with evidence of both higher and lower energy intake after exercise compared with a resting control condition in both men and women, which supports previous acute exercise and appetite regulation studies in healthy weight [78] and overweight and obese [62] women. Although the authors reported no significant change in energy intake after acute exercise in men or women, it is worth noting that mean ad libitum energy intake was higher in men after exercise (Figure 2) [14]. A closer examination of the mean differences and estimated standardised effect sizes revealed that energy intake after the exercise bout was 432 kcal higher than control in men (effect size = 0.68 indicating a moderate to large effect) compared with a 1 kcal increase after exercise in women (effect size = 0.004 indicating a trivial effect) (Figure 2). While this opposes the hypothesis that women are more likely to compensate for acute exercise-induced energy deficits by increasing energy intake, the conclusion that energy intake was unchanged in men should perhaps be interpreted with caution.

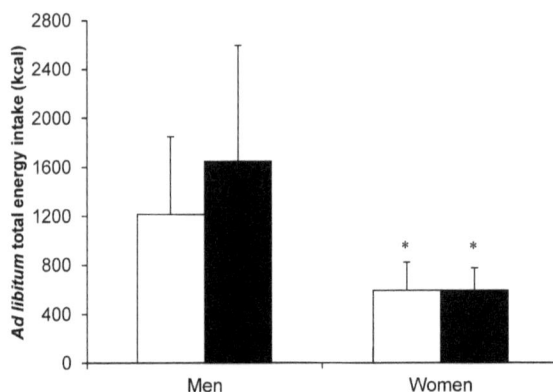

Figure 2. Total ad libitum energy intake during a single laboratory-based buffet meal in the control (□) and exercise (■) conditions in 11 men and 10 women. Exercise involved a single bout of cycling performed at 70% peak oxygen uptake until 30% of total daily energy expenditure was expended. * Significant difference between women and men $p \leq 0.05$. Values are mean (SD). Data from reference [14]. © 2008 Canadian Science Publishing or its licensors. Reproduced with permission.

Subsequent studies investigating potential sex-based differences have reported no change in absolute energy intake in response to a single bout of running [15] and accumulating short bouts of walking to break up sedentary time [66]. Furthermore, these studies have consistently reported a lower relative energy intake after acute exercise compared with control in both sexes, suggesting that acute exercise suppressed relative energy intake independent of sex [14,15,66].

5. Chronic Effects of Exercise on Appetite, Appetite-Regulatory Hormones and Energy Intake

Although acute exercise studies provide important information regarding appetite regulation, exercise training studies are required to discern the long-term effects of exercise on energy balance and weight control. Exercise training studies are now reviewed with continued focus on appetite sensations, appetite-regulatory hormones and energy intake responses between men and women. It should be noted that few well-controlled exercise training studies have been conducted with many studies inherently limited by methodological constraints such as unsupervised exercise, self-reported energy intake, low exercise-induced energy expenditure and a lack of objective measures to quantify exercise energy expenditure.

5.1. Appetite and Appetite-Regulatory Hormones

Alterations in ghrelin concentrations after chronic exercise have been reported in conjunction with favourable changes in body weight. Specifically, weight loss in response to an exercise intervention has been shown to elevate total ghrelin concentrations in healthy weight and overweight and obese women in the fasted state and postprandially (reviewed by [40]). In contrast, Guelfi and colleagues [80] reported no effect of 12 weeks of aerobic or resistance exercise on fasting and postprandial hunger and concentrations of acylated ghrelin and PYY in overweight and obese men, despite a reduction in body fat mass in both exercise interventions. However, the authors reported lower fasting and postprandial leptin concentrations after exercise, which has been observed in other studies with men and women after exercise-induced weight loss [81,82]. Furthermore, chronic exercise studies resulting in weight loss in women appear to reduce fasting insulin concentrations [83,84], but have little effect on fasting total PYY and GLP-1_{7-36} concentrations [84,85].

Several exercise and appetite training studies recruiting both men and women have presented findings with the data for men and women combined [36,86,87]. Although these studies are informative, it is not possible to elucidate the direct effect of sex on the observed responses. Nevertheless, short-term exercise training without weight loss (1 h of daily walking at 70% $\dot{V}O_{2peak}$ for 15 days) resulted in no changes in appetite or circulating concentrations of total PYY and insulin in obese men and women [87]. Martins and colleagues [36,86] have performed two studies investigating appetite and appetite-regulatory hormone responses to standardised meals in overweight and obese men and women undertaking 12 weeks of supervised aerobic exercise resulting in weight loss. The exercise intervention reduced fasting insulin concentrations but resulted in an increase in fasting acylated ghrelin concentrations and hunger perceptions [36]. In the postprandial state, circulating insulin was reduced along with a greater suppression in acylated ghrelin and a tendency for increased PYY and GLP-1 concentrations compared with levels before the intervention [36]. Furthermore, fasting and postprandial concentrations of leptin were reduced after the exercise intervention [86]. These findings led the authors to conclude that in response to chronic exercise, overweight individuals may balance the increased drive to eat with a concomitant increase in the satiety response to a meal, which supports previous findings in overweight and obese men [38].

In many of the studies discussed thus far, participants maintained their usual diet and subsequently lost body mass and fat mass by the end of the chronic exercise intervention. Therefore, it is difficult to determine whether the reported exercise-induced changes in appetite control are attributable to weight loss or to exercise training *per se*. In this regard, the study by Kanaley and colleagues [87] discussed previously did not report changes in appetite or appetite-regulatory hormones (total PYY, and insulin) in response to short-term exercise training without weight loss. Furthermore, total ghrelin concentrations were unchanged after exercise training in women who did not experience weight loss [85,88], and a study conducted in overweight adolescents observed no changes in fasting acylated ghrelin when body weight remained stable during the eight-month supervised exercise intervention [89]. Therefore, it is likely that alterations in appetite-regulatory hormones arise as a secondary consequence to changes in body mass.

Early evidence of exercise-induced sex differences in appetite hormones was provided by Hickey and colleagues [90]. In this study, 12 weeks of aerobic exercise training, without a change in body mass or body fat, significantly reduced fasting insulin and leptin concentrations in women but not in men. Subsequently, Hagobian and colleagues [13] examined appetite hormone responses to meal intake before and after four consecutive days of exercise in previously sedentary overweight and obese men and women. Daily aerobic exercise was performed on a treadmill at 50%–65% $\dot{V}O_{2peak}$ resulting in an energy expenditure equivalent to ~30% of total daily energy expenditure and was completed with and without dietary replacement of the exercise-induced energy deficit. The authors reported that acylated ghrelin concentrations were higher and insulin concentrations were lower after both exercise interventions in women (Figure 3). In contrast, although men demonstrated lower insulin concentrations in the energy deficit condition, this effect was eliminated with energy replacement and acylated ghrelin was not different after exercise regardless of energy status (Figure 3). These findings suggest that women experience perturbations in appetite-regulatory hormones conducive to appetite stimulation in response to the initiation of exercise training. This is consistent with the hypothesis that the mechanisms governing energy balance are more tightly regulated in women than men.

However, in the Midwest Exercise Trial, lower insulin concentrations were observed in men but not women after the 16-month exercise training intervention [32]. This was accompanied by a divergent weight loss response to exercise training (discussed previously) which, coupled with the greater exercise energy expenditure in men, is likely to explain the differential insulin findings between this investigation and that of Hagobian and colleagues [13].

Although replacing the exercise-induced energy deficit suppressed appetite perceptions in men but not women, appetite was not altered when the energy deficit was maintained in either sex [13]. This supports a previous study reporting no change in postprandial appetite in response to 14 days of moderate- or high-intensity exercise training in lean men and women [91]. In another study, sex-based differences in body weight and appetite were examined in response to a 12-week supervised aerobic exercise intervention in overweight and obese men and women [8]. The 12-week exercise program resulted in similar reductions in body mass and body fat in the male and female participants. Furthermore, although fasting hunger ratings were elevated after the exercise training intervention, the magnitude of change was similar between the sexes and this difference did not translate to altered hunger responses in the postprandial period.

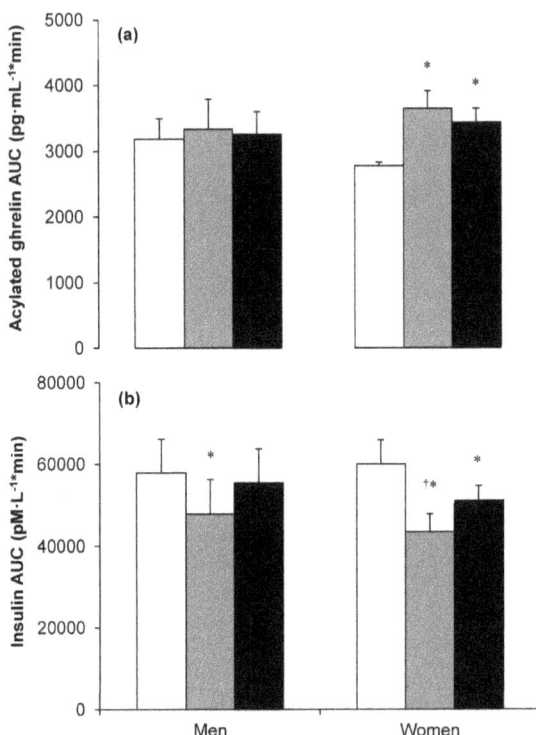

Figure 3. Total area under the curve (AUC) for plasma acylated ghrelin (**a**) and insulin (**b**) concentrations in the control (□), exercise with energy deficit (▨) and exercise with energy balance (■) conditions in nine men and nine women. Exercise involved four consecutive days of treadmill exercise at 50%–65% peak oxygen uptake until 30% of total daily energy expenditure was expended. * Significant difference between exercise intervention and control; † Significant difference between exercise with energy deficit and exercise with energy balance. Values are mean (error bars not stated in original article). Data reproduced from reference [13]. © The American Physiological Society. Reproduced with permission.

5.2. Energy Intake

Current evidence suggests that increasing energy expenditure during short-term exercise training (3 to 14 days) elicits partial compensations in energy intake [91–94]. Furthermore, a recent systematic review concluded that longer term exercise training studies (>2 weeks to 18 months) typically observe no change in energy intake across the training intervention [95]. However, the authors recognised that the available literature is prone to various methodological shortcomings as highlighted previously (e.g., unsupervised exercise, self-reported energy intake) which makes it difficult to interpret the findings with confidence.

A recent study directly comparing isoenergetic three-day energy deficits imposed by diet or exercise reported that dietary restriction stimulated a compensatory increase in ad libitum energy intake that was not observed in response to exercise [96]. This supports the findings from acute studies demonstrating rapid compensatory changes (appetite, appetite-regulatory hormones, energy intake) in response to diet-, but not exercise-induced energy deficits in men [71] and women [15]. These findings suggest that dietary restriction may represent a greater challenge to appetite regulation and energy balance than exercise, highlighting the importance of exercise to facilitate weight management in men and women [3].

A potential sex difference in energy intake responses during short-term exercise training was uncovered in two separate studies by Stubbs and colleagues [93,97]. Specifically, the authors reported that increasing energy expenditure through exercise training (seven days daily moderate- or high-intensity exercise) resulted in a partial compensation in energy intake in healthy women that equated to ~33% of the additional exercise-induced energy expenditure [93]. In contrast, there was no compensation in the energy intake response to an identical training stimulus in healthy men [97]. However, it is worth noting that energy intake was self-recorded in these studies through subjective dietary records and self-weighed intakes. This method of recording energy intake is particularly susceptible to participant bias, which makes it challenging to reconcile self-reported food intake with actual intake [98].

In a subsequent study adopting objective measures of both energy intake and energy expenditure, evidence of partial compensations in energy intake emerged after 14 days of supervised daily exercise which was equivalent to ~30% of the exercise-induced energy deficit [91]. This response was observed when energy intake data were combined for men and women, but only reached significance in men when analysed independently by sex [91]. This is consistent with an early study demonstrating that men, but not women, increase energy intake in response to five days of daily exercise, yet neither sex fully compensated for the imposed exercise energy expenditure [92]. Consequently, these findings refute the hypothesis that women compensate for chronic exercise-induced energy deficits by increasing energy intake.

When data is combined for men and women, studies investigating the effect of 12 weeks of supervised exercise (five days·week^{-1}, 500 kcal·session^{-1}) on body composition and appetite control have reported no exercise-induced change in energy intake assessed using self-reported food diaries [36] or laboratory-based test meals [99]. Furthermore, Westerterp and colleagues [5] reported no significant change in energy intake assessed using a self-reported seven-day weighed diary in men or women after 40 weeks of endurance training. In the Midwest Exercise Trials, energy intake was assessed using a combination of ad libitum meals in the University cafeteria and 24 h recall in overweight and obese men and women undergoing a supervised aerobic exercise program for 10 [9] or 16 months [6]. Similarly, no difference in energy intake was reported after the exercise training interventions in either sex [6,9].

When exercise is supervised and energy intake is quantified objectively using laboratory-based ad libitum meals, no changes in daily energy intake were observed in overweight and obese men or women after a 12-week aerobic exercise intervention (Figure 4) [8]. The authors of this study also highlighted the large variability in individual weight loss responses, both in magnitude and direction, which may afford some insight into why many individuals do not achieve their predicted changes in body composition with chronic exercise. Such heterogeneity in response to alterations in energy balance has been recognised previously [8,9,29,35,37,38]. Interestingly and pertinent to this review, overweight and obese men and women typically demonstrate a similar degree of individual variability when the exercise-induced energy expenditure is equivalent between the sexes [8,38]. For example, Caudwell and colleagues [8] reported body mass changes ranging from −14.7 to 2.0 kg in men and −10.0 to 4 kg in women. Furthermore, when participants are retrospectively classified as "responders" or "non-responders" (based on their actual weight loss relative to their predicted weight loss), there is some evidence supporting higher ad libitum energy intake in individuals experiencing lower than their predicted weight loss [29,37,38].

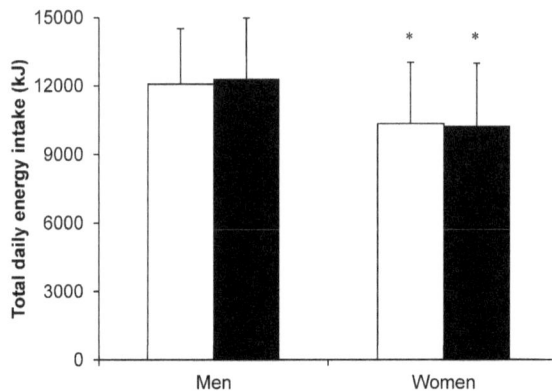

Figure 4. Total daily energy intake before (□) and after (■) a 12-week aerobic exercise training intervention in overweight and obese men (*n* = 35) and women (*n* = 72). Total daily energy intake was quantified objectively using laboratory-based test meal days at Weeks 0 and 12. On each day, participants were provided with an individualised fixed-energy breakfast (ad libitum at Week 0), fixed-energy lunch, ad libitum dinner and evening snack box. * Significant difference between women and men $p \leq 0.05$. Values are mean (SD). Data from reference [8]. © Wolters Kluwer Health, Inc. Reproduced with permission.

6. Implications and Future Directions

Scientific interest in potential sex-based differences in appetite regulation stems from initial evidence suggesting that men experience greater body mass and body fat reductions after exercise training than women [5,6]. Furthermore, evidence from an evolutionary biology perspective suggesting that women have evolved to store body fat to preserve energy balance and reproductive function has also driven research endeavour in this regard [10,12]. However, more recent experimental work has questioned the prevailing view that exercise is less effective for inducing weight loss in women, with several studies showing equivalent effects of exercise training on body composition in both sexes when the exercise-induced energy expenditure is matched [8,9]. Collectively, the balance of findings' presented in this review suggest that men and women do not exhibit different responses (appetite, appetite-regulatory hormones, energy intake) to acute or chronic exercise-induced energy deficits. This has important implications for men and women engaging in exercise for health, and supports the promotion of exercise as a weight management tool for all. However, it is likely that women will need to exercise for a longer duration and/or at a higher intensity to achieve a similar exercise energy expenditure as men.

The findings provided within the current literature from experiments focussing on weight loss can be useful in informing individuals about exercise and dietary approaches for health. In this regard, it has been established that exercise-induced energy deficits stimulate smaller changes in appetite, appetite-regulatory hormones and energy intake compared with dietary restriction in both men [71,96] and women [15]. This may assist in informing an individuals' decision regarding their preferred method of inducing an energy deficit for weight loss and also provide information regarding the anticipated homeostatic responses (i.e., greater appetite stimulation with food restriction).

Considering that exercise training appears to elicit at most a partial, but incomplete, compensation in energy intake in both sexes, it seems that men and women can endure prolonged periods in an exercise-induced energy deficit which may facilitate the development of a negative energy balance. Such incomplete compensation also supports evidence that larger exercise-induced energy deficits promote greater weight loss during an exercise intervention [34,35]. However, it is worth reiterating the considerable variability in responses (albeit to a similar degree in men and women), with some individuals appearing susceptible to increased hunger and energy intake with exercise training that attenuates the degree of weight loss [29,37,38]. Nevertheless, exercise training triggers marked improvements in other important outcomes in the absence of weight loss (e.g., cardiorespiratory fitness, body composition, insulin sensitivity) [26], which is important for those undertaking exercise for health benefits.

Although a considerable body of literature has developed understanding of the relationship between exercise, appetite and weight control, there are only a few studies which have directly focused on sex-based differences. Additional research is required to expand the evidence base before definitive conclusions can be drawn. This should include different types of exercise and insights into the mechanisms governing appetite control, both of which appear sparse in the current literature. Studies investigating a wider array of appetite parameters, particularly appetite hormones beyond the initiation of exercise training, between men and women would also be welcomed. Furthermore, considering potential sex-based differences in non-homeostatic factors governing energy balance (e.g., neuronal responses [100], and cognitive/behavioural cues [101]) is another important line of scientific inquiry and will provide a more holistic insight into appetite regulation in men and women. Future research into the appetite, appetite-regulatory hormone and energy intake responses of elite athletes to exercise and dietary interventions also represents an important future research direction to better understand energy balance and the consequences of energy manipulation in this population. It is imperative that acute and chronic investigations adopt mixed-measures designs and utilise objective measures of energy balance components when examining interactions among appetite, appetite-regulatory hormones and energy intake between men and women.

7. Conclusions

This review has demonstrated that appetite, appetite-regulatory hormone and energy intake responses to acute exercise-induced energy deficits are similar between men and women. Specifically, the consensus of evidence suggests that acute exercise transiently suppresses appetite, and does not stimulate compensatory changes in appetite, appetite-regulatory hormones or energy intake in the hours after acute exercise in either sex. Evidence derived from exercise training studies appear less conclusive, with limited evidence that women, but not men, respond to the initiation of exercise training with compensatory changes in appetite-regulatory hormones conducive to appetite stimulation. However, it is not known whether this change translates into long-term differences after a more sustained period of exercise training. Furthermore, evidence does not support a sex dimorphism in appetite or energy intake when assessed objectively, and increasing energy expenditure through exercise elicits at most a partial energy compensation in both sexes. Few studies have directly compared appetite, appetite-regulatory hormone and energy intake responses to acute and chronic exercise interventions between men and women. Therefore, these conclusions are supported by evidence drawn from the limited studies directly comparing the sexes and supplemented by those conducted in men and women separately. A better understanding of whether appetite, appetite-regulatory hormone and energy intake responses to exercise-induced energy deficits differ by sex may contribute to the development of more effective weight management strategies.

Acknowledgments: This work is supported by the National Institute for Health Research (NIHR) Diet, Lifestyle & Physical Activity Biomedical Research Unit based at University Hospitals of Leicester and Loughborough University. The views expressed are those of the authors and not necessarily those of the NHS, the NIHR or the Department of Health.

Author Contributions: A.E.T. and D.J.S. conceived and designed the review content. A.E.T. wrote the manuscript. K.D., J.A.K. and D.J.S. provided critical revisions to the manuscript. All authors approved the final manuscript.

Conflicts of Interest: The authors declare no conflict of interest.

References

1. Wang, Y.C.; McPherson, K.; Marsh, T.; Gortmaker, S.L.; Brown, M. Health and economic burden of the projected obesity trends in the USA and the UK. *Lancet* **2011**, *378*, 815–825. [CrossRef]
2. Ng, M.; Fleming, T.; Robinson, M.; Thomson, B.; Graetz, N.; Margono, C.; Mullany, E.C.; Biryukov, S.; Abbafati, C.; Abera, S.F.; et al. Global, regional, and national prevalence of overweight and obesity in children and adults during 1980–2013: A systematic analysis for the Global Burden of Disease Study 2013. *Lancet* **2014**, *384*, 766–781. [CrossRef]
3. Donnelly, J.E.; Blair, S.N.; Jakicic, J.M.; Manore, M.M.; Rankin, J.W.; Smith, B.K. American College of Sports Medicine Position Stand. Appropriate physical activity intervention strategies for weight loss and prevention of weight regain for adults. *Med. Sci. Sports Exerc.* **2009**, *41*, 459–471. [CrossRef] [PubMed]
4. Schubert, M.M.; Sabapathy, S.; Leveritt, M.; Desbrow, B. Acute exercise and hormones related to appetite regulation: A meta-analysis. *Sports Med.* **2014**, *44*, 387–403. [CrossRef] [PubMed]
5. Westerterp, K.R.; Meijer, G.A.L.; Janssen, E.M.E.; Saris, W.H.M.; Ten Hoor, F. Long-term effect of physical activity on energy balance and body composition. *Br. J. Nutr.* **1992**, *68*, 21–30. [CrossRef] [PubMed]
6. Donnelly, J.E.; Hill, J.O.; Jacobsen, D.J.; Potteiger, J.; Sullivan, D.K.; Johnson, S.L.; Heelan, K.; Hise, M.; Fennessey, P.V.; Sonko, B.; et al. Effects of a 16-month randomized controlled exercise trial on body weight and composition in young, overweight men and women: The Midwest Exercise Trial. *Arch. Intern. Med.* **2003**, *163*, 1343–1350. [CrossRef] [PubMed]
7. Irving, B.A.; Weltman, J.Y.; Patrie, J.T.; Davis, C.K.; Brock, D.W.; Swift, D.; Barrett, E.J.; Gaesser, G.A.; Weltman, A. Effects of exercise training intensity on nocturnal growth hormone secretion in obese adults with the metabolic syndrome. *J. Clin. Endocrinol. Metab.* **2009**, *94*, 1979–1986. [CrossRef] [PubMed]
8. Caudwell, P.; Gibbons, C.; Hopkins, M.; King, N.; Finlayson, G.; Blundell, J. No sex difference in body fat in response to supervised and measured exercise. *Med. Sci. Sports Exerc.* **2013**, *45*, 351–358. [CrossRef] [PubMed]
9. Donnelly, J.E.; Honas, J.J.; Smith, B.K.; Mayo, M.; Gibson, C.A.; Sullivan, D.K.; Lee, J.; Herrmann, S.D.; Lambourne, K.; Washburn, R.A. Aerobic exercise alone results in clinically significant weight loss for men and women: Midwest Exercise Trial 2. *Obesity* **2013**, *21*, E219–E228. [CrossRef] [PubMed]
10. Wade, G.N.; Jones, J.E. Neuroendocrinology of nutritional infertility. *Am. J. Physiol. Regul. Integr. Comp. Physiol.* **2004**, *287*, R1277–R1296. [CrossRef] [PubMed]
11. Hagobian, T.A.; Braun, B. Physical activity and hormonal regulation of appetite: Sex differences and weight control. *Exerc. Sport Sci. Rev.* **2010**, *38*, 25–30. [CrossRef] [PubMed]
12. Lieberman, D.E. Is exercise really medicine? An evolutionary perspective. *Curr. Sports Med. Rep.* **2015**, *14*, 313–319. [CrossRef] [PubMed]
13. Hagobian, T.A.; Sharoff, C.G.; Stephens, B.R.; Wade, G.N.; Silva, J.E.; Chipkin, S.R.; Braun, B. Effects of exercise on energy-regulating hormones and appetite in men and women. *Am. J. Physiol. Regul. Integr. Comp. Physiol.* **2009**, *296*, R233–R242. [CrossRef] [PubMed]
14. Hagobian, T.A.; Yamashiro, M.; Hinkel-Lipsker, J.; Streder, K.; Evero, N.; Hackney, T. Effects of acute exercise on appetite hormones and ad libitum energy intake in men and women. *Appl. Physiol. Nutr. Metab.* **2013**, *38*, 66–72. [CrossRef] [PubMed]
15. Alajmi, N.; Deighton, K.; King, J.A.; Reischak-Oliveira, A.; Wasse, L.K.; Jones, J.; Batterham, R.L.; Stensel, D.J. Appetite and energy intake responses to acute energy deficits in females versus males. *Med. Sci. Sports Exerc.* **2016**, *48*, 412–420. [CrossRef] [PubMed]
16. Karra, E.; Batterham, R.L. The role of gut hormones in the regulation of body weight and energy homeostasis. *Mol. Cell. Endocrinol.* **2010**, *316*, 120–128. [CrossRef] [PubMed]
17. Hussain, S.S.; Bloom, S.R. The regulation of food intake by the gut-brain axis: Implications for obesity. *Int. J. Obes.* **2013**, *37*, 625–633. [CrossRef] [PubMed]
18. Wynne, K.; Stanley, S.; McGowan, B.; Bloom, S. Appetite control. *J. Endocrinol.* **2005**, *184*, 291–318. [CrossRef] [PubMed]
19. Cummings, D.E.; Overduin, J. Gastrointestinal regulation of food intake. *J. Clin. Investig.* **2007**, *117*, 13–23. [CrossRef] [PubMed]

20. Ghigo, E.; Broglio, F.; Arvat, E.; Maccario, M.; Papotti, M.; Muccioli, G. Ghrelin: More than a natural GH secretagogue and/or an orexigenic factor. *Clin. Endocrinol.* **2005**, *62*, 1–17. [CrossRef] [PubMed]
21. Cummings, D.E.; Frayo, R.S.; Marmonier, C.; Aubert, R.; Chapelot, D. Plasma ghrelin levels and hunger scores in humans initiating meals voluntarily without time- and food-related cues. *Am. J. Physiol. Endocrinol. Metab.* **2004**, *287*, E297–E304. [CrossRef] [PubMed]
22. Batterham, R.L.; Cohen, M.A.; Ellis, S.M.; Le Roux, C.W.; Withers, D.J.; Frost, G.S.; Ghatei, M.A.; Bloom, S.R. Inhibition of food intake in obese subjects by peptide YY$_{3-36}$. *N. Engl. J. Med.* **2003**, *349*, 941–948. [CrossRef] [PubMed]
23. Verdich, C.; Flint, A.; Gutzwiller, J.P.; Näslund, E.; Beglinger, C.; Hellström, P.M.; Long, S.J.; Morgan, L.M.; Holst, J.J.; Astrup, A. A meta-analysis of the effect of glucagon-like peptide-1 (7–36) amide on ad libitum energy intake in humans. *J. Clin. Endocrinol. Metab.* **2001**, *86*, 4382–4389. [CrossRef] [PubMed]
24. Blundell, J.E.; Caudwell, P.; Gibbons, C.; Hopkins, M.; Naslund, E.; King, N.; Finlayson, G. Role of resting metabolic rate and energy expenditure in hunger and appetite control: A new formulation. *Dis. Model. Mech.* **2012**, *5*, 608–613. [CrossRef] [PubMed]
25. Blundell, J.E.; Gibbons, C.; Caudwell, P.; Finlayson, G.; Hopkins, M. Appetite control and energy balance: Impact of exercise. *Obes. Rev.* **2015**, *16*, 67–76. [CrossRef] [PubMed]
26. King, N.A.; Hopkins, M.; Caudwell, P.; Stubbs, R.J.; Blundell, J.E. Beneficial effects of exercise: Shifting the focus from body weight to other markers of health. *Br. J. Sports Med.* **2009**, *43*, 924–927. [CrossRef] [PubMed]
27. Shaw, K.A.; Gennat, H.C.; O'Rourke, P.; Del Mar, C. Exercise for overweight or obesity. *Cochrane Database Syst. Rev.* **2006**, *18*. [CrossRef]
28. Catenacci, V.A.; Wyatt, H.R. The role of physical activity in producing and maintaining weight loss. *Nat. Clin. Pract. Endocrinol. Metab.* **2007**, *3*, 518–529. [CrossRef] [PubMed]
29. King, N.A.; Hopkins, M.; Caudwell, P.; Stubbs, R.J.; Blundell, J.E. Individual variability following 12-weeks of supervised exercise: Identification and characterization of compensation for exercise-induced weight loss. *Int. J. Obes.* **2008**, *32*, 177–184. [CrossRef] [PubMed]
30. Donnelly, J.E.; Smith, B.K. Is exercise effective for weight loss with ad libitum diet? Energy balance, compensation, and gender differences. *Exerc. Sport Sci. Rev.* **2005**, *33*, 169–174. [CrossRef] [PubMed]
31. Després, J.P.; Bouchard, C.; Savard, R.; Tremblay, A.; Marcotte, M.; Thériault, G. The effect of a 20-week endurance training program on adipose-tissue morphology and lipolysis in men and women. *Metabolism* **1984**, *33*, 235–239. [CrossRef]
32. Potteiger, J.A.; Jacobsen, D.J.; Donnelly, J.E.; Hill, J.O. Glucose and insulin responses following 16 months of exercise training in overweight adults: The Midwest Exercise Trial. *Metabolism* **2003**, *52*, 1175–1181. [CrossRef]
33. Caudwell, P.; Gibbons, C.; Finlayson, G.; Näslund, E.; Blundell, J. Exercise and weight loss: No sex differences in body weight response to exercise. *Exerc. Sport Sci. Rev.* **2014**, *42*, 92–101. [CrossRef] [PubMed]
34. Jakicic, J.M.; Marcus, B.H.; Lang, W.; Janney, C. Effect of exercise on 24-month weight loss maintenance in overweight women. *Arch. Intern. Med.* **2008**, *168*, 1550–1559. [CrossRef] [PubMed]
35. Barwell, N.D.; Malkova, D.; Leggate, M.; Gill, J.M.R. Individual responsiveness to exercise-induced fat loss is associated with change in resting substrate utilization. *Metabolism* **2009**, *58*, 1320–1328. [CrossRef] [PubMed]
36. Martins, C.; Kulseng, B.; King, N.A.; Holst, J.J.; Blundell, J.E. The effects of exercise-induced weight loss on appetite-related peptides and motivation to eat. *J. Clin. Endocrinol. Metab.* **2010**, *95*, 1609–1616. [CrossRef] [PubMed]
37. Caudwell, P.; Hopkins, M.; King, N.A.; Stubbs, R.J.; Blundell, J.E. Exercise alone is not enough: Weight loss also needs a healthy (Mediterranean) diet? *Public Health Nutr.* **2009**, *12*, 1663–1666. [CrossRef] [PubMed]
38. King, N.A.; Caudwell, P.P.; Hopkins, M.; Stubbs, J.R.; Naslund, E.; Blundell, J.E. Dual-process action of exercise on appetite control: Increase in orexigenic drive but improvement in meal-induced satiety. *Am. J. Clin. Nutr.* **2009**, *90*, 921–927. [CrossRef] [PubMed]
39. Stensel, D. Exercise, appetite and appetite-regulating hormones: Implications for food intake and weight control. *Ann. Nutr. Metab.* **2010**, *57*, 36–42. [CrossRef] [PubMed]
40. King, J.A.; Wasse, L.K.; Stensel, D.J.; Nimmo, M.A. Exercise and ghrelin. A narrative overview of research. *Appetite* **2013**, *68*, 83–91. [CrossRef] [PubMed]

41. Schubert, M.M.; Desbrow, B.; Sabapathy, S.; Leveritt, M. Acute exercise and subsequent energy intake. A meta-analysis. *Appetite* **2013**, *63*, 92–104. [CrossRef] [PubMed]

42. Deighton, K.; Stensel, D.J. Creating an acute energy deficit without stimulating compensatory increases in appetite: Is there an optimal exercise protocol? *Proc. Nutr. Soc.* **2014**, *73*, 352–358. [CrossRef] [PubMed]

43. Hazell, T.J.; Islam, H.; Townsend, L.K.; Schmale, M.S.; Copeland, J.L. Effects of exercise intensity on plasma concentrations of appetite-regulating hormones: Potential mechanisms. *Appetite* **2016**, *98*, 80–88. [CrossRef] [PubMed]

44. King, N.A.; Burley, V.J.; Blundell, J.E. Exercise-induced suppression of appetite: Effects on food intake and implications for energy balance. *Eur. J. Clin. Nutr.* **1994**, *48*, 715–724. [PubMed]

45. Broom, D.R.; Stensel, D.J.; Bishop, N.C.; Burns, S.F.; Miyashita, M. Exercise-induced suppression of acylated ghrelin in humans. *J. Appl. Physiol.* **2007**, *102*, 2165–2171. [CrossRef] [PubMed]

46. Broom, D.R.; Batterham, R.L.; King, J.A.; Stensel, D.J. Influence of resistance and aerobic exercise on hunger, circulating levels of acylated ghrelin, and peptide YY in healthy males. *Am. J. Physiol. Regul. Integr. Comp. Physiol.* **2009**, *296*, R29–R35. [CrossRef] [PubMed]

47. Ueda, S.; Yoshikawa, T.; Katsura, Y.; Usui, T.; Nakao, H.; Fujimoto, S. Changes in gut hormone levels and negative energy balance during aerobic exercise in obese young males. *J. Endocrinol.* **2009**, *201*, 151–159. [CrossRef] [PubMed]

48. King, J.A.; Miyashita, M.; Wasse, L.K.; Stensel, D.J. Influence of prolonged treadmill running on appetite, energy intake and circulating concentrations of acylated ghrelin. *Appetite* **2010**, *54*, 492–498. [CrossRef] [PubMed]

49. King, J.A.; Wasse, L.K.; Broom, D.R.; Stensel, D.J. Influence of brisk walking on appetite, energy intake, and plasma acylated ghrelin. *Med. Sci. Sports Exerc.* **2010**, *42*, 485–492. [CrossRef] [PubMed]

50. Martins, C.; Morgan, L.M.; Bloom, S.R.; Robertson, M.D. Effects of exercise on gut peptides, energy intake and appetite. *J. Endocrinol.* **2007**, *193*, 251–258. [CrossRef] [PubMed]

51. Becker, G.F.; Macedo, R.C.O.; Cunha, G.S.; Martins, J.B.; Laitano, O.; Reischak-Oliveira, A. Combined effects of aerobic exercise and high-carbohydrate meal on plasma acylated ghrelin and levels of hunger. *Appl. Physiol. Nutr. Metab.* **2012**, *37*, 184–192. [CrossRef] [PubMed]

52. Deighton, K.; Barry, R.; Connon, C.E.; Stensel, D.J. Appetite, gut hormone and energy intake responses to low volume sprint interval and traditional endurance exercise. *Eur. J. Appl. Physiol.* **2013**, *113*, 1147–1156. [CrossRef] [PubMed]

53. Deighton, K.; Karra, E.; Batterham, R.L.; Stensel, D.J. Appetite, energy intake, and PYY_{3-36} responses to energy-matched continuous exercise and submaximal high-intensity exercise. *Appl. Physiol. Nutr. Metab.* **2013**, *38*, 947–952. [CrossRef] [PubMed]

54. King, J.A.; Wasse, L.K.; Stensel, D.J. The acute effects of swimming on appetite, food intake, and plasma acylated ghrelin. *J. Obes.* **2010**, *2011*. [CrossRef] [PubMed]

55. Balaguera-Cortes, L.; Wallman, K.E.; Fairchild, T.J.; Guelfi, K.J. Energy intake and appetite-related hormones following acute aerobic and resistance exercise. *Appl. Physiol. Nutr. Metab.* **2011**, *36*, 958–966. [CrossRef] [PubMed]

56. Metcalfe, R.S.; Koumanov, F.; Ruffino, J.S.; Stokes, K.A.; Holman, G.D.; Thompson, D.; Vollaard, N.B.J. Physiological and molecular responses to an acute bout of reduced-exertion high-intensity interval training (REHIT). *Eur. J. Appl. Physiol.* **2015**, *115*, 2321–2334. [CrossRef] [PubMed]

57. Malkova, D.; McLaughlin, R.; Manthou, E.; Wallace, A.M.; Nimmo, M.A. Effect of moderate-intensity exercise session on preprandial and postprandial responses of circulating ghrelin and appetite. *Horm. Metab. Res.* **2008**, *40*, 410–415. [CrossRef] [PubMed]

58. Sim, A.Y.; Wallman, K.E.; Fairchild, T.J.; Guelfi, K.J. High-intensity intermittent exercise attenuates *ad-libitum* energy intake. *Int. J. Obes.* **2014**, *38*, 417–422. [CrossRef] [PubMed]

59. Howe, S.M.; Hand, T.M.; Larson-Meyer, D.E.; Austin, K.J.; Alexander, B.M.; Manore, M.M. No effect of exercise intensity on appetite in highly-trained endurance women. *Nutrients* **2016**, *8*, 223. [CrossRef] [PubMed]

60. Tiryaki-Sonmez, G.; Ozen, S.; Bugdayci, G.; Karli, U.; Ozen, G.; Cogalgil, S.; Schoenfeld, B.; Sozbir, K.; Aydin, K. Effect of exercise on appetite-regulating hormones in overweight women. *Biol. Sport* **2013**, *30*, 75–80. [CrossRef] [PubMed]

61. Tsofliou, F.; Pitsiladis, Y.P.; Malkova, D.; Wallace, A.M.; Lean, M.E.J. Moderate physical activity permits acute coupling between serum leptin and appetite-satiety measures in obese women. *Int. J. Obes. Relat. Metab. Disord.* **2003**, *27*, 1332–1339. [CrossRef] [PubMed]
62. Unick, J.L.; Otto, A.D.; Goodpaster, B.H.; Helsel, D.L.; Pellegrini, C.A.; Jakicic, J.M. Acute effect of walking on energy intake in overweight/obese women. *Appetite* **2010**, *55*, 413–419. [CrossRef] [PubMed]
63. King, N.A.; Snell, L.; Smith, R.D.; Blundell, J.E. Effects of short-term exercise on appetite responses in unrestrained females. *Eur. J. Clin. Nutr.* **1996**, *50*, 663–667. [PubMed]
64. Larson-Meyer, D.E.; Palm, S.; Bansal, A.; Austin, K.J.; Hart, A.M.; Alexander, B.M. Influence of running and walking on hormonal regulators of appetite in women. *J. Obes.* **2011**, *2012*. [CrossRef] [PubMed]
65. Kawano, H.; Motegi, F.; Ando, T.; Gando, Y.; Mineta, M.; Numao, S.; Miyashita, M.; Sakamoto, S.; Higuchi, M. Appetite after rope skipping may differ between males and females. *Obes. Res. Clin. Pract.* **2012**, *6*, e121–e127. [CrossRef] [PubMed]
66. Bailey, D.P.; Broom, D.R.; Chrismas, B.C.R.; Taylor, L.; Flynn, E.; Hough, J. Breaking up prolonged sitting time with walking does not affect appetite or gut hormone concentrations but does induce an energy deficit and suppresses postprandial glycaemia in sedentary adults. *Appl. Physiol. Nutr. Metab.* **2016**, *41*, 324–331. [CrossRef] [PubMed]
67. Geiker, N.R.; Ritz, C.; Pedersen, S.D.; Larsen, T.M.; Hill, J.O.; Astrup, A. A weight-loss program adapted to the menstrual cycle increases weight loss in healthy, overweight, premenopausal women: A 6-mo randomized controlled trial. *Am. J. Clin. Nutr.* **2016**, *104*, 15–20. [CrossRef] [PubMed]
68. Sung, E.; Han, A.; Hinrichs, T.; Vorgerd, M.; Manchado, C.; Platen, P. Effects of follicular versus luteal phase-based strength training in young women. *Springerplus* **2014**, *3*, 668. [CrossRef] [PubMed]
69. Buffenstein, R.; Poppitt, S.D.; McDevitt, R.M.; Prentice, A.M. Food intake and the menstrual cycle: A retrospective analysis, with implications for appetite research. *Physiol. Behav.* **1995**, *58*, 1067–1077. [CrossRef]
70. Brennan, I.M.; Feltrin, K.L.; Nair, N.S.; Hausken, T.; Little, T.J.; Gentilcore, D.; Wishart, J.M.; Jones, K.L.; Horowitz, M.; Feinle-Bisset, C. Effects of the phases of the menstrual cycle on gastric emptying, glycemia, plasma GLP-1 and insulin, and energy intake in healthy lean women. *Am. J. Physiol. Gastrointest. Liver Physiol.* **2009**, *297*, G602–G610. [CrossRef] [PubMed]
71. King, J.A.; Wasse, L.K.; Ewens, J.; Crystallis, K.; Emmanuel, J.; Batterham, R.L.; Stensel, D.J. Differential acylated ghrelin, peptide YY$_{3-36}$, appetite, and food intake responses to equivalent energy deficits created by exercise and food restriction. *J. Clin. Endocrinol. Metab.* **2011**, *96*, 1114–1121. [CrossRef] [PubMed]
72. Kelly, P.J.; Guelfi, K.J.; Wallman, K.E.; Fairchild, T.J. Mild dehydration does not reduce postexercise appetite or energy intake. *Med. Sci. Sports Exerc.* **2012**, *44*, 516–524. [CrossRef] [PubMed]
73. Wasse, L.K.; Sunderland, C.; King, J.A.; Batterham, R.L.; Stensel, D.J. Influence of rest and exercise at a simulated altitude of 4000 m on appetite, energy intake, and plasma concentrations of acylated ghrelin and peptide YY. *J. Appl. Physiol.* **2012**, *112*, 552–559. [CrossRef] [PubMed]
74. Bilski, J.; Mańko, G.; Brzozowski, T.; Pokorski, J.; Nitecki, J.; Nitecka, E.; Wilk-Frańczuk, M.; Ziółkowski, A.; Jaszcur-Nowicki, J.; Kruczkowski, D.; et al. Effects of exercise of different intensity on gut peptides, energy intake and appetite in young males. *Ann. Agric. Environ. Med.* **2013**, *20*, 787–793. [PubMed]
75. Westerterp-Plantenga, M.S.; Verwegen, C.R.T.; Ijedema, M.J.W.; Wijckmans, N.E.G.; Saris, W.H.M. Acute effects of exercise or sauna on appetite in obese and nonobese men. *Physiol. Behav.* **1997**, *62*, 1345–1354. [CrossRef]
76. George, V.A.; Morganstein, A. Effect of moderate intensity exercise on acute energy intake in normal and overweight females. *Appetite* **2003**, *40*, 43–46. [CrossRef]
77. Maraki, M.; Tsofliou, F.; Pitsiladis, Y.P.; Malkova, D.; Mutrie, N.; Higgins, S. Acute effects of a single exercise class on appetite, energy intake and mood. Is there a time of day effect? *Appetite* **2005**, *45*, 272–278. [CrossRef] [PubMed]
78. Finlayson, G.; Bryant, E.; Blundell, J.E.; King, N.A. Acute compensatory eating following exercise is associated with implicit hedonic wanting for food. *Physiol. Behav.* **2009**, *97*, 62–67. [CrossRef] [PubMed]
79. Pomerleau, M.; Imbeault, P.; Parker, T.; Doucet, E. Effects of exercise intensity on food intake and appetite in women. *Am. J. Clin. Nutr.* **2004**, *80*, 1230–1236. [PubMed]

80. Guelfi, K.J.; Donges, C.E.; Duffield, R. Beneficial effects of 12 weeks of aerobic compared with resistance exercise training on perceived appetite in previously sedentary overweight and obese men. *Metabolism* **2013**, *62*, 235–243. [CrossRef] [PubMed]

81. Okazaki, T.; Himeno, E.; Nanri, H.; Ogata, H.; Ikeda, M. Effects of mild aerobic exercise and a mild hypocaloric diet on plasma leptin in sedentary women. *Clin. Exp. Pharmacol. Physiol.* **1999**, *26*, 415–420. [CrossRef] [PubMed]

82. Thong, F.S.L.; Hudson, R.; Ross, R.; Janssen, I.; Graham, T.E. Plasma leptin in moderately obese men: Independent effects of weight loss and aerobic exercise. *Am. J. Physiol. Endocrinol. Metab.* **2000**, *279*, E307–E313. [PubMed]

83. Garcia, J.M.; Iyer, D.; Poston, W.S.C.; Marcelli, M.; Reeves, R.; Foreyt, J.; Balasubramanyam, A. Rise of plasma ghrelin with weight loss is not sustained during weight maintenance. *Obesity* **2006**, *14*, 1716–1723. [CrossRef] [PubMed]

84. Ueda, S.; Miyamoto, T.; Nakahara, H.; Shishido, T.; Usui, T.; Katsura, Y.; Yoshikawa, T.; Fujimoto, S. Effects of exercise training on gut hormone levels after a single bout of exercise in middle-aged Japanese women. *Springerplus* **2013**, *2*, 83. [CrossRef] [PubMed]

85. Scheid, J.L.; De Souza, M.J.; Leidy, H.J.; Williams, N.I. Ghrelin but not peptide YY is related to change in body weight and energy availability. *Med. Sci. Sports Exerc.* **2011**, *43*, 2063–2071. [CrossRef] [PubMed]

86. Martins, C.; Kulseng, B.; Rehfeld, J.F.; King, N.A.; Blundell, J.E. Effect of chronic exercise on appetite control in overweight and obese individuals. *Med. Sci. Sports Exerc.* **2013**, *45*, 805–812. [CrossRef] [PubMed]

87. Kanaley, J.A.; Heden, T.D.; Whaley-Connell, A.T.; Chockalingam, A.; Dellsperger, K.C.; Fairchild, T.J. Short-term aerobic exercise training increases postprandial pancreatic polypeptide but not peptide YY concentrations in obese individuals. *Int. J. Obes.* **2014**, *38*, 266–271. [CrossRef] [PubMed]

88. Leidy, H.J.; Gardner, J.K.; Frye, B.R.; Snook, M.L.; Schuchert, M.K.; Richard, E.L.; Williams, N.I. Circulating ghrelin is sensitive to changes in body weight during a diet and exercise program in normal-weight young women. *J. Clin. Endocrinol. Metab.* **2004**, *89*, 2659–2664. [CrossRef] [PubMed]

89. Jones, T.E.; Basilio, J.L.; Brophy, P.M.; McCammon, M.R.; Hickner, R.C. Long-term exercise training in overweight adolescents improves plasma peptide YY and resistin. *Obesity* **2009**, *17*, 1189–1195. [CrossRef] [PubMed]

90. Hickey, M.S.; Houmard, J.A.; Considine, R.V.; Tyndall, G.L.; Midgette, J.B.; Gavigan, K.E.; Weidner, M.L.; McCammon, M.R.; Israel, R.G.; Caro, J.F. Gender-dependent effects of exercise training on serum leptin levels in humans. *Am. J. Physiol.* **1997**, *272*, E562–E566. [PubMed]

91. Whybrow, S.; Hughes, D.A.; Ritz, P.; Johnstone, A.M.; Horgan, G.W.; King, N.; Blundell, J.E.; Stubbs, R.J. The effect of an incremental increase in exercise on appetite, eating behaviour and energy balance in lean men and women feeding ad libitum. *Br. J. Nutr.* **2008**, *100*, 1109–1115. [CrossRef] [PubMed]

92. Staten, M.A. The effect of exercise on food intake in men and women. *Am. J. Clin. Nutr.* **1991**, *53*, 27–31. [PubMed]

93. Stubbs, R.J.; Sepp, A.; Hughes, D.A.; Johnstone, A.M.; King, N.; Horgan, G.; Blundell, J.E. The effect of graded levels of exercise on energy intake and balance in free-living women. *Int. J. Obes. Relat. Metab. Disord.* **2002**, *26*, 866–869. [PubMed]

94. Farah, N.M.F.; Malkova, D.; Gill, J.M.R. Effects of exercise on postprandial responses to ad libitum feeding in overweight men. *Med. Sci. Sports Exerc.* **2010**, *42*, 2015–2022. [CrossRef] [PubMed]

95. Donnelly, J.E.; Herrmann, S.D.; Lambourne, K.; Szabo, A.N.; Honas, J.J.; Washburn, R.A. Does increased exercise or physical activity alter ad-libitum daily energy intake or macronutrient composition in healthy adults? A systematic review. *PLoS ONE* **2014**, *9*, e83498. [CrossRef] [PubMed]

96. Cameron, J.D.; Goldfield, G.S.; Riou, M.È.; Finlayson, G.S.; Blundell, J.E.; Doucet, É. Energy depletion by diet or aerobic exercise alone: Impact of energy deficit modality on appetite parameters. *Am. J. Clin. Nutr.* **2016**, *103*, 1008–1016. [CrossRef] [PubMed]

97. Stubbs, R.J.; Sepp, A.; Hughes, D.A.; Johnstone, A.M.; Horgan, G.W.; King, N.; Blundell, J. The effect of graded levels of exercise on energy intake and balance in free-living men, consuming their normal diet. *Eur. J. Clin. Nutr.* **2002**, *56*, 129–140. [CrossRef] [PubMed]

98. Dhurandhar, N.V.; Schoeller, D.; Brown, A.W.; Heymsfield, S.B.; Thomas, D.; Sørensen, T.I.A.; Speakman, J.R.; Jeansonne, M.; Allison, D.B.; Energy Balance Measurement Working Group. Energy balance measurement: When something is not better than nothing. *Int. J. Obes.* **2015**, *39*, 1109–1113. [CrossRef] [PubMed]

99. Bryant, E.J.; Caudwell, P.; Hopkins, M.E.; King, N.A.; Blundell, J.E. Psycho-markers of weight loss. The roles of TFEQ disinhibition and restraint in exercise-induced weight management. *Appetite* **2012**, *58*, 234–241. [CrossRef] [PubMed]

100. Evero, N.; Hackett, L.C.; Clark, R.D.; Phelan, S.; Hagobian, T.A. Aerobic exercise reduces neuronal responses in food reward brain regions. *J. Appl. Physiol.* **2012**, *112*, 1612–1619. [CrossRef] [PubMed]

101. Blundell, J.; de Graaf, C.; Hulshof, T.; Jebb, S.; Livingstone, B.; Lluch, A.; Mela, D.; Salah, S.; Schuring, E.; van der Knaap, H.; et al. Appetite control: Methodological aspects of the evaluation of foods. *Obes. Rev.* **2010**, *11*, 251–270. [CrossRef] [PubMed]

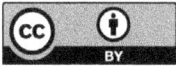

nutrients

MDPI

Article

Effect of 12-Week Vitamin D Supplementation on 25[OH]D Status and Performance in Athletes with a Spinal Cord Injury

Joelle Leonie Flueck [1,*], Max Walter Schlaepfer [2] and Claudio Perret [1]

[1] Institute of Sports Medicine, Swiss Paraplegic Centre Nottwil, Nottwil 6207, Switzerland; claudio.perret@paraplegie.ch
[2] Institute of Human Movement Sciences and Sport, ETH Zurich, Zurich 8092, Switzerland; maxwschlaepfer@gmail.com
* Correspondence: joelle.flueck@paraplegie.ch; Tel.: +41-41-939-6617

Received: 18 August 2016; Accepted: 17 September 2016; Published: 22 September 2016

Abstract: (1) Background: studies with able-bodied athletes showed that performance might possibly be influenced by vitamin D status. Vitamin D seems to have a direct impact on neuromuscular function by docking on vitamin D receptors in the muscle tissue. Additionally, a high prevalence of vitamin D deficiency was shown not only in infants and in the elderly but also in healthy adults and spinal cord injured individuals. Therefore, the aim of our study was to investigate whether a vitamin D dose of 6000 IU daily over 12 weeks would be sufficient to increase vitamin D status in indoor wheelchair athletes to a normal or optimal vitamin D level and whether vitamin D deficiency is associated with an impairment in muscle performance in these individuals; (2) Methods: vitamin D status was assessed in indoor elite wheelchair athletes in order to have a baseline measurement. If vitamin D status was below 75 nmol/L, athletes were supplemented with 6000 IU of vitamin D daily over 12 weeks. A vitamin D status over 75 nmol/L was supplemented with a placebo supplement. Vitamin D status, as well as a Wingate test and an isokinetic dynamometer test, were performed at baseline and after six and 12 weeks; (3) Results: 20 indoor elite wheelchair athletes participated in this double-blind study. All of these athletes showed an insufficient vitamin D status at baseline and were, therefore, supplemented with vitamin D. All athletes increased vitamin D status significantly over 12 weeks and reached an optimal level. Wingate performance was not significantly increased. Isokinetic dynamometer strength was significantly increased but only in the non-dominant arm in isometric and concentric elbow flexion; (4) Conclusion: a dose of 6000 IU of vitamin D daily over a duration of 12 weeks seems to be sufficient to increase vitamin D status to an optimal level in indoor wheelchair athletes. It remains unclear, whether upper body performance or muscle strength and vitamin D status are associated with each other.

Keywords: 25[OH]D; spinal cord injuries; anaerobic performance test; dynamometer test

1. Introduction

A high prevalence of vitamin D deficiency was shown not only in infants [1,2] and in the elderly [3], but also in young and healthy adults [4,5]. As vitamin D is primarily produced by ultraviolet radiation through sunlight exposure, a deficiency can possibly develop in healthy people as well. Such a deficiency may not only increase the risk for several different diseases, such as cancer [6,7], cardiovascular disease [8,9], and dementia [10], but also decrease neuromuscular function [11]. Such a neuromuscular impairment might be explained by the existence of vitamin D receptors (VDR) in human muscle tissue [12]. Thus, vitamin D deficiency might also lead to muscle weakness and pain. Further, vitamin D seems to influence not only muscle growth and cell differentiation, but also increase sarcoplasmic calcium uptake resulting in a higher muscle contractility [13]. Therefore, it is not surprising that positive effects of vitamin D supplementation on muscle function were found [14–18]. Studies showed a reduction in falls and a beneficial effects on muscle strength, balance, and gait performance in the elderly [19]. Other studies found an increase in upper and lower body muscle strength after vitamin D supplementation [18]. Nonetheless, the impact of vitamin D supplementation on muscular performance in athletes remains controversial. Some studies found no effect on performance [20,21], whereas others found a significantly increased isometric quadriceps strength, vertical jump, and sprint time after vitamin D supplementation [22,23].

Similar to the studies with able-bodied individuals, a high prevalence of vitamin D deficiency or insufficiency was found in patients [24] and athletes [25,26] with a spinal cord injury. Due to the impairment of the spinal cord, muscle strength might already be decreased and an additional impairment through vitamin D deficiency needs to be avoided. Only one study investigated the effect of vitamin D supplementation in athletes with a spinal cord injury on vitamin D status [27]. In this study, a vitamin D supplementation with 5000 IU daily increased vitamin D status over wintertime.

Therefore, the aim of our study was to investigate the effect of vitamin D supplementation on muscle strength and performance in indoor wheelchair athletes. Firstly, the objective was to detect whether a dose of 6000 IU daily is sufficient to increase vitamin D status to a normal level over 12 weeks in athletes suffering from a deficiency. Another goal was to investigate the relationship between vitamin D status and muscle strength.

2. Materials and Methods

2.1. Study Participants

Swiss male elite wheelchair indoor athletes, 18 to 60 years old and physically active for at least 45 min twice a week were recruited for this study. They had to perform their sport for more than two years and suffer from a chronic spinal cord injury or from cerebral palsy. The intervention study took place during the winter months (November–April) and the follow-up during spring (April–June) in Nottwil, Switzerland (47° north latitude). Any participant being abroad below the 37th parallel during the study phase or shortly before the start of the study was withdrawn from participating. Participants already supplementing with a vitamin D dose higher than 400 IU daily were also excluded from the study. Other exclusion criteria were suffering from a respiratory or cardiovascular disease, kidney insufficiency, or parathyroid gland ailment. All participants were asked to sign written informed consent and had to maintain their regular training schedule as well as to refrain from taking any additional supplements. The study was approved by the local ethics committee (Ethikkommission Nordwest-und Zentralschweiz (EKNZ), Basel, Switzerland) (Project #2015-344, clinicaltrials.gov NCT02621320).

2.2. Study Design

The double-blind, non-randomized intervention study took place at the Institute of Sports Medicine in Nottwil, Switzerland. Participants visited the institute on five different occasions during the intervention phase and on two additional occasions for those participating in the follow up. On the first visit, the screening questionnaire was completed and the medical history was checked to ensure that all criteria were fulfilled. The second visit was conducted in order to familiarize the participants with the performance tests. All participants performed and isokinetic dynamometer test (see Section 2.4) followed by a fifteen minute recovery break. Subsequently, a 30 s Wingate test on an arm crank ergometer (see Section 2.5) was performed.

Each participant replicated this test procedure on three occasions during the intervention phase and on two additional occasions during the follow up phase (only vitamin D concentration and the Wingate test). The tests took place at the same time of the day and were separated by six weeks. Before each session, the fulfillment of the test requirements was checked (i.e., no exercise twelve hours and no intense exercise 48 h before testing, at least seven hours of sleep during the previous night, no caffeine intake and replicated food intake prior to each session). After completion of this checklist, two venous blood samples were drawn in order to analyze the vitamin D and the calcium status. All participants with an insufficient vitamin D status (<75 nmol/L) received a vitamin D supplement during the intervention phase and all participants with a sufficient vitamin D status (>75 nmol/L) received a placebo supplement during the intervention phase (see Section 2.3). After the blood withdrawal, a Disabilities of the Arm, Shoulder and Hand (DASH) questionnaire [28] was completed.

2.3. Vitamin D Supplementation

Vitamin D3 (cholecalciferol) supplement (Vi-De 3®, Wild and Co. AG, Muttenz, Switzerland) was given in a dose of 6000 IU daily over twelve weeks (intervention phase). The tolerable upper limit intake level of the Endocrine Practice Guidelines Committee of 10,000 IU daily was not exceeded and, therefore, no side effects were expected [29]. The placebo supplement was based on the same alcohol solution (65% ethanol, Dr. Wild and Co. AG, Muttenz, Switzerland). The supplements were handed over in identical bottles and were ingested dropwise (either 60 drops or 1.3 mL daily). Bottles and solutions were not distinguishable for the participants in smell and color.

Self-reported compliance was assessed by regularly asking the frequency of taking vitamin D or placebo supplementation over the last two weeks. To achieve a high compliance, each participant installed a mobile app (Medisafe, Medisafe Inc., Boston, MA, USA) and set a daily reminder.

To assess tolerance, participants were asked every two weeks how they tolerate the supplement.

2.4. The Isokinetic Dynamometer Test

An isokinetic dynamometer (Cybex Norm II, Lumex Inc., Ronkomkoma, NY, USA) was used to measure peak torque of elbow flexion strength at different velocities for isometric ($0°/s$) and concentric ($60°/s$ and $180°/s$) exercise. The device was connected to the software (Humac 2015, CSMi, Stroughton, MA, USA) and calibration was performed in monthly intervals as proposed by the manufacturer. Participants were placed in a supine position fixed with straps and with a pillow under their knees. The shoulder joint was abducted in $45°$ and the wrist was strapped proximal with the hand in a neutral position to the lever arm of the dynamometer. The axis of rotation was aligned with the lateral epicondyle. Testing was limited between $20°$ and $120°$ of elbow flexion. Strong verbal encouragement was used during maximal effort.

A standardized warm-up with 10 repetitions at $120°/s$ was performed before the data collection. Subsequently, data collection started with the measurement of concentric work at 60 and $180°/s$ followed by isometric work.

Test-re-test reliability was checked prior to the start of the study in 10 able-bodied participants. Isometric, as well as both concentric measurements, showed "high" to "very high" reliability according to Munro's classification of the intra-class correlation coefficient (ICC) [30]. The ICC ranged between 0.843 and 0.925 for the different test settings (Table S1).

2.5. The Wingate Test

Participants performed a Wingate test using a rotational speed-dependent arm crank ergometer (Angio V2, Lode B.V., Groningen, The Netherlands) which was connected to the software (Wingate, Lode B.V., Groningen, The Netherlands). This Wingate test on the arm crank ergometer was shown to be highly reliable in individuals with a paraplegia [31] and tetraplegia [32]. Participants were seated in an adapted office chair, which was positioned to allow a slight bend of the elbows. The height of the crank and the distance between the chair and the crank were recorded to replicate the conditions in the next test session. In some participants hand fixations and chest straps were needed to fix them to the crank or the chair. A resistance load of 1%–3% was applied in individuals with a tetraplegia [32]. In individuals with paraplegia, a resistance load of 4% was used. These settings were tested during the familiarization trials and adjusted for the intervention sessions where needed.

Five minutes of a standardized warm-up at 20 W and 60 rpm was performed before the start of the test. Subsequently, the resistance load was applied and the Wingate test was started. After the test, participants stopped to crank immediately and blood lactate concentrations were measured at 0, 2, 4, 6, 8, and 10 min after the end of the test using an enzymatic amperometric chip sensor system (Biosen C-Line Clinic, EKF diagnostic GmbH, Cardiff, UK). Blood samples were taken from the earlobe. A heart rate monitor (S610i, Polar Electro Oy, Kempele, Finland) was used to measure maximal heart rate during the test. These data were analyzed with the Polar Pro Trainer 5 software (Polar Electro Oy, Kempele, Finland). Rated perceived exertion (RPE) was assessed during warm-up and at the end of the test by using a Borg scale ranging from 6 to 20 [33]. Maximal power (P_{peak}), average power (P_{mean}) and fatigue index (FI) during the Wingate test were analyzed.

2.6. Blood Parameters

Blood samples were drawn from the antecubital vein using a blood collection system (S-Monovette® 4.9 mL Z, Sarestedt, Nümbrecht, Germany). Samples were immediately packed into an opaque plastic tube to protect them from any ultraviolet radiation. The samples were then immediately centrifuged at 20 °C at 3000 rpm for 10 min (Rotina 380, Hettich GmbH, Tuttlingen, Germany) in the in-house laboratory of the Swiss Paraplegic Centre, Nottwil, Switzerland. After centrifugation, the samples were stored at −25 °C for later analysis.

Serum 25-hydroxyvitamin D (25[OH]D) was analyzed with an automated benchtop immunoanalyzer (Vidas®, bioMérieux, Marcy l'Etoile, France) using enzyme-linked fluorescent assay (ELFA). Serum calcium concentration was assayed with a photometric technique method (Cobas c501, Roche Diagnostic GmbH, Mannheim, Germany).

2.7. DASH Questionnaire

The Disabilities of the Arm, Shoulder and Hand (DASH) questionnaire was used to assess upper extremity function and symptoms (non-specific for wheelchair users) [28]. The DASH questionnaire was completed at the laboratory previously to the start of the Wingate test.

2.8. Data Analysis

Statistical analysis was performed using the software IBM SPSS Statistics Version 23.0 for Windows (IBM, Armonk, NY, USA). Statistical significance was set at an α-level of 0.05. Distribution of our data was tested by using the Kolmogorov-Smirnov, the Shapiro-Wilk test and the Q-Q plot. The results indicated, that all of your data was normally distributed except for the isokinetic dynamometer test and for the analysis of the follow up phase. For normally distributed data mean ± standard deviation (SD) was used. Not normally distributed data is presented as median [minimum; maximum]. To analyze differences in the mean of the outcome parameters between different time points, a one-way repeated-measurement ANOVA was performed for normally distributed data and the Brunner model [34] was applied for nonparametric data. Pairwise *t*-tests and Wilcoxon post hoc test were performed as post hoc analysis in normal and nonparametric data, respectively. In the case of multiple testing, Bonferroni corrections were applied. Tests six weeks after supplementation were called "intermediate" whereas tests after 12 weeks were called "post". The first measurement during the follow up after six weeks is called "follow up 1" and the second follow up tests after 12-week placebo supplementation are called "follow up 2". Spearman correlation was used to correlate the increase in vitamin D with the difference of peak elbow flexion at baseline and post. Pearson correlation was used to correlate the increase in vitamin D with the difference in peak power and mean power from baseline to post.

3. Results

Twenty-one healthy, male Swiss elite wheelchair indoor athletes participated in this study. Athletes were competing in wheelchair rugby (n = 15), basketball (n = 4), or table tennis (n = 2). One participant had to be excluded from data analysis due to non-compliancy. Therefore, twenty participants were included into data analysis. Ten out of these twenty participants agreed to take part in the follow up study (Table 1).

Table 1. Participants' characteristics.

Participant	Training (h/Week)	Age (Years)	Height (cm)	Weight (kg)	Lesion Level	AIS	Sport	Classification	Follow up
1	3.5	37	185	103	C7	D	WR	2.0	Yes
2	11.0	20	170	54	C6	A	WR	1.5	No
3	4.0	24	179	58	C6	B	WR	0.5	Yes
4	3.5	35	187	97	T4	A	WB	1.0	No
5	4.0	47	185	63	T1	A	WR	2.5	No
6	2.5	27	180	70	T4	A	WB	1.0	Yes
7	3.5	27	181	61	C6	B	WR	2.5	No
8	5.0	48	186	67	C6	B	WR	1.0	Yes
9	5.0	44	176	80	C6	A	WR	0.5	Yes
10	12.0	35	193	92	T1	C	WB	2.5	Yes
11	8.0	38	172	70	C7	D	WR	2.0	Yes
12	4.0	26	188	90	C6	A	WR	0.5	No
13	5.0	30	182	65	C6	B	WR	0.5	No
14	8.0	34	180	85	C5	C	WR	1.5	No
15	6.5	50	185	83	L3	A	WB	3.0	Yes
16	13.5	21	184	63	C7	D	WR	2.5	Yes
17	3.5	65	175	65	C6	C	WR	1.5	No
18	15.0	33	180	60	C6	A	PT	class 1	No
19	4.0	26	155	52	CP	-	WR	1.5	Yes
20	5.0	57	170	72	T5	D	PT	class 4	No
Mean ± SD	6.3 ± 3.7	36 ± 12	180 ± 8	72 ± 15	-	-	-	-	-

AIS = American Spinal Injury Association Impairment Scale; T = thoracic; L, lumbar; C = cervical, CP = cerebral palsy, WB = wheelchair basketball, WR = wheelchair rugby, PT = para table tennis.

3.1. Vitamin D and Calcium Status

All participants enrolled into the study showed an insufficient or deficient vitamin D status at the baseline measurement (Figure 1). Therefore, no placebo group could be formed. Nineteen out of twenty athletes reached an optimal vitamin D status (100 to 220 nmol/L) after six weeks, and no one showed a toxic level (>375 nmol/L). Vitamin D status for the participants taking part in the follow up is shown in Figure 2. Significant differences were found between all different time points ($p < 0.05$). Calcium concentration was not significantly different between the three time points in the intervention study ($p = 0.16$) nor in the five time points, including the follow up data ($p = 0.39$). All calcium concentrations were within the normal physiological range (2.15 to 2.55 mmol/L).

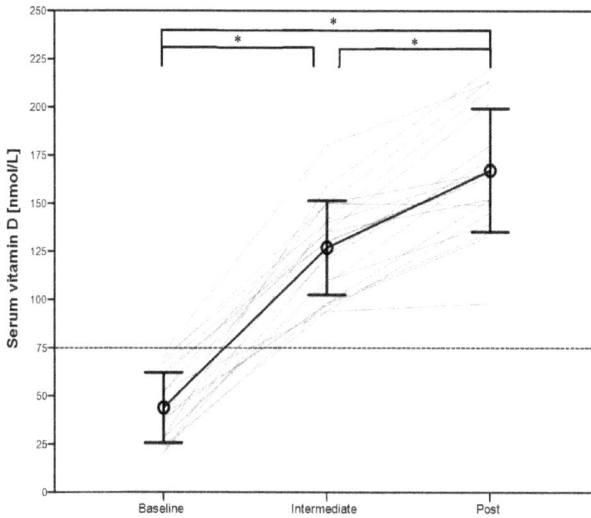

Figure 1. Serum vitamin D concentration at baseline, after six (intermediate) and 12 (post) weeks following vitamin D supplementation. * = significant difference ($p < 0.05$), data presented as mean and standard deviation, grey lines represent individual data.

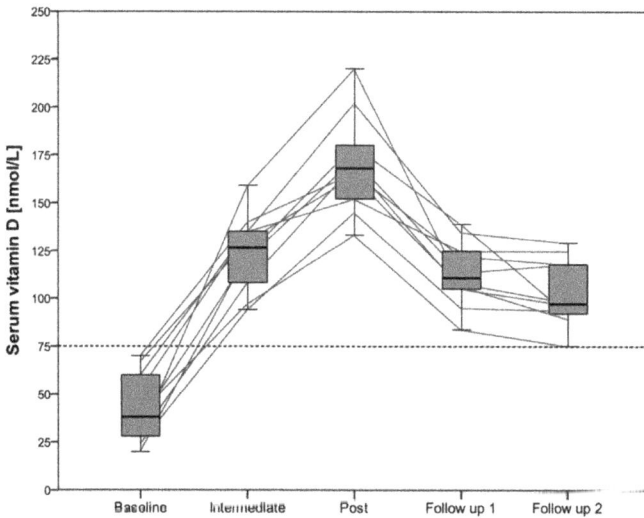

Figure 2. Serum vitamin D concentrations during the intervention and the follow up in 10 participants. Grey lines represents individuals' data, data presented as median with interquartile range.

3.2. Performance Tests

Significant improvements in the non-dominant arm were shown in isometric and 180°/s concentric exercise (Table 2).

Table 2. Peak elbow flexion [Nm] reached during isokinetic dynamometer measurements.

Mode	Arm	Baseline	Intermediate	Post	p-Value
isometric	dominant	65 [46; 96]	71 [46; 98]	72 [50; 100]	0.071
	non-dominant	64 [49; 104]	68 [46; 106] *	71 [49; 106] *	0.019
concentric 60°/s	dominant	46 [30; 77]	47 [35; 71]	47 [37; 73]	0.197
	non-dominant	47 [30; 73]	50 [33; 71]	49 [37; 75]	0.078
concentric 180°/s	dominant	34 [24; 61]	31 [24; 58]	33 [27; 61]	0.269
	non-dominant	34 [24; 53]	37 [24; 54] **	35 [26; 53] **	0.001

Data presented as median [minimum; maximum] from 20 participants. Significant differences compared to baseline measurement * $p < 0.05$ and ** $p < 0.01$.

No significant differences in peak power were found over the three measurements during the intervention study ($p = 0.09$), nor during the follow-up study ($p = 0.53$). The same findings were shown for average power in the intervention ($p = 0.13$) and in the follow-up ($p = 0.71$) study. No significant differences were found in fatigue index ($p = 0.15$), maximal heart rate ($p = 0.92$), RPE ($p = 0.76$), and maximal lactate concentrations ($p = 0.58$) for the intervention study at the different time points (Table S2). Individual absolute and relative changes in peak power from baseline to post measurement in the intervention study are shown in Figure 3. The data for peak power in the follow up study is shown in Figure 4. Spearman correlation showed a significant correlation between the difference in the non-dominant arm at 60°/s and the increase of vitamin D from baseline to post ($p = 0.01$; $r_s = 0.564$). This correlation coefficient (r_s) reflects only "moderate" correlation. No other correlation for the dominant arm or the other exercise velocities showed any significant correlation. The increase in vitamin D status was significantly correlated with the difference in peak power from baseline to post ($p = 0.044$, $r = 0.455$). Again Pearson's r reflects medium correlation. No significant correlation between the increase of vitamin D and mean power from baseline to post was found ($p = 0.27$; $r = 0.258$).

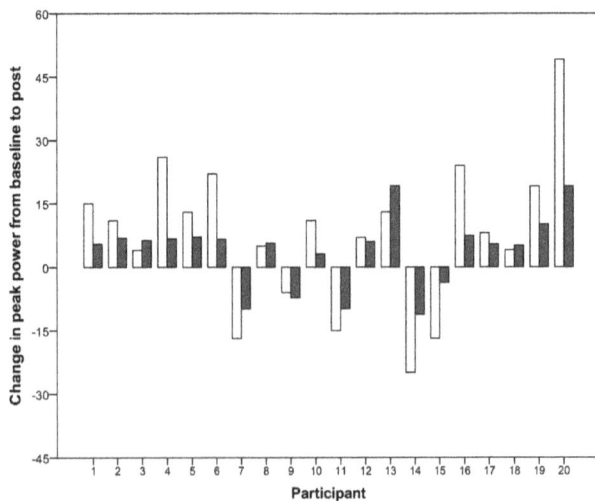

Figure 3. Individual changes in absolute (white bars in [W]) and relative (grey bars in [%]) of peak power from baseline to post measurement in the intervention study.

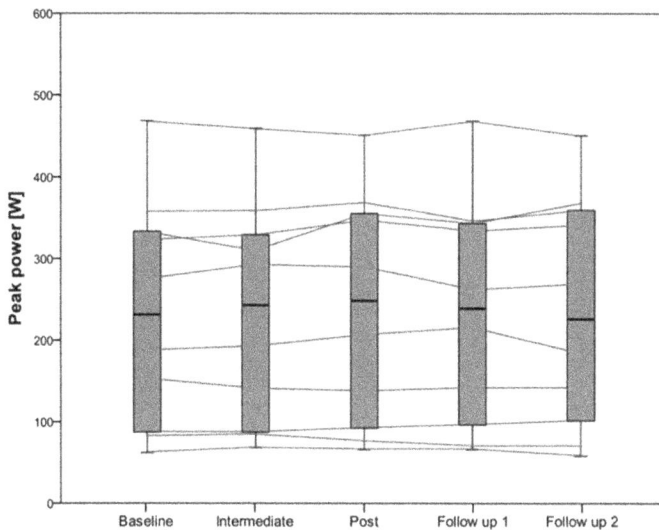

Figure 4. Peak power in 10 participants during the five measurements including the follow up study.

3.3. Other Outcome Parameters

No significant changes over time were found in the DASH score (p = 0.20) nor in the DASH sport score (p = 0.94) during the intervention phase. The participants reported a compliance of 97.3% over twelve weeks of vitamin D supplementation. Three out of twenty participants reported gastrointestinal side effects, such as a higher frequency of bowel movement and loose stool during vitamin D supplementation. Two out of the three showed the lowest compliance (75% and 82.1%) of all participants, and only one had a positive change in peak power from baseline to post measurement.

4. Discussion

A daily supplementation dosage of 6000 IU vitamin D seems to be sufficient to reach an optimal vitamin D status after 12 weeks in indoor athletes with an insufficient vitamin D status at baseline (Figure 1). After a 12 weeks follow up period with placebo supplementation, vitamin D status still was over 75 nmol/L but decreased significantly compared to the value at the end of the 12-week vitamin D supplementation period (Figure 2). The real effect of vitamin D supplementation on upper body exercise performance in athletes with a spinal cord injury still remains unclear due to a lack of a placebo group in our study.

4.1. Vitamin D Status

It is already well-known that a high amount of able-bodied and disabled Swiss athletes suffer from vitamin D deficiency or insufficiency during winter months [25,35]. The prevalence of vitamin D deficiency was even higher in indoor wheelchair athletes compared to outdoor athletes [25]. Nevertheless, it was surprising that all recruited athletes in the present study showed a deficient vitamin D status at baseline (44 ± 18 nmol/L). Oral vitamin D supplementation of 6000 IU daily over a 12-week time period was sufficient to increase vitamin D status to an optimal level (167 ± 24 nmol/L). The calculated slope of the relation between the vitamin D change and the supplementation was 2.05 nmol/L per 100 IU in the present study. This is slightly higher than the proposed slopes of 1.48 nmol/L per 100 IU [36] or 1.75 nmol/L per 100 IU [37]. The lower baseline vitamin D status in our study might explain this slight discrepancy.

Only a few other studies investigated the effect of vitamin D supplementation on vitamin D status in individuals with a spinal cord injury [27,38,39]. Most of these studies failed to achieve a sufficient vitamin D status after the supplementation period [39,40]. In one study [39], over 80% of the participants remained insufficient after vitamin D supplementation with 2000 IU daily over a two-week period. Similar findings were shown with a supplementation of 800 IU daily over a duration of one year [39], and in a study where the compliance for taking vitamin D supplements was only at 72% [40]. Our study showed not only a high compliance but also that a dosage of 6000 IU vitamin D daily over six weeks would be sufficient to increase vitamin D status to a normal level. Nevertheless, an individual approach needs to be applied, as a large individual variability occurred in the intermediate and post measurement of vitamin D status. Concerns whether such a high dose of vitamin D might be problematic were eliminated by the fact that calcium concentration remained in the normal range in our study. In addition, Heaney, Davies, Chen, Holick, and Barger-Lux [37] showed that a dose of 10,000 IU daily over five months was a safe intervention. Therefore, the Endocrine Society set their tolerable upper limit of 10,000 IU daily [29].

The dose of 6000 IU daily over 12 weeks seems to be sufficient and safe for its application in athletes with a spinal cord injury. Due to the fact that vitamin D status decreased during the 12-week follow up under placebo supplementation, we recommend to re-evaluate vitamin D status after a certain time period (e.g., 18 week after the end of the supplementation period).

4.2. Vitamin D and Muscle Performance

The present study did not find any significant increase in anaerobic Wingate test performance, although vitamin D status significantly increased over these 12 weeks. Fifteen out of twenty athletes showed an increase in peak power over this period (Figure 3). A significant increase in isokinetic strength in the non-dominant arm was found comparing baseline and post supplementation measurement (Table 2). Even though this increase was significant, it is not obvious, whether it was due to a training adaptation or due to the increased vitamin D status. The lack of a placebo or control group prevents drawing further conclusions. Similar results were shown by Pritchett, Pritchett, Ogan, Bishop, Broad, and LaCroix [26], whereas vitamin D status did not correlate with 20 m sprint or handgrip strength in wheelchair athletes. A recent meta-analysis [18] found a significant increase in upper limb strength in able-bodied participants favoring the supplementation compared to the placebo intervention. Two of these studies applied a relatively high dose (60,000 and 14,000 IU vitamin D per week) over four to six months [23,41]. A single bolus of 150,000 IU vitamin D increased quadriceps muscle strength of elite judokas significantly after eight days [42]. In contrast, a dose of 2000 IU vitamin D daily over 12 weeks did not significantly increase swimming performance as well as arm-grip strength and one-legged balance in adolescent swimmers [20]. Thus, no conclusive results were found for upper body muscle strength after vitamin D supplementation.

Similar to our results, Hamilton, et al. [43] found a significantly increased peak torque in the non-dominant leg in professional soccer players, but no increase in the dominant leg. Overall, no consistent association between vitamin D and isokinetic strength was found in this study. It remains unclear why, in the non-dominant leg in this study, and the non-dominant arm in our study, muscle strength improved in contrast to the dominant one. Further studies are needed to elucidate this issue as well as to investigate the effects of vitamin D on upper body muscle strength and handgrip function.

In addition, it is known that vitamin D binds to vitamin D receptors in the muscle tissue in order to turn up gene expression of type II muscle fibers [13]. A study performed with an elderly vitamin D deficient population showed a decreased atrophy of type II muscle fibers under vitamin D supplementation [44]. The relative number and size of type II muscle fibers was increased and muscle strength was improved. In addition, a reduction of falls and hip fractures occurred in the intervention group. This study showed, that the type II muscle fibers are possibly more affected compared to type I fibers. Knowing that, in individuals with a spinal cord injury type I muscle fibers are more predominant in the upper body [45], a smaller impact of vitamin D supplementation on these muscles might be expected. Again, such a speculation has to be further investigated in the future by means of muscle biopsies in order to determine the change in muscle fiber size and number after vitamin D supplementation.

4.3. Other Parameters

Our study did not find any significant change in the DASH score outcome over the supplementation period. This result suggests that the upper body impairment did not change over time and no additional injury occurred. Of course, due to the lack of a placebo group, this finding cannot be compared. A recent systematic review performed in healthy adults [46] revealed a small, but positive, effect on reducing the incidence of injuries when supplemented with vitamin D. Wyon, Koutedakis, Wolman, Nevill, and Allen [23] found a similar result in elite ballet dancers, who sustained significantly fewer injuries compared to the placebo group. Much more data is needed to finally conclude the impact of vitamin D supplementation on injury rate and severity of the injury. It is yet not clear whether there exists a positive association in general.

4.4. Limitations

The aim was to conduct a placebo-controlled intervention study. Unfortunately, all recruited participants showed an insufficient vitamin D status and were enrolled into the vitamin D supplementation group. The number of participants was limited due to the lack of further elite wheelchair athletes and due to the stringent inclusion or exclusion criteria. Even though an a priori power analysis showed a high power with 10 participants, this study might have been slightly underpowered due to a high variability in muscle force in athletes with a paraplegia or a tetraplegia. Therefore, it seems very difficult to draw final conclusions on how an insufficient vitamin D status impairs upper body performance or how a vitamin D supplementation might help to improve neuromuscular function. Nevertheless, this study showed clearly how vitamin D status increased over 12 weeks after supplementation and to which extent it decreased during the follow up. Further research is needed to investigate the relationship of vitamin D deficiency and neuromuscular performance in athletes with a spinal cord injury.

5. Conclusions

The present finding show, that a dose of 6000 IU vitamin D daily over 12 weeks is safe and sufficient to reach an optimal vitamin D level in indoor wheelchair athletes. Due to the lack of a placebo group, no final conclusion can be drawn whether vitamin D influences neuromuscular performance in athletes with a spinal cord injury. Isokinetic strength seems to have improved in the non-dominant arm over 12 weeks, but this finding might also result from continuous training.

Supplementary Materials: The following are available online at http://www.mdpi.com/2072-6643/8/10/586/s1, Table S1: Test-retest reliability of the isokinetic dynamometer test in 10 able-bodied participants, Table S2: Parameters measured during the Wingate test at baseline, intermediate and post supplementation.

Acknowledgments: We thank Ruth Heller, Seline Magron and Eliane Arnold-Küng from the Institute of Sports Medicine Nottwil, Switzerland for their help with blood sampling and the laboratory of the Swiss Paraplegic Centre Nottwil, Switzerland for vitamin D analysis. We highly appreciate the support of Wild & Co. AG, Muttenz, Switzerland by providing the vitamin D and placebo solutions for this study.

Author Contributions: J.L.F., M.W.S. and C.P. conceived and designed the experiments; M.W.S. performed the experiments; J.L.F. and M.W.S. analyzed the data; C.P. contributed reagents/materials/analysis tools; J.L.F. and C.P. wrote the paper.

Conflicts of Interest: The authors declare no conflict of interest.

References

1. Ward, K.A.; Das, G.; Berry, J.L.; Roberts, S.A.; Rawer, R.; Adams, J.E.; Mughal, Z. Vitamin D status and muscle function in post-menarchal adolescent girls. *J. Clin. Endocrinol. Metab.* **2009**, *94*, 559–563. [CrossRef] [PubMed]
2. Carroll, A.; Onwuneme, C.; McKenna, M.J.; Mayne, P.D.; Molloy, E.J.; Murphy, N.P. Vitamin D status in irish children and adolescents: Value of fortification and supplementation. *Clin. Pediatr. (Phila.)* **2014**, *53*, 1345–1351. [CrossRef] [PubMed]
3. Bruyere, O.; Cavalier, E.; Souberbielle, J.C.; Bischoff-Ferrari, H.A.; Beaudart, C.; Buckinx, F.; Reginster, J.Y.; Rizzoli, R. Effects of vitamin D in the elderly population: Current status and perspectives. *Arch. Public Health* **2014**, *72*, 32. [CrossRef] [PubMed]
4. Constantini, N.W.; Arieli, R.; Chodick, G.; Dubnov-Raz, G. High prevalence of vitamin D insufficiency in athletes and dancers. *Clin. J. Sport Med.* **2010**, *20*, 368–371. [CrossRef] [PubMed]
5. Farrokhyar, F.; Tabasinejad, R.; Dao, D.; Peterson, D.; Ayeni, O.R.; Hadioonzadeh, R.; Bhandari, M. Prevalence of vitamin D inadequacy in athletes: A systematic-review and meta-analysis. *Sports Med.* **2015**, *45*, 365–378. [CrossRef] [PubMed]
6. Garland, C.F.; Gorham, E.D.; Mohr, S.B.; Grant, W.B.; Giovannucci, E.L.; Lipkin, M.; Newmark, H.; Holick, M.F.; Garland, F.C. Vitamin D and prevention of breast cancer: Pooled analysis. *J. Steroid Biochem. Mol. Biol.* **2007**, *103*, 708–711. [CrossRef] [PubMed]
7. Wong, G.; Lim, W.H.; Lewis, J.; Craig, J.C.; Turner, R.; Zhu, K.; Lim, E.M.; Prince, R. Vitamin D and cancer mortality in elderly women. *BMC Cancer* **2015**, *15*, 106. [CrossRef] [PubMed]
8. Berridge, M.J. Vitamin D cell signalling in health and disease. *Biochem. Biophys. Res. Commun.* **2015**, *460*, 53–71. [CrossRef] [PubMed]
9. Mandarino, N.R.; Junior, F.; Salgado, J.V.; Lages, J.S.; Filho, N.S. Is vitamin D deficiency a new risk factor for cardiovascular disease? *Open Cardiovasc. Med. J.* **2015**, *9*, 40–49. [CrossRef] [PubMed]
10. Annweiler, C.; Rolland, Y.; Schott, A.M.; Blain, H.; Vellas, B.; Herrmann, F.R.; Beauchet, O. Higher vitamin D dietary intake is associated with lower risk of alzheimer's disease: A 7-year follow-up. *J. Gerontol. A Biol. Sci. Med. Sci.* **2012**, *67*, 1205–1211. [CrossRef] [PubMed]
11. Larson-Meyer, D.E.; Willis, K.S. Vitamin D and athletes. *Curr. Sports Med. Rep.* **2010**, *9*, 220–226. [CrossRef] [PubMed]
12. Norman, A.W.; Okamura, W.H.; Bishop, J.E.; Henry, H.L. Update on biological actions of 1alpha,25(OH)2-vitamin D3 (rapid effects) and 24R,25(OH)2-vitamin D3. *Mol. Cell. Endocrinol.* **2002**, *197*, 1–13. [CrossRef]
13. Girgis, C.M.; Clifton-Bligh, R.J.; Hamrick, M.W.; Holick, M.F.; Gunton, J.E. The roles of vitamin D in skeletal muscle: Form, function, and metabolism. *Endocr. Rev.* **2013**, *34*, 33–83. [CrossRef] [PubMed]
14. Beaudart, C.; Buckinx, F.; Rabenda, V.; Gillain, S.; Cavalier, E.; Slomian, J.; Petermans, J.; Reginster, J.Y.; Bruyere, O. The effects of vitamin D on skeletal muscle strength, muscle mass, and muscle power: A systematic review and meta-analysis of randomized controlled trials. *J. Clin. Endocrinol. Metab.* **2014**, *99*, 4336–4345. [CrossRef] [PubMed]
15. Ceglia, L.; Harris, S.S. Vitamin D and its role in skeletal muscle. *Calcif. Tissue Int.* **2013**, *92*, 151–162. [CrossRef] [PubMed]
16. Muir, S.W.; Montero-Odasso, M. Effect of vitamin D supplementation on muscle strength, gait and balance in older adults: A systematic review and meta-analysis. *J. Am. Geriatr. Soc.* **2011**, *59*, 2291–2300. [CrossRef] [PubMed]
17. Stockton, K.A.; Mengersen, K.; Paratz, J.D.; Kandiah, D.; Bennell, K.L. Effect of vitamin D supplementation on muscle strength: A systematic review and meta-analysis. *Osteoporos. Int.* **2011**, *22*, 859–871. [CrossRef] [PubMed]
18. Tomlinson, P.B.; Joseph, C.; Angioi, M. Effects of vitamin D supplementation on upper and lower body muscle strength levels in healthy individuals. A systematic review with meta-analysis. *J. Sci. Med. Sport* **2015**, *18*, 575–580. [CrossRef] [PubMed]
19. Halfon, M.; Phan, O.; Teta, D. Vitamin D: A review on its effects on muscle strength, the risk of fall, and frailty. *BioMed Res. Int.* **2015**, *2015*, 953241. [CrossRef] [PubMed]

20. Dubnov-Raz, G.; Livne, N.; Raz, R.; Cohen, A.H.; Constantini, N.W. Vitamin D supplementation and physical performance in adolescent swimmers. *Int. J. Sport Nutr. Exerc. Metab.* **2015**, *25*, 317–325. [CrossRef] [PubMed]
21. Jastrzebska, M.; Kaczmarczyk, M.; Jastrzebski, Z. The effect of vitamin D supplementation on training adaptation in well trained soccer players. *J. Strength Cond. Res.* **2016**, *30*, 2648–2655. [CrossRef] [PubMed]
22. Close, G.L.; Leckey, J.; Patterson, M.; Bradley, W.; Owens, D.J.; Fraser, W.D.; Morton, J.P. The effects of vitamin D(3) supplementation on serum total 25[OH]D concentration and physical performance: A randomised dose-response study. *Br. J. Sports Med.* **2013**, *47*, 692–696. [CrossRef] [PubMed]
23. Wyon, M.A.; Koutedakis, Y.; Wolman, R.; Nevill, A.M.; Allen, N. The influence of winter vitamin D supplementation on muscle function and injury occurrence in elite ballet dancers: A controlled study. *J. Sci. Med. Sport* **2014**, *17*, 8–12. [CrossRef] [PubMed]
24. Nemunaitis, G.A.; Mejia, M.; Nagy, J.A.; Johnson, T.; Chae, J.; Roach, M.J. A descriptive study on vitamin D levels in individuals with spinal cord injury in an acute inpatient rehabilitation setting. *PM&R* **2010**, *2*, 202–208.
25. Flueck, J.L.; Hartmann, K.; Strupler, M.; Perret, C. Vitamin D deficiency in swiss elite wheelchair athletes. *Spinal Cord* **2016**. [CrossRef] [PubMed]
26. Pritchett, K.; Pritchett, R.; Ogan, D.; Bishop, P.; Broad, E.; LaCroix, M. 25(OH)D status of elite athletes with spinal cord injury relative to lifestyle factors. *Nutrients* **2016**, *8*. [CrossRef] [PubMed]
27. Magee, P.J.; Pourshahidi, L.K.; Wallace, J.M.; Cleary, J.; Conway, J.; Harney, E.; Madigan, S.M. Vitamin D status and supplementation in elite irish athletes. *Int. J. Sport Nutr. Exerc. Metab.* **2013**, *23*, 441–448. [CrossRef] [PubMed]
28. Germann, G.; Harth, A.; Wind, G.; Demir, E. Standardisation and validation of the german version 2.0 of the disability of arm, shoulder, hand (DASH) questionnaire. *Unfallchirurg* **2003**, *106*, 13–19. [CrossRef] [PubMed]
29. Holick, M.F.; Binkley, N.C.; Bischoff-Ferrari, H.A.; Gordon, C.M.; Hanley, D.A.; Heaney, R.P.; Murad, M.H.; Weaver, C.M. Evaluation, treatment, and prevention of vitamin D deficiency: An endocrine society clinical practice guideline. *J. Clin. Endocrinol. Metab.* **2011**, *96*, 1911–1930. [CrossRef] [PubMed]
30. Plichta, S.B.; Kelvin, E.A.; Munro, B.H. *Munro's Statistical Methods for Health Care Research*, 6th ed.; Wolters Kluwer: Philadelphia, PA, USA, 2013; p. 567.
31. Jacobs, P.L.; Mahoney, E.T.; Johnson, B. Reliability of arm wingate anaerobic testing in persons with complete paraplegia. *J. Spinal Cord Med.* **2003**, *26*, 141–144. [CrossRef] [PubMed]
32. Jacobs, P.L.; Johnson, B.; Somarriba, G.A.; Carter, A.B. Reliability of upper extremity anaerobic power assessment in persons with tetraplegia. *J. Spinal Cord Med.* **2005**, *28*, 109–113. [CrossRef] [PubMed]
33. Borg, G.A. Psychophysical bases of perceived exertion. *Med. Sci. Sports Exerc.* **1982**, *14*, 377–381. [CrossRef] [PubMed]
34. Brunner, E.; Langer, F. *Nichtparametrische Analyse Longitudinaler Daten*; R. Oldenbourg Verlag: München, Germany, 1999; p. 237S.
35. Quadri, A.; Gojanovic, B.; Noack, P.; Fuhrer, C.; Steuer, C.; Huber, A.; Kriemler, S. *Seasonal Variation of Vitamin D Levels in Swiss Athletes*; Swiss Sports & Exercise Medicine: Bern, Switzerland, 2016; Volume 64, p. 24.
36. Barger-Lux, M.J.; Heaney, R.P.; Dowell, S.; Chen, T.C.; Holick, M.F. Vitamin D and its major metabolites: Serum levels after graded oral dosing in healthy men. *Osteoporos Int.* **1998**, *8*, 222–230. [CrossRef] [PubMed]
37. Heaney, R.P.; Davies, K.M.; Chen, T.C.; Holick, M.F.; Barger-Lux, M.J. Human serum 25-hydroxycholecalciferol response to extended oral dosing with cholecalciferol. *Am. J. Clin. Nutr.* **2003**, *77*, 204–210. [PubMed]
38. Bauman, W.A.; Emmons, R.R.; Cirnigliaro, C.M.; Kirshblum, S.C.; Spungen, A.M. An effective oral vitamin d replacement therapy in persons with spinal cord injury. *J. Spinal Cord Med.* **2011**, *34*, 455–460. [CrossRef] [PubMed]
39. Bauman, W.A.; Morrison, N.G.; Spungen, A.M. Vitamin D replacement therapy in persons with spinal cord injury. *J. Spinal Cord Med.* **2005**, *28*, 203–207. [CrossRef] [PubMed]
40. Oleson, C.V.; Seidel, B.J.; Zhan, T. Association of vitamin D deficiency, secondary hyperparathyroidism, and heterotopic ossification in spinal cord injury. *J. Rehabil. Res. Dev.* **2013**, *50*, 1177–1186. [CrossRef] [PubMed]
41. Gupta, R.; Sharma, U.; Gupta, N.; Kalaivani, M.; Singh, U.; Guleria, R.; Jagannathan, N.R.; Goswami, R. Effect of cholecalciferol and calcium supplementation on muscle strength and energy metabolism in vitamin D-deficient asian indians: A randomized, controlled trial. *Clin. Endocrinol. (Oxf.)* **2010**, *73*, 445–451. [CrossRef] [PubMed]

42. Wyon, M.A.; Wolman, R.; Nevill, A.M.; Cloak, R.; Metsios, G.S.; Gould, D.; Ingham, A.; Koutedakis, Y. Acute effects of vitamin D3 supplementation on muscle strength in judoka athletes: A randomized placebo-controlled, double-blind trial. *Clin. J. Sport Med.* **2016**, *26*, 279–284. [CrossRef] [PubMed]

43. Hamilton, B.; Whiteley, R.; Farooq, A.; Chalabi, H. Vitamin D concentration in 342 professional football players and association with lower limb isokinetic function. *J. Sci. Med. Sport* **2014**, *17*, 139–143. [CrossRef] [PubMed]

44. Sato, Y.; Iwamoto, J.; Kanoko, T.; Satoh, K. Low-dose vitamin D prevents muscular atrophy and reduces falls and hip fractures in women after stroke: A randomized controlled trial. *Cerebrovasc. Dis.* **2005**, *20*, 187–192. [CrossRef] [PubMed]

45. Schantz, P.; Sjoberg, B.; Widebeck, A.M.; Ekblom, B. Skeletal muscle of trained and untrained paraplegics and tetraplegics. *Acta Physiol. Scand.* **1997**, *161*, 31–39. [CrossRef] [PubMed]

46. Redzic, M.; Lewis, R.M.; Thomas, D.T. Relationship between 25-hydoxyvitamin D, muscle strength, and incidence of injury in healthy adults: A systematic review. *Nutr. Res.* **2013**, *33*, 251–258. [CrossRef] [PubMed]

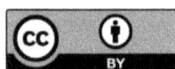

![nutrients logo] *nutrients*

MDPI

Article

Dietary Intake of Athletes Seeking Nutrition Advice at a Major International Competition

Sarah J. Burkhart * and Fiona E. Pelly

School of Health and Sport Sciences, University of the Sunshine Coast, Sippy Downs 4556, Queensland, Australia; fpelly@usc.edu.au
* Correspondence: sburkhar@usc.edu.au; Tel.: +61-7-5456-5046

Received: 8 September 2016; Accepted: 5 October 2016; Published: 14 October 2016

Abstract: International travel and short-term residence overseas is now a common feature of an elite athlete's competition schedule, however, food choice away from home may be challenging and potentially impact on performance. Guidelines for dietary intake specific to competition exist for athletes, however, there is little evidence available to ascertain if athletes meet these recommendations during competition periods, particularly when food is provided in-house. During the Delhi 2010 Commonwealth Games, dietitians based in the dining hall recorded 24 h dietary recalls with all athletes who visited the nutrition kiosk. Analysis of dietary intake was conducted with FoodWorks (Xyris Pty Ltd., Brisbane, Australia). Overall, athletes reported consuming a median total daily energy intake of 8674 kJ (range 2384–18,009 kJ), with carbohydrate within the range of 1.0–9.0 g per kg of bodyweight (g/kg) (median = 3.8) and contributing to 50% total energy (TE) (range 14%–79%). Protein and fat intake ranged from 0.3–4.0 g/kg (median = 1.7) to 10–138 g (median = 67 g), and contributed to 21% TE (range 8%–48%) and 24% TE (range 8%–44%), respectively. Athletes reported consuming between 4 and 29 different food items (median = 15) in the previous 24 h period, with predominately discretionary, grains/cereals, meats, poultry, fish, eggs, and meat alternative items. This suggests that dairy, fruit, and vegetable intake may be suboptimal and intake of the micronutrients iron, zinc, calcium, and vitamins A and C may be of concern for a number of athletes.

Keywords: dietary intake; athlete; international competition

1. Introduction

International travel and short-term residence overseas is now a common feature of an athlete's competition schedule, however, differing eating arrangements and food options when away from home may influence an athlete's food choice, and potentially their performance. An athlete needs to consume suitable food and fluid prior to, during, and after competition in order to maximise performance [1,2]. While sport-specific recommendations exist for athletes to ensure that they consume sufficient total energy (TE) to meet requirements, carbohydrate (CHO) to replenish glycogen stores, protein to aid in muscle repair and growth, as well as fluid to stay adequately hydrated [1,3–9], very little evidence is available to ascertain if athletes meet these recommendations in residence during major international competitions.

While appropriate nutrition is important for performance, investigation into the dietary intake of high performance athletes is limited. Although there appears to be considerable individual variability in dietary intake, the majority of studies to date show that athletes tend on average to meet current evidence-based recommendations for protein, but not CHO [10–14]. This is particularly evident in females [15]. A number of studies have reported that TE intake may also be below expected requirements [14,16,17]. However, these studies are limited by the difficulties experienced when attempting to accurately measure dietary intake. Discrepancies exist between methods of data collection (for example a 24 h recall vs. 7 days weighed food diaries), whether the athlete is in a competition or training phase (or a combination of both), if the athlete is living at home or in a training camp, differing physiological requirements (e.g., strength and power athletes vs. endurance athletes), level of competition, and specific behaviours that may be associated with a particular sport (e.g., methods to make weight in weight-category sports). Assessing dietary intake is further made difficult by the practice of underreporting, where individuals report consuming less food than actual intake [18].

Additionally, the majority of research on dietary intake in athletic populations primarily focuses on quantifying dietary intake in regards to energy and macronutrient content; however, this does not guarantee that the athlete is selecting foods that contribute to a high quality diet. Diet quality is a concept based on the variety and type of foods in an entire diet, the relationship between health status and food groups, and is usually assessed by comparison to national dietary guidelines or similar, and the diversity of choices apparent within the diet [19]. To date, very little research on diet quality within the athletic population exists, with the exception of a comparison of the diets of a select group of Polish athletes to the Swiss Food Pyramid. This study found that athletes did not meet the recommendations for a number of food groups within the food pyramid guide [20]. Sufficient variety of foods from all core food groups is not only important for sports performance; it is often indicative of micronutrient intake and thus linked to prevention of deficiency and decreased risk of chronic disease [21], and therefore warrants investigation.

While literature to date provides some information on dietary intake of athletes during both training and competition phases, limited data is available regarding intake while in residence at international competition events. At major events such as the Olympic (OG) and Commonwealth Games (CG), the majority of athletes and their support team live in a village residence and dine in a large communal dining hall. An extensive range of food is provided free of charge, 24 h a day, for the duration of the competition. While recent data shows that athletes attending these events are generally satisfied with the food provided [22,23], data on actual dietary intake is limited. Only one study has investigated the types of diets (regimens) that are followed by these athletes [24]. Apart from records collected in 1949 [25] and 1964 [26], the most recent and relevant data on dietary intake in this type of environment was collected at the Sydney 2000 OG [23]. This data on apparent consumption within the dining hall suggested that athletes were consuming on average 592 g of carbohydrate (46% TE and on average 7–10 g/kg BM), 202 g (16% TE) of protein and 197 g (35% TE) of fat daily [23], however, no data on individual consumption was collected. Additionally, no data is available on the variety of foods consumed. Therefore, the aim of this research was to describe the self-reported food and dietary intake of athletes who sought professional guidance in regards to their competition diet immediately prior to or during competition at a major international competition.

2. Materials and Methods

2.1. Data Collection

Australian dietitians (*n* = 4) based at the main dining hall nutrition kiosk at the Delhi 2010 Commonwealth Games recorded consultations with athletes who requested assistance with their competition dietary intake from 23 September to 14 October 2010. Athletes were asked to provide demographic details including gender, sport (and event if appropriate), country representing, country of birth, and highest level of education (no schooling, primary/middle school, senior school, or University or other tertiary institution). Information about past experience at similar events, stage of competition (more than 2 days before event, day before event, day of event, between events, or event completed) and previous nutrition support was also collected. Athletes were asked to report if they had a nutrition competition plan to follow specifically for this event. Dietitians also recorded the purpose of the athletes visit to the kiosk (e.g., weight loss/making weight, weight gain, training or performance nutrition, and clinical issues such as food intolerance/allergy).

The dietitian then collected a recall of quantity and timing of all food, fluids and supplements consumed by the athlete over the previous 24 h period on a standard proforma, and verified intake of all food groups from a provided checklist as per the USDA five-step multiple pass method [27]. General questions about usual intake as per standard diet history were collected. The 24 h recall template was piloted and reviewed by a panel of expert dietitians prior to use at this competition. This was based on a similar template used in other settings [28]. Upon completion of the interview, dietitians were asked to subjectively rate the athlete regarding their expert opinion of the athletes' dietary intake and nutrition knowledge on a Likert scale of 1 (very poor) to 5 (very good).

2.2. Data Analysis

Participants were classified into a sport category (power/sprint, weight category, endurance, racquet, skill, and team) based on the physiological requirements of their sport, and a region/country (western: Including Australia and the British Isles, and non-western: Africa, Caribbean, India and Sri Lanka, and Southeast Asia and the Pacific Islands) based on location and cultural style of eating [22]. Athletes were also grouped based on the reason for requesting advice at the kiosk including: General weight loss and making weight, weight gain, performance/training nutrition, and clinical issues (for example, food allergy/intolerance, gastrointestinal issues).

The 24 h recall data was coded and input into FoodWorks Premium Edition (Version 7, Xyris software, Brisbane, Australia 2013) (FoodWorks) by the primary researcher. Foods consumed within the dining hall were matched to the nutritional analysis for the specific menu items that had previously been coded in FoodWorks. If not consumed from the menu, the item was coded against the most appropriate matching food. As FoodWorks is a database of Australian and New Zealand foods, items were coded into the 2013 Australian Dietary Guidelines (ADG) five core food groups (1) Grains—grain and cereal based foods; (2) Vegetables—vegetables and legumes/beans; (3) Fruit; (4) Dairy—milk, yoghurt, cheese and/or alternatives; (5) Meat and alternatives—lean meats, poultry, fish, eggs, tofu, nuts and seeds) and discretionary foods [21] for the analysis of diet variety (number of choices from each group). Discretionary foods were defined as per the ADG as containing high amounts of saturated fat, added sugars and/or salt, and alcohol (for example, potato chips, biscuits, pizza and fried foods) [21]. Some items were coded as both discretionary and a core food due to the contribution of macro- and micronutrients to the athlete's diet. For example, a number of discretionary foods were included in the calculation of the main food groups. Cakes/biscuits ($n = 11$), pizza ($n = 6$), Coco-pops™ ($n = 2$), and a muffin ($n = 1$) were included in the calculation of the grains group, as the predominant ingredient is a cereal grain and thus are a source of CHO. All data were cross-checked to ensure consistency and accuracy of coding.

Data were further coded and input into IBM SPSS Statistics (Version 21, IBM Corp., Armonk, NY, USA, 2012) for analysis. Data associations were calculated with the Kruskal–Wallis test, Mann–Whitney *U* test, independent *t* test or ANOVA, depending on normality of data. Statistical significance was considered to be $p \leq 0.05$ a priori. Results on nutrient intake are presented as median and range of g per kg of bodyweight (g/kg) and as a percentage of total energy intake (% TE). Micronutrient results were compared to the estimated average requirement (EAR), which is the "daily nutrient level estimated to meet the requirements of half the healthy individuals in a particular life stage and gender group" [29] or adequate intake (AI) which is the average daily nutrient intake level based on observed or experimentally-determined approximations or estimates of nutrient intake by a group (or groups) of apparently healthy people that are assumed to be adequate [29]. Each athlete's 24 h recall data was also compared to recommendations [3–7,9,30] for CHO, protein, and fat intake, specific to type of sport and demographic information (for example, height, weight, age, and gender). Diet variety and dietitians' rating of dietary intake and nutrition knowledge is presented as a median score and range.

2.3. Ethical Approval

Ethical approval was granted by the University of the Sunshine Coast Human Ethics Committee (A/10/253). Participation was voluntary and participants were considered to have given consent to participate by taking part in a consultation.

3. Results

3.1. Participant Characteristics

A total of 44 athletes completed a 24 h dietary recall at the nutrition kiosk, representing 1% of the total number of athletes who competed at this event (n = 4352). However, not all athletes reside in the village, eat within the dining hall, and thus have access to the nutrition kiosk. This cohort was the entire sample of athletes that sought dietary advice. Athletes were predominately from non-western regions and reported competing in 13 specific sports (Table 1). Over half of the athletes reported being in a precompetition stage (n = 30, 68%), with the majority of these athletes greater than 2 days away from competition (n = 28, 82%). The mean self-reported body weight of the male and female athletes was 74 kg (range 56–113 kg) and 65 kg (range 49–101 kg), respectively. Six athletes (14%) reported that they had received nutrition education prior to attending this event. While four athletes (10%) reported having a competition plan to follow, only two of these reported nutrition education prior to this event.

3.2. Dietary Intake and Eating Behaviours

Overall, athletes reported consuming a median total daily energy intake of 8674 kJ (range 2384–18,009 kJ), with CHO within the range of 1.0–9.0 g/kg (median = 3.8 g/kg) and contributing to 50% TE (range 14%–79%). Protein intake ranged from 0.3 to 4.0 g/kg (median = 1.7 g/kg) and contributed to 21% TE (range 8%–48%), while total fat intake ranged from 10 to 138 g (median = 67 g) and contributed to 24% TE (range 8%–44%). Dietary intake varied according to reason for requesting assistance at the kiosk and gender of athletes (Table 2). Those competing in racquet (n = 6) and power/sprint sports (n = 9) reported consuming the greatest energy (median = 11,298 kJ, range 7032–13,485 kJ and 10,149 kJ, range 2472–18,009 kJ, respectively). Athletes competing in skill and power/sprint sports reported consuming the highest protein intake (median = 1.8 g/kg, range 1–3 g/kg, and median = 1.7 g/kg, range 0.5–4 g/kg, respectively), while athletes in team sports (n = 2) reported the lowest energy intake (median = 7274 kJ, range 5953–8596 kJ). Athletes in team (n = 2) and weight category sports (n = 13) reported the lowest contribution of energy from CHO (median = 2.5 g/kg, range 1.7–3.3 g/kg, 39% TE, and median = 3.0 g/kg, range 1.0–6.0 g/kg, 46% TE), while athletes competing in endurance sports (n = 4) reported consuming the lowest amount of fat (median = 51 g, range 35–72 g, 21% TE). There was no significant difference in nutrient intake between those in the pre-versus postcompetition phases.

Three main meals were consumed by the majority of athletes (*n* = 23, 77%). Overall, the greatest median contribution to total energy intake was from breakfast (29%) to lunch (31%). Carbohydrate contributed a greater proportion to total energy at breakfast (56%) and to snacks (69%) than lunch and dinner. Protein contribution was predominately from meals consumed at lunch and dinner. Fourteen athletes reported consuming sports drinks as a snack, with these drinks contributing to over half of the TE consumed between meals. Five athletes reported not consuming any snacks in the precompetition period. The average contribution of macronutrients to the total daily intake was similar between genders (Table 3).

Dietary analysis showed that 80% of all athletes did not meet the estimated average requirement (EAR) for at least one micronutrient in the previous 24 h, with 25% not meeting the EAR/AI for 5 or more nutrients. Greater than 80% of both genders did not meet the EAR for iron and phosphorus, and vitamin B1–B3 and vitamin C. A greater proportion of women and men did not meet the EAR for vitamin A and magnesium, and zinc respectively (Figure 1). Over two-thirds (*n* = 39, 90.5%) did not meet the EAR for iron (female M = 13.66 mg, range 3.8–28; male M = 12.32 mg, range 4.2–25 mg). Overall, *n* = 22 (50%) reported using at least one type of supplement, with almost half (*n* = 19, 43%) of all athletes reporting the use of a vitamin or multivitamin supplement. Multivitamin supplements were not disclosed in the 24 h recall by any athletes, and therefore were not included in the calculation of dietary intake. Five athletes (11%) reported that they had been previously diagnosed with a nutrient deficiency (one from each of team, skill, power/sprint, weight, and endurance), of which 4 of these reported as iron deficiency anaemia (*n* = 1, unknown).

Table 1. Demographic information of all athletes who took part in a 24 h recall.

Demographic	TOTAL *n* = 44	Gender		Reason for Consultation [@]			
		Female *n* = 18 (41%)	Male *n* = 26 (59%)	Making Weight or Weight Loss *n* = 26 (59%)	Weight Gain *n* = 4 (9%)	Performance *n* = 9 (21%)	Clinical [#] *n* = 5 (11%)
Age (years) (M ± SD)	26.6 (8)	27.6 (10)	25.9 (7)	25.9 (7)	24 (9)	30.9 (9)	24 (9)
Region * (*n*, %)							
Non-Western ^	36 (86)	14 (78)	24 (92)	26	4	9	2
Western $	8 (14)	4 (22)	2 (8)	-	-	-	3
Sport (*n*, %) ~							
Endurance	4 (9)	2 (11)	2 (8)	2	-	1	1
Power/Sprint	9 (21)	7 (39)	2 (8)	6	-	1	2
Racquet	6 (14)	2 (11)	4 (15)	1	1	3	1
Skill	10 (23)	4 (22)	6 (23)	6	-	3	1
Team	2 (5)	2 (11)	-	1	-	1	-
Weight	13 (30)	1 (6)	12 (46)	10	3	-	-
Education (*n*, %)							
Middle/Senior School	7 (17)	2 (12)	5 (20)	4	1	-	2
Completed Senior School	17 (40)	6 (35)	11 (44)	12	1	4	-
Attended University	18 (43)	9 (53)	9 (36)	9	1	5	3
Experience (*n*, %)							
First CG/OG	34 (79)	15 (83)	19 (73)	21	3	5	5
First athletes village	30 (70)	14 (78)	16 (62)	18	2	5	5
Previous nutrition assistance (*n*, %)	6 (14)	2 (12)	4 (16)	5 (20)	0	0	1 (20)

* 2 responses unknown for region and level of education; [#] Clinical consultations included Coeliac disease, corn allergy, nut allergy and reflux; ^ Bahamas, Bangladesh, Belize, Gambia, India, Kenya, Malawi, Sierra Leone, Sri Lanka, St Vincent, Tanzania, Tonga, Trinidad and Tobago; $ Australia, England, Falkland Islands, Guernsey; [@] Proportions not calculated for region, sport, education or assistance as numbers in most categories are <10; ~ Endurance includes; athletic events 800 m and over, cycling and swimming distance events; Power/Sprint includes; athletic events under 400 m, athletic field events and swimming sprint events; Racket includes; badminton, table tennis and squash; Skill includes; archery and shooting; Team includes hockey; Weight includes; boxing, weight lifting and wrestling.

Table 2. Energy and macronutrient intake of athletes.

Energy and Macronutrients	TOTAL (All Athletes) Median, Range	Gender Median, Range		Reason for Consultation Median, Range			
		Female (n = 18)	Male (n = 26)	Making Weight or Weight Loss (n = 26)	Weight Gain (n = 4)	Performance (n = 9)	Clinical # (n = 5)
Energy							
kilojoules/day	8674, 2473–18,009	8484, 2473–18,008	9369, 2384–15,175	8632, 2384–18,009	11542, 9622–14,560 *	10798, 5953–14,908	7795, 2473–8091 *
Carbohydrate							
g/day	241, 68–576	244, 81–576	230, 68–512	239, 68–576	342, 208–512	317, 133–478	198, 81–258
g/kg **	3.8, 1.0–9.0	4.2, 1–9	3.5, 0.1–7	3.6, 0.1–9.0	4.3, 4.3–6.2	4.8, 1.7–7.4	3, 1.3–4.6
% TE	50, 14–79	49, 35–64	51, 14–79	50, 14–79	49, 36–57	52, 36–62	49, 38–53
Protein							
g/day	121, 20–276	109, 30–276	127, 20–231	115, 20–276	164, 129–232	120, 55–169	109, 30–163
g/kg **	1.7, 0.3–4	1.7, 0.5–4	1.6, 0.3–3.0	1.6, 0.3–4	1.8, 1.7–2.1	1.6, 0.8–2.1	1.7, 0.5–1.8
% TE	21, 8–48	20, 8–40	22, 9–48	21, 8–48	23, 17–41	18, 10–38	24, 19–40
Fat							
g/day	67, 10–138	65, 13–129	67, 10–138	70, 10–138	79, 57–91	74, 28–115	36, 13–56
% TE	24, 8–44	25, 17–43	22, 8–44	25, 8–44	22, 21–31	25, 16–39	20, 17–27

* Energy, kilojoules/day and reason for consultation (Kruskal–Wallis test, $p = 0.047$); ** $n = 41$ as weight unknown for three athletes; # Clinical consultations included coeliac disease, corn allergy, nut allergy, and reflux.

Table 3. Distribution of energy and macronutrient contribution at meal periods.

Distribution of Energy at Meal Time	TOTAL (All Athletes) Median, Range	Gender Median, Range		Reason for Consultation Median, Range			
		Female (n = 18)	Male (n = 26)	Making Weight or Weight Loss (n = 26)	Weight Gain (n = 4)	Performance (n = 9)	Clinical # (n = 5)
Breakfast							
% TE	29, 8–84	26, 8–55	33, 8–84	33, 8–84	34, 16–35	27, 18–40	19, 15–38
% E CHO	56, 22–87	63, 36–87	54, 22–82	55, 22–87	54, 41–59	55, 28–70	71, 63–83
% E PRO	16, 5–39	15, 6–37	16, 5–39	14, 5–39	18, 12–24	17, 13–23	13, 6–18
% E FAT	23, 2–54	22, 3–46	25, 2–54	23, 2–54	32, 12–35	27, 9–50	11, 3–13
Lunch							
% TE	31, 0–72	32, 2–45	30, 0–72	30, 0–72	28, 4–33	32, 18–51	36, 11–45
% E CHO	48, 4–94	45, –81	51, 5–94	46, 5–81	52, 17–94	48, 14–74	35, 4–62
% E PR	26, 2–66	22, 4–55	26, 2–66	28, 4–58	29, 2–66	21, 8–51	34, 7–55
% E FAT	22, 2–48	26, 5–48	17, 2–46	23, 5–45	15, 12–35	17, 11–46	25, 7–48
Dinner							
% TE	26, 0–49	28, 0–49	24, 0–44	25, 0–48	22, 0–42	28, 0–40	28, 0–49
% E CHO	46, 12–85	43, 15–76	49, 12–85	45, 12–85	23, 21–70	50, 15–61	33, 26–76
% E PR	22, 5–62	25, 8–55	22, 5–62	22, 5–49	58, 17–62	19, 15–55	30, 8–44
% E FAT	25, 2–53	28, 5–53	18, 2–50	26, 2–53	16, 7–17	27, 10–43	25, 5–38
Snacks							
% TE	9, 0–54	10, 0–39	9, 0–54	9, 0–39	21, 9–54	7, 0–50	17, 0–31
% E CHO	69, 35–100	72, 35–100	66, 35–100	69, 35–100	54, 41–80	69, 36–100	71, 57–73
% E PR	8, 0–30	6, 0–20	8, 0–30	6, 0–30	10, 5–15	7, 0–13	9, 6–14
% E FAT	18, 0–56	18, 0–53	18, 0–56	18, 0–56	32, 9–41	18, 0–50	14, 8–30

Clinical consultations included coeliac disease, corn allergy, nut allergy and reflux.

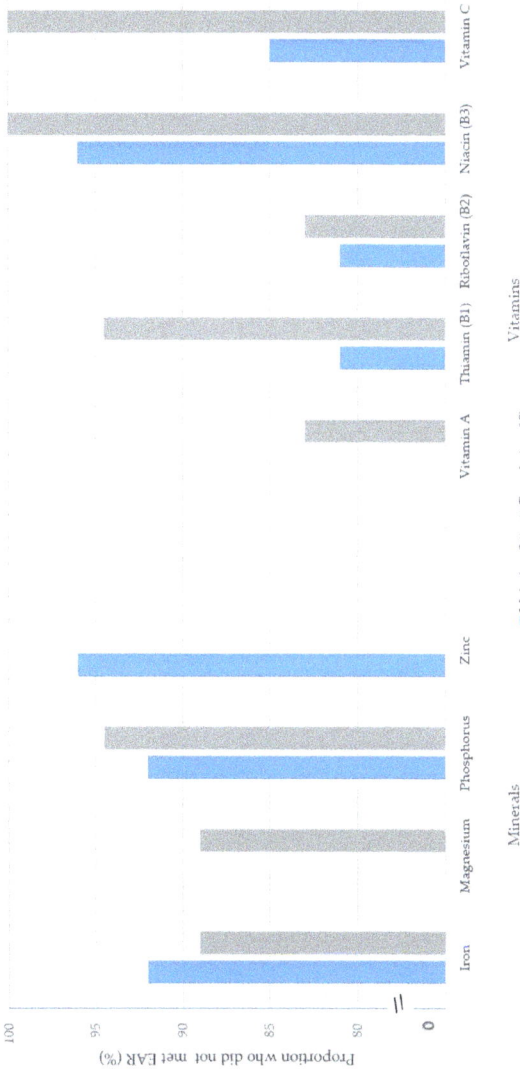

Figure 1. Proportion of male and female athletes who did not meet the micronutrient Estimated Average Requirement (EAR) # . # Micronutrients displayed are those where greater than 80% of the cohort were below the EAR. The following EAR for 19–50 years old were used: iron male = 6 mg/day , iron female = 8 mg/day; magnesium male 330 mg/day (19–30 years of age), 350 mg/day (31–50 years of age), female 255 mg/day (19–30 years of age), 265 mg/day (31–50 years of age); phosphorus male = 580 mg/day, female = 580 mg/day; zinc male = 12.5 mg/day, female = 6.5 mg/day; vitamin A male = 625 µg/day, female = 500 µg/day; thiamine (B1) male = 1.0 mg/day, female = 0.9 mg/day; riboflavin (B2) male = 0.9 mg/day, female = 0.9 mg/day; niacin (B3) male = 12 mg/day, female = 11 mg/day; vitamin C male = 30 mg/day, female = 30 mg/day. 2 athletes missing data to calculate EAR.

3.3. Food Variety

3.3.1. Number of Total Food Items Consumed

Overall, athletes reported consuming between 4 and 29 different food items (median = 15, range 4–29) in the previous 24 h period, with a broad range of items chosen from the discretionary (median = 4, range 0–10), grain (median = 3.5, range 0–7), and meat (median = 3, range 0–7) groups. Athletes from racquet (median = 20, range 15–24) and team sports (median = 18, range 16–20) reported consuming a greater number of food items than other sports in the previous 24 h (Kruskal–Wallis test, $p = 0.034$).

3.3.2. Number and Variety of Items from Each Food Group

Females reported consuming a greater number (median 3.5 vs. 2.0) and variety (3 vs. 1.5) of fruit choices than males ($p = 0.005$ and $p = 0.001$, respectively). Athletes requesting advice for weight gain reported consuming significantly less variety of fruit items than athletes requesting advice for clinical issues ($p = 0.038$) (Table 4). In addition, athletes competing in weight category sports reported consuming less items from the grains group (median 1.0, range 0–5, $p = 0.028$), as well as a lower variety of grains (median 1.0, range 0–3, Kruskal–Wallis test, $p = 0.017$) compared to other sports. There was no significant difference between athletes from western and non–western regions.

Table 4. Variety of items consumed from each food group and dietitians rating of diet and nutrition knowledge based on gender and reason for requesting assistance.

Variety of Items from Each Food Group &	TOTAL Median (Range)	Gender Median (Range)		Reason for Consultation Median (Range)			
		Female (*n* = 18)	Male (*n* = 26)	Making Weight or Weight Loss (*n* = 26)	Weight Gain (*n* = 4)	Performance (*n* = 9)	Clinical # (*n* = 5)
Grains	2 (0–6)	2 (0–5)	2 (0–6)	2 (0–5)	2.5 (2–5)	3 (1–6)	2 (0–3)
Vegetables	2 (0–9)	2 (0–9)	2 (0–8)	2 (0–9)	4 (2–8)	4 (0–5)	2 (0–8)
Fruit *	3 (0–8)	3 (0–8)	1.5 (0–4)	2 (0–7)	1.5 (0–2)	2 (0–8)	4 (3–7)
Dairy	1 (0–2)	1 (0–2)	1 (0–2)	1 (0–2)	1 (1–2)	1 (0–2)	1 (0–2)
Meats	2 (0–7)	2 (0–6)	2 (0–7)	2 (0–7)	2.5 (2–4)	3 (1–6)	2 (1–2)
Discretionary	3 (0–7)	3 (1–7)	3 (0–6)	3 (0–7)	4.5 (3–6)	2 (0–6)	3 (1–3)
TOTAL	15 (4–49)	16.5 (7–29)	13.5 (4–24)	13 (4–21)	15.5 (14–24)	16 (8–29)	15 (9–22)

Clinical consultations included coeliac disease, corn allergy, nut allergy, and reflux; ˙ Discretionary foods included: cakes/biscuits/muffin/pastries, pizza, coco-pops™, soft drinks, ice cream, desserts, and chocolate spread; * Significant difference in fruit variety between genders (Mann–Whitney U test $p = 0.001$) and reason for consultation (Kruskal–Wallis test, $p = 0.038$).

3.3.3. Dietitians Rating of Dietary Intake and Nutrition Knowledge

Overall, dietitians rated the dietary intake and nutrition knowledge of athletes as "average" (median 3, range "very poor–good") and "poor" (median 2, range "very poor–good"), respectively (Table 4). There were no significant differences in international regions or gender. Differences in rating were observed depending on reason for requesting assistance (Table 4). Athletes who requested assistance for weight gain and making weight/weight loss (both median 3 "average", range "very poor–good") were rated as having a significantly poorer dietary intake than those requesting performance nutrition (median 3.5 "average–good", range "poor–good") and clinical advice (median 3 "average", range "very poor–good") (Kruskal–Wallis test, $p = 0.03$).

4. Discussion

This research provides a unique insight into the food selection and dietary intake of athletes at a major competition. Although this is based on the results of a small selection of athletes, this is the entire sample of those who actively sought expert advice from dietitians at this event. Our results indicate that there is considerable variability in the dietary intake of these athletes, and despite representing a single day of intake, many report consuming inadequate total energy and CHO for both basic health requirements and athletic performance. The large variation in intake seen in our results may have to do with differing cultural background, sport category, gender, stage of competition and previous professional advice on dietary intake. In addition, our results indicate that many athletes did not consume a varied diet, with some athletes consuming as little as four or five different items in the previous 24 h period, with many not eating items from a range of food groups. While an athlete can appear to meet macronutrient recommendations based on quantifying intake, the variety of food that is consumed may not provide adequate intake of the micronutrients, fibre, and other food components. Inadequate dietary intake was conferred by the dietitians' general subjective perception of the nutrition knowledge of athletes as poor and dietary intake as average.

In general, we found that the CHO intake of athletes in this study was similar to that observed previously in similar samples [10,11,31], and supports other literature reporting that athletes from varying sports may not consume enough CHO to meet current recommendations for performance [10–14]. While our results are based on one 24 h recall, and we recognise that this may not be indicative of actual habitual intake, there are a number of potential implications on an athlete's performance, as inadequate CHO may compromise storage of muscle and liver glycogen, and may in turn affect physical and/or mental performance. Athletes in this study appeared to consume an adequate amount of protein based on a g/kg BW measure, however as we did not investigate the quantity and timing of protein intake in relation to competition, and this would be worth further investigation. The average contribution of fat to dietary intake varied considerably, but can be considered acceptable for general health [1]. It is also similar to that seen in other athletic populations [10,15,31–33]. The high consumption of discretionary food items appears to have contributed to fat intake, with foods such as pizza, ice cream, biscuits, cake, and muffin commonly consumed by these athletes. The main gender differences appeared to be around the consumption of a variety of fruit, which is not surprising as it is recognised that males typically consume less servings of fruits and vegetables per day than females [34].

We found those athletes that were attempting to make or lose weight were the predominant group to seek advice on their dietary intake. These athletes reported the lowest TE intake of all sports groups and, while not significantly different, appeared to consume less variety of foods with some individuals reporting no foods consumed from a range of food groups. These athletes are required to weigh in at a certain weight in order to participate in their event, and have been reported to reduce their CHO, protein, and fluid intake before competition in a similar environment [23]. A number of these athletes specifically requested assistance for making weight, suggesting that they were under pressure to lose weight within a short time period, and may therefore have already limited their consumption of food. Athletes, particularly those attempting to make weight, may also have inadequate intramuscular stores of CHO after restricting intake, and an insufficient time period in which to try and restore these before competition for maximal performance. It is possible that this may be linked to a lack of professional guidance on dietary intake, as we found that only 5 of the 26 athletes requesting assistance for making weight had reported having dietary advice prior to this event and a nutrition plan to follow. Furthermore, nutrition knowledge of these athletes was rated as poor by the dietitians.

Given the varied intake of TE and macronutrients, and the poor variety of foods consumed in our sample, it is not surprising that a large number of athletes did not meet the EAR/AI for various micronutrients based on their intake in the previous 24 h period. Previous research suggests that athletes generally tend to consume sufficient food to have an adequate intake of most micronutrients with some exceptions in specific athletic groups for vitamin E [11,33], zinc [14], vitamin A, and iron [17]. Interestingly, we found that iron, phosphorus, vitamin C, and the B vitamins were below the EAR in most athletes in this sample. It is likely that our sample had a poorer intake than the rest of the athlete population, as suggested by their reason for seeking a consultation and the dietitians' subjective assessment of their intake. No athlete reported consuming supplements in the previous 24 h, however, half of the athletes reported generally consuming a multivitamin (MV) supplement as part of their normal routine. Clearly, some athletes had poor dietary intake and nutrition knowledge, and a lack of variety in their diet. This may place the athletes at increased risk of illness, particularly when combined with the stress of travel and competition in a foreign country.

While we did not detect any differences in athletes' diet pre- and postcompetition, the phase of competition may actually change eating behaviours. It is plausible that an athlete will be more focused on meeting nutritional goals prior to, as compared to after, competition [35]. Anecdotally, athletes have been known to "relax" their attitude to eating for performance once their event is over, and have been seen to indulge, or consume foods that they may have avoided prior to competition. While this was not apparent in our sample, this may be due to the characteristics of the athletes who participated in this study.

The unique environment of the athlete's village and the location of training/competition venues at this event may have also influenced our results. The majority of athletes must leave the village and travel to different locations to train or compete. Anecdotally, we noted that a number of comments were made about unsuitable food and snack items being available at various training and competition venues. This may have also led athletes to consume more food before travelling away from the village. There may also be differences in the TE consumed at the dinner meal, as a number of competition events were held at night and this may have influenced when, or if, an athlete could eat this meal.

Additionally, while we asked athletes about stage of competition, we did not ask how long the athlete had been based in the athlete's village. If the athlete had recently arrived in the athlete's village, they may have been experiencing jet lag or a loss of appetite on arrival [36]. Conversely, an athlete who has been based in the athlete's village for a longer period of time may be experiencing menu boredom [22] which may influence food choice. Athletes may also vary from their usual intake as the novelty of attending an elite competition event and living in an athlete's village may distract them from focusing on nutritional goals [36]. A large proportion of athletes (79%) reported that this was their first experience at this type of event. It is possible that athletes with previous experience in this environment may find it easier to locate appropriate items and deal with the challenges of eating in a communal setting. Another important characteristic of the dining hall is the influence of other individuals on the athletes food choice [35,37,38]. Research shows individuals who are dining with strangers will consume less food than usual, while those who dine with familiar individuals tend to consume more [38]. Further research on the influences on food choice in this environment would provide valuable information to those who work with athletes competing at these events.

It is important to note that this sample of athletes were recruited when they approached the nutrition kiosk for assistance, thus may not have known how to choose appropriate foods for their particular sport. A large proportion of the athletes who took part in this study were from less westernised countries. Previous research at this [39,40], and similar events [23,41] has demonstrated that athletes from these regions are more likely to seek nutritional support in this environment. We noted that only six athletes had received professional nutrition advice prior to this event, so a lack of sports-specific nutrition knowledge may also be a reason for the variability in dietary intake. Interestingly, the dietitians did not rate the dietary intake of athletes from western and non-western regions differently.

There are a number of limitations in this research that need to be acknowledged. Our results are specifically focused on athletes who approached the kiosk for a consultation and therefore do not represent every athlete present at this event. While the dietitians used a predesigned form to conduct the 24 h recall, there may have been differences in recording methods, and the subjective rating given for both the assessment of dietary intake and nutrition knowledge. As with any collection of dietary intake data, there are limitations with the use of the 24 h recall method. While this method is quick and can provide in-depth information about dietary intake [42], it is only a measure of a single day, and does not represent usual intake [18,43]. There is also the potential for underreporting, as some individuals may report consuming less than their actual intake [18]. It is also feasible that the menu items did not reflect the original recipe, resulting in inaccurate nutritional analysis. Due to the nature of the data that was collected, we were not able to score diet quality nor determine exact servings of each food group, but were able to provide an indication of variety of items consumed in the diet, and variety of items from within each food group.

Future Directions

Based on the results of this study, further research on the dietary intake of athletes in this type of environment is warranted. It would be of interest to investigate what athletes consume over a longer period (both before and during competition) with more detailed methods of data collection. Further research with a larger sample would be beneficial, particularly regarding dietary intake and eating behaviours (e.g., snacking, use of sports drinks, diet quality). As food choice is complex, further research on the factors which influence food choice in this environment would provide insight for caterers and dietitians working with individual athlete.

5. Conclusions

Athletes who requested assistance at the nutrition kiosk at a major international competition generally had a poor variety of foods, distribution of, and in some cases inadequate intake of, energy, macro-, and micronutrients. Of particular concern was the dietary intake of athletes who were attempting to make weight or lose weight in the days prior to competition. While this data is limited in that it is only a measure of one day's intake and is based on the athletes recall, this highlights that these athletes may not be consuming a diet that will assist with maximising performance, and if the same dietary habits are followed over a prolonged period of time, health may also be compromised. Further research is required to examine the dietary habits of athletes in this unique environment.

Acknowledgments: This project was supported by Delaware North Companies Pty Ltd. and internal university higher degree by research funding.

Author Contributions: For research articles with several authors, a short paragraph specifying their individual contributions must be provided. The following statements should be used "F.E. Pelly and S.J. Burkhart conceived and designed the experiments; performed the experiments; S.J. Burkhart analyzed the data; S.J. Burkhart and F.E. Pelly interpreted the data and wrote the paper". Authorship must be limited to those who have contributed substantially to the work reported.

Conflicts of Interest: The authors declare no conflict of interest.

References

1. Rodriquez, N.R.; DiMarco, N.M.; Langley, S. Position of the American Dietetic Association, Dietitians of Canada, and the American College of Sports Medicine: Nutrition and Athletic Performance. *J. Am. Diet. Assoc.* **2009**, *109*, 509–527.
2. International Olympic Committee (IOC). IOC consensus statement on sports nutrition 2010. *J. Sports Sci.* **2011**, *29* (Suppl. 1), S3–S4.
3. Thomas, D.T.; Erdman, K.A.; Burke, L.M. Position of the Academy of Nutrition and Dietetics, Dietitians of Canada, and the American College of Sports Medicine: Nutrition and Athletic Performance. *J. Am. Diet. Assoc.* **2016**, *116*, 501–528. [CrossRef] [PubMed]
4. Burke, L.M.; Hawley, J.A.; Wong, S.H.S.; Jeukendrup, A.E. Carbohydrates for training and competition. *J. Sports Sci.* **2011**, *29* (Suppl. 1), S17–S27. [CrossRef] [PubMed]
5. Burke, L.M.; Millet, G.; Tarnopolsky, M.A. Nutrition for distance events. *J. Sports Sci.* **2007**, *25*, 29–38. [CrossRef] [PubMed]
6. Jeukendrup, A.E. Nutrition for endurance sports: Marathon, triathlon, and road cycling. *J. Sports Sci.* **2011**, *29* (Suppl. 1), S91–S99. [CrossRef] [PubMed]
7. Slater, G.; Phillips, S.M. Nutrition guidelines for strength sports: Sprinting, weightlifting, throwing events, and bodybuilding. *J. Sports Sci.* **2011**, *29* (Suppl. 1), S67–S77. [CrossRef] [PubMed]
8. Stellingwerff, T.; Boit, M.K.; Res, PT. Nutritional strategies to optimize training and racing in middle-distance athletes. *J. Sports Sci.* **2007**, *25*, 17–28. [CrossRef] [PubMed]
9. Tipton, K.D.; Jeukendrup, A.E.; Hespel, P. Nutrition for the sprinter. *J. Sports Sci.* **2007**, *25*, 5–15. [CrossRef] [PubMed]

10. Lun, V.; Erdman, K.A.; Reimer, R.A. Evaluation of nutritional intake in Canadian high-performance athletes. *Clin. J. Sport Med.* **2009**, *19*, 405–411. [CrossRef] [PubMed]

11. Schroder, H.; Navarro, E.; Mora, J.; Seco, J.; Terregrosa, J.M.; Tramullas, A. Dietary habits and fluid intake of a group of elite Spanish basketball players: A need for professional advice? *Eur. J. Sport Sci.* **2007**, *4*, 1–15. [CrossRef]

12. Burke, L.M.; Gollan, R.A.; Read, R.S.D. Dietary intakes and food use of groups of elite Australian male athletes. *Int. J. Sport Nutr. Exerc. Metab.* **1991**, *1*, 378–394. [CrossRef]

13. DeLoach, J.; Meyer, N.; Askew, A.E.; Walker, J. Energy, macronutrient, fluid and dietary supplement intake in Olympic-Level winter sport athletes. In Proceedings of the 10th Annual Congress of the European College of Sports Science, Belgrade, Serbia, 13–16 July 2005; p. 13341.

14. Felder, J.M.; Burke, L.M.; Lowdon, B.J.; Cameron-Smith, D.; Collier, G.R. Nutritional practices of elite female surfers during training and competition. *Int. J. Sport Nutr.* **1998**, *8*, 36–48. [CrossRef] [PubMed]

15. Burke, L.M.; Slater, G.; Broad, E.M.; Haukka, J.; Modulon, S.; Hopkins, W.G. Eating Patterns and Meal Frequency of Elite Australian Athletes. *Int. J. Sport Nutr. Exerc. Metab.* **2003**, *13*, 521–538. [CrossRef] [PubMed]

16. Onywera, V.O.; Kiplami, F.K.; Tuitoek, P.J.; Boit, M.K.; Pitsiladis, Y.P. Food and macronutrient intake of elite Kenyan distance runners. *Int. J. Sport Nutr. Exerc. Metab.* **2004**, *14*, 709–719. [CrossRef] [PubMed]

17. Martin, L.; Lambeth, A.; Scott, D. Nutritional Practices of National Female Soccer Players: Analysis and Recommendations. *J. Sports Sci. Med.* **2006**, *5*, 130–137. [PubMed]

18. Burke, L.M.; Cox, G.R.; Cummings, N.K.; Desbrow, B. Guidelines for daily carbohydrate intake—Do athletes achieve them? *Sports Med.* **2001**, *31*, 267–299. [CrossRef] [PubMed]

19. Wirt, A.; Collins, C.E. Diet quality—What is it and does it matter? *Public Health Nutr.* **2009**, *12*, 2473–2492. [CrossRef] [PubMed]

20. Fraczek, B.; Gacek, M. Frequency of consumption of food products by a group of Polish athletes in relationship to the qualitative recommendations included in the Swiss Food Pyramid. *Med. Sport.* **2013**, *17*, 13–17. [CrossRef]

21. National Health and Medical Research Council. *Australian Dietary Guidelines*; National Health and Medical Research Council: Canberra, Australia, 2013.

22. Burkhart, S.J.; Pelly, F.E. Athletes' opinions of food provision at the 2010 Delhi Commonwealth Games: The influence of culture and sport. *Int. J. Sport Nutr. Exerc. Metab.* **2013**, *23*, 11–23. [CrossRef] [PubMed]

23. Pelly, F. *A Comprehensive Environmental Nutrition Intervention for Athletes Competing at the Sydney 2000 Olympic Games*; University of Sydney: Sydney, Australia, 2007.

24. Pelly, F.; Burkhart, S.J. Dietary Regimens of Athletes Competing at the Delhi 2010 Commonwealth Games. *Int. J. Sport Nutr. Exerc. Metab.* **2014**, *24*, 28–36. [CrossRef] [PubMed]

25. Berry, W.T.; Beveridge, J.B.; Bransby, E.R.; Chalmers, A.K.; Needham, B.M.; Magee, H.R.; Townsend, H.S.; Daubney, C.G. The diet, haemoglobin values, and blood pressures of Olympic athletes. *Br. Med. J.* **1949**, *1*, 300–304. [CrossRef] [PubMed]

26. Jokl, E. *Physiology of Exercise*; Charles C Thomas: Springfield, IL, USA, 1964.

27. United States Department of Agriculture. AMPM—Features, 5 Step Multiple-Pass Approach: USDA, 2016. Available online: https://www.ars.usda.gov/northeast-area/beltsville-md/beltsville-human-nutrition-research-center/food-surveys-research-group/docs/ampm-features/ (accessed on 9 August 2016).

28. Conway, J.M.; Ingwersen, L.A.; Vinyard, B.T.; Moshfegh, A.J. Effectiveness of the US Department of Agriculture 5-step multiple-pass method in assessing food intake in obese and nonobese women. *Am. J. Clin. Nutr.* **2003**, *77*, 1171–1178. [PubMed]

29. The Australian National Health and Medical Research Council (NHMRC). *Nutrient Reference Values for Australia and New Zealand Including Recommended Dietary Intakes*; NHMRC: Canberra, Australia, 2006.

30. Stellingwerff, T.; Maughan, R.J.; Burke, L.M. Nutrition for power sports: Middle-distance running, track cycling, rowing, canoeing/kayaking, and swimming. *J. Sports Sci.* **2011**, *29*, S79–S89. [CrossRef] [PubMed]

31. Garcia-Roves, P.M.; Terrados, N.; Fernandez, S.; Patterson, A.M. Comparison of dietary intake and eating behaviour of professional road cyclists during training and competition. *Int. J. Sport Nutr. Exerc. Metab.* **2000**, *10*, 82–98. [CrossRef] [PubMed]

32. Hassapidou, M.N.; Manstrantoni, A. Dietary intakes of elite female athletes in Greece. *J. Hum. Nutr. Diet.* **2001**, *14*, 391–396. [CrossRef] [PubMed]

33. Mullins, V.A.; Houtkooper, L.B.; Howell, W.H.; Going, S.B.; Brown, C.H. Nutritional status of US elite female heptathletes during training. *Int. J. Sport Nutr. Exerc. Metab.* **2001**, *11*, 299–314. [CrossRef] [PubMed]

34. Baker, A.H.; Wardle, J. Sex differences in fruit and vegetable intake in older adults. *Appetite* **2003**, *40*, 269–275. [CrossRef]

35. Smart, L.R.; Bisogni, C.A. Personal food systems of male college hockey players. *Appetite* **2001**, *37*, 57–70. [CrossRef] [PubMed]

36. Reilly, T.; Waterhouse, J.; Burke, L.M.; Alonso, J.M. Nutrition for travel. *J. Sports Sci.* **2007**, *25* (Suppl. 1), 125–134. [CrossRef] [PubMed]

37. Herman, P.C.; Roth, D.A.; Polivy, J. Effects of the presence of others on food intake: A normative interpretation. *Psychol. Bull.* **2003**, *129*, 873–886. [CrossRef] [PubMed]

38. De Castro, J.M. Family and friends produce greater social facilitation of food intake than other companions. *Physiol. Behav.* **1994**, *56*, 445–455. [CrossRef]

39. Burkhart, S.J.; Pelly, F.E. Beyond sports nutrition: The diverse role of dietitians at the Delhi 2010 Commonwealth Games. *J. Hum. Nutr. Diet.* **2013**, *27*, 639–647. [CrossRef] [PubMed]

40. Burkhart, S.J.; Pelly, F.E. Athlete use and opinion of point of choice nutrition labels at a major international competition. *Appetite* **2013**, *70*, 6–13. [CrossRef] [PubMed]

41. Pelly, F.; Inge, K.; King, T.; O'Connor, H. Provision of a nutrition support service at the Melbourne 2006 Commonwealth Games. In Proceedings of the 2nd Australian Association for Exercise and Sports Science, Sydney, Australia, 28 September–1 October 2006.

42. Dodd, K.W.; Guenther, P.M.; Freedman, L.S.; Subar, A.F.; Kipnis, V.; Midthune, D.; Tooze, J.A.; Krebs-Smith, S.M. Statistical Methods for Estimating Usual Intake of Nutrients and Foods: A Review of the Theory. *J. Am. Diet. Assoc.* **2006**, *106*, 1640–1650. [CrossRef] [PubMed]

43. Grandjean, A.C. Macronutrient intake of US athletes compared with the general population and recommendations made for athletes. *Am. J. Clin. Nutr.* **1989**, *49*, 1070–1076. [PubMed]

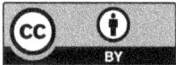

nutrients

MDPI

Article

Time of Day and Training Status Both Impact the Efficacy of Caffeine for Short Duration Cycling Performance

James C. Boyett [1], Gabrielle E. W. Giersch [1], Christopher J. Womack [1], Michael J. Saunders [1], Christine A. Hughey [2], Hannah M. Daley [2] and Nicholas D. Luden [1,*]

[1]   Human Performance Lab, Department of Kinesiology, James Madison University, Harrisonburg, VA 22807, USA; boyettjc@dukes.jmu.edu (J.C.B.); gierscge@dukes.jmu.edu (G.E.W.G.); womackcx@jmu.edu (C.J.W.); saundemj@jmu.edu (M.J.S.)
[2]   Department of Chemistry, James Madison University, Harrisonburg, VA 22807, USA; hugheyca@jmu.edu (C.A.H.); daleyhm@dukes.jmu.edu (H.M.D.)
*   Correspondence: ludennd@jmu.edu; Tel.: +1-540-568-4069

Received: 26 August 2016; Accepted: 7 October 2016; Published: 14 October 2016

Abstract: This project was designed to assess the effects of time of day and training status on the benefits of caffeine supplementation for cycling performance. Twenty male subjects (Age, 25 years; Peak oxygen consumption, 57 mL·kg^{-1}·min^{-1}) were divided into tertiles based on training levels, with top and bottom tertiles designated as 'trained' ($n = 7$) and 'untrained' ($n = 7$). Subjects completed two familiarization trials and four experimental trials consisting of a computer-simulated 3-km cycling time trial (TT). The trials were performed in randomized order for each combination of time of day (morning and evening) and treatment (6mg/kg of caffeine or placebo). Magnitude-based inferences were used to evaluate all treatment effects. For all subjects, caffeine enhanced TT performance in the morning (2.3% ± 1.7%, 'very likely') and evening (1.4% ± 1.1%, 'likely'). Both untrained and trained subjects improved performance with caffeine supplementation in the morning (5.5% ± 4.3%, 'likely'; 1.0% ± 1.7%, 'likely', respectively), but only untrained subjects rode faster in the evening (2.9% ± 2.6%, 'likely'). Altogether, our observations indicate that trained athletes are more likely to derive ergogenic effects from caffeine in the morning than the evening. Further, untrained individuals appear to receive larger gains from caffeine in the evening than their trained counterparts.

Keywords: exercise time of day; caffeine supplementation; training history; diurnal; training status

1. Introduction

Caffeine use in sport is widespread due to its reputed performance benefits. There is consistent evidence that caffeine enhances cycling performance in events lasting longer than a few minutes [1–5]. While not unanimous [6–8], caffeine intake can also improve peak anaerobic power and speed [9–11] as well as peak muscle function (strength, power, and endurance) under certain conditions [6,7,12,13]. Although caffeine has the capacity to improve physical performance, there are a number of unresolved factors that may impact the magnitude of the effect of caffeine, such as time of day and training status.

Only two studies have investigated the potential interaction between time of day and caffeine on performance outcomes, and both suggest that the value of caffeine is heightened in the morning. In the first study, caffeine increased peak squat power in the morning but not in the evening [13]. Caffeine appeared to compensate for underperformance in the morning placebo trial such that squat power was elevated to levels observed in both evening trials (caffeine and placebo). We recently investigated whether time of day influenced the effects of caffeine on cycling performance, using a post-hoc analysis in which cyclists who completed trials early in the day (prior to 10 a.m.) were compared to those who performed later in the day (after 10 a.m.) [5]. In line with Mora-Rodríguez et al., caffeine ingestion improved performance among subjects that completed their trials early in the day but had an unclear effect on performance in those who performed later trials. Based on these preliminary results, the primary purpose of the present study was to use a crossover design to test the hypothesis that caffeine would elicit larger improvements in 3-km time trial (TT) performance in the morning compared to the evening.

Like time of day, training status may also mediate the magnitude of caffeine's ergogenic effect. A 2010 meta-analysis indicated that caffeine tended ($p = 0.08$) to enhance muscle endurance in untrained more so than trained subjects [14]. However, this conclusion was largely reached by comparing effect sizes derived from studies with trained subjects to other studies with untrained individuals. Regardless of the performance measure, we are aware of only four investigations that included both trained and untrained subjects in the same experimental design, the first of which reported that caffeine improved 100 m swim performance more so in trained than untrained swimmers [10]. Though this is in contrast to the meta-analysis, it may not be fair to use swimming as a model to determine the effects of training status, as the technical nature of swimming mechanics likely made it difficult for the untrained swimmers to take full advantage of potential improvements in whole muscle function. The only other study to compare trained and untrained subjects in the same design, that also observed caffeine-induced improvements in performance, reported that untrained and trained subjects experienced similar improvements in 10-km cycling performance [15], which again is in contrast to the prior mentioned meta analysis. The other two studies concluded that training status had no effect on time-to-fatigue [16] or peak strength [17], although there was no main effect of caffeine in either study. The lack of a significant ergogenic effect of caffeine in these studies (i.e., experimental models that did not detect a beneficial effect of caffeine) makes it impossible to tease out the impact of training levels. We recruited participants that were accustomed to cycling exercise and ultimately enrolled subjects that had a wide range of cycling experience and fitness levels. This allowed us to examine a separate factor (other than time of day) that may alter the magnitude of benefit conferred by caffeine ingestion. Specifically, in addition to time of day, we tested the hypothesis that untrained cyclists would receive more of a performance benefit from caffeine compared to their trained counterparts.

The outcomes of this investigation have marked practical relevance. Athletes and coaches make training/competition decisions based on risk and reward. It is therefore worthwhile to establish whether or not time trial performance is differentially impacted by time of day and/or training status, as this will instruct best practices for caffeine use as an ergogenic aid. There can be downsides to caffeine consumption, particularly in the evening. For instance, caffeine intake later in the day can interfere with quantity and quality of sleep [18], thereby possibly impairing recovery from heavy exercise [19] and subsequent performance [20]. Our collective hypothesis was that trained subjects supplementing with caffeine in the evening will experience the least improvement in performance and therefore should reconsider caffeine as an ergogenic aid late in the day.

2. Materials and Methods

2.1. Subjects

Twenty-two healthy male subjects from James Madison University and the surrounding area volunteered for the study. Two subjects withdrew for reasons unrelated to the study, resulting in complete data from eleven trained and nine untrained cyclists. Descriptive data are shown in Table 1. Subjects were required to have performed, at minimum, either "occasional" cycling (one day/month) for the untrained cyclists or "consistent" cycling (four days/week) in their weekly exercise routine over the past three months for trained cyclists. Cycling frequency and duration were self-reported. Trained and untrained cyclists were determined by the number of hours cycling per week, with comparison based on the top (trained) vs. bottom (untrained) tertiles. The categorization of untrained and trained subjects is generally supported by individual peak oxygen consumption

(VO$_{2peak}$) values (Table 1). The notable exception is that one 'untrained' subject possessed a VO$_{2peak}$ of 61.3 mL·kg^{-1}·min^{-1}. However, this subject was only performing 1.5 h of weekly cycling. Subjects provided information about their resistance training routines and this information was used as a covariate for all analyses (data reported in Table 1). Subjects were informed of the experimental procedures and risks prior to giving written consent. The study was approved by the James Madison University Institutional Review Board (IRB #15-0559). We also implemented a questionnaire asking about caffeine habits (coffee, tea, soda, chocolate, etc.); daily caffeine intake was calculated by assigning typical caffeine values to each respective item. Caffeine levels are reported in Table 1. Only one subject regularly consumed >300 mg/day, the previously established benchmark for 'high' caffeine intake (400 mg/day). Therefore, any differences in caffeine intake between subjects likely had a negligible impact on our performance outcomes.

Table 1. Descriptive Data for All Subjects and the Upper and Lower Cycle Training Tertiles.

	All Subjects (*n* = 20)	Trained (*n* = 7)	Untrained (*n* = 7)
Height (m)	1.75 ± 0.07	1.75 ± 0.07	1.76 ± 0.08
Body Mass (kg)	73.6 ± 10.9	70.2 ± 10.7	76.0 ± 10.6
Age (year)	22 [18–44]	22 [18–39]	21 [19–44]
V̇O$_{2peak}$ (mL·kg^{-1}·min^{-1})	57.2 ± 9.3	64.8 ± 7.9	49.2 ± 5.6
Caffeine Intake (mg/day)	32 [0–407]	100 [8–407]	2 [0–204]
Cycle Training (h/week)	4.0 [1.5–10.0]	8.0 [5.0–10.0]	2.3 [1.5–3.5]
Resistance Training (h/week)	1.0 [0–22.5]	1.5 [0–22.5]	3.5 [0–9]

Age, caffeine intake, cycle training, and resistance training are expressed as medians [range] because data did not display a normal distribution. All other variables are expressed as means ± SD. VO$_{2peak}$ and cycling volume were higher in Trained vs. Untrained (*p* < 0.05).

2.2. Cardiovascular Fitness Testing

Following height and body weight measurements, subjects performed an incremental exercise test to exhaustion on a bicycle ergometer (Velotron, Racermate, Inc., Seattle, WA, USA) to determine peak oxygen consumption (VO$_{2peak}$). The test began at a workload of 100 W (untrained) or 150 W (trained), and was increased by 25 W every minute until volitional fatigue. Metabolic measurements were assessed using a Moxus Modular Metabolic System (AEI Technologies, Pittsburgh, PA, USA) throughout the test and VO$_{2peak}$ was determined by the highest 30-s mean oxygen uptake.

2.3. Experimental Design

A randomly counterbalanced, double blind, placebo controlled design was implemented to compare the effects of the four different treatment conditions. Subjects performed four trials: two morning trials starting between 6:00 a.m. and 10:00 a.m. (but with consistent starting times within each subject), and two evening trials starting between 4:00 p.m. and 8:00 p.m., with an eight-hour minimum separation between morning and evening start times for each subject. During the experimental trials, subjects ingested a capsule one hour prior to exercise containing either 6 mg/kg body weight anhydrous caffeine or all-purpose flour (placebo). Only ad libitum water consumption was permitted following capsule consumption. The four treatment conditions were designated as: 1 Morning placebo (AM$_{PLA}$); 2 Morning caffeine (AM$_{CAF}$); 3 Evening placebo (PM$_{PLA}$); and 4 Evening caffeine (PM$_{CAF}$).

2.4. Performance Trials

Each subject performed six exercise trials (two familiarization trials followed by four experimental trials) on both an isokinetic dynamometer (Biodex Multi-Joint System—PRO, Biodex Medical Systems, Inc., Shirley, NY, USA), and cycle ergometer, with 6 (2.5–17) days between each experimental trial. Venous blood samples were obtained immediately upon arrival to the laboratory and again prior to exercise (one-hour following capsule consumption). Subjects then began each trial with a 5-min treadmill warm-up at 3.5 mph. Following the warm-up, subjects completed two sets of four leg extension repetitions on an isokinetic dynamometer (two warm up repetitions followed by two peak torque measurements) at 30 degrees/s with the right leg. Each set was separated by 60 s. This protocol was repeated at 120 degrees/s and 240 degrees/s, respectively (grand total of 24 repetitions; 12 total warm-up repetitions (4 at each speed) and 12 total maximum repetitions (4 at each speed)). After a ~3 min transition, subjects performed a flat 3-km time trial on the cycle ergometer. The familiarization trials were identical to the experimental trials, with the exception of the supplementation protocol. Cycling power output (and consequently cycling velocity) was self-controlled by adjusting both resistance on the flywheel using a simulated gear shifter and pedaling cadence. Subjects were instructed to treat each trial as a competition prior to the beginning of each trial, but subjects did not receive verbal feedback or encouragement from the investigators during testing. Further, no visual feedback from the time trial was provided, with the exception of elapsed distance. 3-km time trial time was used as the performance measure.

2.5. Serum Caffeine Levels

Blood samples were obtained from the antecubital vein. After 30 min of coagulations, samples were centrifuged at 2500 rpm for 15 min. Serum was stored at -80 °C until analysis. Serum caffeine levels were subsequently determined via mass spectrometry.

2.5.1. Sample Preparation for Liquid Chromatography/Mass Spectrometry Analysis

Serum samples were stored at -80 °C prior to extraction. 200 μL of serum was extracted by vortexing with 5 mL of ethyl acetate for 5 min. The extract was then centrifuged for 10 min at $4000 \times g$ to separate the organic and aqueous layers. The top ethyl acetate layer was transferred to a tube, the extraction repeated and the organic fractions combined. The extract was then lyophilized in a CentriVap (Labconco, Kansas City, MO, USA) and reconstituted in 200 μL of 96:4 water:methanol for quantitation by LC/MS.

2.5.2. LC/MS Analysis

An Agilent 1290 ultra-high performance liquid chromatograph (UHPLC) coupled to a 6224 time of flight mass spectrometer (TOF MS) (Agilent Technologies, Santa Clara, CA, USA) was used to separate caffeine from other metabolites and measure its concentration in the serum extracts. Gradient elution with an Agilent Zorbax Eclipse Plus C18 column (2.1 mm × 150 mm, 1.8 μm particles) held at 35 °C was performed with mobile phase A (water, 0.1% v/v formic acid) and B (acetonitrile, 0.1% v/v) at 0.45 mL/min. as follows: B was held at 4% for 7 min and increased to 70% by 12 min. At 14.5 min the gradient was returned to the initial conditions. Five microliters of serum extract were injected in duplicate. Caffeine was ionized by positive ion electrospray (ESI) as follows: capillary, +3500 V; drying gas, 350 °C and 10 L/min; nebulizer 30 psig. Mass spectral data was acquired in profile and centroid mode at 3 specta/s over 100–1700 m/z. TOF ion optics were: fragmentor, 115 V; skimmer, 65 V and octopole retardation factor V_{p-p}, 750 V. An internal reference mass (IRM) solution (purine and HP-921, Agilent Technologies, Santa Clara, CA, USA) was delivered to the ESI source to ensure high mass accuracy (<15 ppm).

A caffeine stock solution (1000 ppm, water) was serially diluted to yield a minimum of seven calibration levels that ranged from 0.01 to 20 ppm. Agilent's Mass Hunter Quantitative Analysis software (B.06) (Agilent, Santa Clara, CA, USA) was used to generate external calibration curves and calculate the concentrations of caffeine in ppm.

2.6. Dietary and Exercise Control

Subjects were provided with instructions for recording food intake so dietary intake could be replicated across trials. All subjects recorded food intake for 24 h prior to all experimental trials. Subjects were provided with a copy of food records from the 24 h preceding the initial experimental trials to be used to facilitate dietary replication for the 24-h time period preceding subsequent trials. Subjects were also instructed to abstain from any alcohol (24 h), caffeine (12 h), and food intake (4 h; post-absorptive state) prior to each experimental trial. Our intent was to collect performance data in the morning and evening under similar feeding conditions. The most feasible way to accomplish this was to study subjects in a post-absorptive state, so as to avoid early waking and feeding prior to the morning trial. However, this leads to discrepancies in fasting duration prior to the morning and evening trials; the morning trials were conducted after an overnight fast (~7–10 h of fasting) whereas the evening trials were performed after a 4-h fast. While it is conceivable that this variance could impact performance, performance (both strength and 3-km TT) was virtually identical between the morning and evening under placebo conditions, suggesting that any error variance due to different fasting durations was likely negligible. Subjects were instructed to maintain consistent exercise habits between trials and to abstain from any heavy and/or unaccustomed exercise 48 h prior to each experimental trial. Subjects submitted physical activity logs for verification.

2.7. Statistical Analysis

All data were log transformed to diminish the effects of nonuniformity. Magnitude-based inferences about the data were derived using methods described by Hopkins and colleagues [21]. A previously established 'smallest worthwhile change' in performance was used as the threshold value for a substantial treatment effect (separate treatment conditions vs. placebo) [22]. The smallest worthwhile change in performance was defined as $0.3 \times$ the within-subject variability of a similar group of cyclists previously studied in our laboratory [5] (Coefficient of Variation = 2.7% for time) which translates to a difference of 0.8% or 2.4 s in the current project [23]. As recommended by Hopkins, for the isokinetic data, $0.2 \times$ SD of the AM_{PLA} trial was used to determine smallest worthwhile change [22]. The coefficient of variation for peak strength measurements (derived from placebo conditions) was: 3.9% at 30 degrees/s, 3.2% at 120 degrees/s, and 4.6% at 240 degrees/s. The coefficient of variation for 3-km TT performance was: 1.1% for all subjects, 1.1% for trained, and 0.8% for untrained.

A published spreadsheet [24] was then used to determine the likelihood of the true treatment effect (of the population) reaching the substantial change threshold ($0.3 \times$ CV); these were classified as <1% almost certainly no chance, 1%–5% = very unlikely, 5%–25% = unlikely, 25%–75% = possible, 75%–95% = likely, 95%–99% = very likely, and >99% = almost certain. If the percent chance of the effect reaching the substantial change threshold was <25% and the effect was clear, it was classified as a 'trivial' effect. If 90% confidence intervals included values exceeding the substantial change threshold for both a positive and negative effect, effects were classified as unclear (>5% chance of reaching the substantial threshold for both a positive and negative effect). To test the effects of time of day, the outcomes derived for each group using the spreadsheet mentioned above [24] were compared using a second spreadsheet [25]. Likewise, the effects of training status were compared using this same method. All data reported as mean ± 90% Confidence Interval unless noted otherwise.

We estimated the statistical power of our experimental design using a publicly available spreadsheet created for magnitude-based inferences [26]. Data derived from a subset of male subjects (n = 24) using a similar measurement protocol in our laboratory was used to estimate within-subject variability [5]. With a sample size of 20, the current design and statistical methods had the statistical power of 0.99 to detect changes in time trial performance of 1.5% and 0.7 to detect a performance change of 0.8%. For leg extension an effect of 4.05% (smallest meaningful effect derived from $0.2 \times$ within subject standard deviation under placebo conditions) could be detected with a power of 0.96. The between subject comparisons (trained vs. untrained) were associated with low power thereby increasing the likelihood of making a type II error. However, we detected magnitude-based differences in 3-km TT performance (caffeine vs. placebo) between trained and untrained subjects and these data are reported; peak strength data specific to each training group are omitted because of the lack of power and lack of clear statistical outcomes.

3. Results

3.1. Serum Caffeine Levels

Serum caffeine levels in AM were: All Subjects—Pre 0.7 ± 1.3 ppm, Post 13.8 ± 2.4 ppm; Trained—Pre 0.6 ± 0.9 ppm, Post 13.1 ± 2.0; Untrained—Pre 0.2 ± 0.3 ppm, Post 13.6 ± 2.3 ppm. Caffeine levels in PM were: All Subjects—Pre 0.7 ± 0.8, Post 14.7 ± 3.1 PPM; Trained—Pre 0.6 ± 0.7 ppm, Post 13.1 ± 3.9 ppm; Untrained—Pre 0.6 ± 0.5 ppm, Post 15.0 ± 2.8 ppm. There were no differences between trained and untrained subjects, nor were there any differences between AM and PM caffeine levels following caffeine ingestion.

3.2. The 3-km Time Trial Performance

3.2.1. All Subjects

All 3-km performance data are displayed in Figure 1. Individual performance data are displayed in Figure 2. In all subjects, AM_{CAF} 3-km time trial performance (3-km TT) was 'very likely' better than AM_{PLA} ($2.9\% \pm 1.7\%$), while PM_{CAF} 'possibly' improved performance vs. PM_{PLA} ($1.1\% \pm 1.1\%$). AM_{CAF} 'likely' improved 3-km TT performance to a greater extent than PM_{CAF} ($1.7\% \pm 2.0\%$) when compared to the respective placebo condition (PLA).

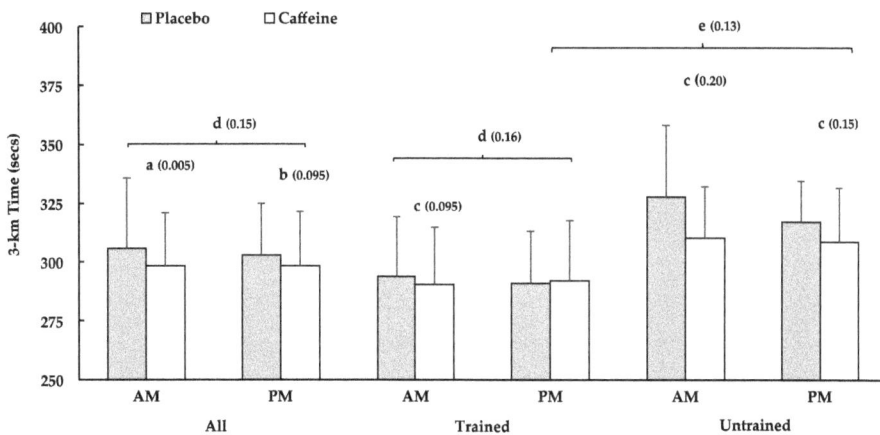

Figure 1. The 3-km Time Trial Performance. Bars depict mean finishing time in seconds ($\pm$SD). AM, morning; PM, afternoon; (**a**) 'very likely' faster than PLA; (**b**) 'possibly' faster than PLA; (**c**) 'likely' faster than PLA; (**d**) 'likely' different response to caffeine between AM and PM; (**e**) 'likely' different response to caffeine between Trained and Untrained in PM. *p*-values derived from pairwise comparisons are displayed in parentheses.

3.2.2. Trained Subjects

AM_{CAF} performance was 'likely' faster than AM_{PLA} ($1.8\% \pm 1.9\%$), whereas caffeine's effect was 'unclear' in the evening (PM_{CAF} vs. PM_{PLA}: $-1.0\% \pm 3.1\%$). Additionally, AM_{CAF} 'likely' improved performance more than PM_{CAF} (AM_{CAF} vs. PM_{CAF}: $2.8\% \pm 3.4\%$), when compared to PLA.

3.2.3. Untrained Subjects

AM_{CAF} and PM_{CAF} 'likely' improved time trial performance vs. AM_{PLA} ($5.5\% \pm 8.0\%$) and PM_{PLA} ($3.2\% \pm 3.8\%$), respectively. The time of day (AM vs. PM) comparison was 'unclear'.

3.2.4. Training Status

It was 'unclear' whether trained or untrained benefited more from caffeine in the AM condition, but untrained subjects 'likely' benefited more from caffeine supplementation than trained in the PM condition (trained: $-1.0\% \pm 3.2\%$, untrained: $3.2\% \pm 3.8\%$, AM_{CAF} vs. PM_{CAF}: $4.2\% \pm 4.5\%$).

3.3. Peak Muscle Torque

All peak skeletal muscle torque data are presented in Table 2. Knee extension torque at 30 degrees/s (30EXT) was 'possibly' improved by caffeine in PM when compared to PM_{PLA}, but all other PM measures were 'likely' trivial. PM Caffeine 'possibly' increased PM_{CAF} torque more than AM_{CAF} torque in the 30EXT condition when compared to PLA. All other time of day comparisons were 'trivial' or 'unclear'.

Bars depict mean finishing time in seconds ($\pm$SD). (a) 'Very likely' faster than PLA; (b) 'possibly' faster than PLA; (c) 'likely' faster than PLA; (d) 'Likely' different response to caffeine between AM and PM; (e) 'Likely' different response to caffeine between Trained and Untrained in PM. *p*-Values derived from pairwise comparisons are displayed in parentheses.

Data are reported as individual 3-km finishing times under all four experimental conditions, grouped by training tertiles. Numbers below the horizontal axis (x-axis) represent each individual subject.

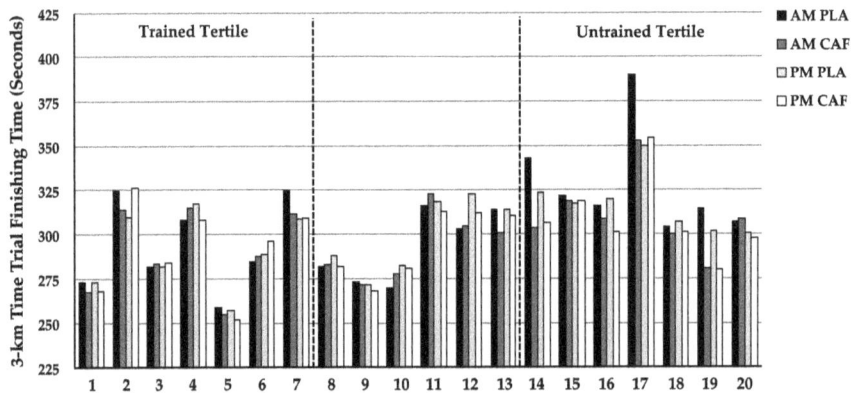

Figure 2. Individual 3-km Time Trial Performances. AM, morning; PM, afternoon; PLA, placebo; CAF, caffeine.

Table 2. Peak Muscle Strength Data.

Velocity	30 Degrees/s		120 Degrees/s		240 Degrees/s	
Time	AM	PM	AM	PM	AM	PM
PLA	192.7 ± 39.1	190.7 ± 38.7	171.3 ± 31.7	171.7 ± 29.5	154.6 ± 28.6	157.9 ± 29.9
CAF	194.1 ± 47.5	202.3 ± 41.8	171.3 ± 33.0	174.7 ± 29.2	158.4 ± 33.6	160.0 ± 26.1
PLA vs. CAF	0.9 ± 4.4 (-0.3 ± 4.3) 12/85/3 Likely Trivial	5.2 ± 3.6 (5.94 ± 3.5) 72/28/0 Possible; $p = 0.07$	-0.3 ± 3.5 (-0.1 ± 3.3) 4/91/6 Likely Trivial	1.3 ± 3.1 (1.9 ± 2.9) 10/90/1 Likely Trivial	2.0 ± 3.1 (2.0 ± 2.9) 18/81/0 Likely Trivial	0.8 ± 3.6 (1.8 ± 3.6) 9/89/2 Likely Trivial
AM vs. PM	-4.3 ± 5.5 (-6.19 ± 5.4) 1/46/53; Possible; $p = 0.06$		-1.6 ± 4.6 (-2.0 ± 4.3) 3/75/22; Likely Trivial		1.3 ± 4.6 (0.2 ± 4.5) 19/77/4; Likely Trivial	

Values for Placebo (PLA) and Caffeine (CAF) reported as Mean $\pm$ SD. AM, morning; PM, afternoon. Comparison values reported as adjusted (actual in parenthesis). Mean $\pm$ 90% CI for differences between change scores (i.e., AM vs. PM), % likelihoods of positive effect/trivial effect/negative effect and semantic inferences.

4. Discussion

The purpose of the current study was to investigate how the benefit of caffeine for 3-km cycling TT performance was influenced by time of day and training status. Caffeine enhanced 3-km TT performance more in the morning than in the evening (all subjects and trained subjects). Caffeine also improved cycling performance among untrained subjects in the morning and evening, whereas the benefit for trained subjects was 'likely' in the morning and 'unclear' in the evening. Further, caffeine intake enhanced 3-km performance more among untrained- than trained subjects, in the evening. Secondarily, we assessed peak muscle strength at three separate angular velocities prior to the time trials. Caffeine has been shown to increase peak strength [6,7,12,13,27] and there is some evidence that strength may contribute to the ergogenic properties of caffeine for cycling performance [28]. Therefore, we measured peak strength in an attempt to provide some physiological insight into the time trial outcomes. However, caffeine only increased strength at the slowest velocity (30 degrees/s) in the evening, which does not align with the TT performance results. This suggests that the gains in time trial performance were not mediated by improvements in strength.

Consistent with our general hypothesis, caffeine enhanced 3-km TT performance among trained subjects in the morning but not the evening. This supports results from a recent study, in which we reported that caffeine supplementation elicited the largest improvements in 3-km cycling TT performance among subjects that completed trials prior to 10:00 a.m. [5]. Importantly, prior observations made in strength-trained participants that caffeine elevates performance in the morning but not the evening [13] can now be extended to include longer sustained efforts. To our knowledge there are no other data from which to directly compare our findings.

The scant information on this topic also makes it difficult to provide a well-founded explanation for why caffeine appears to deliver a more pronounced benefit in the morning. We suspected that the time of day differences in performance could be related to varying rates of caffeine metabolism throughout the day. Cytochrome P450 1A2, the enzyme responsible for caffeine metabolism, has been shown to have higher activity levels during sleeping hours and directly after waking, when compared to the rest of day [29]. Considering that caffeine metabolites appear to be more potent than caffeine itself, faster caffeine metabolism could lead to a higher concentration of metabolites in the morning thereby delivering a stronger effect [30]. However, this was not the case in the current study. Caffeine levels were virtually identical between AM and PM trials (reported in Section 3.1). An alternative hypothesis is that the greater gains with caffeine in the morning are related to slower time trial performances in the morning compared to the evening, in the absence of caffeine. Though the physiology is largely unknown, there is good evidence that somatic control and physical performance (peak muscle strength, power, and swimming) can be impaired in the morning compared to the evening [20,31–33], perhaps providing an opportune time to utilize performance enhancing agents. This idea is supported by Mora-Rodriguez et al. where physical performance was worse in the morning compared to the evening, and caffeine raised morning performance to the levels achieved in the afternoon trials. The current data does not seem to support systematic somatic deficits in the morning, as only 9 of 20 subjects (2 of 7 trained tertile and 5 of 7 untrained tertile) performed slower in the AM_{PLA} than the PM_{PLA}. However, 5 of these 9 subjects (1 trained; 4 untrained) had much slower times under AM_{PLA} conditions, which had a large effect on the overall outcomes (i.e., larger gains in AM vs. PM). These slower times may represent a true time of day effect or may reflect individual circadian rhythms. Unfortunately, we do not have chronotype data from which to test this possibility.

While training status did not affect the response to caffeine in the morning, the untrained tertile did experience a more favorable response to caffeine than trained subjects in the evening. This aligns with a recent meta-analysis on this topic that concluded that caffeine tended to improve muscle endurance more in untrained than in trained subjects [14]. The current data are an important addition to our understanding since, as highlighted in the introduction, this conclusion was largely deduced by comparing effect sizes derived from separate studies conducted on trained vs. untrained cohorts. The differential impact that training status had on the caffeine benefits in the evening is a function of both the lack of improvement among the trained subjects and a 'likely' beneficial effect among untrained subjects. The physiological mechanisms responsible for this result are unknown and beyond the scope of this investigation. However, the concentration of adenosine receptors (the presumed primary target of caffeine) do appear to be higher in trained compared to untrained individuals [34]. And though highly speculative, the higher concentration of adenosine receptors may increase tissue sensitivity to any given concentration of adenosine, thereby requiring larger doses of caffeine to elicit a desirable effect. This may especially be an issue when the effects of caffeine are expected to be relatively small (i.e., the evening).

The current project revealed that caffeine's effect on 3-km TT performance was partially mediated by time of day and training status. However, peak muscle torque was largely unaffected by caffeine except 'possibly' at the slowest speed of contraction (30 degrees/s). There is some precedent for null strength findings [35–37], but most of the literature suggests that peak muscle function is heightened with caffeine [6,7,12,13,27]. Interestingly, as angular velocity increases, so do the number of trivial outcomes, indicating that movement velocity may impact the effects of caffeine. This could possibly be related to caffeine's role as an adenosine antagonist, a mechanism responsible for its ergogenic effects [38]. Adenosine receptor density has been shown to be greater in slow-twitch muscle fibers [39]. However, higher movement velocities require a greater reliance on force output (and power) from fast twitch fibers due to reductions in slow twitch fiber power production secondary to shifting the velocity × power curve to the right [40]. Therefore, at the higher movement velocities, it is possible that the fiber type most responsive to caffeine supplementation (slow twitch fibers) would contribute a smaller proportion to whole muscle power output, resulting in a smaller measurable effect of caffeine. This would explain why no ergogenic effects of caffeine were observed for peak strength at speeds greater than 30 degrees/s. In support of this idea, Jacobson et al. [41] reported improvements in isokinetic knee extension strength with caffeine consumption which were greater at slower movement speeds.

5. Conclusions

The primary weaknesses of the current study include the relatively small sample size, the lack of mechanistic insight (RPE, muscle pain, etc.), and as discussed in Section 2.6, the markedly different fasting durations preceding the morning and evening trials. Specific to the latter, it seems possible that the different fasting durations preceding the morning and evening trials could have influenced performance in both placebo and caffeine conditions. However, performance was virtually identical across placebo trials (morning vs. evening). Further, despite evidence that feeding status can influence the pharmacokinetics of caffeine ingestion [42], caffeine levels were similar in both caffeine conditions, suggesting that the 4 h of fasting, regardless of duration, likely leads to similar rates of caffeine absorption/metabolism. Notwithstanding these potential issues, the findings of this study support the idea that time of day and training status influence caffeine ergogenics and that these are probably not mediated by peak strength. This suggests that caffeine may be a suitable supplement for use during morning competition, but with less noticeable results in the evening. The current results also indicate that trained subjects supplementing with caffeine in the evening did not benefit from caffeine. Because of the potential detrimental effects that evening caffeine consumption has on sleep, we recommend that athletes confirm that caffeine is effective on an individual basis before using in the evening. The research on external factors that may alter how an individual performs with caffeine supplementation is still sparse, and more information is needed before personalized prescription for optimal performance outcomes can be provided.

Author Contributions: James Boyett, Gabrielle Giersch, Michael Saunders, Christopher Womack and Nicholas Luden conceived and designed the experiments; James Boyett and Gabrielle Giersch performed the experiments; Gabrielle Giersch, Christine Hughey and Hannah Daley analyzed the blood samples; James Boyett and Nicholas Luden analyzed the data; Christopher Womack, Michael Saunders and Nicholas Luden contributed to reagents/materials/analysis tools; James Boyett wrote the paper; Michael Saunders, Christopher Womack, Nicholas Luden, Christine Hughey and Hannah Daley contributed to the major edits; James Boyett,

Gabrielle Giersch, Christopher Womack, Michael Saunders, Christine Hughey, Hannah Daley and Nicholas Luden gave their approval for the final version.

Conflicts of Interest: The authors declare no conflict of interest.

References

1. Kovacs, E.M.; Stegen, J.H.C.H.; Brouns, F. Effect of caffeinated drinks on substrate metabolism, caffeine excretion, and performance. *J. Appl. Physiol.* **1998**, *85*, 709–715. [PubMed]
2. Womack, C.J.; Saunders, M.J.; Bechtel, M.K.; Bolton, D.J.; Martin, M.; Luden, N.D.; Dunham, W.; Hancock, M. The influence of a CYP1A2 polymorphism on the ergogenic effects of caffeine. *J. Int. Soc. Sports Nutr.* **2012**, *9*, 7. [CrossRef] [PubMed]
3. Ivy, J.L.; Costill, D.L.; Fink, W.J.; Lower, R.W. Influence of caffeine and carbohydrate feedings on endurance performance. *Med. Sci. Sports* **1979**, *11*, 6–11. [CrossRef] [PubMed]
4. Wiles, J.D.; Bird, S.R.; Hopkins, J.; Riley, M. Effect of caffeinated coffee on running speed, respiratory factors, blood lactate and perceived exertion during 1500-m treadmill running. *Br. J. Sports Med.* **1992**, *26*, 116–120. [CrossRef] [PubMed]
5. Pataky, M.W.; Womack, C.J.; Saunders, M.J.; Goffe, J.L.; D'Lugos, A.C.; El-Sohemy, A.; Luden, N.D. Caffeine and 3-km cycling performance: Effects of mouth rinsing, genotype, and time of day. *Scand. J. Med. Sci. Sports* **2015**, *26*, 613–619. [CrossRef] [PubMed]
6. Beck, T.W.; Housh, T.J.; Schmidt, R.J.; Johnson, G.O.; Housh, D.J.; Coburn, J.W.; Malek, M.H. The acute effects of a caffeine-containing supplement on strength, muscular endurance, and anaerobic capabilities. *J. Strength Cond. Res.* **2006**, *20*, 506–510. [CrossRef] [PubMed]
7. Forbes, S.C.; Candow, D.G.; Little, J.P.; Magnus, C.; Chilibeck, P.D. Effect of Red Bull energy drink on repeated Wingate cycle performance and bench-press muscle endurance. *Int. J. Sport Nutr. Exerc. Metab.* **2007**, *17*, 433–444. [CrossRef] [PubMed]
8. Greer, F.; McLean, C.; Graham, T.E. Caffeine, performance, and metabolism during repeated Wingate exercise tests. *J. Appl. Physiol.* **1998**, *85*, 1502–1508. [PubMed]
9. Doherty, M.; Smith, P.; Hughes, M.; Davison, R. Caffeine lowers perceptual response and increases power output during high-intensity cycling. *J. Sports Sci.* **2004**, *22*, 637–643. [CrossRef] [PubMed]
10. Collomp, K.; Ahmaidi, S.; Chatard, J.C.; Audran, M.; Préfaut, C. Benefits of caffeine ingestion on sprint performance in trained and untrained swimmers. *Eur. J. Appl. Physiol. Occup. Physiol.* **1992**, *64*, 377–380. [CrossRef] [PubMed]
11. Wiles, J.D.; Coleman, D.; Tegerdine, M.; Swaine, I.L. The effects of caffeine ingestion on performance time, speed and power during a laboratory-based 1 km cycling time-trial. *J. Sports Sci.* **2006**, *24*, 1165–1171. [CrossRef] [PubMed]
12. Goldstein, E.; Jacobs, P.L.; Whitehurst, M.; Penhollow, T.; Antonio, J. Caffeine enhances upper body strength in resistance-trained women. *J. Int. Soc. Sports Nutr.* **2010**, *7*, 18. [CrossRef] [PubMed]
13. Mora-Rodríguez, R.; Pallarés, J.G.; López-Gullón, J.M.; López-Samanes, A.; Fernández-Elías, V.E.; Ortega, J.F. Improvements on neuromuscular performance with caffeine ingestion depend on the time-of-day. *J. Sci. Med. Sport* **2015**, *18*, 338–342. [CrossRef] [PubMed]
14. Warren, G.L.; Park, N.D.; Maresca, R.D.; McKibans, K.I.; Millard-Stafford, M.L. Effect of caffeine ingestion on muscular strength and endurance: A meta-analysis. *Med. Sci. Sports Exerc.* **2010**, *42*, 1375–1387. [CrossRef] [PubMed]
15. Astorino, T.A.; Cottrell, T.; Lozano, A.T.; Aburto-Pratt, K.; Duhon, J. Ergogenic Effects of Caffeine on Simulated Time-Trial Performance Are Independent of Fitness Level. *J. Caffeine Res.* **2011**, *1*, 179–185. [CrossRef]
16. Porterfield, S.; Linderman, J.; Laubach, L.; Daprano, C. Comparison of the Effect of Caffeine Ingestion on Time to Exhaustion between Endurance Trained and Untrained Men. *J. Exerc. Physiol. Online* **2013**, *16*, 90–98.
17. Brooks, J.H.; Wyld, K.; Chrismas, B.C.R. Acute Effects of Caffeine on Strength Performance in Trained and Untrained Individuals. *J. Athl. Enhanc.* **2015**, *4*. [CrossRef]
18. Drake, C.; Roehrs, T.; Shambroom, J.; Roth, T. Caffeine effects on sleep taken 0, 3, or 6 h before going to bed. *J. Clin. Sleep Med.* **2013**, *9*, 1195–1200. [CrossRef] [PubMed]
19. Skein, M.; Duffield, R.; Edge, J.; Short, M.J.; Mündel, T. Intermittent-sprint performance and muscle glycogen after 30 h of sleep deprivation. *Med. Sci. Sports Exerc.* **2011**, *43*, 1301–1311. [CrossRef] [PubMed]

20. Souissi, N.; Bessot, N.; Chamari, K.; Gauthier, A.; Sesboüé, B.; Davenne, D. Effect of time of day on aerobic contribution to the 30-s Wingate test performance. *Chronobiol. Int.* **2007**, *24*, 739–748. [CrossRef] [PubMed]

21. Hopkins, W.G.; Marshall, S.W.; Batterham, A.M.; Hanin, J. Progressive statistics for studies in sports medicine and exercise science. *Med. Sci. Sports Exerc.* **2009**, *41*, 3–13. [CrossRef] [PubMed]

22. Hopkins, W.G. How to Interpret Changes in an Athletic Performance Test. *Sportscience* **2004**, *8*, 1–7.

23. Paton, C.C.D.; Hopkins, W.G.W. Variation in performance of elite cyclists from race to race. *Eur. J. Sport Sci.* **2006**, *6*, 25–31. [CrossRef]

24. Hopkins, W. Spreadsheets for analysis of controlled trials, with adjustments for a subject characteristic. *Sportscience* **2004**, *10*, 46–50.

25. Hopkins, W.G. A spreadsheet for combining outcomes from several subject groups. *Sportscience* **2006**, *10*, 51–53.

26. Hopkins, W. Estimating Sample Size for Magnitude-Based Inferences. *Sportscience* **2006**, *10*, 63–70.

27. Timmins, T.D.; Saunders, D.H. Effect of caffeine ingestion on maximal voluntary contraction strength in upper- and lower-body muscle groups. *J. Strength Cond. Res.* **2014**, *28*, 3239–3244. [CrossRef] [PubMed]

28. Black, C.D.; Waddell, D.E.; Gonglach, A.R. Caffeine's ergogenic effects on cycling: Neuromuscular and perceptual factors. *Med. Sci. Sports Exerc.* **2015**, *47*, 1145–1158. [CrossRef] [PubMed]

29. Kalow, W.; Tang, B.K. Use of caffeine metabolite ratios to explore CYP1A2 and xanthine oxidase activities. *Clin. Pharmacol. Ther.* **1991**, *50*, 508–519. [CrossRef] [PubMed]

30. Orrú, M.; Guitart, X.; Karcz-Kubicha, M.; Solinas, M.; Justinova, Z.; Barodia, S.K.; Zanoveli, J.; Cortes, A.; Lluis, C.; Casado, V.; et al. Psychostimulant pharmacological profile of paraxanthine, the main metabolite of caffeine in humans. *Neuropharmacology* **2013**, *67*, 476–484. [CrossRef] [PubMed]

31. Atkinson, G.; Todd, C.; Reilly, T.; Waterhouse, J. Diurnal variation in cycling performance: Influence of warm-up. *J. Sports Sci.* **2005**, *23*, 321–329. [CrossRef] [PubMed]

32. Kline, C.E.; Durstine, J.L.; Davis, J.M.; Moore, T.A.; Devlin, T.M.; Zielinski, M.R.; Youngstedt, S.D. Circadian variation in swim performance. *J. Appl. Physiol.* **2007**, *102*, 641–649. [CrossRef] [PubMed]

33. Pallarés, J.G.; López-Samanes, Á.; Moreno, J.; Fernández-Elías, V.E.; Ortega, J.F.; Mora-Rodríguez, R. Circadian rhythm effects on neuromuscular and sprint swimming performance. *Biol. Rhythm Res.* **2014**, *45*, 51–60. [CrossRef]

34. Mizuno, M.; Kimura, Y.; Tokizawa, K.; Ishii, K.; Oda, K.; Sasaki, T.; Nakamura, Y.; Muraoka, I.; Ishiwata, K. Greater adenosine A_{2A} receptor densities in cardiac and skeletal muscle in endurance-trained men: A [^{11}C]TMSX PET study. *Nucl. Med. Biol.* **2005**, *32*, 831–836. [CrossRef] [PubMed]

35. Astorino, T.A.; Martin, B.J.; Schachtsiek, L.; Wong, K.; Ng, K. Minimal effect of acute caffeine ingestion on intense resistance training performance. *J. Strength Cond. Res.* **2011**, *25*, 1752–1758. [CrossRef] [PubMed]

36. Astorino, T.A.; Rohmann, R.L.; Firth, K. Effect of caffeine ingestion on one-repetition maximum muscular strength. *Eur. J. Appl. Physiol.* **2008**, *102*, 127–132. [CrossRef] [PubMed]

37. Woolf, K.; Bidwell, W.K.; Carlson, A.G. The effect of caffeine as an ergogenic aid in anaerobic exercise. *Int. J. Sport Nutr. Exerc. Metab.* **2008**, *18*, 412–429. [CrossRef] [PubMed]

38. Snyder, S.H.; Katims, J.J.; Annau, Z.; Bruns, R.F.; Daly, J.W. Adenosine receptors and behavioral actions of methylxanthines. *Proc. Natl. Acad. Sci. USA* **1981**, *78*, 3260–3264. [CrossRef] [PubMed]

39. Lynge, J.; Hellsten, Y. Distribution of adenosine A_1, A_{2A} and A_{2B} receptors in human skeletal muscle. *Acta Physiol. Scand.* **2000**, *169*, 283–290. [CrossRef] [PubMed]

40. Sargeant, A.J. Structural and functional determinants of human muscle power. *Exp. Physiol.* **2007**, *92*, 323–331. [CrossRef] [PubMed]

41. Jacobson, B.H.; Weber, M.D.; Claypool, L.; Hunt, L.E. Effect of caffeine on maximal strength and power in élite male athletes. *Br. J. Sports Med.* **1992**, *26*, 276–280. [CrossRef] [PubMed]

42. Skinner, T.L.; Jenkins, D.G.; Folling, J.; Leveritt, M.D.; Coombes, J.S.; Taaffe, D.R. Influence of carbohydrate on serum caffeine concentrations following caffeine ingestion. *J. Sci. Med. Sport* **2013**, *16*, 343–347. [CrossRef] [PubMed]

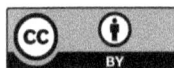

nutrients

MDPI

Article

The Effect of a 20 km Run on Appetite Regulation in Long Distance Runners

Chihiro Kojima [1], Aya Ishibashi [1,2], Kumiko Ebi [1] and Kazushige Goto [1,*]

[1] Graduate School of Sport and Health Science, Ritsumeikan University, Kusatsu, Shiga 525-8577, Japan; sh0007ek@ed.ritsumei.ac.jp (C.K.); aya.ishibashi@jpnsport.go.jp (A.I.); ab@fc.ritsumei.ac.jp (K.E.)

[2] Department of Sports Science, Japan Institute of Sports Science, Nishigaoka, Kitaku, Tokyo 115-0056, Japan

* Correspondence: kagoto@fc.ritsumei.ac.jp; Tel./Fax: +81-77-599-4127

Received: 15 September 2016; Accepted: 14 October 2016; Published: 26 October 2016

Abstract: The purpose of the present study was to investigate appetite-related hormonal responses and energy intake after a 20 km run in trained long distance runners. Twenty-three male long-distance runners completed two trials: either an exercise trial consisting of a 20 km outdoor run (EX) or a control trial with an identical period of rest (CON). Blood samples were collected to determine plasma acylated ghrelin, peptide YY_{3-36} (PYY_{3-36}) and other hormonal and metabolite concentrations. Energy intake during a buffet test meal was also measured 30 min after the exercise or rest periods. Although plasma acylated ghrelin concentrations were significantly decreased after the 20 km run ($p < 0.05$), plasma PYY_{3-36} did not change significantly following exercise. Absolute energy intake during the buffet test meal in EX (1325 ± 55 kcal) was significantly lower than that in CON (1529 ± 55 kcal), and there was a relatively large degree of individual variability for exercise-induced changes in energy intake (-40.2% to 12.8%). However, exercise-induced changes in energy intake were not associated with plasma acylated ghrelin or PYY_{3-36} responses. The results demonstrated that a 20 km run significantly decreased plasma acylated ghrelin concentrations and absolute energy intake among well-trained long distance runners.

Keywords: appetite-related hormones; energy intake; long distance run; athletes

1. Introduction

Appetite regulation is closely associated with circulating hormones secreted from digestive organs. Plasma ghrelin, secreted from the stomach, is known to be the only hormone that promotes hunger and food intake [1]. In contrast, peptide YY_{3-36} (PYY_{3-36}) and glucagon-like peptide-1 (GLP-1) are produced in the gastrointestinal tract. These hormones have the opposite role of ghrelin, resulting in attenuation of appetite [2–5]. Recently, attention to the influence of acute exercise on feeding behavior and its related endocrine regulations has increased. King et al. [6] showed that plasma ghrelin concentrations and subjective feelings of hunger were significantly impaired by 90 min of running at 70% of maximal oxygen uptake ($\dot{V}O_{2max}$). Moreover, Martins et al. [7] demonstrated that plasma GLP-1 and PYY_{3-36} concentrations were significantly increased by 60 min of endurance exercise at 65% of $\dot{V}O_{2max}$. Jokisch et al. [8] suggested that energy intake during a buffet test meal was reduced significantly after exercise compared with rest conditions for sedentary males. Although some inconsistent results still exist [9,10], the attenuating effect of exercise on hunger and energy intake is well established [6,7,11,12]. These findings could contribute to the design of optimal exercise prescriptions for health promotion and protection against obesity.

In contrast to the abundant studies on untrained individuals, appetite regulation after high-intensity (above 80% of $\dot{V}O_{2max}$) and prolonged (>60 min) exercise, which is commonly incorporated into the daily training program of trained athletes, remains under exploration. Sim et al. [13] showed that high-intensity interval training (HIIT, 15 s sprint at 170% of $\dot{V}O_{2max}$ with 60 s active recovery at 32% of $\dot{V}O_{2max}$) suppressed subsequent ad libitum energy intake and ghrelin concentrations in obese individuals. Deighton et al. [14] investigated the influence of HIIT (30 s all-out sprint with 4 min active recovery at 30 W) on appetite regulation in young untrained males, with the results suggesting that subjective feelings of appetite, as well as ghrelin concentrations, were markedly suppressed following HIIT. However, previous studies which investigated the effects of prolonged exercise (>60 min) on appetite regulation are limited. In particular, the majority of previous studies were conducted in a laboratory setting. To our knowledge, no study found any influence from prolonged exercise among well-trained athletes during actual training in the field. Since trained athletes experience greater exercise-induced metabolic and endocrine responses compared with individuals with lower fitness levels [15], their levels of exercise-induced appetite suppression may be more profound. Reduction of energy intake by exercise (exercise-induced anorexia) may be beneficial for weight management. However, athletes are commonly required to facilitate recovery of energy substrates (e.g., muscle glycogen, intramyocellular lipid) and promote muscle protein synthesis after training. Impaired energy intake after strenuous exercise is thought to delay recovery of exercise capacity and to promote accumulated fatigue. Levenhagent et al. [16] demonstrated that nutrient intake immediately after exercise enhanced glucose uptake and protein synthesis in the leg and whole body muscles when compared with consuming the same meal 3 h after exercise. Considering the importance of nutrient intake during the early phase of the post-exercise period, elucidation of appetite regulation during the early phase of prolonged high-intensity exercise in athletes is valuable.

In the present study, we investigated the time course of changes in appetite-related hormonal responses and spontaneous energy intake after a 20 km outdoor run (approximately 78 min in duration) in trained long distance runners. We hypothesized that the run would result in decreased spontaneous energy intake during a subsequent meal, with lowered plasma acylated ghrelin concentrations and elevated plasma PYY_{3-36} concentrations.

2. Materials and Methods

2.1. Subjects

Twenty-three male, college endurance runners (age, 20.0 ± 0.3 (mean $\pm$ standard error) years; height, 171.2 ± 1.9 cm; weight, 56.3 ± 1.0 kg; BMI, 19.3 ± 0.4 kg/m^2; and $\dot{V}O_{2max}$, 67.1 ± 1.0 mL/kg/min) participated in this study. All subjects belonged to the same running team, which specialized in long-distance running and maintained regular practice (2.5 h/day) 6 times a week. Subjects were informed of the purpose, experimental procedures, and risks of the study, and written informed consent was obtained from all participants. The study was approved by the Ethics Committee for Human Experiments of Ritsumeikan University (BKC-IRB-2014-015), Japan.

2.2. Experimental Design

Prior to conducting experiments, $\dot{V}O_{2max}$ was determined using incremental running test. Subjects started running at 14 km/h and running velocity was increased by 2 km/h every 4 min until 18 km/h. Once the running velocity reached 18 km/h, it was increased by 0.6 km/h every 1 min until exhaustion. Respiratory gases were collected and analyzed using an automatic gas analyzer (AE310S, Minato Medical Science Co., Ltd., Tokyo, Japan). The collected data were averaged every 30 s.

All subjects completed two trials on different days. The first visit was designed as an exercise trial (EX), and the second visit consisted of a trial without exercise (CON). Each trial was separated by 1 week. Due to experimental setting with performing 20 km outdoor run, the present study was conducted without crossover-design to match environmental factor within subjects during a 20 km run. We selected a 20 km run because it was actually incorporated into the training program in long distance runners. Exercise-induced metabolic and hormonal responses, subjective appetite, and energy intake after exercise or rest were compared between the two trials. On the day prior to the trials, the content of regular practice and calories consumed during dinner were matched to avoid any influence on metabolic and appetitive responses on the following day. Dinner was provided between 8:00 p.m. and 9:00 p.m. and consisted of regular Japanese food. The total calories consumed (1331 ± 50 kcal) were identical in each trial. Subjects stayed in accommodations at the university, and their scheduled sleep time was set from 11:00 p.m. to 6:30 a.m.

On the measurement days, the subjects arrived at the laboratory at 7:00 a.m. following an overnight fast, and they rested for at least 20 min before blood collection. On the EX day, all subjects completed a 20 km outdoor run between 7:30 a.m. and 10:30 a.m. They were instructed to run at a prescribed pace and their elapsed time was monitored. Heart rate was recorded continuously every 15 s during exercise using a heart rate monitor (Polar RCX5, Polar Electro Oy, Kempele, Finland). Subjects were allowed to consume a total of 400 mL of water during the exercise period. The ambient temperature during the run was 12.1 °C. On the CON day, the subjects did not engage in exercise, and instead rested in the laboratory for a period of time identical to that taken to complete the run. During this period, they were allowed to read books and were required to consume the same amount of water (400 mL) they had consumed on the day of EX. The room temperature was set at 19 °C.

Blood sampling, evaluation of subjective feelings of appetite using a visual analog scale (VAS), and respiratory gas sampling were conducted several times before and after exercise or rest, and 30 min following the 20 km outdoor run or rest period. Thirty min after the run or the rest period, energy and macronutrient intake during a buffet test meal were evaluated.

2.3. Blood Parameters

On the experimental trial days, subjects arrived at the laboratory at 7:00 a.m. following an overnight fast. After resting for 20 min, a baseline blood sample was obtained. A series of blood samples were subsequently collected immediately after exercise or rest, and 30 min following the exercise or rest period. Serum and plasma samples were obtained by centrifugation (10 min, 4 °C) and stored at −80 °C until analysis. From the obtained samples, plasma acylated ghrelin and PYY_{3-36}, serum growth hormone (GH), free fatty acids (FFA), creatine kinase (CK), and myoglobin (Mb) concentrations were measured. Blood glucose and lactate concentrations were measured immediately after blood collection using a glucose analyzer (Free Style, Nipro Co., Osaka, Japan) and a lactate analyzer (Lactate Pro, ARKRAY Co., Kyoto, Japan), respectively. Blood glucose measurements were performed in duplicate and the average values were used. Serum GH concentration was measured using electrochemiluminescence immunoassay. Serum FFA concentration was measured using enzymatic methods. Serum CK and Mb concentrations were measured at a clinical laboratory (SRL Inc., Tokyo, Japan). The intra-assay coefficients of variation (CV) were 1.9% for GH, 1.3% for FFA, 2.8% for CK, and 2.4% for Mb.

For the measurement of plasma acylated ghrelin and PYY_{3-36} concentrations, blood was drawn into a chilled tube containing EDTA, dipeptidyl peptidase-4 (DPP-IV), protease, and esterase inhibitors. After obtaining plasma by centrifugation at 4 °C, hydrochloric acid (1 mmol/L) was immediately added to the micro tube for acylated ghrelin analysis, following the manufacturer's instructions. Plasma acylated ghrelin concentration was measured using an enzyme-linked immunosorbent assay (ELISA) kit (Mitsubishi Chemical Medicine Corp., Tokyo, Japan). The intra-assay CV was 4.6%. The plasma PYY_{3-36} concentration was measured using an ELISA kit (Phoenix Pharmaceuticals, Inc., Burlingame, CA, USA) and the intra-assay CV was 6.1%. All ELISAs were performed in duplicate.

2.4. Subjective Feelings of Hunger, Appetite, Perceived Food Consumption, Satiety, and Fatigue

Ratings of subjective hunger, appetite, perceived food consumption, satiety, and fatigue were evaluated using a 100 mm VAS [17] before exercise (or rest), immediately after exercise (or rest), at 15 and 30 min after exercise (or rest), and after the buffet test meal.

2.5. Respiratory Parameters

A resting expired gas sample was collected 20 min after completing the 20 km run or rest. The subjects sat on a comfortable chair, and a respiratory gas sample was collected for 3 min and analyzed using an automatic gas analyzer (AE310S, Minato Medical Science Co., Ltd., Tokyo, Japan) to evaluate oxygen uptake ($\dot{V}O_2$), carbon dioxide output ($\dot{V}CO_2$), ventilatory volume ($\dot{V}E$), and the respiratory exchange ratio (RER). The values were averaged every 30 s. Appropriate calibrations of O_2 and CO_2 sensors and the volume transducer were performed using calibration gases and a 2 L syringe immediately before measurements were taken.

2.6. Ad Libitum Buffet Meal

A buffet test meal was started 30 min after the 20 km run or rest to evaluate energy and macronutrient intake. The meal lasted 30 min; however, the participants were not informed of the elapsed time during the test. All subjects were instructed to "eat until they felt comfortable satiety" in a separate environment from other subjects. The buffet meal consisted of abundant food items eaten regularly in standard Japanese breakfasts and included rice balls, bread, jam, grilled salmon, boiled beef, ham, sausages, boiled eggs, potato salad, natto (fermented soybean), boiled spinach, miso soup, milk, yogurt, cheese, oranges, apples, bananas, green tea, orange juice, and vegetable juice. The energy intake was determined by counting number of plates (calorie for each plate is already known) and by weighting remaining foods after eating. A dietary analysis program (Excel Eiyou-kun version 6.0, Kenpakusha, Tokyo, Japan) was also used to calculate energy intake and macronutrient content.

2.7. Statistical Analysis

Data are expressed as means ± SE. For all variables, normal distribution was confirmed using Kolmogorov-Smirnov test. Time courses of changes in blood parameters and subjective feelings of appetite were compared using a two-way repeated-measures analysis of variance (ANOVA) to determine interaction (trial × time) and main effects (trial, time). When ANOVA revealed a significant interaction or main effect, a Tukey-Kramer post hoc test was performed. Energy intake and respiratory gas parameters were compared between the two conditions using a paired *t*-test. The relationship between the exercise-induced relative change in energy intake and each blood parameter was determined using Pearson correlation coefficients. Statistical significance was accepted as a *p*-value < 0.05.

3. Results

3.1. Exercise Duration and Heart Rate Response during the 20 km Run

The average time taken to complete the 20 km run was 77.9 ± 0.3 min. The average heart rate (HR) during exercise was 157 ± 3 beats/min. The estimated percentage for maximum HR was $78.0\% \pm 1.3\%$.

3.2. Scores for Subjective Appetite and Fatigue

Table 1 shows the time-course changes in subjective scores for appetite and fatigue. A significant interaction (trial × time), as well as main effects of trial and time, were observed for hunger and appetite ($p < 0.05$). Hunger scores were significantly lower in EX than in CON immediately and 15 min after exercise ($p < 0.05$); however, this significant difference was not observed between the trials 30 min after exercise. Similarly, scores of appetite were significantly lower in EX compared with CON immediately and 15 min after exercise ($p < 0.05$). A two-way ANOVA revealed a significant interaction (trial × time) effect, and a main effect of time for perceived food consumption ($p < 0.05$). Perceived food consumption was significantly lower in EX compared with CON immediately after exercise ($p < 0.05$). Significant main effects of trial and time for satiety were observed ($p < 0.05$). Satiety scores were significantly higher in EX than in CON immediately, 15 min and 30 min after the exercise period ($p < 0.05$). Two-way ANOVA revealed a significant interaction effect (trial × time), as well as main effects of trial and time, for fatigue. In EX, scores for fatigue were significantly increased immediately and 15 min after exercise ($p < 0.05$). In addition, fatigue scores were significantly higher in EX than in CON at all time points after the exercise period ($p < 0.05$).

Table 1. Change in scores of subjective feeling of appetite and fatigue.

		Pre	Post 0 min	Post 15 min	Post 30 min	After Meal
Hunger (mm)	EX	57 ± 4	$51 \pm 6^{\dagger}$	$60 \pm 5^{\dagger}$	68 ± 4	$11 \pm 1^{*}$
	CON	60 ± 3	$70 \pm 3^{*}$	$71 \pm 3^{*}$	$72 \pm 3^{*}$	$16 \pm 3^{*}$
Appetite (mm)	EX	59 ± 5	$52 \pm 7^{\dagger}$	$62 \pm 5^{\dagger}$	68 ± 5	$18 \pm 4^{*}$
	CON	58 ± 4	$70 \pm 3^{*}$	$72 \pm 3^{*}$	$72 \pm 3^{*}$	$23 \pm 4^{*}$
Prospective food consumption (mm)	EX	63 ± 4	$54 \pm 6^{\dagger}$	61 ± 5	$69 \pm 4^{*}$	$20 \pm 4^{*}$
	CON	58 ± 4	$67 \pm 3^{*}$	$70 \pm 2^{*}$	68 ± 3	$22 \pm 3^{*}$
Satiety (mm)	EX	30 ± 4	$29 \pm 5^{\dagger}$	$32 \pm 5^{\dagger}$	$31 \pm 5^{\dagger}$	$82 \pm 4^{*,\dagger}$
	CON	26 ± 3	20 ± 3	18 ± 5	18 ± 3	$70 \pm 5^{*}$
Fatigue (mm)	EX	$43 \pm 4^{\dagger}$	$58 \pm 4^{*,\dagger}$	$55 \pm 4^{*,\dagger}$	$52 \pm 4^{\dagger}$	$41 \pm 4^{\dagger}$
	CON	29 ± 3	26 ± 3	$23 \pm 3^{*}$	24 ± 4	26 ± 4

Values are means ± SE. *: $p < 0.05$ vs. pre, †: $p < 0.05$ vs. CON.

3.3. Blood Parameters

Table 2 shows the time-course of changes in blood glucose, lactate, serum GH, FFA, Mb, and CK concentrations. No significant differences between the trials were observed at baseline (before exercise or rest) for any blood parameters, expect for blood glucose concentrations. A significant interaction (trial × time) and a main effect of time were observed. Blood glucose concentrations were significantly increased immediately after the exercise period compared with CON ($p < 0.05$). However, blood glucose concentrations were significantly lower in EX compared with those in CON 30 min after exercise ($p < 0.05$). No significant interaction (trial × time), or main effects of time or trial were observed for blood lactate concentrations ($p < 0.05$). Blood lactate concentrations did not significantly change from baseline values in either trial. Two-way ANOVA revealed a significant interaction (trial × time), as well as main effects of time and trial, for serum GH, FFA, and Mb concentrations. Serum GH concentrations were significantly increased after exercise in EX ($p < 0.05$). Thirty min after exercise, serum GH concentrations remained significantly higher in EX compared with CON ($p < 0.05$). Serum FFA concentrations were markedly increased after exercise ($p < 0.05$), and were significantly different to those in CON ($p < 0.05$). Serum Mb concentrations were significantly increased immediately and 30 min after exercise ($p < 0.05$), and were also significantly different between EX and CON ($p < 0.05$). Lastly, a significant interaction (trial × time) as well as main effects of time for serum CK concentrations were observed. Although serum CK increased significantly with exercise ($p < 0.05$), there was no significant difference between the trials at any point (main effect of trial; $p > 0.05$).

Figure 1 shows the changes in plasma acylated ghrelin concentrations. Significant main effects of time and trial were observed for plasma acylated ghrelin ($p < 0.05$). Plasma acylated ghrelin concentrations at baseline were significantly lower in EX compared with CON ($p < 0.05$) and exercise significantly decreased plasma acylated ghrelin concentrations immediately after the exercise period (before exercise, 20.2 ± 1.4 fmol/mL; immediately after exercise, 17.3 ± 1.7 fmol/mL, $p < 0.05$) with a significant reduction relative to CON ($p < 0.05$). Thirty minutes after exercise, plasma acylated ghrelin concentrations remained significantly lower in EX than in CON ($p < 0.05$). In contrast, the CON trial did not show significant change in acylated ghrelin concentration over time.

Figure 2 shows the time-course change of plasma PYY_{3-36} concentrations. Two-way ANOVA revealed a significant main effect of the trial for plasma PYY_{3-36} concentration. Although plasma PYY_{3-36} concentrations at baseline were significantly lower in EX than in CON ($p < 0.05$), there was no significant difference between the trials after exercise. Furthermore, plasma PYY_{3-36} concentration did not change significantly from baseline values in either EX or CON.

Table 2. Change in blood variables.

		Pre	Post 0 min	Post 30 min
Glucose (mmol/L)	EX	4.92 ± 0.05 [†]	5.30 ± 0.12 [*,†]	4.64 ± 0.08 [*,†]
	CON	4.78 ± 0.05	4.84 ± 0.05	4.93 ± 0.04 [*]
Lactate (mmol/L)	EX	1.6 ± 0.2	1.6 ± 0.2	1.6 ± 0.1
	CON	1.4 ± 0.1	1.5 ± 0.1	1.4 ± 0.1
GH (ng/mL)	EX	1.8 ± 0.5	8.9 ± 1.8 [*,†]	4.1 ± 0.8 [†]
	CON	2.5 ± 0.6	2.1 ± 0.4	1.3 ± 0.3
FFA (mmol/L)	EX	0.42 ± 0.05	1.22 ± 0.08 [*,†]	0.90 ± 0.08 [*,†]
	CON	0.38 ± 0.03	0.35 ± 0.03	0.55 ± 0.04 [*]
Mb (ng/mL)	EX	36 ± 2	136 ± 26 [*,†]	140 ± 22 [*,†]
	CON	37 ± 3	36 ± 2	35 ± 2
CK	EX	349 ± 27	457 ± 30 [*]	436 ± 29 [*]
(U/L)	CON	402 ± 74	389 ± 68 [*]	385 ± 70 [*]

Values are means $\pm$ SE. [*]: $p < 0.05$ vs. pre, [†]: $p < 0.05$ vs. CON.

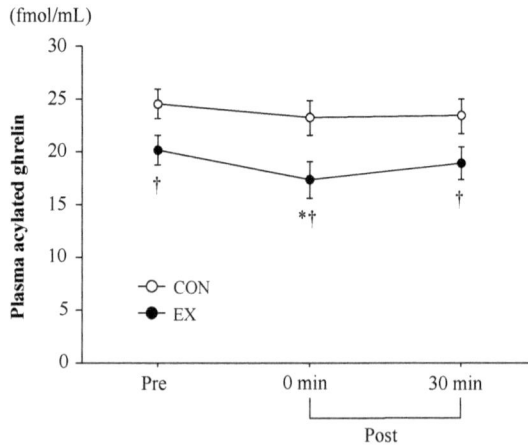

Figure 1. Change in plasma acylated ghrelin concentrations. Values are means $\pm$ SE. [*] $p < 0.05$ vs. pre, [†] $p < 0.05$ vs. CON.

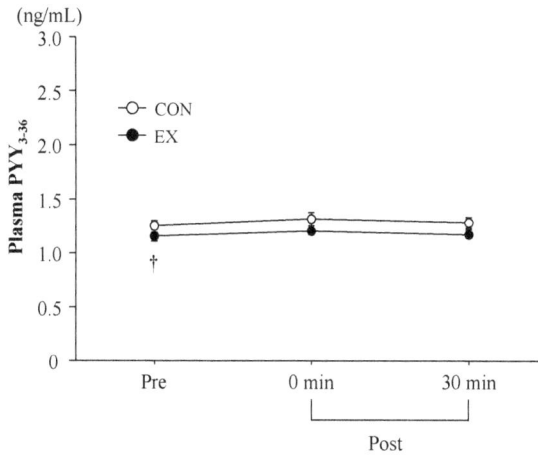

Figure 2. Change in plasma $PYY_{3\text{-}36}$ concentrations. Values are means $\pm$ SE. † $p < 0.05$ vs. CON.

3.4. Respiratory Parameters

Resting $\dot{V}O_2$ and $\dot{V}CO_2$ after exercise were significantly higher in EX than in CON ($\dot{V}O_2$, 271 ± 5 mL/min in EX vs. 233 ± 8 mL/min in CON; $\dot{V}CO_2$, 202 ± 6 mL/min in EX vs. 182 ± 6 mL/min in CON, $p < 0.05$). Moreover, there was a trend toward lower RER in EX than in CON (0.75 ± 0.02 in EX vs. 0.78 ± 0.02 in CON, $p = 0.056$) and toward higher $\dot{V}E$ in EX than in CON (8.7 ± 0.4 L/min in EX vs. 7.9 ± 0.3 L/min in CON, $p = 0.057$).

3.5. Energy and Macronutrient Intake

Table 3 shows the energy intake, macronutrient intake ratios, and types of menu selected during the buffet test meal. The time required to finish eating was not significantly different between EX and CON. Energy intake was significantly lower in EX (1325 ± 55 kcal) compared to CON (1529 ± 55 kcal, $p < 0.05$); the exercise-induced relative change in energy intake was $-12.9\% \pm 2.8\%$. With regard to macronutrient distribution, fat intake was significantly lower in EX than in CON ($p < 0.05$), while carbohydrate intake was significantly higher in EX than in CON ($p < 0.05$). Moreover, comparing the caloric intake within four categories of food (staple foods, others, fruits, and drinks) among the 21 different menus indicated that calories consumed from staple foods, including carbohydrates (e.g., rice, bread) and others (e.g., fish, meat) were significantly lower in EX ($p < 0.05$). In contrast, calories consumed from drinks including tea, juice, milk, and soups were slightly but significantly greater in EX ($p < 0.05$).

Table 3. Energy intake, macronutrient intake ratio and categories of selected menus.

		EX	CON
General information			
Duration of eating	(min)	22 ± 1	23 ± 1
Energy intake	(kcal)	1325 ± 55 [†]	1529 ± 55
Detailed information			
Macronutrient intake			
Protein	(%)	14.6 ± 0.5	15.3 ± 0.5
	(g)	49 ± 3 [†]	58 ± 2
Fat	(%)	26.2 ± 1.4 [†]	29.8 ± 1.2
	(g)	39 ± 3	51 ± 3
Carbohydrate	(%)	59.2 ± 1.9 [†]	54.9 ± 1.5
	(g)	190 ± 9	202 ± 10
Categories of selected menus			
Staple food (rice and bread)	(kcal)	545 ± 34 [†]	659 ± 45
Others	(kcal)	553 ± 38 [†]	694 ± 28
Fruits	(kcal)	101 ± 15	75 ± 12
Drinks (tea, juice milk and soup)	(kcal)	126 ± 11 [†]	101 ± 16

Values are means ± SE. [†]: $p < 0.05$ vs. CON.

3.6. Inter-Individual Variability in Exercise-Induced Changes in Energy Intake

Figure 3 shows the individual data of exercise-induced relative changes in energy intake [(energy intake in EX − energy intake in CON)/energy intake in CON × 100]. A relatively large individual difference in energy intake was observed (ranging from −40.2% to 12.8%). In total, 3 of 23 subjects (13.0%) had increased energy intake after the exercise period compared with rest, while there were no differences in intake between the trials in 2 subjects (8.7%). However, 18 subjects (78.3%) had reduced energy intake after exercise compared with rest.

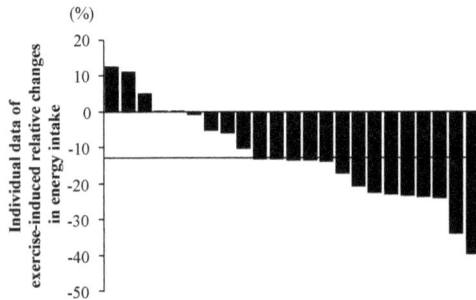

Figure 3. Individual data of exercise-induced relative change in energy intake. The line indicates the average value of relative change in exercise-induced energy intake (−12.9% ± 2.8%).

3.7. Correlation between Exercise-Induced Relative Changes in Energy Intake and Blood Variables

When the relationship between the exercise-induced relative change in energy intake and blood variables was determined, changes in energy intake showed a significant inverse correlation with serum Mb concentrations 30 min ($r = -0.477$, $p < 0.05$) after exercise. Moreover, there was an inverse trend of correlation between exercise-induced relative change in energy intake and serum Mb concentrations immediately after exercise ($r = -0.372$, $p = 0.08$). Exercise-induced absolute change in energy intake showed an inverse trend of correlation with that in area under the curve (AUC) of serum Mb ($r = -0.393$, $p = 0.06$). However, plasma acylated ghrelin concentrations immediately ($r = 0.11$, $p = 0.61$) and 30 min

($r = 0.20$, $p = 0.37$) after exercise did not correlate significantly with exercise-induced relative changes in energy intake. Similarly, plasma PYY_{3-36} concentrations immediately ($r = 0.12$, $p = 0.58$) and 30 min ($r = 0.03$, $p = 0.90$) after exercise were not correlated with exercise-induced relative changes in energy intake. No significant relationship was observed between exercise-induced absolute change in energy intake and AUCs of ghrelin ($r = -0.05$, $p = 0.81$) or PYY_{3-36} ($r = -0.34$, $p = 0.11$).

4. Discussion

The present study was designed to determine the impact of a 20 km run on appetite regulation in well-trained long distance runners. We found that absolute energy intake during a buffet test meal after the exercise period was significantly reduced compared with that after a rest period of identical duration. However, this reduction in energy intake was not associated with exercise-induced acylated ghrelin or PYY_{3-36} responses.

4.1. Exercise-Induced Ghrelin and PYY_{3-36} Responses

Plasma acylated ghrelin concentrations were significantly decreased after exercise, in agreement with previous studies [6,18,19]; however, the magnitude of the reduction in plasma acylated ghrelin concentrations (14% reduction) was smaller compared to previously reported values [14,18,20]. A relatively small reduction in plasma acylated ghrelin could be due to a moderate GH response, as exercise-induced GH elevations suppress ghrelin [21–23]. In the present study, because the magnitude of the exercise-induced GH response was modest (pre-exercise, 1.8 ± 0.5 ng/mL; immediately after exercise, 8.9 ± 1.8 ng/mL), it may have resulted in a relatively small ghrelin response. Furthermore, plasma PYY_{3-36} concentrations were not significantly elevated after the exercise period. There have been inconsistencies in the reported effect of acute exercise on PYY_{3-36} response [12–14,24]. These inconsistencies may be due to whether breakfast was consumed prior to exercising or not. In fact, two studies that demonstrated exercise-induced PYY_{3-36} elevations provided a standard breakfast before the exercise period [12,14], while exercise in the present study was completed following an overnight fast.

4.2. Energy Intake Following 20 km Run

The most important finding in the present study was a significant reduction in energy intake after a 20 km run in well-trained long distance runners. In addition, a detailed analysis of the selected menus during the buffet test meal indicated that lowered energy intake in EX was due to a reduction in calories consumed from staple foods (e.g., rice and bread) and other foods (e.g., fish or meat), and not from fruits or drinks. Previous reports investigating the effect of acute exercise on appetite regulation among well-trained athletes ($\dot{V}O_{2max}$ above 65 mL/kg/min) are quite limited. Moreover, this is the first study, to our knowledge, demonstrating that acute exercise decreased absolute energy intake in well-trained athletes. Exercise-induced decreases in appetite have been generally accepted to be dependent on exercise intensity [25]. However, the average HR (157 ± 3 bpm) during the 20 km run did not reach a maximal level (78.0% $\pm$ 1.3% of estimated maximal HR). Moreover, blood lactate concentrations did not change significantly from baseline, suggesting that exercise intensity was moderate. Resting $\dot{V}O_2$, which was determined after the 20 km run, was significantly elevated 20 min after the exercise period, and resting energy expenditure was increased during the post-exercise period. Therefore, reduction of absolute energy intake with a concomitant increase in resting energy expenditure might promote a negative energy balance. However, caution is necessary since energy expenditure during a 20 km run was not evaluated in the present study. Further investigations need to determine energy expenditure during exercise and post-exercise for confirming energy availability. In addition, the influence of low energy availability on post-exercise recovery and training adaptations is required to explore.

4.3. Inter-Individual Variability of Exercise-Induced Reduction of Energy Intake

The relatively larger sample size of this study ($n = 23$) enabled us to perform additional statistical analyses. Although energy intake in EX was significantly lower than in CON, a relatively large degree of individual variability was observed (-40.2% to 12.8%); a similar trend was also reported in previous studies [24,26–28]. To clarify the association between appetite-related hormonal responses and exercise-induced reductions in energy intake, we divided all subjects into two groups (a group with greater reductions in energy intake and a group with smaller reductions in energy intake) based on the average value of the exercise-induced relative change in energy intake ($-12.9\% \pm 2.8\%$). There were no significant differences between the two groups for acylated ghrelin ($p = 0.78$) or PYY$_{3-36}$ ($p = 0.53$) concentrations 30 min after the exercise period (immediately before the buffet test meal), suggesting that reduced energy intake after a 20 km run was not associated with exercise-induced acylated ghrelin or PYY$_{3-36}$ responses. Thus, a plausible factor contributing to the reduction in energy intake after the 20 km run may be an exercise-induced elevation of GLP-1, as GLP-1 has anorexigenic effects. Ellingsgaard et al. [29] suggested that GLP-1 secretion was stimulated by exercise-induced interleukin-6 (IL-6) production in skeletal muscle in rats. IL-6 is an inflammatory cytokine, and long distance running markedly increases IL-6 production in skeletal muscle, as well as in the blood [30]. Ueda et al. [12] also observed a significant inverse correlation between the decrease in energy intake after exercise and an incremental GLP-1 response. Therefore, the impact of GLP-1 concentration mediated by IL-6 elevation after a 20 km run on reduced energy intake should be considered. Furthermore, we found that exercise-induced elevations of Mb concentrations were significantly correlated with exercise-induced relative changes in energy intake. Currently, we are unsure whether increased Mb concentrations directly affected exercise-induced reductions in energy intake. However, future investigations to study the influence of muscle damage and the inflammatory response on appetite regulation would be informative. Another possible factor contributing to the reduction of energy intake might be an exercise-induced elevation of core temperature, since this has been demonstrated to lower energy intake after exercise [31]. However, it is unlikely that an elevation of core temperature had a strong impact in our study, since the 20 km run was completed in a cold environment during winter (ambient temperature: 12.1 °C).

4.4. Macronutrient Intake Following a 20 km Run

The influence of exercise on macronutrient intake distribution remains unclear [10,32,33]. Blundell et al. [34] suggested that acute exercise may alter food preference, which is associated with replenishment of short-term energy stores. In the present study, carbohydrate intake during the buffet test meal was significantly higher in EX than in CON. Considering that fat oxidation (evaluated by RER) was significantly enhanced during the post-exercise period in EX, replenishment of muscle glycogen appeared to be augmented after the 20 km run. Therefore, the increased proportion of carbohydrate is reasonable. Dehydration and thirst may have also contributed to altered macronutrient intake [33]. However, it is unlikely that dehydration occurred since the run was performed in a cold outdoor environment, and a total of 400 mL of water was provided to each participant. Furthermore, body weight did not change significantly after the exercise period (pre: 56.3 ± 1.0 kg, post: 55.8 ± 1.0 kg, $p > 0.05$).

4.5. Limitations

Several limitations should be considered in the present study. First, there were slight, but significant differences in baseline acylated ghrelin and PYY$_{3-36}$ concentrations between the two trials. The reason for this difference is unclear as training volume, dinner before the testing day, and accommodations the night prior to the trial were controlled and matched between the two trials. However, there was no significant correlation between energy intake and acylated ghrelin or PYY$_{3-36}$ concentrations at baseline (acylated ghrelin, EX: $r = -0.16$, $p = 0.47$, CON: $r = -0.16$, $p = 0.47$;

PYY$_{3-36}$, EX: $r = -0.35$, $p = 0.10$, CON: $r = -0.17$, $p = 0.45$). In addition, in the EX trial, the lower acylated ghrelin concentration (anorexigenic effect) might be offset by the lower PYY$_{3-36}$ concentration (orexigenic effect). Therefore, the influence of different acylated ghrelin and PYY$_{3-36}$ concentrations at baseline would have been negligible; Second, the present study was conducted without using randomized counter-balanced design to match environmental condition during 20 km outdoor run, and all subjects completed firstly EX. Unick et al. [35] revealed that energy intake during the meal was similar in spite of the order of exercise trial and rest trial (exercise trial followed by rest trial or rest trial followed by exercise trial). Therefore, it is assumed that the present experimental design without crossover design had little influence on energy intake during buffet test meal; Third, exercise intensity during the 20 km run may have been lower than during a competition. Therefore, the reduction of energy intake after exercise may have been underestimated. Finally, information on energy intake during the rest of the trial day, and on following day, was not recorded. Previous studies reported that a compensatory increase in energy intake after an ad libitum meal was not observed over such a time period [6,13,36]. However, caution is necessary because subjects of above studies [6,13,36] were not competitive endurance athletes. Further investigations are needed to confirm whether compensatory increase in energy intake will happen.

5. Conclusions

A 20 km run significantly decreased subjective hunger, plasma acylated ghrelin concentrations, and absolute energy intake in well-trained long distance runners. However, the exercise-induced reduction of energy intake was not associated with acylated ghrelin or PYY$_{3-36}$ responses.

Acknowledgments: We wish to thank the all of athletes and coach for commitment to the research. We thank laboratory members for help the excellent technical support during the experiment. Especially, we would like to thank nutritionists Aya Kaizaki, Aoi Ikedo, Saori Matsumiya and Ai Sato for preparation and production of the buffet meal in the experiment.

Author Contributions: The present study was designed by C.K., and K.G.; data were collected and analyzed by C.K., A.I., and K.G.; data interpretation and manuscript preparation were undertaken by C.K., K.E., and K.G. All authors approved the final version of the paper. The present study was partially supported by a research grant form Ritsumeikan University and Grant-in-Aid for Scientific Research from the Japan Society for the Promotion of Science.

Conflicts of Interest: The authors declare no conflict of interest.

Abbreviations

PYY	peptide YY
GLP-1	glucagon-like peptide-1
$\dot{V}O_{2max}$	maximal oxygen uptake
HIIT	high-intensity interval training
VAS	visual analog scale
GH	growth hormone
FFA	free fatty acid
Mb	myoglobin
CK	creatine kinase
CV	coefficients of variation
IL-6	interleukin-6

References

1. Kojima, M.; Kanagawa, K. Ghrelin: Structure and function. *Physiol. Rev.* **2005**, *85*, 495–522. [CrossRef] [PubMed]
2. Batterham, R.L.; Broom, S.R. The gut hormone peptide YY regulates appetite. *Ann. N. Y. Acad. Sci.* **2003**, *994*, 162–168. [CrossRef] [PubMed]

3. Battrerham, R.L.; Cowley, M.A.; Small, C.J.; Herzog, H.; Cohen, M.A.; Dakin, C.L.; Wren, A.M.; Brynes, A.E.; Low, M.J.; Ghatei, M.A.; et al. Gut hormone PYY$_{3-36}$ physiologically inhibits food intake. *Nature* **2002**, *418*, 650–654. [CrossRef]

4. Batterham, R.L.; Cohen, M.A.; Ellis, S.M.; Le Roux, C.W.; Withers, D.J.; Frost, G.S.; Ghatei, M.A.; Bloom, S.R. Inhibition of food intake in obese subjects by peptide YY$_{3-36}$. *N. Engl. J. Med.* **2003**, *349*, 941–948. [CrossRef] [PubMed]

5. Kreymann, B.; Williams, G.; Ghatei, M.A.; Bloom, S.R. Glucagon-like peptide-1 7-36: A physiological incretin in man. *Lancet* **1987**, *2*, 1300–1304. [CrossRef]

6. King, J.A.; Miyashita, M.; Wasse, L.K.; Stensel, D.J. Influence of prolonged treadmill running on appetite, energy intake and circulating concentrations of acylated ghrelin. *Appetite* **2010**, *54*, 492–498. [CrossRef] [PubMed]

7. Martins, C.; Morgan, L.M.; Bloom, S.R.; Robertson, M.D. Effect of exercise on gut peptides, energy intake and appetite. *J. Endocrinol.* **2007**, *193*, 251–258. [CrossRef] [PubMed]

8. Jokisch, E.; Coletta, A.; Raynor, H.A. Acute energy compensation and macronutrient intake following exercise in active and inactive males who are normal weight. *Appetite* **2012**, *58*, 722–729. [CrossRef] [PubMed]

9. Hubert, P.; King, N.A.; Blundell, J.E. Uncoupling the effects of energy expenditure and energy intake: Appetite pesponse to short-term energy deficit induced by meal omission and physical activity. *Appetite* **1998**, *31*, 9–19. [CrossRef] [PubMed]

10. Pomerleau, M.; Imbeault, P.; Parker, T.; Doucet, E. Effects of exercise intensity on food intake and appetite in women. *Am. J. Clin. Nutr.* **2004**, *80*, 1230–1236. [PubMed]

11. Broom, D.R.; Batterham, R.L.; King, J.A.; Stensel, D.J. Influence of resistance and aerobic exercise on hunger, circulating levels of acylated ghrelin, and peptide YY in healthy males. *Am. J. Physiol. Regul. Integr. Comp. Physiol.* **2009**, *269*, R29–R35. [CrossRef] [PubMed]

12. Ueda, S.; Yoshikawa, T.; Katsura, Y.; Usui, T.; Fujimoto, S. Comparable effects of moderate intensity exercise on changes in anorectic gut hormone levels and energy intake to high intensity exercise. *J. Endocrinol.* **2009**, *203*, 357–364. [CrossRef] [PubMed]

13. Sim, A.K.; Wallman, K.E.; Fairchild, T.J.; Guelfi, K.J. High-intensity intermittent exercise attenuates ad-libitum energy intake. *Int. J. Obes. (Lond.)* **2014**, *38*, 417–422. [CrossRef] [PubMed]

14. Deighton, K.; Barry, R.; Connon, C.E.; Stensel, D.J. Appetite, gut hormone and energy intake response to low volume sprint interval and traditional endurance exercise. *Eur. J. Appl. Physiol.* **2013**, *113*, 1147–1156. [CrossRef] [PubMed]

15. Schubert, M.M.; Desbrow, B.; Sabapathy, S.; Leveritt, M. Acute exercise and subsequent energy intake. A meta-analysis. *Appetite* **2013**, *63*, 92–104. [CrossRef] [PubMed]

16. Levenhagen, D.K.; Gresham, J.D.; Carlson, M.G.; Maron, D.J.; Borel, M.J.; Flakoll, O.J. Postexersie nutrient intake timing in humans is critical to recovery of leg glucose and protein homeostasis. *Am. J. Physiol. Endocrinol. Metab.* **2001**, *280*, E982–E993. [PubMed]

17. Flint, A.; Raben, A.; Blundell, J.E.; Astrup, A. Reproducibility, power and validity of visual analogue scales in assessment of appetite sensations in single test meal studies. *Int. J. Obes. Relat. Metab. Disord.* **2000**, *24*, 38–48. [CrossRef] [PubMed]

18. Broom, D.R.; Stensel, D.J.; Bishop, N.C.; Bruns, S.F.; Miyashita, M. Exercise-induced suppression of acylated ghrelin in humans. *J. Appl. Physiol.* **2007**, *102*, 2165–2171. [CrossRef] [PubMed]

19. Kawano, H.; Mineta, M.; Asaka, M.; Miyashita, M.; Numao, S.; Gando, Y.; Ando, T.; Sakamoto, S.; Higuchi, M. Effects of different modes of exercise on appetite and appetite-regulating hormones. *Appetite* **2013**, *66*, 26–33. [CrossRef] [PubMed]

20. Shiiya, T.; Ueno, H.; Toshinai, K.; Kawagoe, T.; Naito, S.; Tobina, T.; Nishida, Y.; Shindo, M.; Kangawa, K.; Tanaka, H.; et al. Significant lowering of plasma ghrelin but not des-acyl ghrelin in response to acute exercise in men. *Endocr. J.* **2011**, *58*, 335–342. [CrossRef] [PubMed]

21. Dall, R.; Kanaley, J.; Hansen, T.K.; Møller, N.; Christiansen, J.S.; Hosoda, H.; Kangawa, K.; Jørgensen, J.O. Plasma ghrelin levels during exercise in healthy subjects and in growth hormone-deficient patients. *Eur. J. Endocrinol.* **2002**, *147*, 65–70. [CrossRef] [PubMed]

22. Gholipour, M.; Kordi, M.R.; Taghikhani, M.; Ravasi, A.A.; Gaeini, A.A.; Tabrizi, A. Possible role for growth hormone in suppressing acylated ghrelin and hunger ratings during and after intermittent exercise of different intensities in obese individuals. *Acta Med. Iran.* **2014**, *52*, 29–37. [PubMed]

23. Vestergaad, E.T.; Dall, R.; Lange, K.H.; Kjaer, M.; Christiansen, J.S.; Jorgensen, J.O. The ghrelin responses to exercise before and after growth hormone administration. *J. Clin. Endocrinol. Metab.* **2007**, *92*, 297–303. [CrossRef] [PubMed]

24. Hagobian, T.A.; Yamashiro, M.; Hinkel-Lipsker, J.; Streder, K.; Evero, N.; Hackney, T. Effects of acute exercise on appetite hormones and ad libitum energy intake in men and women. *Appl. Physiol. Nutr. Metab.* **2013**, *38*, 66–72. [CrossRef] [PubMed]

25. Deighton, K.; Stensel, D.J. Creating an acute energy intake deficient without stimulating compensatory increases in appetite: Is there an optimal exercise protocol? *Proc. Nutr. Soc.* **2014**, *73*, 352–358. [CrossRef] [PubMed]

26. Finlayson, G.; Bryant, E.; Blundell, J.E.; King, N.A. Acute compensatory eating following exercise is associated with implicit hedonic wanting for food. *Physiol. Behav.* **2009**, *97*, 62–67. [CrossRef] [PubMed]

27. Hopkins, M.; Blundel, J.E.; King, N.A. Individual variability in compensatory eating following acute exercise in overweight and obese women. *Br. J. Sports Med.* **2014**, *48*, 1472–1476. [CrossRef] [PubMed]

28. Unick, J.L.; Otto, A.D.; Goodpaster, B.H.; Helsel, D.L.; Pellegrini, C.A.; Jakicic, J.M. Acute effects of walking on energy intake in overweight/obese women. *Appetite* **2010**, *55*, 413–419. [CrossRef] [PubMed]

29. Eliingsgaard, H.; Hauselmann, I.; Schuler, B.; Habib, A.M.; Baggio, L.L.; Meier, D.T.; Eppler, E.; Bouzakri, K.; Wueest, S.; Muller, Y.D.; et al. Interleukin-6 enhance insulin secretion by increasing glucagon-like peptide-1 secretion from L cells and alpha cell. *Nat. Med.* **2011**, *17*, 1481–1489. [CrossRef] [PubMed]

30. Fischer, C.P. Interleukin-6 in acute exercise and training: What is the biological relevance? *Exerc. Immunol. Rev.* **2009**, *12*, 6–33.

31. Shorten, A.L.; Wallman, K.E.; Guelfi, K.J. Acute effect of environment temperature during exercise on subsequent energy in active men. *Am. J. Clin. Nutr.* **2009**, *90*, 1215–1221. [CrossRef] [PubMed]

32. Elder, S.J.; Roberts, S.B. The effects of exercise on food intake and body fatness: A summary of published studies. *Nutr. Rev.* **2007**, *65*, 1–19. [CrossRef] [PubMed]

33. Westerterp-plantenga, M.S.; Verwegen, C.R.; Ijedema, M.J.; Wijckmans, N.E.; Saris, W.H. Acute effects of exercise or sauna on appetite in obese and nonobese men. *Physiol. Behav.* **1997**, *62*, 1345–1354. [CrossRef]

34. Blundell, J.E.; Stubbs, R.J.; Hughes, D.A.; Whybrow, S.; King, N.A. Cross talk between physical activity and appetite control: does physical activity stimulate appetite? *Proc. Nutr. Soc.* **2003**, *62*, 651–661. [CrossRef] [PubMed]

35. Unick, J.L.; O'Leary, K.C.; Dorfman, L.; Thomas, J.G.; Strohacker, K.; Wing, R.R. Consistency in compensatory eating responses following acute exercise in inactive, overweight and obese women. *Br. J. Nutr.* **2015**, *113*, 1170–1177. [CrossRef] [PubMed]

36. Beaulieu, K.; Olver, T.D.; Abbott, K.C.; Lemon, P.W. Energy intake over 2 days is unaffected by acute sprint interval exercise despite increased appetite and energy expenditure. *Appl. Physiol. Nutr. Metab.* **2014**, *40*, 79–86. [CrossRef] [PubMed]

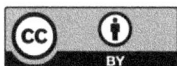

nutrients

Article

Investigating the Cellular and Metabolic Responses of World-Class Canoeists Training: A Sportomics Approach

Wagner Santos Coelho [1,2], Luis Viveiros de Castro [1], Elizabeth Deane [1], Alexandre Magno-França [1], Adriana Bassini [1,2] and Luiz-Claudio Cameron [1,2,*]

[1] Laboratory of Protein Biochemistry, Federal University of State of Rio de Janeiro, Rio de Janeiro 22290-240, Brazil; wagscoelho@hotmail.com (W.S.C.); luisviveirosdecastro@gmail.com (L.V.d.C.); bethcataldi@gmail.com (E.D.); amvfranca@gmail.com (A.M.-F.); abassini@me.com (A.B.)

[2] Department of Biochemistry and Sportomics, Olympic Laboratory, Brazil Olympic Committee, Rio de Janeiro 22631-910, Brazil

* Correspondence: cameron@unirio.br; Tel.: +552-198-225-2007

Received: 26 August 2016; Accepted: 29 October 2016; Published: 11 November 2016

Abstract: (1) Background: We have been using the Sportomics approach to evaluate biochemical and hematological changes in response to exercise. The aim of this study was to evaluate the metabolic and hematologic responses of world-class canoeists during a training session; (2) Methods: Blood samples were taken at different points and analyzed for their hematological properties, activities of selected enzymes, hormones, and metabolites; (3) Results: Muscle stress biomarkers were elevated in response to exercise which correlated with modifications in the profile of white blood cells, where a leukocyte rise was observed after the canoe session. These results were accompanied by an increase in other exercise intensity parameters such as lactatemia and ammonemia. Adrenocorticotropic hormone and cortisol increased during the exercise sessions. The acute rise in both erythrocytes and white blood profile were probably due to muscle cell damage, rather than hepatocyte integrity impairment; (4) Conclusion: The cellular and metabolic responses found here, together with effective nutrition support, are crucial to understanding the effects of exercise in order to assist in the creation of new training and recovery planning. Also we show that Sportomics is a primal tool for training management and performance improvement, as well as to the understanding of metabolic response to exercise.

Keywords: metabolism; biochemistry of exercise; ammonia; urate; exercise intensity biomarkers; physical stress response

1. Introduction

Physical stress response due to a sport challenge is implicated in many metabolic modifications which affect the equilibrium of the biochemical internal environment [1,2]. This includes changes in the amount and kinetics of diverse biomarkers that are correlated with exercise intensity and muscle damage [3,4]. Some of these changes in metabolism can be assessed using blood as a biological matrix. For more than one decade, our group has dedicated research efforts towards understanding changes in metabolism using exercise as an induced-stress metabolic model [3,5–16]. The Sportomics approach targets metabolic and signaling molecule evaluations during either mimicked or real conditions faced in sports situations; it combines "-omics" technique with classic clinical laboratory analyses in order to understand sport-induced modifications [16]. These approaches represent a powerful tool to understand changes in physical and metabolic stress [17–19] and allow researchers to propose interventions in order to optimize athletes' performance [5,20,21]. The approach is also a useful investigation tool for studying the effects of nutrition supplementation on physical training in different physiological or clinical conditions, such as type 2 diabetes mellitus [22]. Therefore, the analysis of world-class athletes in a field perspective allows us the possibility of understanding metabolic and signaling responses during high metabolic stress. Similar to a personalized-medicine approach, the Sportomics method allows us to better understand individual changes and to propose individualized interventions.

Several recent investigations have focused on the ammonemia changes resulting from a physical effort, which may be modified due to different causes [23–25]. Amino acids play a central metabolic role as an energetic source during exercise, which requires their deamination in order to be transduced into chemical energy. Increased muscle contraction rate also can contribute to changes in ammonemia, through adenosine monophosphate (AMP) deamination [26–29]. During intense or prolonged exercise, the reduced ability to resynthesize ATP promotes accumulation of ammonia and inosine monophosphate (IMP) which is metabolized to urate [30]. An intensity relationship has been proposed between ammonemia and exercise, as ammonia rapidly increases at intensities greater than 50%–60% of VO_{2max} [31,32]. However, ammonia production and release is not solely restricted to intense exercise. During prolonged (>1 h) submaximal exercise (60%–75% VO_{2max}), ammonia could be produced through the breakdown of branched chain amino acid (BCAA) for additional energy provision [33–35].

Ammonia may cross the blood brain barrier causing neurotoxic effects including neuropsychiatric disorders, convulsion, and death [36], and may be implicated in central fatigue [25]. Therefore, ammonia accumulation may be avoided through a detoxification system. Humans convert ammonia to urea mainly in hepatocytes, and different cells can decrease ammonemia by synthesizing amino acids as a mechanism for further excretion of urea [9,11,37]. Therefore, an increase in urea levels reflects both AMP and amino acid deamination. On the other hand, urate is the final metabolite of the purine metabolism; hence, its measure can be stoichiometrically related to IMP deamination. Since urea and urate are, respectively, the final products of ammonia and purine metabolism, the study of the kinetics of those blood analytes leads to a better understanding of the metabolic pathways of ammonia origin and the response to exercise [37]. For this reason, our group has proposed nutritional and training interventions to promote metabolic adaptations in elite athletes to enhance their performance in training and competitions [3,10].

Canoeing has been featured as an Olympic sport since the Summer Olympic Games of 1936 in Berlin. Currently, men's and women's competitions cover distances of 200 m, 500 m, and 1000 m either solo, in pairs, or in crews of four. Canoeing contests are sprint events requiring sustained bursts of speed and power, leading to intense mechanical and metabolic stress. Little is known about these athletes' metabolic responses during training sessions or competitions, therefore, the aim of this study was to evaluate four world-class canoeists during a training session through a Sportomics approach. As far as we know, this is the first metabolic investigation in the field, coming from our unique opportunity to investigate world-class athletes. This investigation will help enlighten us about the metabolism behavior in elite athletes.

2. Materials and Methods

This study assessed the metabolic response of four male world-class canoeists during a combined training session. All athletes were currently engaged in international elite competitions (including world championships, Pan-American, and Olympic games). During the trials, the athletes were instructed to maintain their typical hydration and food ingestion habits. Additionally, clinical evaluation, anthropometric measurements, and laboratory tests of collected blood samples were performed to assess health status. A Sportomics evaluation and analysis was performed to understand the metabolic effects of a training session. Subjects were fully instructed about the testing procedures and each signed a written informed consent. This study was conducted according to all procedures involving human subjects approved by the Ethics Committee for Human Research at the Federal University of the State of Rio de Janeiro (117/2007, renewed in 2011, 2013 and 2016) and met the requirements regulating research on human subjects (Health National Council, Brazil, 1996) the proper written informed consent was read and signed by the athletes.

2.1. Experimental Designs

After a regular warm up, the athletes were subjected to a training protocol that consisted of several canoe sprint bouts, with three minute intervals between each bout, covering different distances and intensities. The total distance totaled 16 kilometers. This first part of the protocol had a duration of 210 min followed by a rest period of 20 min during which they ingested a 500 mL beverage consisting of about 20% carbohydrate (short and medium absorption); 2% lipids; 5% proteins (casein and whey proteins). Next, they performed a weight lifting training session for 50 min focusing on exercises that recruit large muscle groups for both upper and lower body, followed by a 70 min of recovery. See the experimental trial depicted (Figure 1).

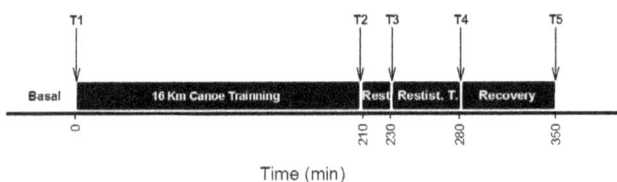

Figure 1. Experimental trial. Blood samples of the athletes were collected at the time points indicted in the Figure and as described in materials and methods.

2.2. Blood Collection

Blood samples were collected following an antecubital vein puncture before (T1) and after (T2) the 16 km canoe training session; before (T3) and after (T4) the resistance training; and after the recovery period (T5) (Figure 1). Samples for hematological analysis assays were collected into tubes with K_2-EDTA (Vacuette, Greiner Bio-One, Frickenhausen, Germany). White blood cell (total and differential), erythrocyte, and thrombocyte counts were measured in whole blood within a two-hour time frame after collection. Blood was immediately centrifuged to obtain either plasma or serum that was aliquoted, centrifuged ($3000\times g$; 10 min; 4 °C), and stored in liquid nitrogen for later analysis (never more than eight hours). Samples were analyzed in duplicate or triplicate, when necessary, and measured against a standard curve with no less than five points.

2.3. Blood Analysis

A range of hematological and biochemical analyses was carried out totalizing around 100 analytes. The large amount of data generated was used in a non-target analysis linked to an ex-post facto study design. We chose near 20 analytes that could be relevant for our study of the athlete's performance. Among others, our data set included a broad spectrum of metabolites and biomarkers related to different cellular and systemic signaling processes like inflammation and both muscle and hepatic injury.

Alanine aminotransferase (ALT), aspartate aminotransferase (AST), alkaline phosphatase (ALP), lactate dehydrogenase (LDH), γ-glutamyltransferase (γGT), creatine phosphokinase muscle-brain fraction (CKMB), creatine phosphokinase (CK), ammonia, urea, blood urea nitrogen (BUN), creatinine, urate, glucose, lactate, and 2-hydroxybutyrate were measured by the enzymatic kinetic method [38] in an automatic analyzer (ADVIA 1200—SIEMENS, Erlangen, Germany/Autolab 18 Boehringer Mannheim, Ingelheim am Rhein, Germany). Myoglobin was evaluated by the Hybridization Signal Amplification Method [39]. Albumin and total protein were assessed by electrophoretic analysis [40]. High-density lipoprotein (HDL), low-density lipoprotein (LDL), very-low-density lipoprotein (VLDL), total lipids, triacylglycerols (TG), and total cholesterol were assessed by the Chabrol & Charonnat method [41]. Amino acids were measured by high performance liquid chromatography (HPLC) [42]. CKMB-mass, insulin, adrenocorticotropic hormone (ACTH), and cortisol levels were assessed by chemiluminescence (Immulite 2000 Siemens, Erlangen, Germany) [43].

2.4. Statistical Analysis

Statistical analyses were performed using the software SigmaPlot 11.0 integrated with SigmaStat 3.5 packages (Systat, Santa Clara, CA, USA). Due to the nature of the experiment, including the similarity of subjects and the controlled experimental conditions (diet, sleep, training and major physical condition variables), the data were expressed as mean ± standard error (SEM). Data were normalized to pre-training results (T1) for clarity and analyzed by Analysis of Variance (ANOVA) using the condition and time as the repeated measured variables, which were confirmed using Tukey's post hoc test. $p < 0.05$ was defined as the limit for statistically different mean values.

3. Results

Anthropometric characteristics of the individuals are presented on Table 1. Approximate averages of the values measured were as follows: 1.77 m of height, 82.9 kg of weight, 9.8 kg of fat weight, 73 kg of fat-free mass, 11.5% of body fat percentage, indicating that all tested individuals presented typical body composition, fat distribution, and weight profiles. We assessed the lipid profiles and serum protein levels of the individuals to characterize their nutritional status. As observed in Table 2, the assessed lipid profiles were in accordance with the healthy status of the general population. Table 3 presents the results regarding serum protein levels. Despite the fact that these data are considered normal values for the general population, it is worth noting that the assessed albuminemia was low considering a world-class team of athletes. Due to the lack of knowledge of world-class biomarker levels we chose to show all the data as a reference for future studies [3,5,10,21].

Table 1. Anthropometric parameters of the athletes were measured and are shown here as mean ± standard error.

Anthropometry	
Height (m)	1.77 ± 0.02
Weight (Kg)	82.9 ± 5.0
Fat weight (Kg)	9.8 ± 2.4
Fat-free mass (Kg)	73.0 ± 2.6
Fat percentage (%)	11.5 ± 2.0
BMI (Kg/m^2)	26.2 ± 1.2

Table 2. Lipid panel values–high-density lipoprotein (HDL); low-density lipoprotein (LDL); very low-density lipoprotein (VLDL)-were assessed as described in materials and methods and are shown here as mean ± standard error.

Lipid Panel (mg/dL)	
Serum cholesterol	173.6 ± 24.2
Serum triacylglycerol	83.3 ± 20.0
HDL	55.3 ± 5.0
LDL	95.0 ± 26.5
VLDL	16.6 ± 3.8
Cholesterol/HDL ratio	3.2 ± 0.7
LDL/HDL ratio	1.9 ± 0.6
Non cholesterol lipids	118.3 ± 28.9

Table 3. Protein fractions were assessed as described in materials and methods and are shown here as mean ± standard error.

Protein Fractions (g/dL)	
Total proteins	6.7 ± 0.12
Albumin	2.7 ± 1.23
α-1 globulin	0.4 ± 0.14
α-2 globulin	0.5 ± 0.05
β-1 globulin	0.4 ± 0.02
β-2 globulin	0.2 ± 0.003
γ globulin	1.2 ± 0.12

3.1. Muscle Stress Biomarkers

Well-established metabolic stress biomarkers were assessed in order to characterize the training intensity of the proposed trial. Compared to basal levels, AST showed a statistically significant increase after the resistance training (T4) by 30%, and continued to increase by up to 40% after the recovery period. Other biomarkers, such as ALT, ALP, and γGT, did not change throughout the trial (Figure 2, panels A and B). CK activity in blood samples, a classic muscle injury marker, was significantly higher by approximately 60% at T4. Compared to the pre-exercise state, it kept increasing to nearly two-fold at T5 (Figure 3, panel A). Despite the fact that no significant change was observed in CKMB and LDH blood activity, the CKMB mass activity, a very specific muscle injury parameter, reached an increment of 170% at T4 and was up regulated by three-fold at T5 (Figure 3, panel A). Blood levels of myoglobin were significantly increased after the first session of exercise, with an increment of 170%, and kept increasing throughout the trial to reach six-fold values at T5 when compared to basal (Figure 3, panel B).

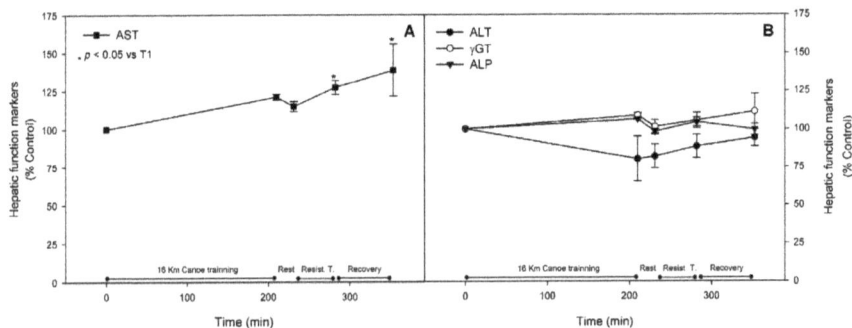

Figure 2. Hepatic injury biomarker. Aspartate aminotransferase (AST), alanine aminotransferase (ALT), γ-glutamyltransferase (γGT), and alkaline phosphatase (ALP) were measured as described in materials and methods and are represented as mean ± standard error of percentage values against control. * Indicates statistical difference against control values ($p < 0.05$). (**Panel A**) shows AST results and ALT, γGT, and ALP results are presented in (**Panel B**).

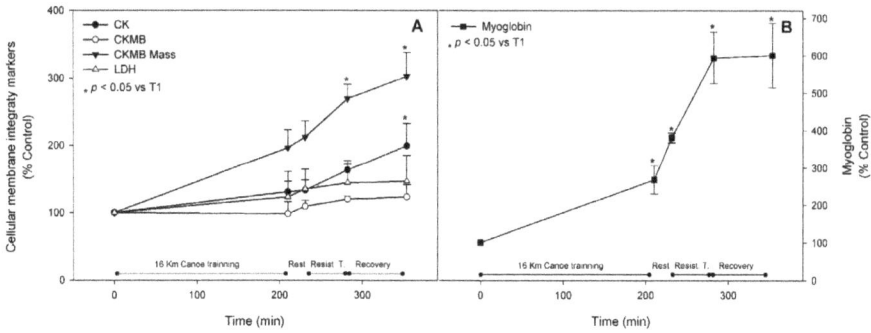

Figure 3. Cellular membrane integrity markers. Creatine phosphokinase (CK), creatine phosphokinase muscle-brain fraction (CKMB) activity and mass, lactate dehydrogenase (LDH) (**A**); and myoglobin (**B**) were measured as described in materials and methods and are represented as mean ± standard error of percentage values against control. * Indicates statistical difference against control values (*p* < 0.05).

3.2. White Blood Cells

During the trial, blood leukocytes rose by 40.0% ± 16.1% and 62.1% ± 26.8% after the canoe (T2) and weight lifting (T4) sessions, respectively, showing a discrete decrease after recovery and reaching levels of 43.2% ± 21.5% higher than basal. These results were mainly due to the increment in the neutrophil count, which showed a significant increase by 54.3% ± 22.3% and 166.2% ± 71.4% after T2 and T4, respectively, and was still 136.0 ± 58.2 higher than basal levels after the recovery. Despite the slight increase after the canoe training, the levels of lymphocytes showed a significant decrease of approximately 40% after the 20 min rest between the training sessions and remained significantly lower until the end of the protocol (Figure 4). Eosinophils measurements tended to accompany the lymphocytes pattern, presenting an increment of approximately 30% at T2 followed by an acute reduction that remained until the trial was terminated. Monocytes acutely responded to exercise stress and the recovery periods, increasing by about 30% after both exercise sessions with a rapid restoration of the original values. Thrombocyte levels responded positively and significantly to the canoe training sessions; they increased 30% compared to the control at T2, acutely returned to basal levels after the 20 min rest prior following resistance training, and remained similar to the original value for the rest of the trial (Figure 5).

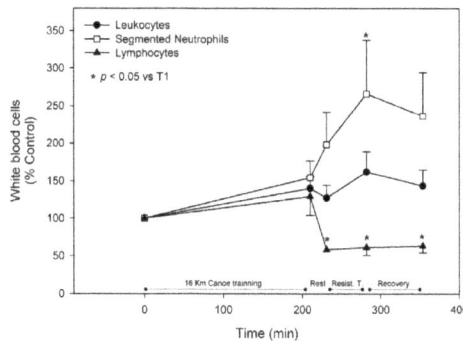

Figure 4. White blood cells. Leukocytes, segmented neuthrophils, and lymphocytes were measured as described in materials and methods and are represented as mean ± standard error of percentage values against control. * Indicates statistical difference against control values (*p* < 0.05).

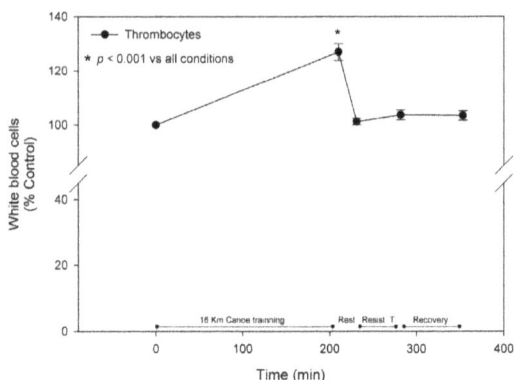

Figure 5. Thrombocytes. Thrombocyte levels were measured as described in materials and methods and are represented as mean ± standard error of percentage values against control. * Indicates statistical difference against any other condition ($p < 0.05$).

3.3. Branched Chain Amino Acids

Plasma branched chain amino acids (BCAA), which are important substrates either as metabolic fuel or as protein synthesis precursors, decreased right after both physical stimuli. Leucine showed the most prominent, significant decrease after the canoe training, reaching almost 50% of the basal value, and continued to decrease by approximately 22% after the resistance training. These decreases did not return to the original values, even after the recovery period. Both isoleucine and valine plasma concentrations seemed to be down regulated after canoe training, however, this decrease was not significantly different. After the 20 min rest between training sessions their levels returned to original values (Figure 6, panel A).

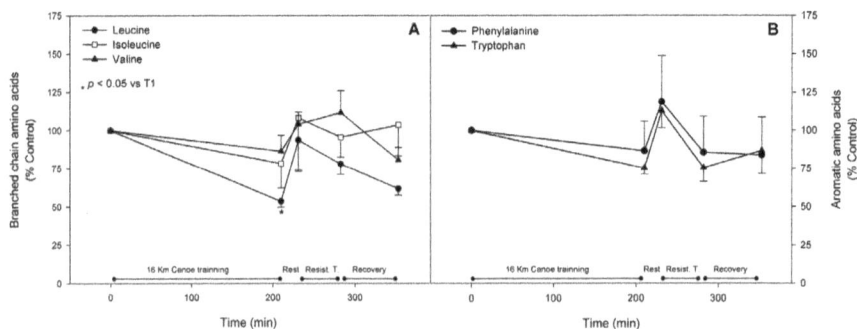

Figure 6. Branched chain (**A**) and aromatic (**B**) amino acids. Amino acid parameters were assessed as described in materials and methods and are represented as mean ± standard error of percentage values against control. * Indicates statistical difference against control values ($p < 0.05$).

3.4. Aromatic Amino Acids

The three amino acids comprising the aromatic amino acids (AAA), phenylalanine, tryptophan and tyrosine, are ketoglucogenic amino acids that may be deviated to the gluconeogenic pathway in hepatocytes. Our results showed that these amino acids decreased in the range of 15%–25% after both the canoe and the weight lifting exercises (Figure 6, panel B).

3.5. Gluconeogenic Amino Acids

Many amino acids may serve as both substrates in anaplerotic reactions replenishing intermediates of the tricarboxylic cycle and as gluconeogenic substrates. Hence, many amino acids serve as energy sources in metabolic pathways. Interestingly, the plasma concentration of some of these amino acids increased right after the first exercise bout. Alanine showed a two-fold increment after the canoe training and also showed a slighter increment of approximately 20% at T4, after resistance training. Glutamate was up regulated by 63% at T2, but regained the original levels at T4. Ornithine plasma levels were enhanced by approximately 20% at T2. Methionine was elevated by approximately 86% after the canoe training session and decreased for the remainder of the trial. Taurine followed the methionine response, which is one of its precursors, rising 56% at T2. Glycine showed a later increase, with levels elevated by about 35% at T3 and with measurements similar to control at all other time points. On the other hand, arginine blood levels were down regulated to 60% of control values at T2 and 69% at T4. Glutamine presented a similar but slighter response, reaching 85% of basal values at T2 and returning to control levels thereafter. Lysine showed an approximately 30% decremented level at T2 when compared to control. Other assessed amino acids, such as asparagine, aspartate, serine, and threonine, did not fluctuate throughout the trial.

3.6. Metabolic Pathway Substrates, Intermediates, and Products

The metabolism of amino acids results in the production of nitrogen compounds, including ammonia; the increase in the levels of these compounds in the blood is tightly related to exercise intensity and duration. Ammonemia was significantly up regulated after the canoe training session by 78% and remained significantly enhanced (by about 71%) even after the recovery period. Urea blood level was slightly higher by about 21% at T4 and tended to reach normal values after the recovery period. Urea concentration may reflect total ammonia excretion. IMP production is correlated to urate appearance in the blood, which is the final product of purine catabolism. Urate blood concentration rose significantly in blood by 24% and 20% at T4 and T5, respectively, when compared to the control. Blood levels of creatinine, a muscle damage indicator that may also suggest hemoconcentration alteration, responded acutely to both exercise sessions, augmenting significantly by 24% at T2. This was followed by a restoration of control values at T3, then a significant enhancement right after resistance training by 20% when compared to the control, and then a return to normal values at the end of the recovery period (Figure 7). BUN concentration remained unchanged throughout the trial.

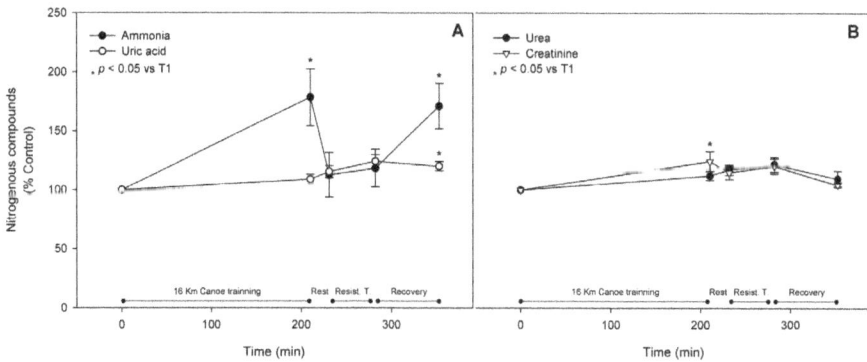

Figure 7. Nitrogenous compounds. Ammonia and uric acid are shown in (**Panel A**). Urea and creatinine fluctuations are presented in (**Panel B**). Nitrogenous compounds were evaluated as reported in materials and methods and are shown as mean ± standard error of percentage values against control. * Indicates statistical difference against control values ($p < 0.05$).

Serum glucose, insulin, ACTH, and cortisol fluctuations during exercise are also related to the destinations of amino acid metabolites and, therefore, were measured. Due to the stress caused by the canoe training session, the hypothalamus activated the production of Corticotropin Releasing Hormone (CRH), which in turn stimulated the anterior pituitary gland to produce ACTH, and then the adrenal gland to produce cortisol. While ACTH serum levels increased by 82% at T2, cortisol rose only 12% in comparison to initial levels. After exercise, the HPA axis was suppressed, and blood levels of both hormones diminished significantly when ACTH reached values of 36% at T4, and measured cortisol was 39% at T5 when compared to T2 (Figure 8).

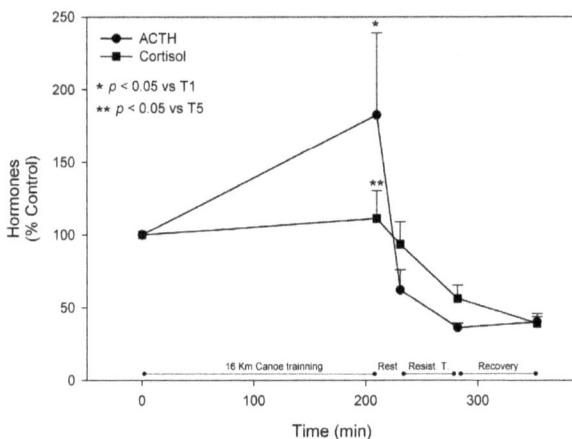

Figure 8. Hypothalamic-pituitary adrenal axis hormones. Adrenocorticotropic hormone (ACTH) and cortisol were measured as described in materials and methods and are represented as mean ± standard error of percentage values against control. * Indicates statistical difference against control values ($p < 0.05$). ** Indicates statistical significance when compared to T5 values ($p < 0.05$).

Insulin presented a slight decrease in response to the canoe exercise by about 10% and a significant increase of 137% after the 20 min of rest due to the food and hydro-electrolyte reposition; it returned to the approximate basal levels after the resistance training session and presented a drop by 50% of the original concentration. Glycemia was significantly enhanced by 78% after the canoe bout and tended to decrease progressively throughout the trial while maintaining its blood level slightly higher than basal. The ketone body 2-hydroxybutyrate blood levels were also significantly augmented after the canoe bout by 29%, followed by a slighter increment of 11% after the second exercise training session (Figure 9, panels A and B). It is well known that the lactate blood levels increase according to the exercise intensity. Our results showed a significant increment of 360% and 255% after the canoe and resistance training sessions, respectively (Figure 9, panel A).

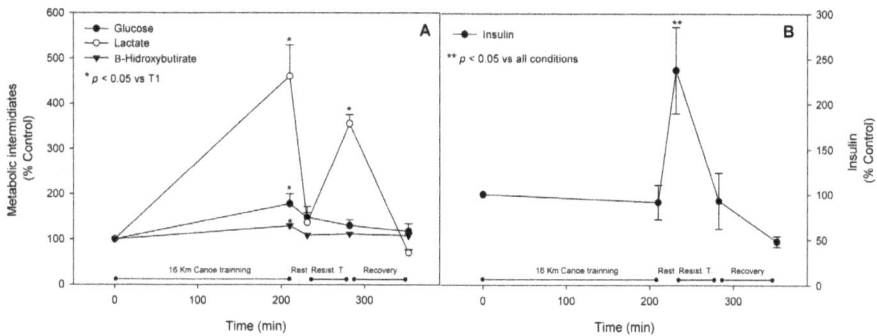

Figure 9. Metabolic intermediates and Insulin. Glucose, lactate, 2-hidroxybutirate (A), and insulin (B) were assessed as described in materials and methods and are represented as mean ± standard error of percentage values against control. * Indicates statistical difference against control values ($p < 0.05$). ** Indicates statistical significance when compared to all conditions ($p < 0.05$).

4. Discussion

Canoeing competitions are sprint events requiring sustained bursts of speed and power, leading to intense biochemical and metabolic stress. Many metabolites produced due to physical effort may be implicated in fatigue and impairment of physical performance, hence, the understanding of these responses is crucial to upgrade training sessions and optimize athlete performance. Here, we applied a Sportomics approach to study and evaluate different metabolic and cellular responses during a training session of world-class canoe athletes. Sportomics can help us in the understanding of the metabolism and signaling events that occur in response to exercise and allow us to perform interventions increasing both metabolic and sportive performances [10,16,19].

We measured serum levels of known exercise intensity biomarkers to characterize the applied training protocol magnitude and assure the possibility of correlating exercise intensity to the metabolic responses. Exercise intensity can be inferred by increases in plasma levels of CK, CKMB mass, CKMB, and LDH [3,44–46]. Several studies have investigated the increase in CK in response to exercise [3,5,10,21]. In this study, CK and CKMB mass blood levels increased continuously throughout the exercise trial, rising significantly at T4 and T5 when compared to basal levels. This suggests that the exercise stress and duration represented enough stimuli to cause such changes; a similar result was described by Siegel et al. [47]. Despite these observations, CKMB levels did not elevate significantly at any time point throughout the exercise session. However, it is worth noting that the blood basal levels of this enzyme were higher than expected due to exercise accumulation along the regular training season of the athletes, and this fact may have limited the furthest increment along the executed protocol. Additionally, immune assays show more analytical sensitivity when compared to enzymatic activity measurements. Therefore, it is necessary to separate immune assays from enzymatic assays. It is important to emphasize that most protocols measure the enzymatic activity of CK (also LDH and others) as a way to understand its increase or decline in response to exercise. These enzymes are also being subjected to blood environment changes that can lead to an increase in the specific activity (i.e., the ability to an enzyme to catalyze a reaction in a given unit of time), so it is our understanding that the preferable way to measure muscle cellular injury is to use a direct measurement of the enzyme content using immunological quantitative methods (such as ELISA or Western blot or mass spectrometry). For us, this is an important statement because we believe that researchers should carefully analyze the results of any increase of enzymes during exercise by the way of enzymatic activity.

Blood levels of LDH also remained constant throughout the exercise trial, and this result is in accordance with other studies which have shown a classic delayed response of LDH blood levels to strenuous exercise [48–50]. Myoglobin release from muscle to blood is a well-known biochemical marker of muscle injury [51]. In our study, myoglobin significantly increased due to the exercise stress, confirming skeletal muscle damage induced by the exercise protocol. This confirms the CK findings and corroborates our interpretation concerning the difference in the CK and CKMB increase.

Classical biochemical hepatic damage markers such as AST, ALT, ALP, and γGT can be increased as a result of liver and/or muscle injury after strenuous exercise [52,53]. In the present study, the only enzyme that presented a significant increase throughout the protocol was AST, while the serum level of the other enzymes remained unchanged throughout the exercise. Since these enzymes are also present in muscles, the origin of this increase could not be differentiated between muscle or liver cell disruption. However, we have recently proposed that muscle damage can be distinguished from liver damage by using the more specific liver biomarkers such as ALT and γGT [5], which remained constant in the present study. These data together suggest that the increases of these proteins are more likely from muscle rather than liver cellular injury.

White blood cell counts increase after many types of exercise and the release of neutrophils is directly correlated with exercise intensity and duration [3,17,18]. In this study, we reported an increment in total leukocytes in response to both exercise sessions, which can be attributed to the release of neutrophils. Interestingly, after a discrete increment in lymphocyte levels at T2, it returned to basal values and continued decreasing reaching a significant reduction between the training sessions. Previous studies indicated that the response of white blood cells to exercise is dependent on both cytokine and myokines modulation [54–56]. Taken together these results may suggest that white blood cell mobilization is due not to a non-specific exercise-induced spleen release, but rather to a specific signal. Additionally, we reported an increase in platelet count without any change in erythrocyte count, indicating that this effect occurs in a spleen-independent manner. As previously suggested, these results may indicate that both thrombocytosis and leucocytosis observed during the exercise bout are induced by either muscle cell damage or differential cell signaling [3,18].

Muscle cell damage is known to stimulate immune cell mobilization to the bloodstream and migration to muscle tissue [5]. Exercise has been proposed to be a physiological way to modulate immunity; while acute severe exercise usually impedes immunity, chronic moderate exercise improves it [57,58]. Although the evidence to support these concepts is inconclusive, it supports the idea that exercise-induced immune suppression increases susceptibility to symptoms of infection, particularly around time of competition [59]. Moreover, metabolic stress is correlated with exercise induced white blood cell response, as carbohydrate supplementation and availability have been proposed to affect neutrophil count after intense exercise [60–62]. We previously described that a combination of training, rest and nutritional intervention could have an important impact in amino acid availability, muscle cellular injury, and immune response in another world-class athlete [10]. Therefore, the immune responses reported here may be directly correlated with the alterations in the nutritional status and metabolic availability as observed during the present experimental trial.

In this sense, it is important to maintain plasma level amino acids during training sessions, since many amino acids serve both as anabolic and energetic precursors. In addition, it has been proposed that blood fluctuations in the concentration of BCAAs may affect its ratio in the brain [63]. In our study, the levels of many amino acids presented a blood concentration decrease during the sport trial. Leucine showed the most important decrease after the canoe training session. Isoleucine and valine concentration also decreased in a smaller range. Aromatic amino acids, which are generally metabolized in the liver, were slightly consumed during the canoe exercise session; similar results were described before [10]. Glutamine levels presented a similar response; they decreased after the canoe trial and were restored after the recovery period. This could be the result of two processes: glutamine exportation from muscle to decrease its ammonia levels; and the use of glutamine as both a gluconeogenic substrate and a urea cycle feeder in the liver. On the other hand, alanine was up regulated after the first exercise bout, showing a two-fold increment at T2. This response may be attributed to a metabolic attempt to offer gluconeogenic substrates for further oxidation. The depletion of glycogen storage is related to exercise intensity, duration, and nutritional status, which in turn may increase the use of amino acids as energy substrates, thereby increasing ammonia and the production of other nitrogen compounds [64]. Both glutamine and alanine are anaplerotic and gluconeogenic substrates and contribute to ATP and glucose synthesis. The ergogenic properties of glutamine have been extensively studied [6,62,65], and we have recently reported the metabolic effects of alanine in comparison to long-term glutamine supplementation during an intermittent exercise protocol. Long term administration of glutamine is capable of reducing ammonia production during intermittent exercise, hence, it is postulated to be a protector against an increase in blood ammonia in an exercise intensity-dependent manner [21].

Many studies have indicated that ammonia is a useful physiological marker of prolonged intense exercise, and its appearance in blood is positively correlated with exercise intensity [1,10,30]. High ammonemia can be toxic to both muscles and the central nervous system (CNS). Such changes are believed to contribute to the disturbances in neuropsychological function and motor control deficits and are also observed in patients with cirrhosis and, therefore, could induce central and peripheral fatigue [25,60,66]. Therefore, measuring ammonia production during a sport session may represent an important tool to control exercise intensity and to understand the metabolic response of a given athlete. The canoe athletes experienced an increase in their blood ammonia levels during the exercise trial due to both stimuli, which remained up regulated even after the recovery period. This effect was followed by an increase in other measured nitrogenous compounds, such as urea, urate and creatinine. These responses may have occurred as a result of an increased demand for ATP by muscle contraction, leading to adenosine monophosphate (AMP) deamination and, subsequently, the production of ammonia and urate [26–29]. Many studies have shown that ammonia production and release represents the exercise effort intensity, rapidly increasing in intensities greater than 50%–60% of VO_{2max} up to maximal exhaustion [31,32]. Ammonia plasma concentration is also up regulated during prolonged (greater than one hour) submaximal exercise (60%–75% VO_{2max}). In these conditions, ammonia could be produced in increasing amounts through the breakdown of branched chain amino acid (BCAA) prior to oxidation for additional energy provision [33–35].

The response of the other nitrogen metabolites may shed light on understanding the protein and amino acid oxidation response during exercise. Urea and urate blood concentration is indirectly correlated with the myokinase (adenylate kinase, ADK) contribution to ATP synthesis. Under a resting physiological state, approximately 90% of the skeletal muscle adenosine monophosphate deaminase (AMPD) is in a sarcoplasmic position and in an inactive form. However, a significant change occurs as intense muscle contraction begin, when approximately 50%–60% of AMPD becomes bound to the myofibrils [28]. Binding of the enzyme increases its activity causing an increased rate of degradation of AMP to IMP. This is correlated with the appearance of urate in the blood which is a final metabolite of purine metabolism [30]. This increased breakdown of AMP will affect the equilibrium of the ADK reaction by creating additional ATP from ADP to increase the cellular energy charge and maintain contractions under conditions of increasing stress [29]. During intense exercise, when AMP production and deamination are high, ADP levels also increase as utilization of ATP exceeds re-phosphorylation [67]. Therefore, any strategies, such as diet adequacies and supplementations, to protect against hyperammonemia or an increment of any nitrogenous compound could enhance physical performance or prevent CNS injuries, as previously reported by our group [6,10,21].

During the canoe trial, glycemia rose significantly, which may be a result of the HPA axis activation. Exercise is known to be a potent activator of this endocrine system, resulting in the release of ACTH, as confirmed here. This ultimately culminates with glucocorticoids production and release into blood circulation, which may lead to gluconeogenesis activation and promotion of an adrenergic stimulus, providing glucose to blood from hepatic glycogenolysis [68–70]. Nevertheless, afferent neural feedback signals from contracting muscle and feedback signals mediated via the blood stream can stimulate glucose production to maintain glycemia. Therefore, central mechanisms coupled with the degree of motor center activity can be responsible for part of the increase in glucose mobilization, especially during intense exercise where hepatic glucose release exceeds peripheral glucose uptake, and plasma glucose rises [71]. Furthermore, cortisol is implicated in exercise induced lymphocyte apoptosis, via glucocorticoid dependent-pathways [72], which might affect immune function and protect the organism from an overreaction of the immune system in the face of exercise-induced muscle damage [73].

Hepatic glucose production increases during exercise, to cope with the augmented demand, as a product of liver glycogenolysis and gluconeogenesis. Whereas the former predominates during high intensity exercise, the latter contributes substantially with prolonged exercise and the concomitant decline in liver glycogen stores and with increased gluconeogenic precursor supply. In fact, it has been postulated that the increase in glucose production with exercise intensity in healthy subjects can be entirely attributed to increases in net hepatic glycogenolysis [74]. This pathway is also supported by our data. On the other hand, a decline in plasma insulin is important for the rise in glucose production during exercise [71], due to the fact that insulinemia tends to decrease in response to prolonged exercise, with a more pronounced effect on athletes than untrained individuals [75], which is in agreement with the results reported here.

5. Conclusions

The data presented here allow us to consider hormonal, metabolic, and signaling response together with the knowledge of nutrition and training environment. This combined information permits a better understanding of the individual responses of exercise and sport stress. Our group developed the concept of Sportomics with a focus on bridging the same existent gap between translational and personalized medicine [76]. As stated by Liebman et al. [77], the workflow bench to bedside approach is being refined in the face of a new bedside-bench-bedside approach. Sportomics is useful to evaluate the unprecedented kinetics of some metabolites [3,5,10,11,13,14,16,37,78] and to shed light on the importance of in-field metabolic analyses to the understanding of the inter-individual response to exercise. Besides an effective nutritional support, collecting physiological data during training and competition can provide important information about an athlete's clinical condition, bringing strategies to modify metabolism during exercise as well as supporting coaches to prescribe their sessions and recovery time. Therefore, and due to the uniqueness of this study, we believe Sportomics is a primal tool for training management and performance improvement, as well as for preserving health and increasing the quality of life of athletes.

Acknowledgments: The authors acknowledge the Comitê Olimpíco do Brasil (BOC); Conselho Nacional de Desenvolvimento Científico e Tecnológico (CNPq); Coordenação de Aperfeiçoamento de Pessoal de Nível Superior (CAPES); Financiadora de Estudos e Projetos (FINEP); Fundação Carlos Chagas Filho de Amparo à Pesquisa do Estado do Rio de Janeiro (FAPERJ); Merck-Sigma-Aldrich; Universidade Federal do Estado do Rio de Janeiro (UNIRIO) and Waters Corporation for the project funding including the costs to publish in open access.

Author Contributions: W.S.C., L.V.C., E.D., A.B. and L.C.C. conceived and designed the experiments; W.S.C., L.V.C., E.D. and A.B. performed the experiments; W.S.C., A.M.F. and L.C.C. analyzed the data; A.B. contributed reagents/materials/analysis tools; W.S.C., A.M.F. and L.C.C. wrote the paper.

Conflicts of Interest: The authors declare no conflict of interest.

References

1. Ament, W.; Verkerke, G.J. Exercise and fatigue. *Sports Med.* **2009**, *39*, 389–422. [CrossRef] [PubMed]
2. Rose, A.J.; Richter, E.A. Regulatory mechanisms of skeletal muscle protein turnover during exercise. *J. Appl. Physiol.* **2009**, *106*, 1702–1711. [CrossRef] [PubMed]
3. Bessa, A.; Nissenbaum, M.; Monteiro, A.; Gandra, P.G.; Bassini-Cameron, A.; Werneck-de-Castro, J.P.S.; Vaz de Macedo, D.; Cameron, L.-C. High-intensity ultraendurance promotes early release of muscle injury markers. *Br. J. Sports Med.* **2008**, *42*, 889–893. [CrossRef] [PubMed]
4. Burd, N.A.; Tang, J.E.; Moore, D.R.; Phillips, S.M. Exercise training and protein metabolism: Influences of contraction, protein intake, and sex-based differences. *J. Appl. Physiol.* **2009**, *106*, 1692–1701. [CrossRef] [PubMed]

5. Bassini-Cameron, A.; Sweet, E.; Bottino, A.; Bittar, C.; Veiga, C.; Cameron, L.-C. Effect of caffeine supplementation on haematological and biochemical variables in elite soccer players under physical stress conditions. *Br. J. Sports Med.* **2007**, *41*, 523–530. [CrossRef] [PubMed]

6. Carvalho-Peixoto, J.; Alves, R.C.; Cameron, L.C. Glutamine and carbohydrate supplements reduce ammonemia increase during endurance field exercise. *Appl. Physiol. Nutr. Metab.* **2007**, *32*, 1186–1190. [CrossRef] [PubMed]

7. Lazarim, F.L.; Antunes-Neto, J.M.F.; da Silva, F.O.C.; Nunes, L.A.S.; Bassini-Cameron, A.; Cameron, L.-C.; Alves, A.A.; Brenzikofer, R.; Vaz de Macedo, D. The upper values of plasma creatine kinase of professional soccer players during the Brazilian National Championship. *J. Sci. Med. Sport* **2009**, *12*, 85–90. [CrossRef] [PubMed]

8. De Souza Martins, S.C.; Romão, L.F.; Faria, G.C.; de Holanda Afonso, R.C.; Murray, S.A.; Pellizzon, C.H.; Mercer, J.A.; Cameron, L.C.; Moura-Neto, V. Effect of thyroid hormone T3 on myosin-Va expression in the central nervous system. *Brain Res.* **2009**, *1275*, 1–9. [CrossRef] [PubMed]

9. De Almeida, R.D.; Prado, E.S.; Llosa, C.D.; Magalhães-Neto, A.; Cameron, L.C. Acute supplementation with keto analogues and amino acids in rats during resistance exercise. *Br. J. Nutr.* **2010**, *104*, 1438–1442. [CrossRef] [PubMed]

10. Resende, N.M.; de Magalhães Neto, A.M.; Bachini, F.; de Castro, L.E.V.; Bassini, A.; Cameron, L.C. Metabolic changes during a field experiment in a world-class windsurfing athlete: A trial with multivariate analyses. *OMICS* **2011**, *15*, 695–704. [CrossRef] [PubMed]

11. Prado, E.S.; de Rezende Neto, J.M.; de Almeida, R.D.; de Melo, M.G.D.; Cameron, L.C. Keto analogue and amino acid supplementation affects the ammonaemia response during exercise under ketogenic conditions. *Br. J. Nutr.* **2011**, *105*, 1729–1733. [CrossRef] [PubMed]

12. Cameron, L.C. Mass Spectrometry Imaging: Facts and perspectives from a non-mass spectrometrist point of view. *Methods* **2012**, *57*, 417–422. [CrossRef] [PubMed]

13. Gonçalves, L.C.; Bessa, A.; Freitas-Dias, R.; Luzes, R.; Werneck-de-Castro, J.P.S.; Bassini, A.; Cameron, L.C. A sportomics strategy to analyze the ability of arginine to modulate both ammonia and lymphocyte levels in blood after high-intensity exercise. *J. Int. Soc. Sports Nutr.* **2012**, *9*, 30. [CrossRef] [PubMed]

14. Bassini, A.; Magalhães-Neto, A.M.; Sweet, E.; Bottino, A.; Veiga, C.; Tozzi, M.B.; Cameron, L.C. Caffeine decreases systemic urea in elite soccer players during intermittent exercise. *Med. Sci. Sports Exerc.* **2013**, *45*, 683–690. [CrossRef] [PubMed]

15. Neto, R.A.; de Souza Dos Santos, M.C.; Rangel, I.F.; Ribeiro, M.B.; Cavalcanti-de-Albuquerque, J.P.; Ferreira, A.C.; Cameron, L.C.; Carvalho, D.P.; Werneck de Castro, J.P. Decreased serum T3 after an exercise session is independent of glucocorticoid peak. *Horm. Metab. Res.* **2013**, *45*, 893–899. [CrossRef] [PubMed]

16. Bassini, A.; Cameron, L.C. Sportomics: Building a new concept in metabolic studies and exercise science. *Biochem. Biophys. Res. Commun.* **2014**, *445*, 708–716. [CrossRef] [PubMed]

17. Reid, S.A.; Speedy, D.B.; Thompson, J.M.D.; Noakes, T.D.; Mulligan, G.; Page, T.; Campbell, R.G.D.; Milne, C. Study of hematological and biochemical parameters in runners completing a standard marathon. *Clin. J. Sport Med.* **2004**, *14*, 344–353. [CrossRef] [PubMed]

18. Wu, H.J.; Chen, K.T.; Shee, B.W.; Chang, H.C.; Huang, Y.J.; Yang, R.S. Effects of 24 h ultra-marathon on biochemical and hematological parameters. *World J. Gastroenterol.* **2004**, *10*, 2711–2714. [CrossRef] [PubMed]

19. Bragazzi, N.L. Nutritional Sciences at the Intersection of Omics Disciplines and Ethics. Available online: http://onlinelibrary.wiley.com/doi/10.1002/9781118930458.ch47/summary (accessed on 11 March 2016).

20. Page, A.J.; Reid, S.A.; Speedy, D.B.; Mulligan, G.; Thompson, J. Exercise-associated hyponatremia, renal function, and nonsteroidal antiinflammatory drug use in an ultraendurance mountain run. *Clin. J. Sport Med.* **2007**, *17*, 43–48. [CrossRef] [PubMed]

21. Bassini-Cameron, A.; Monteiro, A.; Gomes, A.; Werneck-de-Castro, J.P.S.; Cameron, L. Glutamine protects against increases in blood ammonia in football players in an exercise intensity-dependent way. *Br. J. Sports Med.* **2008**, *42*, 260–266. [CrossRef] [PubMed]

22. Liu, Y.; Spreng, T.; Lehr, M.; Yang, B.; Karau, A.; Gebhardt, G.; Steinacker, G.M. The supportive effect of supplementation with α-keto acids on physical training in type 2 diabetes mellitus. *Food Funct.* **2015**, *6*, 2224–2230. [CrossRef] [PubMed]

23. Nybo, L.; Dalsgaard, M.K.; Steensberg, A.; Møller, K.; Secher, N.H. Cerebral ammonia uptake and accumulation during prolonged exercise in humans. *J. Physiol.* **2005**, *563 Pt 1*, 285–290. [CrossRef] [PubMed]

24. Nybo, L.; Secher, N.H. Cerebral perturbations provoked by prolonged exercise. *Prog. Neurobiol.* **2004**, *72*, 223–261. [CrossRef] [PubMed]

25. Wilkinson, D.J.; Smeeton, N.J.; Watt, P.W. Ammonia metabolism, the brain and fatigue; revisiting the link. *Prog. Neurobiol.* **2010**, *91*, 200–219. [CrossRef] [PubMed]

26. Parnas, J.K. Ammonia formation in muscle and its source. *Am. J. Physiol.* **1929**, *90*, 467.

27. Lowenstein, J.M. The purine nucleotide cycle revisited. *Int. J. Sports Med.* **1990**, *11*, S37–S46. [CrossRef] [PubMed]

28. Rundell, K.W.; Tullson, P.C.; Terjung, R.L. AMP deaminase binding in contracting rat skeletal muscle. *Am. J. Physiol.* **1992**, *263*, C287–C293. [CrossRef] [PubMed]

29. Hisatome, I.; Morisaki, T.; Kamma, H.; Sugama, T.; Morisaki, H.; Ohtahara, A.; Holmes, E.W. Control of AMP deaminase 1 binding to myosin heavy chain. *Am. J. Physiol.* **1998**, *275*, C870–C881. [PubMed]

30. Hellsten, Y.; Richter, E.A.; Kiens, B.; Bangsbo, J. AMP deamination and purine exchange in human skeletal muscle during and after intense exercise. *J. Physiol.* **1999**, *520*, 909–920. [CrossRef] [PubMed]

31. Babij, P.; Matthews, S.M.; Rennie, M.J. Changes in blood ammonia, lactate and amino acids in relation to workload during bicycle ergometer exercise in man. *Eur. J. Appl. Physiol. Occup. Physiol.* **1983**, *50*, 405–411. [CrossRef] [PubMed]

32. Buono, M.J.; Clancy, T.R.; Cook, J.R. Blood lactate and ammonium ion accumulation during graded exercise in humans. *J. Appl. Physiol. Respir. Environ. Exerc. Physiol.* **1984**, *57*, 135–139. [PubMed]

33. Kasperek, G.J.; Dohm, G.L.; Snider, R.D. Activation of branched-chain keto acid dehydrogenase by exercise. *Am. J. Physiol.* **1985**, *248 Pt 2*, R166–R171. [PubMed]

34. Wagenmakers, A.J.; Coakley, J.H.; Edwards, R.H. Metabolism of branched-chain amino acids and ammonia during exercise: Clues from McArdle's disease. *Int. J. Sports Med.* **1990**, *11*, S101–S113. [CrossRef] [PubMed]

35. Van Hall, G.; van der Vusse, G.J.; Söderlund, K.; Wagenmakers, A.J. Deamination of amino acids as a source for ammonia production in human skeletal muscle during prolonged exercise. *J. Physiol.* **1995**, *489*, 251–261. [CrossRef]

36. Felipo, V.; Butterworth, R.F. Neurobiology of ammonia. *Prog. Neurobiol.* **2002**, *67*, 259–279. [CrossRef]

37. Camerino, S.R.A.S.; Lima, R.C.P.; França, T.C.L.; de Azevedo Herculano, E.; Rodrigues, D.S.A.; Rodrigues, D.A.S.; de Sousa Gouveia, M.G.; Cameron, L.C.; Prado, E.S. Keto analogues and amino acid supplementation and its effects on ammonemia and performance under thermoneutral conditions. *Food Funct.* **2016**, *7*, 872–870. [CrossRef] [PubMed]

38. Pardue, H.L. A comprehensive classification of kinetic methods of analysis used in clinical chemistry. *Clin. Chem.* **1977**, *23*, 2189–2201. [PubMed]

39. Werner, M.; von Wasielewski, R.; Komminoth, P. Antigen retrieval, signal amplification and intensification in immunohistochemistry. *Histochem. Cell Biol.* **1996**, *105*, 253–260. [CrossRef] [PubMed]

40. Fairbanks, G.; Steck, T.L.; Wallach, D.F. Electrophoretic analysis of the major polypeptides of the human erythrocyte membrane. *Biochemistry* **1971**, *10*, 2606–2617. [CrossRef] [PubMed]

41. Knight, J.A.; Anderson, S.; Rawle, J.M. Chemical basis of the sulfo-phospho-vanillin reaction for estimating total serum lipids. *Clin. Chem.* **1972**, *18*, 199–202. [PubMed]

42. Bayer, E.; Grom, E.; Kaltenegger, B.; Uhmann, R. Separation of amino acids by high performance liquid chromatography. *Anal. Chem.* **1976**, *48*, 1106–1109. [CrossRef] [PubMed]

43. Kohen, F.; Pazzagli, M.; Kim, J.B.; Lindner, H.R. An immunoassay for plasma cortisol based on chemiluminescence. *Steroids* **1980**, *36*, 421–437. [CrossRef]

44. Kumae, T.; Kurakake, S.; Arakawa, H.; Uchiyama, I. A study for prevention of chronic fatigue. part 2. effects of strenuous physical exercise performed in a training camp on serum enzyme activity levels and subjective fatigue. *Environ. Health Prev. Med.* **1998**, *3*, 89–95. [CrossRef] [PubMed]

45. Smith, J.E.; Garbutt, G.; Lopes, P.; Pedoe, D.T. Effects of prolonged strenuous exercise (marathon running) on biochemical and haematological markers used in the investigation of patients in the emergency department. *Br. J. Sports Med.* **2004**, *38*, 292–294. [CrossRef] [PubMed]

46. Rodrigues, B.M.; Dantas, E.; de Salles, B.F.; Miranda, H.; Koch, A.; Willardson, J.M.; Simão, R. Creatine kinase and lactate dehydrogenase responses after upper-body resistance exercise with different rest intervals. *J. Strength Cond. Res.* **2010**, *24*, 1657–1662. [CrossRef] [PubMed]

47. Siegel, A.J.; Verbalis, J.G.; Clement, S.; Mendelson, J.H.; Mello, N.K.; Adner, M.; Shirey, T.; Glowacki, J.; Lee-Lewandrowski, E.; Lewandrowski, K.B. Hyponatremia in marathon runners due to inappropriate arginine vasopressin secretion. *Am. J. Med.* **2007**, *120*, 461.e11–461.e17. [CrossRef] [PubMed]
48. Chen, T.C.; Hsieh, S.S. Effects of a 7-day eccentric training period on muscle damage and inflammation. *Med. Sci. Sports Exerc.* **2001**, *33*, 1732–1738. [CrossRef] [PubMed]
49. Milias, G.A.; Nomikos, T.; Fragopoulou, E.; Athanasopoulos, S.; Antonopoulou, S. Effects of eccentric exercise-induced muscle injury on blood levels of platelet activating factor (PAF) and other inflammatory markers. *Eur. J. Appl. Physiol.* **2005**, *95*, 504–513. [CrossRef] [PubMed]
50. Chatzinikolaou, A.; Fatouros, I.; Gourgoulis, V.; Avloniti, A.; Jamurtas, A.Z.; Nikolaidis, M.G.; Douroudos, I.; Michailidis, Y.; Beneka, A.; Malliou, P.; et al. Time course of changes in performance and inflammatory responses after acute plyometric exercise. *J. Strength Cond. Res.* **2010**, *24*, 1389–1398. [CrossRef] [PubMed]
51. Brancaccio, P.; Lippi, G.; Maffulli, N. Biochemical markers of muscular damage. *Clin. Chem. Lab. Med.* **2010**, *48*, 757–767. [CrossRef] [PubMed]
52. Ohno, H.; Watanabe, H.; Kishihara, C.; Taniguchi, N.; Takakuwa, E. Effect of physical exercise on the activity of GOT isozyme in human plasma. *Tohoku J. Exp. Med.* **1978**, *126*, 371–376. [CrossRef] [PubMed]
53. Fallon, K.E.; Sivyer, G.; Sivyer, K.; Dare, A. The biochemistry of runners in a 1600 km ultramarathon. *Br. J. Sports Med.* **1999**, *33*, 264–269. [CrossRef] [PubMed]
54. Pedersen, B.K.; Åkerström, T.C.A.; Nielsen, A.R.; Fischer, C.P. Role of myokines in exercise and metabolism. *J. Appl. Physiol.* **2007**, *103*, 1093–1098. [CrossRef] [PubMed]
55. Mathur, N.; Pedersen, B.K. Exercise as a mean to control low-grade systemic inflammation. *Mediat. Inflamm.* **2008**, *2008*, 09502. [CrossRef] [PubMed]
56. Haugen, F.; Norheim, F.; Lian, H.; Wensaas, A.J.; Dueland, S.; Berg, O.; Funderud, A.; Skålhegg, B.S.; Raastad, T.; Drevon, C.A. IL-7 is expressed and secreted by human skeletal muscle cells. *Am. J. Physiol. Cell Physiol.* **2010**, *298*, C807–C816. [CrossRef] [PubMed]
57. Syu, G.D.; Chen, H.I.; Jen, C.J. Differential effects of acute and chronic exercise on human neutrophil functions. *Med. Sci. Sports Exerc.* **2012**, *44*, 1021–1027. [CrossRef] [PubMed]
58. Syu, G.D.; Chen, H.I.; Jen, C.J. Severe exercise and exercise training exert opposite effects on human neutrophil apoptosis via altering the redox status. *PLoS ONE* **2011**, *6*, e24385. [CrossRef] [PubMed]
59. Walsh, N.P.; Gleeson, M.; Shephard, R.; Gleeson, M.; Woods, J.A.; Bishop, N.; Fleshner, M.; Green, C.; Pedersen, B.K.; Hoffman-Goete, L.; et al. Position statement. Part one: Immune function and exercise. *Exerc. Immunol. Rev.* **2011**, *17*, 6–63. [PubMed]
60. Castell, L.M.; Newsholme, E.A. The effects of oral glutamine supplementation on athletes after prolonged, exhaustive exercise. *Nutrition* **1997**, *13*, 738–742. [CrossRef]
61. Castell, L.M.; Newsholme, E.A. The relation between glutamine and the immunodepression observed in exercise. *Amino Acids* **2001**, *20*, 49–61. [CrossRef] [PubMed]
62. Castell, L.M.; Poortmans, J.R.; Leclercq, R.; Brasseur, M.; Duchateau, G.; Newsholme, E.A. Some aspects of the acute phase response after a marathon race, and the effects of glutamine supplementation. *Eur. J. Appl. Physiol. Occup. Physiol.* **1997**, *75*, 47–53. [CrossRef] [PubMed]
63. Crowell, P.L.; Block, K.P.; Repa, J.J.; Torres, N.; Nawabi, M.D.; Buse, M.G.; Harper, A.E. High branched-chain alpha-keto acid intake, branched-chain alpha-keto acid dehydrogenase activity, and plasma and brain amino acid and plasma keto acid concentrations in rats. *Am. J. Clin. Nutr.* **1990**, *52*, 313–319. [PubMed]
64. Rohde, T.; MacLean, D.A.; Pedersen, B.K. Effect of glutamine supplementation on changes in the immune system induced by repeated exercise. *Med. Sci. Sports Exerc.* **1998**, *30*, 856–862. [CrossRef] [PubMed]
65. Bowtell, J.L.; Gelly, K.; Jackman, M.L.; Patel, A.; Simeoni, M.; Rennie, M.J. Effect of oral glutamine on whole body carbohydrate storage during recovery from exhaustive exercise. *J. Appl. Physiol.* **1999**, *86*, 1770–1777. [PubMed]
66. Banister, E.W.; Cameron, B.J. Exercise-induced hyperammonemia: Peripheral and central effects. *Int. J. Sports Med.* **1990**, *11*, S129–S142. [CrossRef] [PubMed]
67. Sahlin, K.; Harris, R.C.; Nylind, B.; Hultman, E. Lactate content and pH in muscle obtained after dynamic exercise. *Pflugers Arch.* **1976**, *367*, 143–149. [CrossRef] [PubMed]
68. Few, J.D. Effect of exercise on the secretion and metabolism of cortisol in man. *J. Endocrinol.* **1974**, *62*, 341–353. [CrossRef] [PubMed]

69. Farrell, P.A.; Garthwaite, T.L.; Gustafson, A.B. Plasma adrenocorticotropin and cortisol responses to submaximal and exhaustive exercise. *J. Appl. Physiol.* **1983**, *55*, 1441–1444. [PubMed]

70. Duclos, M.; Gouarne, C.; Bonnemaison, D. Acute and chronic effects of exercise on tissue sensitivity to glucocorticoids. *J. Appl. Physiol.* **2003**, *94*, 869–875. [CrossRef] [PubMed]

71. Kjaer, M. Hepatic glucose production during exercise. *Adv. Exp. Med. Biol.* **1998**, *441*, 117–127. [PubMed]

72. Kruger, K.; Agnischock, S.; Lechtermann, A.; Tiwari, S.; Mishra, M.; Pilat, C.; Wagner, A.; Tweddell, C.; Gramlich, I.; Mooren, F.C. Intensive resistance exercise induces lymphocyte apoptosis via cortisol and glucocorticoid receptor-dependent pathways. *J. Appl. Physiol.* **2011**, *110*, 1226–1232. [CrossRef] [PubMed]

73. Sapolsky, R.M.; Romero, L.M.; Munck, A.U. How do glucocorticoids influence stress responses? Integrating permissive, suppressive, stimulatory, and preparative actions. *Endocr. Rev.* **2000**, *21*, 55–89. [CrossRef] [PubMed]

74. Petersen, K.F.; Price, T.B.; Bergeron, R. Regulation of net hepatic glycogenolysis and gluconeogenesis during exercise: Impact of type 1 diabetes. *J. Clin. Endocrinol. Metab.* **2004**, *89*, 4656–4664. [CrossRef] [PubMed]

75. Viru, A.; Karelson, K.; Smirnova, T. Stability and variability in hormonal responses to prolonged exercise. *Int. J. Sports Med.* **1992**, *13*, 230–235. [CrossRef] [PubMed]

76. Schork, N.J. Personalized medicine: Time for one-person trials. *Nature* **2015**, *520*, 609–611. [CrossRef] [PubMed]

77. Liebman, M.N.; Franchini, M.; Molinaro, S. Bridging the gap between translational medicine and unmet clinical needs. *Technol. Health Care* **2015**, *23*, 109–118. [PubMed]

78. Magno-Franca, A.; Bassini, A.; Bessa, A.O.; Nissenbaum, M.; Vaz de Macedo, D.; Cameron, L.C. A sportomic follow-up of a muscle injury succeeded by acetaminophen hepatotoxicity. *OA Sports Med.* **2013**, *1*, 1–5. [CrossRef]

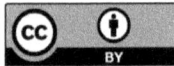

![nutrients logo] *nutrients*

MDPI

Article

Cardiorespiratory Fitness and Peak Torque Differences between Vegetarian and Omnivore Endurance Athletes: A Cross-Sectional Study

Heidi M. Lynch *, Christopher M. Wharton and Carol S. Johnston

Arizona State University, School of Nutrition and Health Promotion, Phoenix, AZ 85004, USA;
Christopher.Wharton@asu.edu (C.M.W.); Carol.Johnston@asu.edu (C.S.J.)
* Correspondence: Hnetland@asu.edu; Tel.: +1-847-828-1332

Received: 1 September 2016; Accepted: 10 November 2016; Published: 15 November 2016

Abstract: In spite of well-documented health benefits of vegetarian diets, less is known regarding the effects of these diets on athletic performance. In this cross-sectional study, we compared elite vegetarian and omnivore adult endurance athletes for maximal oxygen uptake (VO2 max) and strength. Twenty-seven vegetarian (VEG) and 43 omnivore (OMN) athletes were evaluated using VO2 max testing on the treadmill, and strength assessment using a dynamometer to determine peak torque for leg extensions. Dietary data were assessed using detailed seven-day food logs. Although total protein intake was lower among vegetarians in comparison to omnivores, protein intake as a function of body mass did not differ by group (1.2 ± 0.3 and 1.4 ± 0.5 g/kg body mass for VEG and OMN respectively, $p = 0.220$). VO2 max differed for females by diet group (53.0 ± 6.9 and 47.1 ± 8.6 mL/kg/min for VEG and OMN respectively, $p < 0.05$) but not for males (62.6 ± 15.4 and 55.7 ± 8.4 mL/kg/min respectively). Peak torque did not differ significantly between diet groups. Results from this study indicate that vegetarian endurance athletes' cardiorespiratory fitness was greater than that for their omnivorous counterparts, but that peak torque did not differ between diet groups. These data suggest that vegetarian diets do not compromise performance outcomes and may facilitate aerobic capacity in athletes.

Keywords: vegetarian; endurance; VO2 max; dynamometer; protein; sustainability; torque; body composition; Dual X-ray Absorptiometry (DXA)

1. Introduction

Vegetarian diets are increasingly being adopted for a variety of reasons including health, sustainability, and ethics-related concerns. Adherence to a vegetarian diet has been associated with a reduced risk of developing coronary heart disease [1], breast cancer [2], colorectal cancers [3], prostate cancer [4], type 2 diabetes [5], insulin resistance [6], hypertension [7], cataracts [8] and dementia [9]. Vegetarians also typically have a lower body mass index (BMI) [10] and an improved lipid profile [11]. In addition to promoting physical health, reducing or eliminating meat from the diet is environmentally advantageous since producing meat requires more land, water, and energy resources than growing plants for food [12], and producing meat creates more greenhouse gases compared to a plant-based diet [13,14].

In spite of the many health aspects of vegetarian diets some concern has been raised pertaining to the nutrient adequacy of vegetarian diets for supporting athletic performance. Vegetarian diets are typically lower in vitamin B12, protein, creatine, and carnitine [15,16], and iron and zinc from plant sources are less bioavailable than from meat sources [17]. However, vegetarian diets are typically higher in carbohydrate and antioxidants [18,19], which may be advantageous for athletic performance, particularly for endurance activities [20].

Despite these issues, little research directly examining vegetarian diets and athletic performance is available. There have been mixed results regarding hypertrophic potential when comparing vegetarian diets with omnivore diets during resistive exercise training; however, in all cases these differences did not translate to differential strength gains at the completion of the trials [21–24]. Adoption of a lacto-ovo vegetarian (LOV) diet for six weeks did not significantly affect endurance performance among a group of trained, male endurance athletes, in spite of a decrease in total testosterone while on the vegetarian diet [25]. There were also no group differences between 20 participants adopting an LOV diet compared to maintaining their usual omnivorous diet in terms of muscle buffering capacity in conjunction with sprint training for five weeks [26]. These studies provide some insight into the effect of a vegetarian diet on athletic performance. However, a considerable limitation in many of these studies is the inclusion of participants who typically consume meat but subsequently adopt a vegetarian diet only for the duration of the study rather than comparing participants who have adhered to a vegetarian or meat-containing diet long-term.

In a 1986 observational trial, Hanne and colleagues compared athletes who had maintained either an LOV or omnivore diet for at least two years and found no group differences for aerobic or anaerobic capacity [27]. However, aerobic capacity was estimated using cycle ergometry and predicted VO2 max, and strength or torque were not measured. Moreover, body adiposity was estimated using skinfold thickness. Given the current interest in vegetarian diets, in terms of both long-term health and environmental benefits, it is important to reaffirm, using leading-edge technology, that high-level athletic performance is supported by these diets.

The purpose of the present cross-sectional study was to examine body composition and performance measures in vegetarian and omnivore adult endurance athletes who had adhered to their respective diet plans for at least three months. Body composition, including visceral adiposity, was measured using dual-energy X-ray absorptiometry (DXA), leg strength was measured using a dynamometer, and aerobic capacity was determined using the Bruce protocol treadmill test. It was hypothesized that there would be no differences between groups on any parameters.

2. Materials and Methods

2.1. Participant Recruitment

Healthy men and women, both vegetarians and omnivores, were recruited through advertisements on Stevebay.org (a popular website for endurance athletes), Facebook, and through word of mouth. Participants were either on a competitive club sports team at a National Collegiate Athletic Association (NCAA) Division 1 university or training for a major endurance race (such as a marathon, triathlon, cycling race, or other ultra-endurance event). An equal number of omnivore and vegetarian athletes were enrolled in the study between the ages of 21–58 years (35 per group); however, answers to diet questions indicated that eight of the vegetarians ate meat on occasion, and these subjects were reclassified as omnivores. Participants completed a health history questionnaire and were excluded if they had any chronic disease. All participants had the study verbally explained to them and provided their written consent; this study was approved by the Institutional Review Board at Arizona State University, number HS1211008557. Study recruitment and all study measurements took place between August and November 2015.

2.2. Experimental Approach

In this cross-sectional investigation participants completed all study measurements in a single visit. Prior to the visit, participants completed a seven-day food log. Fifty-seven out of seventy participants returned completed food logs, all of which were used in dietary analysis using Food Processor SQL Nutrition and Fitness Software by ESHA Research, Inc. (version 10.11.0, Salem, OR, USA). Height and body mass were measured using a SECA directprint 284 digital measuring station when participants were wearing light clothing and no shoes. Participants also completed a full-body DXA scan (Lunar iDXA, General Electric Company, East Cleavland, OH, USA), which was conducted by a certified radiology technologist.

Maximal oxygen uptake was determined by following the Bruce protocol [28] on a Trackmaster TMX425C treadmill using the Parvo Medics TrueOne 2400 (Sandy, UT, USA) metabolic measurement system. Prior to beginning the test, participants were instructed how to report their fatigue level using the Borg rating of perceived exertion (RPE) scale [29]. When asked by a research assistant, they reported their RPE at the end of each minute of the test by pointing to a printed Borg RPE chart being held by a research assistant. Participants were verbally encouraged by the research team to push as long as they could and to try to reach a true maximal effort. Handrail support was not allowed during the test. Maximal respiratory exchange ratio (RER) was recorded to help determine whether subjects had reached a "true" maximal effort during the test. Maximal RER values of ≥ 1.1 were considered indicative of true maximal oxygen uptake [30,31]. Peak oxygen uptake reported is the highest oxygen uptake measured during the test.

Finally, participants completed a series of leg extensions and flexions on the HumacNorm isokinetic dynamometer (Computer Sports Medicine Inc. (CSMi, Stoughton, MA, USA) at 60 degrees per second (d/s), 180 d/s, and 240 d/s. Participants were familiarized with the protocol and conducted one practice repetition at each speed prior to performing three maximal effort repetitions at each speed. All sets, including practice repetitions, were performed on both legs, and self-reported dominant side was recorded. Participants moved from the VO2 max test immediately into the dynamometer testing, and there were 30 s of rest between sets on the dynamometer.

2.3. Statistical Analyses

Based on the data of Hanne et al. [27], at 80% power and an alpha level of 5%, 15 participants per group would be needed to detect a 10% difference in strength and 80 participants per group would be needed to detect a 10% change in aerobic capacity between groups. Data were analyzed for normality and log transformed if necessary, and outliers (values > 3 standard deviations (SD) from the mean) were removed prior to data analyses. Data reported are the mean $\pm$ SD, and participant characteristics are displayed by gender and diet group. A 2-way analysis of variance (ANOVA) analysis was used to determine differences between diet groups for participant characteristics followed by an independent *t*-test for post-hoc examination by diet within gender if indicated. Dietary data are reported by group, and a general linear model analysis was used to examine differences between groups controlling for gender. Data were analyzed using the Statistical Package for Social Sciences (SPSS) 23.0 for Mac (SPSS, Inc., Chicago, IL, USA).

3. Results

In the vegetarian group, 24 of the 27 participants (89%) had adhered to a vegetarian diet for >2 years. Of the remaining three participants, the diet had been followed for three, six, or eleven months. Fifteen of the vegetarians were vegans (nine men and six women), and twelve were lacto-ovo vegetarians (five men and seven women).

There were no significant age or gender differences between groups (Table 1). Significant differences were noted between diet groups for body mass and for lean body mass (LBM): female vegetarians tended to have a lower total body mass and LBM compared to the female omnivores (-11% and -7% respectively). Adiposity, however, did not differ between diet groups. Physical activity levels, recorded as kcal·kg^{-1}·week^{-1}, were 20% higher for vegetarians compared to omnivores ($p = 0.018$) (Table 1). Maximal oxygen uptake (mL/kg/min) differed significantly between diet groups, and post-hoc analyses revealed a significantly greater aerobic capacity in the female vegetarians in comparison to the female omnivores ($+13\%$, $p < 0.05$) (Table 1); however, absolute maximal oxygen uptake (L/min) did not differ between diet groups. Peak torque when doing leg extensions was not different between diet groups. The 7-day diet records revealed several differences in nutrient intake between diet groups. Although total energy intakes were similar between the diet groups, the vegetarians consumed more carbohydrate, fiber, and iron daily compared to omnivores (Table 2). However, daily intakes for protein, saturated fat, cholesterol, vitamin B12, and selenium were lower among the vegetarians in comparison to the omnivores.

Table 1. Participant characteristics by diet group (vegetarian, VEG; omnivorous, OMN) [1].

	VEG		OMN		p
Measure	Male (14)	Female (13)	Male (26)	Female (17)	
Age, year	36.1 ± 10.2	36.7 ± 7.7	38.0 ± 10.0	37.1 ± 8.7	0.608
Body mass, kg	73.3 ± 14.8	58.3 ± 7.6 **	78.0 ± 11.0	65.4 ± 11.6	**0.043**
BMI, kg/m^2	24.0 ± 4.4	21.8 ± 2.5	24.8 ± 2.6	23.5 ± 3.8	0.123
Lean mass, kg	56.3 ± 7.4	42.0 ± 4.9 **	60.2 ± 7.3	45.4 ± 5.1	**0.026**
Waist, cm	81.6 ± 10.7	69.0 ± 14.8	85.2 ± 7.4	73.8 ± 8.2	0.093
Body fat, %	19.2 ± 6.5	25.5 ± 4.2	19.2 ± 6.4	26.9 ± 8.1	0.659
Visceral fat, cm^3	447.4 ± 419.8	110.4 ± 123.0	538.5 ± 404.3	206.4 ± 254.6	0.656
METS, kcal·kg^{-1}·week^{-1}	108.8 ± 32.9	106.1 ± 36.6 **	91.7 ± 33.2	85.6 ± 20.8	**0.018**
VO2 max, mL/kg/min	62.6 ± 15.4	53.0 ± 6.9 *	55.7 ± 8.4	47.1 ± 8.6	**0.011**
VO2 max, L/min	4.44 ± 0.81	3.21 ± 0.67	4.29 ± 0.59	3.03 ± 0.49	0.295
Peak torque, ft-lbs	114.4 ± 26.2	65.5 ± 12.8	124.2 ± 24.5	73.6 ± 18.6	0.104

[1] Data are the mean $\pm$ SD; n in parentheses; gender distribution did not differ by diet group ($p = 0.460$; Chi Square analysis). p for 2-way ANOVA analyses by diet (non-normal data transformed prior to analysis (visceral fat)). The single asterisk (*) indicates significant difference within gender by diet group ($p < 0.05$); the double asterisk (**) indicates a trend for difference within gender by diet group ($0.05 < p < 0.10$).

Table 2. Nutrient differences by diet group (vegetarian, VEG; omnivorous, OMN) [1].

	VEG (22)	OMN (35)	p	Reference Range [2]
Total kilocalories (kcal)	2443 ± 535	2266 ± 612	0.072	-
Carbohydrate (CHO) (g)	328 ± 70	248 ± 101	**0.001**	-
CHO (% energy)	53 ± 6	48 ± 7	**0.010**	45%–65%
Fiber (g)	38 ± 13	24 ± 9	**<0.001**	38/25 g [M/F]
Protein (g)	78 ± 19	101 ± 35	**0.006**	-
Protein (% energy)	12 ± 2	17 ± 4	**<0.001**	10%–35%
Protein (g/kg body mass)	1.2 ± 0.3	1.4 ± 0.5	0.220	0.8 g/kg
Fat (g)	90 ± 26	83 ± 33	0.901	-
Fat (% energy)	32 ± 5	32 ± 6	0.952	20%–35%
Saturated fat (g)	22.8 ± 11.2	25.7 ± 10.1	0.207	-
Saturated fat (% energy)	8.3 ± 3.1	11.6 ± 6.3	**0.002**	<10%
Cholesterol (mg)	102.8 ± 119.5	301.2 ± 165.6	**<0.001**	-
Vitamin C (mg)	117.0 ± 64.0	83.0 ± 46.5	0.076	90/75 mg [M/F]
Vitamin D (IU)	115.4 ± 111.4	129.0 ± 115.5	0.201	600 IU
Vitamin B12 (mcg)	3.0 ± 3	4.8 ± 4.6	**0.006**	2.4 mcg
Selenium (mcg)	41.8 ± 36.0	62.6 ± 33.6	**0.002**	55 mcg
Sodium (mg)	2931.2 ± 783.1	2972.8 ± 887.5	0.794	<2300 mg
Iron (mg)	19.4 ± 7.8	15.4 ± 5.4	**0.017**	8/18 mg [M/F]
Zinc (mg)	8.5 ± 9.1	8.9 ± 4.9	0.149	11/8 mg [M/F]
Calcium (mg)	971.0 ± 401.6	878.1 ± 314.9	0.378	1000 mg
Phosphorus (mg)	782.0 ± 378.0	831.2 ± 336.4	0.507	700 mg
Omega-3 fatty acid (g)	1.6 ± 2.5	0.9 ± 0.7	0.326	-
Omega-3 fatty acid (% energy)	0.004 ± 0.005	0.004 ± 0.003	0.613	0.6%–1.2%
Omega-6 fatty acid (g)	7.7 ± 5.4	6.1 ± 4.4	0.145	-
Omega-6 fatty acid (% energy)	2.8 ± 1.6	2.4 ± 1.3	0.358	5%–10%

[1] Data are the mean $\pm$ SD; sample size in parentheses. p for general linear model analyses (non-normal data transformed prior to analysis (all variables except carbohydrate variables and fat percentage) and 2 outliers (VEG group) removed prior to analysis for saturated fat); [2] Reference ranges are the Recommended Dietary Allowance or the Acceptable Macronutrient Distribution Range; note the American College of Sports Medicine recommends that athletes consume 1.2–2.0 g protein/kg body mass.

4. Discussion

Results from this study indicate that compared to their omnivore counterparts, vegetarian endurance athletes have comparable strength as indicated by leg extension peak torque, and possibly a greater degree of aerobic capacity, particularly in females, as indicted by a progressive maximal treadmill test to exhaustion. Dietary intake on several key nutrients differed considerably between groups. Some, but not all, results are consistent with previous reports.

Our study is significant for its increased rigor in measurement assessments compared to previous comparisons of vegetarian and omnivore athletes. We determined maximal oxygen uptake by a graded test to exhaustion on a treadmill instead of predicting VO2 max using a cycle ergometer, as recommended by Shepard and colleagues [32]. Additionally, we measured body composition using a DXA scan, currently regarded as the clinical gold standard for body composition assessment, instead of skinfolds [33]. Finally, we assessed both athletic performance and nutrient intake differences between vegetarians and omnivores, whereas most previously published studies focus exclusively on one of these areas.

4.1. Body Mass and BMI

Like other studies of vegetarians in the general population, vegetarian participants in the present study had significantly lower body mass compared to omnivores [10,34]. This is in spite of the fact that our study included participants engaged in considerable endurance activities, which could be very different in multiple ways from the general population. One prior study in athletes, conducted by Hanne et al. compared vegetarians and omnivores anthropometrically and found no significant differences between groups for weight [27]. It is noteworthy that the athletes in the Hanne et al. study included football, basketball, and water polo players in addition to endurance athletes.

4.2. Lean Body Mass

LBM was significantly lower for the vegetarian athletes compared to their omnivore counterparts, a difference which was most prominent among the female participants with female vegetarian athletes possessing 7% less LBM as compared to the female omnivore athletes. In spite of this, there were no significant differences in body fat percentage or BMI between groups. To our knowledge, this is the first study to examine lean body mass differences between vegetarian and omnivore athletes. It is important to note, however, that this difference in lean body mass did not translate into differential peak torque on the leg extension.

Although other studies have not assessed lean body mass of vegetarian athletes specifically, Campbell and colleagues compared resistance-training induced changes in lean body mass and strength between groups assigned to either an omnivorous diet or a lacto-ovo-vegetarian diet for the duration of the study and found that, in spite of differential lean body mass gains, the two groups increased strength similarly [21]. Conversely, a 12-week training study by Haub and colleagues showed no significant differences in strength, body composition, or muscle cross-sectional area between groups assigned to either a lacto-ovo-vegetarian or beef-containing diet.

4.3. Body Fat Percent and Visceral Adipose Tissue (VAT)

Contrary to the female vegetarian athletes in Hanne's group, no significant differences in body fat percentage were found between vegetarian and omnivore athletes in this study. Additionally, there were no significant differences between groups for visceral adipose tissue (VAT). Participants in the present study had VAT values above those reported for similar aged healthy lean sedentary adults (~250 cm^3), both omnivores and vegetarians [35,36], but lower than those noted for older adults (1000–1560 cm^3) [37]. Although there are no standard reference ranges for VAT, values near 1000 cm^3 were associated with BMI values near 25 kg/m^2 and values > 300 cm^3 have been suggested as predictive of risk for metabolic syndrome in young adults [36,37]. As technology permitting quantification of visceral adipose tissue is relatively new for research purposes, this study contributes to the emerging literature by providing VAT values for athletes. VAT and BMI is strongly correlated in this study ($p = 0.742$), a factor that may be important for estimating VAT inexpensively without a DXA scan.

4.4. VO2 Max

Unlike athletes in Hanne's study, vegetarians in the present study had significantly higher maximal oxygen uptake than their omnivore counterparts [27]. This difference was most predominant in the female participants with a 13% greater VO2 max score for the female vegetarians as compared to the female omnivores, but this difference was not observed for absolute VO2 max (L/min), which suggests that body weight factored into this difference. This gender difference is intriguing and merits further investigation in future studies. One potential reason that athletes in the present study had higher VO2 max values than those in Hanne's study may be due to the difference between cycle ergometry and treadmill testing methods. However, it is possible that the athletes in our study simply were more trained and that diet effects on differences in VO2 potential emerge only at higher levels of fitness.

Other work that contributes to our understanding of aerobic and anaerobic performance differences by diet include the study of Hietavala et al. that found no significant difference in time to exhaustion (albeit a higher oxygen uptake at a given percent of maximal oxygen consumption) between participants following a low-protein vegetarian diet compared to a mixed diet [38]. Subjects in this study adhered to the low protein vegetarian diet (0.80 ± 0.11 g of protein per kilogram of body mass (g/kg) vs. 1.59 ± 0.28 g/kg on their normal diet) for four days before being tested on a cycle ergometer. As this study did not use participants who practiced vegetarianism outside of the study, and the amount of protein that subjects were allowed to consume on the vegetarian diet was restricted, true differences between vegetarians and omnivores may not be evident. Baguet et al. found no differences in repeated sprint ability between participants following a vegetarian or mixed diet for five weeks; again, these subjects were not following a vegetarian diet long-term [26]. Raben et al. found no differences in maximal oxygen uptake among subjects after adoption of a lacto-ovo vegetarian diet for six weeks [25]. However, the major disadvantage of interpreting results of these studies for vegetarian athletes is that participants in these studies only adhered to a vegetarian diet briefly for the duration of the study.

4.5. Peak Torque

Similar to the Hanne et al. study that compared the power output of vegetarian and omnivore athletes [27], we found no significant differences by diet in terms of peak torque using leg extensions. Other studies in untrained older men that have examined strength development over time in response to a training program have found mixed results when comparing participants following a vegetarian or mixed diet [21,24]. This is noteworthy, particularly since strength and lean body mass were strongly correlated ($r = 0.764$) in the present study, as well as the fact that omnivores had significantly more lean body mass vs. the vegetarians. A nonsignificant trend for omnivores to produce higher peak torque is observed, however. It is conceivable that the omnivore diet pattern may be preferred for sports that rely on greater lean mass, and subsequently peak torque. To further investigate this, future work ought to examine if strength can be increased similarly by vegetarian and omnivore athletes engaged in strength training (not just by participants following a vegetarian diet for a few weeks).

4.6. Nutrient Intake

Nutrient intake was calculated from food and beverage intakes only and did not include any supplements. There were no significant differences in caloric intake or total fat intake between vegetarians and omnivores. However, vegetarians reported significantly more dietary carbohydrate (both in terms of absolute intake and as a percent of daily calories), fiber, and iron intake.

Omnivores consumed more dietary protein (both in terms of absolute intake and as a percent of daily calories), saturated fat, cholesterol, and vitamin B12. However, when expressed relative to body mass, there were no differences in dietary protein intake.

That vegetarians and omnivores in the present study did not differ in terms of caloric intake is consistent with findings by Janelle and Barr from their comparison of 45 vegetarian and omnivore women [16], yet it is in contrast to results from Calkins and colleagues who compared 50 vegetarian, vegan, and omnivores. They found vegetarians consumed about 200 fewer kcal than omnivores [19]. These studies were both in the general population, not specifically with athletes. Calkins et al. also reported that omnivores consumed more fat than vegetarians, a fact that partially contributed to the higher caloric intake. This too is in contrast to the findings in the present study which found no significant difference either in grams of fat consumed or the percent contribution of fat to the daily calorie intake, even though saturated fat was significantly higher in omnivorous diets. Other studies involving the general population have also reported omnivores eating more energy and total fat than vegetarians [10,39–41].

Higher carbohydrate (when expressed either as an absolute amount or as a percent of total daily calories) and fiber intake among vegetarians in comparison to omnivores in the present study is consistent with findings in other studies [10,39,41–44]. As these studies have been conducted in the general population, the present study contributes to the literature by demonstrating that this dietary pattern can be extended to endurance athletes as well. One study by Janelle and Barr stands in contrast to these findings, as they did not find significant differences in carbohydrate or fiber intake between vegetarian and omnivore women; those participants were not athletes [16]. That vegetarians in the present study consumed more carbohydrates than omnivores is notable since they are all athletes, and the importance of carbohydrates for exercise is well-established [45–47].

Like the present study, other studies have also reported that vegetarians consume less protein (both absolute intake and as a percent of the daily calories) [10,16,39,42] and vitamin B12 [40,48] than omnivores. Our study contributes to the literature since other reports have been in the general population instead of within athletic groups. Of note, though, differences in dietary protein intake are not significant when expressed relative to body mass, which is typically the preferred method for recommending protein for athletes [47]. Nonetheless, dietary protein intake was weakly correlated with peak torque ($r = 0.359$, $p = 0.006$) in the present study, and dietary protein intake was moderately correlated with lean body mass ($r = 0.415$, $p = 0.001$). Expectantly, lean body mass was strongly correlated with peak torque ($r = 0.764$, $p < 0.001$). Hence, it is conceivable that protein intake could influence strength if intakes had been inadequate. In the present evaluation, protein intakes in the vegetarian participants averaged 1.2 g/kg body mass, which falls in the recommended range for athletes [47,49].

There are conflicting findings in the rest of the literature regarding whether omnivores or vegetarians consume more iron. The Wilson et al. study of vegetarian men found that vegetarians consumed more iron [41], but Ball and Bartlett reported no difference in dietary iron intake between female vegetarian and omnivores [50]. Clary et al. compared 1475 vegans, vegetarians, semi-vegetarians, pescetarians, and omnivores and also showed that vegetarians consume more iron than omnivores [39]. Although vegetarians consumed more iron than omnivores in the present study, iron bioavailability was likely reduced as has been shown in other trials [17]. Dietary intakes of zinc did not vary by diet group herein, but generally the literature suggests that vegetarians consume somewhat less dietary zinc than omnivores [16,51–53]. The lower intakes of selenium by vegetarians in comparison to omnivores has also been reported by others and reflects the low levels of selenium in plant foods relative to flesh foods [54,55].

4.7. Limitations

In addition to the small sample size, limitations to the study include the variable level of experience of the athletes for their respective sports, and related fitness levels. Although most participants were training for and competing in races such as marathons, Ironman-distance triathlons, and competitive cycling, there were a few participants who were training for shorter distance races. However, this variation makes results more generalizable to athletes of various fitness levels.

4.8. Future Directions

Future work is needed to compare vegetarian and omnivore endurance athletes' performance on events more similar to actual sporting events (such as time trials or peak power on a cycle ergometer) and probe differences by type of vegetarian diet (lacto-ovo vegetarian or vegan). Additional work is needed to explore the adequacy of long-term adherence to vegetarian and vegan diets for supporting development of lean body mass.

5. Conclusions

Our cross-sectional comparison of vegetarian and omnivore adult endurance athletes shows higher maximal oxygen uptake values among vegetarians and comparable strength, in spite of anthropometric and dietary differences. This study suggests that following a vegetarian diet may adequately support strength and cardiorespiratory fitness development, and may even be advantageous for supporting cardiorespiratory fitness. Certainly many factors affect an athlete's sports performance, and there is no dietary substitute for quality training. However, our study contributes to the literature about cardiorespiratory and strength comparisons between vegetarian and omnivore endurance athletes, and may provide a rationale about the adequacy of vegetarian diets for sport performance. As this was a small cross-sectional study using endurance athletes, larger intervention trials are necessary to bolster conclusions about adequacy of vegetarian diets to support performance in strength and power-focused sports.

Acknowledgments: This study was supported by a grant through the Graduate and Professional Student Association (GPSA) at Arizona State University.

Author Contributions: H.M.L. and C.S.J. conceived and designed the experiments; H.M.L. performed the experiments; H.M.L. and C.S.J. analyzed the data; H.M.L., C.S.J., and C.M.W. wrote the paper.

Conflicts of Interest: The authors declare no conflict of interest. The funding sponsor had no role in the design of the study; in the collection, analyses, or interpretation of data; in the writing of the manuscript, and in the decision to publish the results.

References

1. Fraser, G. A comparison of first event coronary heart disease rates in two contrasting California populations. *J. Nutr. Health Aging* **2004**, *9*, 53–58.
2. Catsburg, C.; Kim, R.S.; Kirsh, V.A.; Soskolne, C.L.; Kreiger, N.; Rohan, T.E. Dietary patterns and breast cancer risk: A study in 2 cohorts. *Am. J. Clin. Nutr.* **2015**, *101*, 817–823. [CrossRef] [PubMed]
3. Orlich, M.J.; Singh, P.N.; Sabaté, J.; Fan, J.; Sveen, L.; Bennett, H.; Knutsen, S.F.; Beeson, W.L.; Jaceldo-Siegl, K.; Butler, T.L.; et al. Vegetarian dietary patterns and the risk of colorectal cancers. *JAMA Int. Med.* **2015**, *175*, 767–776. [CrossRef] [PubMed]
4. Tantamango-Bartley, Y.; Knutsen, S.F.; Knutsen, R.; Jacobsen, B.K.; Fan, J.; Beeson, W.L.; Sabate, J.; Hadley, D.; Jaceldo-Siegl, K.; Penniecook, J.; et al. Are strict vegetarians protected against prostate cancer? *Am. J. Clin. Nutr.* **2016**, *103*, 153–160. [CrossRef] [PubMed]
5. Kahleova, H.; Pelikanova, T. Vegetarian Diets in the Prevention and Treatment of Type 2 Diabetes. *J. Am. Coll. Nutr.* **2015**, *34*, 448–458. [CrossRef] [PubMed]
6. Kim, M.-H.; Bae, Y.-J. Comparative Study of Serum Leptin and Insulin Resistance Levels Between Korean Postmenopausal Vegetarian and Non-vegetarian Women. *Clin. Nutr. Res.* **2015**, *4*, 175–181. [CrossRef] [PubMed]
7. Yokoyama, Y.; Nishimura, K.; Barnard, N.D.; Takegami, M.; Watanabe, M.; Sekikawa, A.; Okamura, T.; Miyamoto, Y. Vegetarian diets and blood pressure: A meta-analysis. *JAMA Int. Med.* **2014**, *174*, 577–587. [CrossRef] [PubMed]

8. Appleby, P.N.; Allen, N.E.; Key, T.J. Diet, vegetarianism, and cataract risk. *Am. J. Clin. Nutr.* **2011**, *93*, 1128–1135. [CrossRef] [PubMed]
9. Giem, P.; Beeson, W.L.; Fraser, G.E. The incidence of dementia and intake of animal products: Preliminary findings from the Adventist Health Study. *Neuroepidemiology* **1993**, *12*, 28–36. [CrossRef] [PubMed]
10. Spencer, E.A.; Appleby, P.N.; Davey, G.K.; Key, T.J. Diet and body mass index in 38000 EPIC-Oxford meat-eaters, fish-eaters, vegetarians and vegans. *Int. J. Obes.* **2003**, *27*, 728–734. [CrossRef] [PubMed]
11. Quiles, L.; Portolés, O.; Sorlí, J.V.; Corella, D. Short Term Effects on Lipid Profile and Glycaemia of a Low-Fat Vegetarian Diet. *Nutr. Hosp.* **2014**, *32*, 156–164.
12. Pimentel, D.; Pimentel, M. Sustainability of meat-based and plant-based diets and the environment. *Am. J. Clin. Nutr.* **2003**, *78*, 660S–663S. [PubMed]
13. Monsivais, P.; Scarborough, P.; Lloyd, T.; Mizdrak, A.; Luben, R.; Mulligan, A.A.; Wareham, N.J.; Woodcock, J. Greater accordance with the Dietary Approaches to Stop Hypertension dietary pattern is associated with lower diet-related greenhouse gas production but higher dietary costs in the United Kingdom. *Am. J. Clin. Nutr.* **2015**, *102*, 138–145. [CrossRef] [PubMed]
14. Masset, G.; Vieux, F.; Verger, E.O.; Soler, L.-G.; Touazi, D.; Darmon, N. Reducing energy intake and energy density for a sustainable diet: A study based on self-selected diets in French adults. *Am. J. Clin. Nutr.* **2014**, *99*, 1460–1469. [CrossRef] [PubMed]
15. Delanghe, J.; De Slypere, J.P.; De Buyzere, M.; Robbrecht, J.; Wieme, R.; Vermeulen, A. Normal reference values for creatine, creatinine, and carnitine are lower in vegetarians. *Clin. Chem.* **1989**, *35*, 1802–1803. [PubMed]
16. Janelle, K.C.; Barr, S.I. Nutrient intakes and eating behavior see of vegetarian and nonvegetarian women. *J. Am. Diet. Assoc.* **1995**, *95*, 180–189. [CrossRef]
17. Hunt, J.R. Bioavailability of iron, zinc, and other trace minerals from vegetarian diets. *Am. J. Clin. Nutr.* **2003**, *78*, 633S–639S. [PubMed]
18. Rauma, A.-L.; Mykkänen, H. Antioxidant status in vegetarians versus omnivores. *Nutrition* **2000**, *16*, 111–119. [CrossRef]
19. Calkins, B.M.; Whittaker, D.J.; Nair, P.P.; Rider, A.A.; Turjman, N. Diet, nutrition intake, and metabolism in populations at high and low risk for colon cancer. Nutrient intake. *Am. J. Clin. Nutr.* **1984**, *40*, 896–905. [PubMed]
20. Nieman, D. Vegetarian dietary practices and endurance performance. *Am. J. Clin. Nutr.* **1988**, *48*, 754–761. [PubMed]
21. Campbell, W.W.; Barton, M.L., Jr.; Cyr-Campbell, D.; Davey, S.L.; Beard, J.L.; Parise, G.; Evans, W.J. Effects of an omnivorous diet compared with a lactoovovegetarian diet on resistance-training-induced changes in body composition and skeletal muscle in older men. *Am. J. Clin. Nutr.* **1999**, *70*, 1032–1039. [PubMed]
22. Haub, M.D.; Wells, A.M.; Tarnopolsky, M.A.; Campbell, W.W. Effect of protein source on resistive-training-induced changes in body composition and muscle size in older men. *Am. J. Clin. Nutr.* **2002**, *76*, 511–517. [PubMed]
23. Wells, A.M.; Haub, M.D.; Fluckey, J.; Williams, D.K.; Chernoff, R.; Campbell, W.W. Comparisons of vegetarian and beef-containing diets on hematological indexes and iron stores during a period of resistive training in older men. *J. Am. Diet. Assoc.* **2003**, *103*, 594–601. [CrossRef] [PubMed]
24. Haub, M.D.; Wells, A.M.; Campbell, W.W. Beef and soy-based food supplements differentially affect serum lipoprotein-lipid profiles because of changes in carbohydrate intake and novel nutrient intake ratios in older men who resistive-train. *Metabolism* **2005**, *54*, 769–774. [CrossRef] [PubMed]
25. Raben, A.; Kiens, B.; Richter, E.A.; Rasmussen, L.B.; Svenstrup, B.; Micic, S.; Bennett, P. Serum sex hormones and endurance performance after a lacto-ovo vegetarian and a mixed diet. *Med. Sci. Sports Exerc.* **1992**, *24*, 1290–1297. [CrossRef] [PubMed]
26. Baguet, A.; Everaert, I.; De Naeyer, H.; Reyngoudt, H.; Stegen, S.; Beeckman, S.; Achten, E.; Vanhee, L.; Volkaert, A.; Petrovic, M.; et al. Effects of sprint training combined with vegetarian or mixed diet on muscle carnosine content and buffering capacity. *Eur. J. Appl. Physiol.* **2011**, *111*, 2571–2580. [CrossRef] [PubMed]
27. Hanne, N.; Dlin, R.; Nrotstein, A. Physical fitness, anthropometric and metabolic parameters in vegetarian athletes. *J. Sports Med. Phys. Fit.* **1986**, *26*, 180–185.

28. Bruce, R.A.; Blackmon, J.R.; Jones, J.W.; Strait, G. Exercising testing in adult normal subjects and cardiac patients. *Pediatrics* **1963**, *32*, 742–756. [CrossRef] [PubMed]

29. Borg, G. *Borg's Perceived Exertion and Pain Scales*; Human Kinetics: Champaign, IL, USA, 1998.

30. Wier, L.T.; Jackson, A.S.; Ayers, G.W.; Arenare, B. Nonexercise models for estimating VO2 max with waist girth, percent fat, or BMI. *Med. Sci. Sports Exerc.* **2006**, *38*, 555–561. [CrossRef] [PubMed]

31. Astorino, T.A.; Robergs, R.A.; Ghiasvand, F.; Marks, D.; Burns, S. Incidence of the oxygen plateau at VO2 max during exercise testing to volitional fatigue. *Methods* **2000**, *3*, 1–12.

32. Shephard, R.J.; Allen, C.; Benade, A.J.S.; Davies, C.T.M.; di Prampero, P.E.; Hedman, R.; Merriman, J.E.; Myhre, K.; Simmons, R. The maximum oxygen intake: An international reference standard of cardio-respiratory fitness. *Bull. World Health Organ.* **1968**, *38*, 757. [PubMed]

33. Andreoli, A.; Garaci, F.; Cafarelli, F.P.; Guglielmi, G. Body composition in clinical practice. *Eur. J. Radiol.* **2016**, *85*, 1461–1468. [CrossRef] [PubMed]

34. Berkow, S.E.; Barnard, N. Vegetarian diets and weight status. *Nutr. Rev.* **2006**, *64*, 175–188. [CrossRef] [PubMed]

35. Knurick, J.R.; Johnston, C.S.; Wherry, S.J.; Aguayo, I. Comparison of correlates of bone mineral density in individuals adhering to lacto-ovo, vegan, or omnivore diets: A cross-sectional investigation. *Nutrients* **2015**, *7*, 3416–3426. [CrossRef] [PubMed]

36. Miazgowski, T.; Krzyżanowska-Świniarska, B.; Dziwura-Ogonowska, J.; Widecka, K. The associations between cardiometabolic risk factors and visceral fat measured by a new dual-energy X-ray absorptiometry-derived method in lean healthy Caucasian women. *Endocrine* **2014**, *47*, 500–505. [CrossRef] [PubMed]

37. Lin, H.; Yan, H.; Rao, S.; Xia, M.; Zhou, Q.; Xu, H.; Rothney, M.P.; Xia, Y.; Wacker, W.K.; Ergun, D.L.; et al. Quantification of visceral adipose tissue using lunar dual-energy X-ray absorptiometry in Asian Chinese. *Obesity* **2013**, *21*, 2112–2117. [CrossRef] [PubMed]

38. Hietavala, E.-M.; Puurtinen, R.; Kainulainen, H.; Mero, A.A. Low-protein vegetarian diet does not have a short-term effect on blood acid–base status but raises oxygen consumption during submaximal cycling. *J. Int. Soc. Sports Nutr.* **2012**, *9*, 50. [CrossRef] [PubMed]

39. Clarys, P.; Deliens, T.; Huybrechts, I.; Deriemaeker, P.; Vanaelst, B.; De Keyzer, W.; Hebbelinck, M.; Mullie, P. Comparison of nutritional quality of the vegan, vegetarian, semi-vegetarian, pesco-vegetarian and omnivorous diet. *Nutrients* **2014**, *6*, 1318–1332. [CrossRef] [PubMed]

40. Alexander, D.; Ball, M.; Mann, J. Nutrient intake and haematological status of vegetarians and age-sex matched omnivores. *Eur. J. Clin. Nutr.* **1994**, *48*, 538–546. [PubMed]

41. Wilson, A.; Ball, M. Nutrient intake and iron status of Australian male vegetarians. *Eur. J. Clin. Nutr.* **1999**, *53*, 189–194. [CrossRef] [PubMed]

42. Key, T.J.; Davey, G.K.; Appleby, P.N. Health benefits of a vegetarian diet. *Proc. Nutr. Soc.* **1999**, *58*, 271–275. [CrossRef] [PubMed]

43. Kennedy, E.T.; Bowman, S.A.; Spence, J.T.; Freedman, M.; King, J. Popular diets: Correlation to health, nutrition, and obesity. *J. Acad. Nutr. Diet.* **2001**, *101*, 411. [CrossRef]

44. Hardinge, M.G.; Chambers, A.C.; Crooks, H.; Stare, F.J. Nutritional studies of vegetarians III. Dietary levels of fiber. *Am. J. Clin. Nutr.* **1958**, *6*, 523–525. [PubMed]

45. Costill, D.; Miller, J. Nutrition for endurance sport: Carbohydrate and fluid balance. *Int. J. Sports Med.* **1980**, *1*, 2–14. [CrossRef]

46. Rodriguez, N.R.; DiMarco, N.M.; Langley, S. Position of the American dietetic association, dietitians of Canada, and the American college of sports medicine: Nutrition and athletic performance. *J. Am. Diet. Assoc.* **2009**, *109*, 509–527. [PubMed]

47. Thomas, D.T.; Erdman, K.A.; Burke, L.M. Position of the academy of nutrition and dietetics, dietitians of canada, and the american college of sports medicine: Nutrition and athletic performance. *J. Acad. Nutr. Diet.* **2016**, *116*, 501–528. [CrossRef] [PubMed]

48. Antony, A.C. Vegetarianism and vitamin B-12 (cobalamin) deficiency. *Am. J. Clin. Nutr.* **2003**, *78*, 3–6. [PubMed]

49. Phillips, S.M.; Van Loon, L.J. Dietary protein for athletes: From requirements to optimum adaptation. *J. Sports Sci.* **2011**, *29* (Suppl. 1), S29–S38. [CrossRef] [PubMed]

50. Ball, M.J.; Bartlett, M.A. Dietary intake and iron status of Australian vegetarian women. *Am. J. Clin. Nutr.* **1999**, *70*, 353–358. [PubMed]

51. Freeland-Graves, J.H.; Bodzy, P.W.; Eppright, M.A. Zinc status of vegetarians. *J. Am. Diet. Assoc.* **1980**, *77*, 655–661. [PubMed]

52. Anderson, B.M.; Gibson, R.S.; Sabry, J.H. The iron and zinc status of long-term vegetarian women. *Am. J. Clin. Nutr.* **1981**, *34*, 1042–1048. [PubMed]

53. Gibson, R.S. Content and bioavailability of trace elements in vegetarian diets. *Am. J. Clin. Nutr.* **1994**, *59*, 1223S–1232S. [PubMed]

54. Larsson, C.L.; Johansson, G.K. Dietary intake and nutritional status of young vegans and omnivores in Sweden. *Am. J. Clin. Nutr.* **2002**, *76*, 100–106. [PubMed]

55. Letsiou, S.; Nomikos, T.; Panagiotakos, D.; Pergantis, S.A.; Fragopoulou, E.; Antonopoulou, S.; Pitsavos, C.; Stefanadis, C. Dietary habits of Greek adults and serum total selenium concentration: The ATTICA study. *Eur. J. Nutr.* **2010**, *49*, 465–472. [CrossRef] [PubMed]

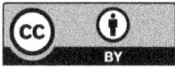

nutrients

MDPI

Article

An Exploratory Investigation of Endotoxin Levels in Novice Long Distance Triathletes, and the Effects of a Multi-Strain Probiotic/Prebiotic, Antioxidant Intervention

Justin D. Roberts [1],*, Craig A. Suckling [1], Georgia Y. Peedle [1], Joseph A. Murphy [2], Tony G. Dawkins [3] and Michael G. Roberts [2]

[1] Department of Life Sciences, Faculty of Science and Technology, Anglia Ruskin University, Cambridge Campus, Cambridge CB1 1PT, UK; craig.suckling@pgr.anglia.ac.uk (C.A.S.); georgia.peedle@student.anglia.ac.uk (G.Y.P.)
[2] College Lane, School of Life and Medical Sciences, University of Hertfordshire, Hatfield, Hertfordshire AL10 9AB, UK; jamurphy123@gmail.com (J.A.M.); m.g.roberts@herts.ac.uk (M.G.R.)
[3] Cardiff School of Sport, Cardiff Metropolitan University, Cyncoed Campus, Cyncoed Road, Cardiff CF23 6XD, UK; tdawkins@cardiffmet.ac.uk
*   Correspondence: justin.roberts@anglia.ac.uk; Tel.: +44-845-196-5154

Received: 22 August 2016; Accepted: 15 November 2016; Published: 17 November 2016

Abstract: Gastrointestinal (GI) ischemia during exercise is associated with luminal permeability and increased systemic lipopolysaccharides (LPS). This study aimed to assess the impact of a multistrain pro/prebiotic/antioxidant intervention on endotoxin unit levels and GI permeability in recreational athletes. Thirty healthy participants (25 males, 5 females) were randomly assigned either a multistrain pro/prebiotic/antioxidant (LAB^4$_{ANTI}$; 30 billion CFU·day^{-1} containing 10 billion CFU·day^{-1} *Lactobacillus acidophilus* CUL-60 (NCIMB 30157), 10 billion CFU·day^{-1} *Lactobacillus acidophillus* CUL-21 (NCIMB 30156), 9.5 billion CFU·day^{-1} *Bifidobacterium bifidum* CUL-20 (NCIMB 30172) and 0.5 billion CFU·day^{-1} *Bifidobacterium animalis* subspecies *lactis* CUL-34 (NCIMB 30153)/55.8 mg·day^{-1} fructooligosaccharides/ 400 mg·day^{-1} α-lipoic acid, 600 mg·day^{-1} *N*-acetyl-carnitine); matched pro/prebiotic (LAB^4) or placebo (PL) for 12 weeks preceding a long-distance triathlon. Plasma endotoxin units (via *Limulus* amebocyte lysate chromogenic quantification) and GI permeability (via 5 h urinary lactulose (L): mannitol (M) recovery) were assessed at baseline, pre-race and six days post-race. Endotoxin unit levels were not significantly different between groups at baseline (LAB^4$_{ANTI}$: 8.20 ± 1.60 pg·mL^{-1}; LAB^4: 8.92 ± 1.20 pg·mL^{-1}; PL: 9.72 ± 2.42 pg·mL^{-1}). The use of a 12-week LAB^4$_{ANTI}$ intervention significantly reduced endotoxin units both pre-race (4.37 ± 0.51 pg·mL^{-1}) and six days post-race (5.18 ± 0.57 pg·mL^{-1}; $p = 0.03$, $\eta p^2 = 0.35$), but only six days post-race with LAB^4 (5.01 ± 0.28 pg·mL^{-1}; $p = 0.01$, $\eta p^2 = 0.43$). In contrast, endotoxin units remained unchanged with PL. L:M significantly increased from 0.01 ± 0.01 at baseline to 0.06 ± 0.01 with PL only ($p = 0.004$, $\eta p^2 = 0.51$). Mean race times (h:min:s) were not statistically different between groups despite faster times with both pro/prebiotoic groups (LAB^4$_{ANTI}$: 13:17:07 ± 0:34:48; LAB^4: 12:47:13 ± 0:25:06; PL: 14:12:51 ± 0:29:54; $p > 0.05$). Combined multistrain pro/prebiotic use may reduce endotoxin unit levels, with LAB^4$_{ANTI}$ potentially conferring an additive effect via combined GI modulation and antioxidant protection.

Keywords: endotoxemia; probiotics; prebiotics; antioxidants; triathlon

1. Introduction

Participation trends, including "recreational athletes", in multi-sport and ultra-endurance events have increased in recent years [1,2]. Symptoms associated with gastrointestinal (GI) distress (e.g., cramping, diarrhoea, nausea, and abdominal pain) are estimated to occur in 25%–90% of endurance athletes, and are often cited as reasons for non-completion [3–5]. In preparation for such events, exercise-related GI symptoms may go unreported, which could impact on training efficiency and race completion. It has been shown that exercise induced GI hypoperfusion may provoke transient damage to the gut epithelium [6], with one study demonstrating that 30 min of running at 80% of peak oxygen uptake (VO_2peak) significantly increased luminal permeability in healthy volunteers [7].

Mechanistically, prolonged or strenuous exercise may increase key phosphorylation enzymes [8], disrupting the tight junction proteins claudin (influenced by protein kinase A) and occludin (influenced by both protein kinase C and tyrosine kinase). Acute changes in tight junction permeability and paracellular transport may lead to a greater prevalence of systemic lipopolysaccharides (LPS). LPS from gram-negative intestinal bacteria may provoke immune responses and endotoxin-associated symptoms characteristic of GI complaints often experienced in runners [8]. Despite this, research is relatively sparse on whether prolonged training or ultra-endurance events actually result in elevated LPS, particularly in more "recreationally active" athletes; or whether targeted nutrition strategies offer beneficial support.

In one study, 68% of highly trained athletes taking part in a long-distance triathlon reported with endotoxin levels of 5–15 $pg \cdot mL^{-1}$ in the first 16 h post-event, corresponding with elevated cytokine responses in the same period [9]. In contrast, 81% of runners requiring medical attention at the end of an ultra-marathon were found to have LPS concentrations >100 $pg \cdot mL^{-1}$ [10], with 80.6% of these athletes reporting GI symptoms (nausea, diarrhoea, and vomiting). LPS concentrations at or above these levels have been more commonly associated in patients with Crohn's disease [11] and sepsis [12].

The term "mild endotoxemia" has been used to depict an acute elevation in LPS from endurance exercise by several authors [9,13,14], but may well reflect normal or transient levels of circulatory LPS. It has also been shown that LPS responses to exertional heat stress may be significantly higher in less trained individuals [13], but still within normal limits. Conversely, one study reported an average increase in resting LPS levels of 60 $pg \cdot mL^{-1}$ across a five-stage ultra-run, with daily (pre–post stage) average LPS changes of 30 $pg \cdot mL^{-1}$ [15]. Despite such diversity, the potential for exercise related endotoxin-mediated cytokinemia may explain individual susceptibility to GI symptoms and recovery from endurance exercise. If prevalent, the presence of, and repeated exposure to, "low grade" LPS (ranging from ~10 to 50 $pg \cdot mL^{-1}$ or higher [16]) may promote a mild inflammatory state which could be detrimental to the longer term health of recreational athletes who regularly engage in exercise.

Probiotic bacteria, particularly the gram-positive genera *Lactobacillus* and *Bifidobacterium* species, are known to modify GI microbiota [17–19], and have been shown to reduce GI episode severity [20] and respiratory tract infections commonly associated with training [21]. However, therapeutic benefits of probiotics are highly strain specific. As example, the use of *Lactobacillus casei* strain Shirota in one study, significantly increased natural killer cell cytolytic activity in healthy volunteers [22], whereas combined *Streptococcus thermophilus* FP4/*Bifidobacterium breve* BR03 was recently shown to reduce circulating IL-6 in response to muscle damaging exercise [23] elsewhere. In clinical trials, a multistrain high dose probiotic (LAB⁴—containing *Lactobacillus acidophilus* CUL60 and CUL21, *Bifidobacterium lactis* CUL34 and *Bifidobacterium bifidum* CUL20), resulted in significant improvements in irritable bowel syndrome responses [24] and prevented an increase in antibiotic resistant enterococci [25]. Chronic multistrain interventions have also been shown to reduce faecal zonulin levels by ~25% in endurance trained athletes, demonstrating improved GI barrier integrity [26]. The inclusion of *Bifidobacterium species* and prebiotics (e.g., fructo-oligosaccharides, inulin, pectin) in such formulas may also play an important role in short-chain fatty acid production, which may also support epithelial integrity [27].

Antioxidants nutrients such as α-lipoic acid, *N*-acetyl-carnitine, vitamin C, quercetin, resveratrol, and curcumin may also provide important roles in minimizing epithelial disruption [28–31], associated with elevated oxidative stress from GI hypoperfusion. Alpha lipoic acid in particular is proposed to act as a multi-functional antioxidant, regenerating endogenous glutathione, and minimising GI mucosal injury [31–33]. The aims of this exploratory study were therefore: (i) to assess endotoxin levels and GI permeability in recreational athletes training for and taking part in their first long distance triathlon; and (ii) to assess the potential benefits of a 12-week multistrain pro/prebiotic/antioxidant strategy on GI symptoms, endotoxin levels and race time compared to a control group.

2. Materials and Methods

2.1. Participants

Following study approval from the University of Hertfordshire Life and Medical Sciences Ethics Committee (LMS/SF/UH/00011), and power calculation assessment for sample size (G*power3, Dusseldorf [34]; using $\alpha = 0.05$; $1 - \beta = 0.80$; based on observed data [9,14]), thirty recreationally active participants (25 males, 5 females; M $\pm$ SE: age 35 ± 1 years; weight: 76.52 ± 2.20 kg; initial VO$_2$max: 48.93 ± 0.99 mL·kg^{-1}·min^{-1}) were randomly invited to take part in an intervention study which took place in the final 12 weeks of a nine month progressive training programme. All participants provided written, informed consent, and satisfactorily completed a general health screen prior to study inclusion. Participant characteristics are displayed in Table 1, with no observed differences between intervention groups for age, height, weight, bodyfat or VO$_2$max.

Table 1. Pre-screening (Month 0) and baseline (Month 6) characteristics for intervention groups.

Variable	LAB^{4}ANTI		LAB^4		PL	
Distribution	(*n* = 10; 7 male, 3 female)		(*n* = 10; 9 male, 1 female)		(*n* = 10; 9 male, 1 female)	
Age (years)	33 $\pm$ 2		35 $\pm$ 2		35 $\pm$ 3	
Height (m)	1.74 $\pm$ 0.34		1.79 $\pm$ 0.27		1.76 $\pm$ 0.16	
	Pre-screening	Baseline	Pre-screening	Baseline	Pre-screening	Baseline
Weight (kg)	75.21 $\pm$ 4.12	73.61 $\pm$ 3.96 *	83.77 $\pm$ 4.71	81.94 $\pm$ 4.44 *	77.42 $\pm$ 3.03	74.56 $\pm$ 2.76
Body fat (%)	22.56 $\pm$ 1.67	19.36 $\pm$ 2.23 *	21.88 $\pm$ 1.68	20.93 $\pm$ 1.52	21.28 $\pm$ 2.38	18.64 $\pm$ 1.93 *
VO$_2$max (L·min^{-1})	3.26 $\pm$ 0.20	3.57 $\pm$ 0.19 *	3.78 $\pm$ 0.28	3.94 $\pm$ 0.27	3.30 $\pm$ 0.14	3.70 $\pm$ 0.10 *
VO$_2$max (mL·kg^{-1}·min^{-1})	42.90 $\pm$ 1.59	48.60 $\pm$ 1.80 *	43.89 $\pm$ 1.75	47.56 $\pm$ 1.69 *	43.40 $\pm$ 2.53	50.50 $\pm$ 1.71 *

Data presented as mean $\pm$ SE No significant differences reported between groups. * denotes significant difference ($p < 0.05$) to pre-screening only within group.

Pre-screening: At the start of the nine month training programme, all participants underwent full screening including suitability assessment from their General Practitioner, a 12-lead electrocardiogram to assess for potential underlying cardiac abnormalities, and completion of a standard incremental maximal stress test (using a Computrainer erogometer system, RaceMate Inc., Seattle, WC, USA) for the assessment of maximal oxygen consumption (using a Metalyser 3B automated gas-analyser; Cortex Biophysik, Leipzig, Germany). In addition, routine assessment of height (Seca 200 stadiometer, Hamburg, Germany), body mass (Seca 780, Hamburg, Germany) and body composition (Tanita Body Segmental Analyser 418-BC, Tokyo, Japan) was undertaken. Participants were required to have no previous experience of long distance triathlons, be recreationally active (defined as general exercise activity 1–3 times per week) and have basic proficiency in swimming, cycling and running disciplines. As a means to further quantify "recreationally active", participants were required to have a relative maximum oxygen uptake of 30–50 mL·kg^{-1}·min^{-1} for women, and 35–55 mL·kg^{-1}·min^{-1} for men during pre-screening testing. Participants were excluded if there was any history (including familial) of cardiovascular abnormalities (including coronary heart disease) and diabetes; or any known blood related disorders.

2.2. Experimental Design and Procedures

In a randomized, repeated-measures, double-blind, placebo controlled study design, participants attended the Human Physiology Laboratory, University of Hertfordshire 12 weeks prior to undertaking a long distance triathlon (Barcelona Challenge Triathlon) comprising a 3.8 km sea swim, 180.0 km road cycle course and a 42.2 km marathon run. Although participants had no prior experience to this triathlon distance, they had all adhered to a standardized training programme for the previous six months as part of a larger training cohort. General training progression ("recreationally trained") from the previous six months was assessed prior to the intervention study using the same incremental test procedure and equipment (including anthropometrical measures) as for pre-screening (see Table 1). Thereafter, participants attended the laboratory on three occasions: baseline (Week 0), pre-race (Week 12) and post-race (six days post) for blood and urine sampling as described below. Due to constraints with field based sampling, and varying participant travel arrangements, the post-race timepoint (six days) was selected for consistency and to assess whether any previous patterns were still evident during the longer term recovery period.

Blood sampling: Participants were requested to rest the day before all test sessions. Upon arrival, a fasted, venous wholeblood sample was collected from participants by a qualified phlebotomist into duplicate 4 mL K_3EDTA vacutainers (Greiner Bio-One GmbH, Kremsmunster, Austria). Samples were centrifuged for 10 min at 3000 rpm, with aliquotted plasma pipetted into sterile, nonpyrogenic, polypropylene cyrovials (Fisherbrand, Fisher Scientific, Loughborough, UK) and immediately frozen at $-80\,^\circ$C for later assessment of resting endotoxin units and IgG endotoxin-core antibodies.

Urine sampling: Assessment of GI permeability was assessed via 5 h recovery of urinary lactulose and mannitol via a standard sugar absorption test [35]. Briefly, upon arrival, participants provided a urine sample with total volume assessed, and then (following blood sampling) consumed a standardized 100 mL test drink containing 5 g lactulose solution (Sandoz Ltd., Camberley, Surrey, UK), 2 g mannitol (Mannitol powder: 99.86% pure certified, Blackburn Distributions Ltd., Nelson, Lancashire, UK) and 40 g of sucrose (Tate and Lyle, London, UK). For the first two hours post consumption, participants were not allowed to eat or drink, and thereafter could eat/ drink as normal (with the exception of refined/sugary products or drinks). Over a five hour period, participants collected total urine output into 3 L polyethylene opaque beakers (Sarstedt, Numbrecht, Germany). With total sample volume assessed, duplicate urine samples were aliquotted into sterile cryovials and immediately frozen at $-80\,^\circ$C for later assessment of saccharide recovery.

2.3. Biochemical Assays

Endotoxin unit assessment: Quantification of endotoxin units was derived from plasma samples using an established endpoint chromogenic assay method (Pierce® LAL Chromogenic Endotoxin Quantitation Kit, Thermo Fisher Scientific, Waltham, MA, US). After thawing to room temperature and sample preparation, 50 µL aliquots were added to an endotoxin-free microtitre plate and incubated at 37 °C for 5 min. Following this, 50 µL aliquots of *Limulus* amoebocyte lysate (LAL) were added to each well, the plate gently shaken for 10 s, and re-incubated at 37 °C for 10 min. At exactly 10 min, 100 µL aliquots of chromogenic substrate solution was added to each well, the plate gently shaken for 10 s, and then further re-incubated at 37 °C for 6 min. At this point, 50 µL aliquots of stop reagent (25% acetic acid) was added to each well, and the plate gently shaken for 10 s. Samples were read on a spectrophotometer at an absorbance of 405 nm (Victor 3 multilabel plate reader, PerkinElmer Inc., Llantrisant, UK) and referenced against a calibration curve based on dilutions of an *Escherichia coli* (*E. coli*) endotoxin standard (011:B4; vial concentration 26 EU·mL^{-1}) with non-incubated mock reaction controls taken into consideration. Values of quantified endotoxin units (EU·mL^{-1}) were then converted to pg·mL^{-1}.

IgG Endotoxin-core Antibody Assessment: IgG endotoxin-core antibodies (IgG anti-EU) were measured from plasma samples via solid-phase ELISA (EndoCab® IgG, Hycult Biotech, Uden, The Netherlands). Reagents were prepared in accordance with the manufacturer's instructions at room temperature. Plasma samples were thawed to room temperature and diluted 200-fold using the supplied dilution buffer. Following this, 100 µL aliquots of the standard or prepared sample were carefully pipetted into microtitre wells coated with endotoxin rough-lipopolysaccharides, the microtitre plate then covered and incubated at 37 °C for 60 min. The plate was then washed four times manually, with 200 µL of supplied washer buffer added to each microtitre well during each wash cycle. Following this, 100 µL of diluted conjugate (streptavidin-peroxidase) was added to each well to bind the captured endotoxin core-antibodies. The plate was then covered and incubated at 37 °C for 60 min, before being manually washed a further four times with washer buffer. Then, 100 µL aliquots of tetramethylbenzidine (TMB) were added to each microtitre well, the plate covered and incubated at room temperature for 30 min avoiding exposure to sunlight. The reaction was then stopped by addition of 100 µL aliquots of oxalic acid to each well. Samples were read on a spectrophotometer at an absorbance of 450 nm (Victor 3 multilabel plate reader, PerkinElmer Inc., Llantrisant, UK) and referenced against a calibration curve (logarithmic scale) based on dilutions of a reconstituted human EndoCab IgG standard. Values are presented in standard median units ($MU \cdot mL^{-1}$).

GI Permeability Assessment: Following sample thawing and preparation, assessment of saccharide recovery was performed via enzymatic method assays for lactulose and mannitol using a Randox RX Monza semi-automated, flow cell based clinical chemistry analyser (Randox Ltd., Country Antrim, UK). Briefly, for lactulose, reagents were prepared in accordance with the manufacturer's instructions at room temperature (INstruchemie BV, Delfzil, Netherlands). Sample preparation involved 50 µL urine aliquots being mixed with 50 µL dissociation buffer and 5 µL galactosidase reagent, incubated at 37 °C overnight, and centrifuged at 2000 rpm for 5 min. Additionally, a non-incubated control was also prepared to account for NADPH already present in the sample. Thereafter, 200 µL of lactulose buffer reagent was carefully pipetted into centrifuge tubes and mixed with 5 µL sample, incubated at 37 °C for 5 min, and read at an absorbance of 340 nm (reading A1). Following this, 50 µL start reagent was added to the sample, mixed and incubated at 37 °C for 10 min and read at an absorbance of 340 nm (reading A2). Recovered lactulose ($mmol \cdot L^{-1}$) was calculated taking into consideration pre-incubated and non-incubated samples against standard, blank and quality control samples.

For mannitol assessment, reagents were prepared in accordance with the manufacturer's instructions at room temperature (INstruchemie BV, Delfzil, The Netherlands); and a reference curve generated from dilutions of a 20 $mmol \cdot L^{-1}$ mannitol standard. Samples were prepared by mixing 3 µL urine aliquots with 200 µL NAD buffer reagent and incubating at 37 °C for 5 min. From this 60 µL diluted start reagent was added to the sample, mixed and incubated for a further 37 °C for 10 min. Samples were read at an absorbance of 340 nm, and recovered mannitol ($mmol \cdot L^{-1}$) calculated against a standard reference taking into consideration blank and quality control samples.

2.4. Nutritional Interventions and Diaries

Nutritional interventions: Following baseline assessment, participants were allocated, in a double-blinded manner, to one of three intervention groups using a random number generator approach. Participants were provided with a 90-day supply of either: capsulated (hydroxypropyl methylcellulose) multistrain probiotic/prebiotic/antioxidant (LAB^4_{ANTI}), matched pro/prebiotic (LAB^4) or placebo (PL) in opaque, sealed pots with instructions for daily ingestion timing. This allocation covered the 12-week pre-race period and the six-day post-race period. Intervention supplementation was provided by Biocare Ltd. (Birmingham, UK) for commercial use, with products pre-capsulated by the manufacturer. Placebo supplements were prepared within our laboratory using the same size hydroxypropyl methylcellulose capsules.

For both LAB^4 and LAB^4_{ANTI}, participants were instructed to consume one multistrain pro/prebiotic capsule daily in the evening with food. Each multistrain capsule contained 150 $mg \cdot day^{-1}$ *Lactobacillus acidophilus* (10 billion $CFU \cdot day^{-1}$, *Lactobacillus acidophilus* CUL-60 [NCIMB 30157] and 10 billion $CFU \cdot day^{-1}$ *Lactobacillus acidophillus* CUL-21 [NCIMB 30156]), 16.8 $mg \cdot day^{-1}$ *Bifidobacterium bifidum* and *lactis* (9.5 billion $CFU \cdot day^{-1}$, *Bifidobacterium bifidum* CUL-20 [NCIMB

30172] and 0.5 billion CFU·day^{-1} *Bifidobacterium animalis subspecies lactis* CUL-34 [NCIMB 30153]), and 55.8 mg·day^{-1} fructooligosaccharides (Bio-Acidophilus Forte, Biocare Ltd., Birmingham, UK). For those assigned to PL, participants were instructed to consume one placebo capsule daily in the evening with food, containing 200 mg cornflour.

For LAB^4$_{ANTI}$, participants additionally consumed two capsules in the morning with breakfast (each capsule contained 200 mg α-lipoic-acid and 300 mg of *N*-acetyl-carnitine hydrochloride; Acetyl Carnitine and Alpha Lipoic Acid formulation, Biocare Ltd., Birmingham, UK). For control consistency between groups, those assigned to LAB^4 and PL were instructed to additionally consume matched cornflour placebo capsules with breakfast. Throughout the study, participants were required to not be consuming any other nutritional supplements other than glucose drinks/gels as part of endurance training. Adherence was checked via nutrition diaries and monthly briefings with all participants.

Nutrition diaries: Participants were requested to maintain habitual dietary intake throughout the intervention and record via weekly food diaries at the beginning and end of each month. Participants were provided with example diaries and individually instructed in diary completion, with emphasis on meal breakdown, portion size and weight, fluid intake and consumption of prescribed supplementation. Dietary analyses were undertaken using Dietplan 6.50 (Forestfield Software Ltd., West Sussex, UK) based on a seven-day representation from each month.

2.5. Training Monitoring, GI Questionnaires and Assessment of Race Times

Training programme: Over the course of the 12-week intervention, participants continued with a triathlon training programme, prescribed by an accredited Sport and Exercise Physiologist, focusing on swimming, cycling and running disciplines, as well as functional training. Training was designed to be flexible around daily activities with a requirement to achieve a minimum of 80% of the total training volume set. Training was monitored via weekly training diaries in which participants recorded exercise duration and overall session rating of perceived exertion (sRPE). Training load, training monotony and training strain were determined from a modified training method previously described (duration × sRPE [36,37]).

GI response questionnaire: Participants completed an overall monthly training GI response questionnaire, adapted from symptoms previously reported [4,9,38]. Participants were asked to subjectively rate their responses across four subsections (general training, endurance training (>3 h), acute (<24 h) and longer term (<72 h) recovery periods). For the training subsections the following symptoms were evaluated: urge to urinate, urge to defecate, bloating, belching, flatulence, nausea, stomach/intestinal pain or discomfort, stomach/intestinal cramping, headaches, and dizziness. For the recovery subsections, the following symptoms were evaluated: constipation and/or diarrhoea, stomach/intestinal pain or discomfort, bloating, flatulence, nausea, stomach/intestinal cramping, headaches, dizziness, mental fatigue, excessive and sweating. Collectively, this resulted in a maximum symptom count of 40. Symptoms were graded for severity according to a category scale (0 = none; 1 = low severity; 2 = moderate severity; 3 = high severity). From this, mean symptom count and symptom severity scores were assessed to evaluate the subjective impact of each intervention.

Race times: All participants, as entrants of the Barcelona Challenge Triathlon, were required to wear official timing chips throughout the race. Overall race times, including triathlon specific stage times (swim, bike, and run) were provided by the race director following confirmation of official final times.

2.6. Statistical Analyses

Statistical analyses were performed using SPSS (v22, IBM, Armonk, NY, USA). Following assessment of normality via a Shapiro–Wilk test, a 3 × 3 factorial design analysis of variance (Anova) was employed to assess treatment and time interactions, using least significant difference (LSD) post hoc evaluation. Where pertinent, within group assessment was undertaken using a general linear repeated measures Anova, with LSD post hoc evaluation. For assessment of race times between groups only, a between-group Anova was performed, with LSD post hoc analysis. GI questionnaires were assessed via chi-squared analysis. An alpha level of ≤ 0.05 was employed for statistical significance. Data are reported as means $\pm$ SE.

3. Results

3.1. Nutrition and Training Data

Dietary analysis comparisons for each month are shown in Table 2. No significant differences were reported between or within groups across the 12-week intervention period for energy, carbohydrate, fat or protein intake ($p > 0.05$). On average across the 12-week intervention, daily energy intake for LAB^4_{ANTI} was 35.10 ± 1.31 kcal·kg^{-1}·day^{-1} compared with 33.97 ± 1.73 kcal·kg^{-1}·day^{-1} for LAB^4 and 35.53 ± 1.66 kcal·kg^{-1}·day^{-1} for PL. Macronutrient intake was also comparable, with an average fat intake of 1.45 ± 0.08 g·kg^{-1}·day^{-1} for LAB^4_{ANTI} compared 1.27 ± 0.08 g·kg^{-1}·day^{-1} for LAB^4 and 1.30 ± 0.07 g·kg^{-1}·day^{-1} for PL. Likewise, average carbohydrate intake was 4.06 ± 0.22 g·kg^{-1}·day^{-1} for LAB^4_{ANTI} compared with 4.02 ± 0.24 g·kg^{-1}·day^{-1} for LAB^4 and 4.37 ± 0.31 g·kg^{-1}·day^{-1} for PL. Similarly, average protein intake was comparable between pro/prebiotic groups at 1.55 ± 0.07 g·kg^{-1}·day^{-1} for LAB^4_{ANTI}, 1.50 ± 0.11 g·kg^{-1}·day^{-1} for LAB^4, and non-significantly higher for PL at 1.72 ± 0.10 g·kg^{-1}·day^{-1}.

Table 2. Dietary analysis comparisons between groups.

Variable	LAB^4_{ANTI}	LAB^4	PL
Energy intake (kcal·kg^{-1}·day^{-1})			
T1	35.96 ± 2.16	33.13 ± 1.16	35.57 ± 2.88
T2	33.88 ± 2.06	33.03 ± 4.66	34.57 ± 2.98
T3	35.42 ± 2.57	35.76 ± 2.43	36.60 ± 2.85
Fat (g·kg^{-1}·day^{-1})			
T1	1.45 ± 0.13	1.28 ± 0.10	1.24 ± 0.14
T2	1.37 ± 0.12	1.27 ± 0.21	1.19 ± 0.08
T3	1.52 ± 0.18	1.26 ± 0.12	1.47 ± 0.11
Carbohydrate (g·kg^{-1}·day^{-1})			
T1	4.29 ± 0.33	3.80 ± 0.30	4.46 ± 0.47
T2	3.95 ± 0.43	3.90 ± 0.59	4.32 ± 0.58
T3	3.93 ± 0.39	4.36 ± 0.36	4.34 ± 0.57
Protein (g·kg^{-1}·day^{-1})			
T1	1.51 ± 0.12	1.43 ± 0.14	1.81 ± 0.18
T2	1.56 ± 0.07	1.39 ± 0.17	1.70 ± 0.14
T3	1.57 ± 0.15	1.68 ± 0.28	1.67 ± 0.19

Data represent average daily intake (mean $\pm$ SE). T1–3 represent Months 1–3 respectively. No significant differences reported between or within groups ($p > 0.05$).

Training load comparisons are shown in Table 3. No significant differences were reported between groups across the intervention for training load, monotony or strain ($p > 0.05$). There was, however, a significant time interaction effect for training load ($F = 16.30$, $p < 0.0001$, $\eta p^2 = 0.38$) and training strain ($F = 4.88$, $p = 0.011$, $\eta p^2 = 0.16$). The training programme was designed to progressively build over the 12 weeks, with a peak training load in Month 2, and an increased training strain in Month 3 leading to a final taper period prior to the race. The target range (particular for training load) represents the generic range set for all participants i.e., to meet a minimum of 80% training load.

Across the intervention, all groups satisfactorily met the minimum training load. Average training loads at Month 2 were all significantly higher than Months 1 and 3, as expected ($p < 0.0001$).

Interestingly, however, peak training loads at Month 2 were all greater than the high end target set at 3278 AU (arbitrary units). For LAB^4 in particular, training load was noted at 4311 ± 348 AU (F = 8.21, $p = 0.006$, $\eta p^2 = 0.58$ compared to Month 1), further reflecting the increased strain (4065 ± 381 AU) in this month (F = 6.79, $p = 0.011$, $\eta p^2 = 0.53$). Training strain in Month 3 was noted as being lower in all groups ($p = 0.003$) compared to Month 2 and in direct comparison to the target range.

Table 3. Training load comparisons.

Variable	Target Range	LAB^4_{ANTI}	LAB^4	PL
Weekly training load (AU)				
T1	2173–2716	2410 ± 242	2851 ± 279	2807 ± 368
T2	2622–3278	3885 ± 558 #	4311 ± 348 *#	3915 ± 516 #
T3	2231–2789	2232 ± 148	2768 ± 498	2263 ± 180
Training monotony (AU)				
T1	1.07–1.33	0.94 ± 0.11	0.98 ± 0.08	1.11 ± 0.08
T2	0.97–1.21	0.88 ± 0.07	0.96 ± 0.08	0.88 ± 0.08
T3	1.27–1.58	0.90 ± 0.12	0.87 ± 0.09	0.72 ± 0.05
Training strain (AU)				
T1	2951–3688	2755 ± 562	2945 ± 450	3224 ± 566
T2	3350–4187	3430 ± 620	4065 ± 381 *#	3293 ± 552
T3	3352–4440	2281 ± 370	2681 ± 650	1946 ± 186

Data represent arbitrary units (AU) and presented as mean $\pm$ SE Target range indicates 80%–100% of training programme. No significant differences reported between groups ($p > 0.05$). * denotes significant difference from T1 within group ($p \leq 0.006$). # denotes significant difference from T3 within group ($p \leq 0.04$).

3.2. Endotoxin Unit (EU) Assessment

Data for endotoxin units (EU) and IgG endotoxin-core antibody assessment are shown in Figure 1a–c for LAB^4_{ANTI}, LAB^4 and PL respectively. A significant interaction effect was reported for endotoxin units over time (F = 4.21, $p = 0.019$, $\eta p^2 = 0.11$) and group (F = 3.50, $p = 0.036$, $\eta p^2 = 0.09$) only. At baseline, whilst EU levels were highest with PL (9.72 ± 2.42 pg·mL^{-1}), no significance was found in comparison to either LAB^4_{ANTI} (8.20 ± 1.60 pg·mL^{-1}) or LAB^4 (8.92 ± 1.20 pg·mL^{-1}, $p > 0.05$). EU concentrations ranged from 3.03 to 27.75 pg·mL^{-1}. Within group, LAB^4_{ANTI} resulted in a significant reduction in endotoxin units both pre-race (4.37 ± 0.51 pg·mL^{-1}) and six days post-race (5.18 ± 0.57 pg·mL^{-1}; F = 4.27, $p = 0.033$, $\eta p^2 = 0.35$). For LAB^4, there was a significant reduction in endotoxin units over time (F = 6.04, $p = 0.011$, $\eta p^2 = 0.43$), with post-hoc analysis indicating EU levels of 5.01 ± 0.28 pg·mL^{-1} six days post-race being significantly lower than baseline ($p = 0.047$) only. Endotoxin unit levels for PL did not significantly differ across the intervention period or six days post-race ($p > 0.05$).

3.3. IgG Endotoxin-Core Antibody (Anti-EU) Assessment

Overall, a significant group interaction effect was reported for IgG anti-EU, with LAB^4_{ANTI} demonstrating lower concentrations of IgG endotoxin core-antibodies in comparison to both LAB^4 and PL (F = 10.82, $p < 0.0001$, $\eta p^2 = 0.25$) at baseline. Whilst IgG anti-EU levels remained significantly lower pre-race with LAB^4_{ANTI} compared to LAB^4 ($p = 0.003$), there was no statistical difference in comparison to PL. By post-race, no significant differences were reported between groups ($p > 0.05$). Within group, IgG anti-EU levels for LAB^4_{ANTI} increased from 40.42 ± 12.39 MU·mL^{-1} at baseline, to 58.83 ± 22.94 MU·mL^{-1} pre-race in contrast to the decrease in endotoxin unit levels observed. However, the overall increase in IgG anti-EU to 77.93 ± 26.03 MU·mL^{-1} post-race was not deemed significant (F = 1.01, $p = 0.387$, $\eta p^2 = 0.11$) overall.

For LAB^4, IgG anti-EU also increased from 209.23 ± 59.73 MU·mL^{-1} at baseline to 251.73 ± 60.72 MU·mL^{-1} pre-race in relative contrast to the decrease in endotoxin unit levels observed for this group. Post-race IgG anti-EU concentrations decreased to 161.61 ± 50.16 MU·mL^{-1}, but overall changes were not deemed statistically significant (F = 1.95, $p = 0.174$, $\eta p^2 = 0.20$) for LAB^4. In a converse manner, average plasma IgG anti-EU concentrations decreased from 223.98 ± 51.46 MU·mL^{-1} at baseline to 181.56 ± 58.19 MU·mL^{-1} pre-race with PL, returning to 207.94 ± 31.96 MU·mL^{-1} six days post-race; however, overall changes in IgG anti-EU for PL were not statistically significant ($F = 0.30$, $p = 0.746$, $\eta p^2 = 0.04$).

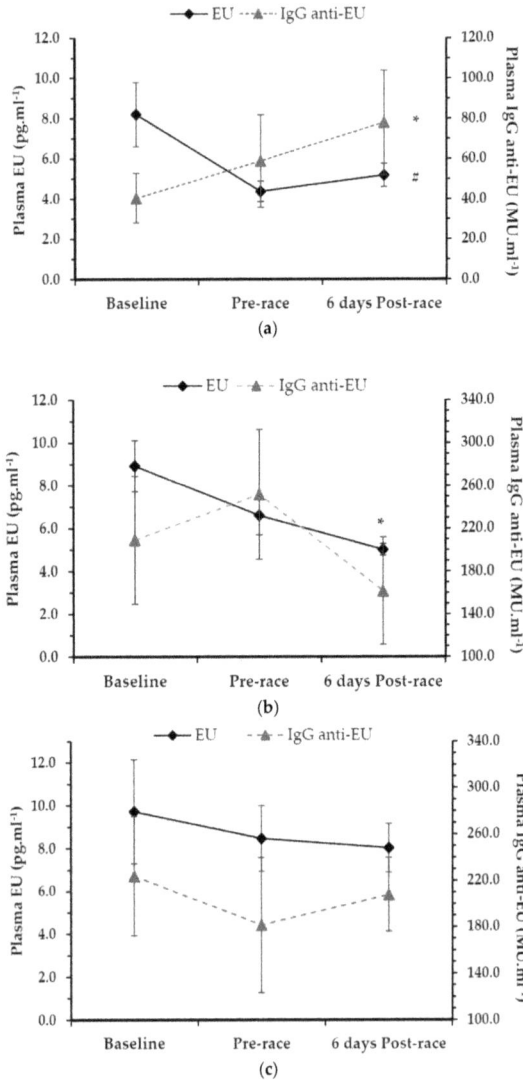

Figure 1. (**a**) Plasma endotoxin unit (EU) concentrations (pg·mL^{-1}) and IgG endotoxin antibodies (anti-EU; MU·mL^{-1}) for LAB^4$_{ANTI}$ group (Mean $\pm$ SE). * denotes lower IgG anti-EU values overall than both LAB^4 and PL conditions ($p < 0.001$); # denotes significant reduction in endotoxin units over time within group ($p = 0.03$); (**b**) Plasma endotoxin unit (EU) concentrations (pg·mL^{-1}) and IgG endotoxin antibodies (anti-EU; MU·mL^{-1}) for LAB^4 group (Mean $\pm$ SE). * denotes significant difference from baseline for endotoxin units within group ($p = 0.047$); (**c**) Plasma endotoxin unit (EU) concentrations (pg·mL^{-1}) and IgG endotoxin antibodies (anti-LPS; MU·mL^{-1}) for PL group (Mean $\pm$ SE). No significant differences reported ($p > 0.05$).

3.4. Intestinal Permeability

Assessment of intestinal permeability from urinary lactulose:mannitol (L:M) ratio measurement is shown in Figure 2. GI permeability generally increased in all groups from baseline to six days post-race (F = 9.66, $p < 0.0001$, $\eta p^2 = 0.21$). No significant differences were reported between groups ($p > 0.05$). Within group, L:M increased marginally from 0.032 ± 0.006 at baseline, to 0.037 ± 0.010 pre-race and 0.054 ± 0.007 six days post-race with LAB^4_{ANTI} ($p > 0.05$) Similarly, there was a non-significant increase in L:M with LAB^4 from 0.028 ± 0.005 at baseline, to 0.039 ± 0.007 and 0.044 ± 0.012 both pre- and six days post-race respectively ($p > 0.05$).

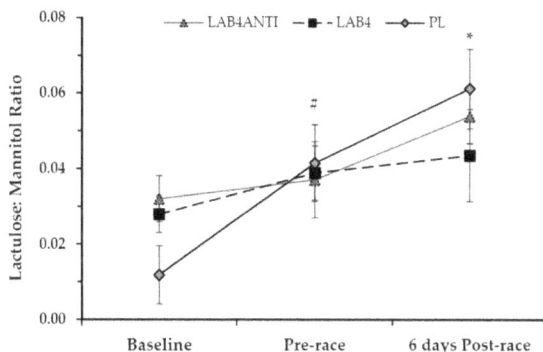

Figure 2. Assessment of intestinal permeability via urinary lactulose:mannitol ratio (Mean ± SE). Values measured in $mmol \cdot L^{-1}$. # denotes significant increase from baseline for PL only ($p = 0.05$); * denotes significant increase from baseline for PL only ($p = 0.002$).

However, for PL, L:M significantly increased over the intervention (F = 8.16, $p = 0.004$, $\eta p^2 = 0.51$) from 0.012 ± 0.008 at baseline to 0.041 ± 0.010 pre-race ($p \leq 0.05$). L:M further increased in PL to 0.061 ± 0.011 six days post-race ($p = 0.002$). A similar interaction effect for time was also observed with the per cent recovery of lactulose (F = 5.66, $p = 0.005$, $\eta p^2 = 0.14$), as shown in Table 4. Within group, for PL only, the per cent recovery of lactulose increased from $0.35\% \pm 0.18\%$ at baseline to $0.94\% \pm 0.12\%$ six days post-race ($p = 0.01$). No significant differences were found for per cent recovery of mannitol either between or within groups ($p > 0.05$).

Table 4. Recovery of urinary lactulose and mannitol (%).

Variable	LAB^4_{ANTI}	LAB^4	PL
% recovery of lactulose			
Baseline	0.71 ± 0.13	0.52 ± 0.07	0.35 ± 0.18
Pre-race	0.55 ± 0.14	0.74 ± 0.10	0.72 ± 0.17
6 days Post-race	0.83 ± 0.11	0.90 ± 0.24	0.94 ± 0.12 *
% recovery of mannitol			
Baseline	29.99 ± 2.87	25.57 ± 2.22	30.61 ± 3.96
Pre-race	23.31 ± 3.60	27.42 ± 3.33	23.51 ± 2.18
6 days Post-race	22.42 ± 3.27	25.01 ± 1.89	23.48 ± 2.64

Data presented as mean ± SE. * denotes significant difference to baseline within group only ($p = 0.01$).

3.5. GI Questionnaire

Overall symptom counts for training related GI issues were significantly lower in both LAB^4 groups at the end of Month 1 (7.80 ± 2.20 for LAB^4_{ANTI} and 6.78 ± 1.31 for LAB^4) compared with PL

(11.90 ± 2.02; $p \leq 0.013$). However, by Month 2, only symptom counts for LAB[4] were significantly lower (8.11 ± 2.18) than PL (13.20 ± 2.72; $p < 0.001$). At Month 2, there was a significant increase in symptom counts for LAB[4]ANTI (10.70 ± 2.88, $p = 0.015$ within group), which was also greater than LAB[4] ($p = 0.036$). By the end of the intervention, there was a similar pattern to Month 1, with both LAB[4] groups reporting lower symptom counts to training GI issues (8.80 ± 2.70 for LAB[4]ANTI and 7.00 ± 2.16 for LAB[4]) compared with PL (13.90 ± 2.42; $p < 0.001$).

Average symptom severity was significantly lower with both LAB[4] groups at Month 1 (9.80 ± 3.05 for LAB[4]ANTI and 7.56 ± 1.56 for LAB[4]) compared to PL (15.50 ± 2.97; $p < 0.001$). This pattern continued throughout the intervention, with severity scores for LAB[4] groups remaining lower than PL (16.70 ± 3.64) at Month 3 (10.10 ± 3.27 for LAB[4]ANTI and 8.00 ± 2.50 for LAB[4]; $p < 0.001$). No differences were reported for average symptom severity within group across the intervention ($p > 0.05$) or between LAB[4] groups ($p > 0.05$).

3.6. Race Times

Mean race finishing times are shown in Figure 3. Overall, no significant differences were found between groups for overall finishing times (F = 2.12, $p = 0.149$), despite faster completion times for both LAB[4]ANTI (13 h 17 min 07 s ± 34 min 48 s) and LAB[4] (12 h 47 min 13 s ± 25 min 06 s) compared with PL (14 h 12 min 51 s ± 29 min 54 s). Faster swim and cycle stage times were also recorded on average for LAB[4] (93.7 ± 4.4 min and 370.7 ± 10.4 min respectively) compared with both LAB[4]ANTI (99.8 ± 6.5 min and 392.5 ± 16.9 min) and PL (103.6 ± 9.9 min and 405.1 ± 14.3 min). However, average stage times were not significantly different between groups for either swim (F = 0.45, $p = 0.642$) or cycle (F = 2.30, $p = 0.129$) stages.

This was further reflected in the marathon stage, despite both LAB[4] groups completing the marathon course in similar times (285.8 ± 13.1 min for LAB[4]ANTI vs. 287.41 ± 16.04 min for LAB[4]) in contrast to PL (320.8 ± 21.1 min; F = 1.06, $p = 0.368$). It was however noted that despite a non-significant interaction effect, post-hoc comparisons indicated a significant difference for the bike stage between LAB[4] and PL groups only ($p = 0.046$), and a strong trend for a significant differences in overall finishing times between these two groups ($p = 0.058$).

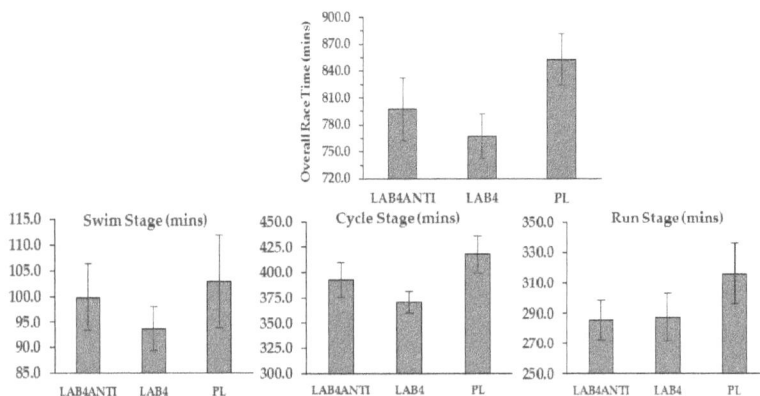

Figure 3. Race time comparisons in minutes (Mean ± SE), including triathlon stage disciplines. No significant differences reported between groups ($p > 0.05$). Converted overall times: LAB[4]ANTI = 13 h 17 min 07 s (±34 min 48 s); LAB[4] = 12 h 47 min 47 s (±25 min 31 s); PL= 14 h 01 min 40 s (±31 min 32 s).

4. Discussion

The concept of exercise-mediated endotoxemia remains contentious, with varying terminology reported in the literature, including methodologies used to assess endotoxin units. Whereas some authors have referred to the term "mild" endotoxemia to reflect relatively small changes in endotoxin levels (5–15 pg·mL^{-1}) along with acute cytokinemia following sustained endurance exercise [9], others have suggested that values ranging from 10 to 50 pg·mL^{-1} are indicative of normal, yet sustained "low grade" endotoxin levels which may modulate a systemic inflammatory response [13,16]. Clinical states of endotoxemia reflect much higher endotoxin concentrations (>80–300 pg·mL^{-1} [11,12]), with only a handful of studies demonstrating that strenuous ultra-endurance exercise actually elicits these levels at the point of exhaustion or during acute recovery [10,15]. Less is known whether repetitive GI provocation from repeated training elevates resting endotoxin levels, and what impact this may have on individuals preparing for, or recovering from, long distance events.

Average resting endotoxin units in the current study remained within normal limits (<10 pg·mL^{-1}), and were comparable to values observed (~11.0 $\pm$ 5.0 pg·mL^{-1}) for healthy volunteers with similar fitness levels [14,39,40]. This is in contrast to our hypothesis that plasma endotoxin units would be raised following repetitive endurance exercise as evidenced elsewhere [13,15]. However, the range for endotoxin units was 3.03–27.75 pg·mL^{-1}, indicating that if "low grade endotoxemia" does occur at values >10–50 pg·mL^{-1}, then some individuals may be susceptible to repeated exposure.

LPS translocation across the GI tract is known to provoke systemic immune reactions with varied consequences [41]. Specifically, LPS attachment to LPS-binding protein and its transference to an MD-2/toll-like receptor (TLR) 4/CD14 complex activates NF-kappa-B and various inflammatory modulators (TNF-α, IL-1β, IL-6 and CRP). This is considered a protective mechanism acting to minimise bacterial entry across the GI tract. Under normal physiological conditions, endotoxins from gram negative bacteria are usually contained locally, with only relatively small quantities entering the systemic circulation. However, when GI defences are either disrupted (i.e., luminal damage from exercise) or LPS "sensing" is "overloaded" a heightened inflammatory response may result which could, in part, relate to GI symptoms associated with exercise [42]. This could have implications to daily recovery mechanisms throughout prolonged training periods, and in the days following ultra-endurance events.

The use of a 12-week LAB^4 strategy reduced average endotoxin units by 26.0%, but was not statistically significant. In contrast, the LAB^4$_{ANTI}$ intervention resulted in a significant 46.6% reduction in endotoxin units, with pre-race levels in this group reducing to 4.37$\pm$ 0.51 pg·mL^{-1}. These levels are comparable to resting values observed in trained athletes elsewhere at ~3.8 $\pm$ 2.0 pg·mL^{-1} [13], and could have important implications for those individuals with previously raised endotoxin levels (e.g., >20 pg·mL^{-1}) or who are more susceptible to training related GI symptoms. Whilst the general trend in IgG anti-EU supported these findings, the inter-individual variability observed resulted in non-significant findings. It was noted that average IgG anti-EU levels for LAB^4$_{ANTI}$ were, however, significantly lower than both LAB^4 and PL. Although this possibly indicates an adaptive response in this group, IgG anti-EU ranges observed were comparable to those reported elsewhere [43] and most likely reflect variance in relation to individual gut microbiota profiles.

Altered GI permeability was only observed in the PL condition, which whilst not reaching clinical significance (i.e., L:M $\geq$ 0.09; [44,45]), represented a 4.2 fold increase over the intervention and recovery periods (compared to a 0.7 fold increase in the L:M ratio for LAB^4$_{ANTI}$ and 0.6 fold increase for LAB^4). Additionally, both GI symptom count and severity were significantly lower in both LAB^4 interventions compared with PL by the end of the training period, observations similar to those reported elsewhere employing probiotic strategies [21,46,47]. Collectively, these results support the contention that a multistrain pro/prebiotic intervention maintains tight junction stability, potentially through interference with phosphorylation processes. Although this supports previous findings [26,48], such strategies may only apply to chronic interventions, as recent research has demonstrated no impact of acute (7 days) probiotic use on endotoxin levels following endurance exercise at 60%VO_2max under ambient or heat-stressed conditions [49].

Studies have demonstrated that regular use of probiotics can improve epithelial resistance by establishing competitive "biofilm" activity. Indeed, as LPS types vary across gram-negative bacteria species, some LPS are poorly sensed by TLR4 and may have more direct impact on NF-κ-B activation [50]. Therefore, direct exclusion of LPS translocation through maintained epithelial integrity and/or increased preponderance of gram-positive genera may offer potential therapeutic benefit [51]. Specifically, the provision of *Lactobacillus* genus may work by activating TLR2 and hence more favourable innate immune responses [52–54]. Additionally the use of a 14 week multistrain probiotic strategy significantly decreased faecal zonulin levels elsewhere, supporting improved tight junction stability [26].

However, effects of probiotics are strain specific. The product used in the current study does not appear to have been used in a training context previously. Clinical trials, however, have demonstrated that the inclusion of the *Lactobacillus* strains CUL-60 and CUL-21 modulated the facultative anaerobes (*Enterobacteriaceae*, *Enteroccus/Streptococcus* and *Staphylococcus* species) during antibiotic therapy [24,55]. Two other papers utilizing similar dosages to the current study also indicate that the CUL-60 and CUL-21 strains prevented an increase in antibiotic resistant *Enterococci* and reduced the incidence of *Clostridium difficile* toxins [25,56]. Future research should address strain specific colonization and impact on gut microbiota, which may explain inter-individual differences particularly in athletes.

The inclusion of *Bifidobacterium* and prebiotics (e.g., inulin, galacto- or fructo-oligosaccharides [FOS]) in such formulas may also provide additional benefits. Studies have demonstrated a significant increase in short-chain fatty acids (SCFA), with prebiotic use additionally supporting increased *Bifidobacteria* growth, and decreased levels of bacteriodes and *Fermicutes* phyla [57–61]. Additionally, prebiotic use has been shown to improve mucosal dendritic cell function associated with TLR2 activity [62], and increase the expression of glucagon-like peptide 2, associated with GI barrier regulation [59]. Although low dose FOS was employed in the current study, the "synbiotic" effect with a multistrain probiotic formula has been shown to confer improvements in gastrointestinal well-being elsewhere [63].

In the current study, a combined antioxidant in conjunction with a multistrain pro/prebiotic strategy appeared to confer an additive effect through reduced endotoxin unit levels at the end of the 12-week training period, as well as six days post-race. Specifically, alpha lipoic acid acts as a multi-functional antioxidant through rapid regeneration of glutathione [64,65]. GI epithelial damage may be directly associated with oxidative stress from GI ischemia (particularly hydrogen peroxide), and in extreme cases may lead to ischemic colitis or infarct tissue [66]. Endogenous glutathione peroxidase may be a crucial enzyme in the protection of the intestinal lumen from repetitive damage [67]. Alpha lipoic acid, along with *N*-acetyl-carnitine, may therefore act in a local antioxidant manner, and via phosphoinositide 3-kinase/Akt signalling may down-regulate LPS stimulation of NF-κ-B [68–70]. Other dietary antioxidants such as ascorbic acid have been shown to blunt the endotoxin response to exercise, but with secondary effects on ascorbate radical production [28]. Various flavonoids (e.g., quercetin found in onions) and isoflavones (e.g., genistein found in soybeans) have been shown to inhibit protein kinase C and protein tyrosine kinases respectively, although the use of 2 g·day^{-1} quercetin for seven days was also shown to block the rise in heat shock protein 70, potentially restricting thermotolerant adaptation [71].

To date, only two studies appear to have assessed endotoxin levels in the hours/days following ultra-endurance events. Subclinical symptoms associated with exercise-mediated endotoxemia may vary in both severity and duration (possibly lasting several days). One study demonstrated raised (but effectively normal) endotoxin levels at 16 h following an ironman triathlon, but did not assess return to baseline levels [9]. A further study demonstrated that endotoxin levels had returned to baseline 1–3 weeks post event, reflecting the exhaustive nature of the event [10]. A limitation of the current study was the logistical difficulty of collecting samples immediately or 24 h post event. With varying individual travel plans, participants were instructed to rest in the 5 days post-race. At six days post-race, endotoxin units remained unchanged with PL (8.02 ± 1.14 pg·mL^{-1}), but were significantly lower for both intervention groups (5.18 ± 0.57 pg·mL^{-1} for LAB$^4_{ANTI}$, and 5.01 ± 0.28 pg·mL^{-1} for LAB^4). This represented an overall reduction in endotoxin units from baseline of 36.8% for LAB$^4_{ANTI}$ and 43.9% for LAB^4 strategies. Although cytokine profiles were not assessed in the current study, a general reduction in endotoxin levels via pro/prebiotic/antioxidant combinations may have important benefits in minimizing low grade cytokinemia from endurance exercise [72,73].

The use of LAB$^4_{ANTI}$ or LAB^4 did not significantly improve times within-race only in direct comparison to PL. This is despite a 6.5% (~56 min) faster overall time for LAB$^4_{ANTI}$ compared to PL, and 10.0% (~86 min) faster for LAB^4 compared to PL. This did not reflect our original hypothesis, and likely reflects the wider variance in capabilities observed with "recreationally trained" individuals. However, it was noted that faster times were reported for LAB^4 during both swim and cycle stages, with a trend towards an overall difference compared to PL ($p = 0.058$). It is acknowledged that exercise performance was not assessed in the current study as baseline measures could not be ascertained. As participants were entering their first long distance triathlon, comparison between groups only provided an insight into whether either intervention strategy offered potential race benefits. Future research should focus on whether combined pro/prebiotic/antioxidant strategies offer direct performance benefits in controlled settings, particularly in individuals more susceptible to GI related issues.

5. Conclusions

Chronic multistrain pro/prebiotic supplementation during periods of endurance training may provide individual support to minimise GI symptoms through maintenance of intestinal permeability. The inclusion of an antioxidant strategy (e.g., α-lipoic acid/N-acetyl carnitine) may confer additive benefits via reductions in training-related endotoxin unit levels. In a recreationally trained cohort, LAB$^4_{ANTI}$ or LAB^4 strategies did not influence race times in direct comparison to a control group also undertaking their first long distance triathlon. Combined pro/prebiotic/antioxidant strategies may have important implications for individuals undertaking endurance training, particularly those more susceptible to GI symptoms.

Acknowledgments: This study was supported by Biocare Ltd. (UK), with provision of nutritional products.

Author Contributions: J.D.R., C.A.S. and M.G.R. conceived and designed the study; all authors were involved with data collection; J.D.R., C.A.S., G.Y.P. and J.A.M. undertook assay analysis; J.D.R. and C.A.S. analysed the data; and J.D.R. wrote the paper. All authors reviewed the paper and approved the final version prior to submission.

Conflicts of Interest: The authors declare no conflict of interest.

References

1. Da Fonseca-Engelhardt, K.; Knechtle, B.; Rüst, C.A.; Knechtle, P.; Lepers, R.; Rosemann, T. Participation and performance trends in ultra-endurance running races under extreme conditions-'Spartathlon' versus 'Badwater'. *Extreme Physiol. Med.* **2013**, *2*, 15. [CrossRef] [PubMed]

2. Hoffman, M.D. Performance trends in 161-km ultramarathons. *Int. J. Sports Med.* **2010**, *31*, 31–37. [CrossRef] [PubMed]

3. De Oliveira, E.P.; Burini, R.C.; Jeukendrup, A. Gastrointestinal complaints during exercise: Prevalence, etiology, and nutritional recommendations. *Sports Med.* **2014**, *44* (Suppl. 1), S79–S85. [CrossRef] [PubMed]

4. Ten Haaf, D.S.M.; van der Worp, M.P.; Groenewould, H.M.M.; Leij-Halfwerk, S.; Nijhuis-van der Sanden, M.W.G.; Verbeek, A.L.M.; Staal, J.B. Nutritional indicators for gastrointestinal symptoms in female runners: The 'Marikenloop study'. *BMJ Open* **2014**, *4*, e005780. [CrossRef] [PubMed]

5. Stuempfle, K.; Hoffman, M.D. Gastrointestinal distress is common during a 161-km ultramarathon. *J. Sports Sci.* **2015**, *33*, 1814–1821. [CrossRef] [PubMed]

6. Van Wick, K.; Lenaerts, K.; van Loon, L.J.C.; Peters, W.H.M.; Buurman, W.A.; Dejong, C.H.C. Exercise-induced splanchnic hypoperfusion results in gut dysfunction in healthy men. *PLoS ONE* **2011**, *6*, e22366. [CrossRef] [PubMed]

7. Pals, K.L.; Ray-Tai, C.; Ryan, A.J.; Gisolfi, C.V. Effect of running intensity on intestinal permeability. *J. Appl. Physiol.* **1997**, *82*, 571–576. [PubMed]

8. Zuhl, M.; Schneider, S.; Lanphere, K.; Conn, C.; Dokladny, K.; Mosely, P. Exercise regulation of intestinal tight junction proteins. *Br. J. Sports Med.* **2014**, *48*, 980–986. [CrossRef] [PubMed]

9. Jeukendrup, A.E.; Vet-Joop, K.; Sturk, A.; Stegen, J.H.J.C.; Senden, J.; Saris, W.H.M.; Wagenmakers, A.J.M. Relationship between gastro-intestinal complaints and endotoxemia, cytokine release and the acute-phase reaction during and after a long-distance triathlon in highly trained men. *Clin. Sci.* **2000**, *98*, 47–55. [CrossRef] [PubMed]

10. Brock-Utne, J.G.; Gaffin, S.L.; Wells, M.T.; Gathiram, P.; Sohar, E.; James, M.F.; Morrell, D.F.; Norman, R.J. Endotoxemia in exhausted runners after a long-distance race. *S. Afr. Med. J.* **1988**, *73*, 533–536. [PubMed]

11. Guo, Y.; Zhou, G.; He, C.; Yang, W.; He, Z.; Liu, Z. Serum levels of lipopolysaccharide and 1,3-β-D-Glucan refer to the severity in patients with Crohn's disease. *Mediat. Inflamm.* **2015**, *2015*, 843089. [CrossRef] [PubMed]

12. Opal, S.M.; Scannon, P.J.; Vincent, J.-E.; White, M.; Carroll, S.F.; Palardy, J.E.; Parejo, N.A.; Pribble, J.P.; Lemke, J.H. Relationship between plasma levels of lipopolysaccharide (LPS) and LPS-binding protein in patients with severe sepsis and septic shock. *J. Infect. Dis.* **1999**, *180*, 1584–1589. [CrossRef] [PubMed]

13. Selkirk, G.A.; McLellan, T.M.; Wright, H.E.; Rhind, S.G. Mild endotoxemia, NF-κB translocation, and cytokine increase during exertional heat stress in trained and untrained individuals. *Am. J. Physiol. Regul. Integr. Comp. Physiol.* **2008**, *295*, R611–R623. [CrossRef] [PubMed]

14. Yeh, Y.J.; Law, L.Y.L.; Lim, C.L. Gastrointestinal response and endotoxemia during intense exercise in hot and cool environments. *Eur. J. Appl. Physiol.* **2013**, *113*, 1575–1583. [CrossRef] [PubMed]

15. Gill, S.K.; Teixeira, A.; Rama, L.; Rosado, F.; Hankey, J.; Scheer, V.; Hemmings, K.; Ansley-Robson, P.; Costa, R.J.S. Circulatory endotoxin concentration and cytokine profile in response to exertional-heat stress during a multi-stage ultra-marathon competition. *Exerc. Immunol. Rev.* **2015**, *21*, 114–128. [PubMed]

16. Maitra, U.; Deng, H.; Glaros, T.; Baker, B.; Capelluto, D.G.S.; Li, Z.; Li, L. Molecular mechanisms responsible for the selective low-grade induction of pro-inflammatory mediators in murine macrophages by lipopolysaccharide. *J. Immunol.* **2012**, *189*, 1014–1023. [CrossRef] [PubMed]

17. Tuohy, K.M.; Probert, H.M.; Smejkal, C.W.; Gibson, G.R. Using probiotics and prebiotics to improve gut health. *Drug Discov. Today* **2003**, *8*, 692–700. [CrossRef]

18. Gareau, M.G.; Sherman, P.M.; Walker, W.A. Probiotics and the gut microbiota in intestinal health and disease. *Nat. Rev. Gastroenterol. Hepatol.* **2010**, *7*, 503–514. [CrossRef] [PubMed]

19. Martin, R.; Miquel, S.; Ulmer, J.; Kechaou, N.; Langella, P.; Bermudez-Humaran, L. Role of commensal and probiotic bacteria in human health: A focus on inflammatory bowel disease. *Microb. Cell Fact.* **2013**, *12*, 71. [CrossRef] [PubMed]

20. West, N.P.; Pyne, D.B.; Cripps, A.W.; Hopkins, W.G.; Eskesen, D.C.; Jairath, A.; Christophersen, C.T.; Conlon, M.A.; Fricker, P.A. *Lactobacillus fermentum* (PCC®) supplementation and gastrointestinal and respiratory-tract illness symptoms: A randomised control trial in athlete. *Nutr. J.* **2011**, *10*, 30. [CrossRef] [PubMed]

21. Gleeson, M.; Bishop, N.C.; Oliveira, M.; Tauler, P. Daily probiotic's (*Lactobacillus casei* Shirota) reduction of infection incidence in athletes. *Int. J. Sports Nutr. Exerc. Metabol.* **2011**, *21*, 55–64. [CrossRef]

22. Nageo, F.; Nakayama, M.; Muto, T.; Okumura, K. Effects of a fermented milk drink containing *Lactobacillus casei* strain Shirota on the immune system in healthy human subjects. *Biosci. Biotechnol. Biochem.* **2000**, *64*, 2706–2708. [CrossRef]

23. Jager, R.; Purpura, M.; Stone, J.D.; Turner, S.M.; Anzalone, A.J.; Eimerbrink, M.J.; Pane, M.; Amoruso, A.; Rowlands, D.S.; Oliver, J.M. Probiotic *Streptococcus thermophilus* FP4 and *Bifidobacterium breve* BR03 supplementation attenuates performance and range-of-motion decrements following muscle damaging exercise. *Nutrients* **2016**, *8*, E642. [CrossRef] [PubMed]

24. Williams, E.A.; Stimpson, J.; Wang, D.; Plummer, S.; Garaiova, I.; Barker, M.E.; Corfe, B.M. Clinical trial: A multistrain probiotic preparation significantly reduces symptoms of irritable bowel syndrome in a double-blind placebo-controlled study. *Aliment. Pharmacol. Ther.* **2008**, *29*, 97–103. [CrossRef] [PubMed]

25. Plummer, S.F.; Garaiova, I.; Sarvotham, T.; Cottrell, S.L.; Le Scouiller, S.; Weaver, M.A.; Tang, J.; Dee, P.; Hunter, J. Effects of probiotics on the composition of the intestinal microbiota following antibiotic therapy. *Int. J. Antimicrob. Agents* **2005**, *26*, 69–74. [CrossRef] [PubMed]

26. Lamprecht, M.; Bogner, S.; Schippinger, G.; Steinbauer, K.; Fankhauser, F.; Hallstroem, S.; Schuetz, B.; Greilberger, J.F. Probiotic supplementation affects markers of intestinal barrier, oxidation, and inflammation in trained men; a randomized, double-blinded, placebo-controlled trial. *J. Int. Soc. Sports Nutr.* **2012**, *9*, 45. [CrossRef] [PubMed]

27. Topping, D.L.; Clifton, P.M. Short-chain fatty acids and human colonic function: Roles of resistant starch and nonstarch polysaccharides. *Physiol. Rev.* **2001**, *81*, 1031–1064. [PubMed]

28. Ashton, T.; Young, I.S.; Davison, G.W.; Rowlands, C.C.; McEneny, J.; Van Blerk, C.; Jones, E.; Peters, J.R.; Jackson, S.K. Exercise-induced endotoxemia: The effect of ascorbic acid supplementation. *Free Radic. Biol. Med.* **2003**, *35*, 284–291. [CrossRef]

29. Suzuki, T.; Hara, H. Quercitin enhances intestinal barrier function through the assembly of zonnula occludens-2, occludin, and claudin-1 and the expression of claudin-4 in caco-2 cells. *J. Nutr.* **2009**, *139*, 965–974. [CrossRef] [PubMed]

30. Bereswill, S.; Munoz, M.; Fischer, A.; Plickert, R.; Haag, L.-M.; Otto, B.; Kuhl, A.A.; Loddenkemper, C.; Gobel, U.B.; Heimsaat, M.M. Anti-inflammatory effects of resveratrol, curcumin and simvastatin in acute small intestinal inflammation. *PLoS ONE* **2010**, *5*, e15099. [CrossRef] [PubMed]

31. Hussein, S.A.; El-Senosy, Y.A.; Hassan, M.F. Gastro protective, antiapoptotic and anti-inflammatory effect of alpha-lipoic acid on ethanol induced gastric mucosal lesions in rats. *Am. J. Biochem. Mol. Biol.* **2014**, *4*, 48–63. [CrossRef]

32. Sung, M.J.; Kim, W.; Ahn, S.Y.; Cho, C.-H.; Koh, G.Y.; Moon, S.-O.; Kim, D.H.; Lee, S.; Kang, K.P.; Jang, K.Y.; et al. Protective effect of α-lipoic acid in lipopolysaccharide-induced endothelial fractalkine expression. *Circ. Res.* **2005**, *97*, 880–890. [CrossRef] [PubMed]

33. Zembron-Lacny, A.; Slowinska-Lisowska, M.; Szygula, Z.; Witkowski, K.; Stefaniak, T.; Dziubek, W. Assessment of the antioxidant effectiveness of α-lipoic acid in healthy men exposed to muscle-damaging exercise. *J. Physiol. Pharmacol.* **2009**, *60*, 139–143. [PubMed]

34. Faul, F.; Erdfelder, E.; Lang, A.-G.; Buchner, A. G*power 3: A flexible statistical power analysis program for the social, behavioral, and biomedical sciences. *Behav. Res. Methods* **2007**, *39*, 175–191. [CrossRef] [PubMed]

35. Johnston, S.D.; Smye, M.; Watson, R.G.P.; McMillan, S.A.; Trimble, E.R.; Love, A.H.G. Lactulose-mannitol intestinal permeability test: A useful screening test for adult coeliac disease. *Ann. Clin. Biochem.* **2000**, *37*, 512–519. [PubMed]

36. Foster, C.; Florhaug, J.A.; Franklin, J.; Gottschall, L.; Hrovatin, L.A.; Parker, S.; Doleshal, P.; Dodge, C. A new approach to monitoring exercise training. *J. Strength Cond. Res.* **2001**, *15*, 109–115. [CrossRef] [PubMed]

37. Comyns, T.; Flanagan, E.P. Applications of the session rating of perceived exertion system in professional rugby union. *Strength Cond. J.* **2013**, *35*, 78–85. [CrossRef]

38. Jentjens, R.L.P.G.; Wagenmakers, A.J.M.; Jeukendrup, A.E. Heat stress increases muscle glycogen use but reduces the oxidation of ingested carbohydrates during exercise. *J. Appl. Physiol.* **2002**, *92*, 1562–1572. [CrossRef] [PubMed]

39. Nadhazi, Z.; Takats, A.; Offenmuller, K.; Bertok, L. Plasma endotoxin level of healthy donors. *Acta Microbiol. Immunol. Hung.* **2002**, *49*, 151–157. [CrossRef] [PubMed]

40. Hurley, J.C. Endotoxemia: Methods of detection and clinical correlates. *Clin. Microbiol. Rev.* **1995**, *8*, 268–292. [PubMed]

41. Flynn, M.G.; McFarlin, B.K. Toll-like receptor 4: Link to the anti-inflammatory effects of exercise? *Exerc. Sport Sci. Rev.* **2006**, *34*, 176–181. [CrossRef] [PubMed]

42. Stuempfle, K.J.; Valentino, T.; Hew-Butler, T.; Hecht, F.M.; Hoffman, M.D. Nausea is associated with endotoxemia during a 161-km ultramarathon. *J. Sports Sci.* **2016**, *34*, 1662–1668. [CrossRef] [PubMed]

43. Sharma, B.; Srivastava, S.; Singh, N.; Sachdev, V.; Kapur, S.; Saraya, A. Role of probiotics on gut permeability and endotoxemia in patients with acute pancreatitis: A double-blind randomised controlled trial. *J. Clin. Gastroenterol.* **2011**, *45*, 442–448. [CrossRef] [PubMed]

44. Greco, L.; D'Adamo, G.; Truscelli, A.; Parrilli, G.; Mayar, M.; Budillon, G. Intestinal permeability after single dose gluten challenge in coeliac disease. *Arch. Dis. Child.* **1991**, *66*, 870–872. [CrossRef] [PubMed]

45. Van Elburg, R.M.; Uil, J.J.; Kokke, F.T.M.; Mulder, A.M.; van de Broek, W.G.M.; Mulder, C.J.J.; Heymans, H.S.A. Repeatability of the sugar-absorption test, using lactulose and mannitol, for measuring intestinal permeability for sugars. *J. Pediatr. Gastroenterol. Nutr.* **1995**, *20*, 184–188. [CrossRef] [PubMed]

46. Rosenfeldt, V.; Benfeldt, E.; Valerius, N.H.; Paerregaard, A.; Michaelsen, K.F. Effect of probiotics on gastrointestinal symptoms and small intestinal permeability in children with atopic dermatitis. *J. Pediatr.* **2004**, *145*, 612–616. [CrossRef] [PubMed]

47. Cox, A.J.; Pyne, D.B.; Saunders, P.U.; Fricker, P.A. Oral administration of the probiotic *Lactobacillus* fermentum VRI-003 and mucosal immunity in endurance athletes. *Br. J. Sports Med.* **2010**, *44*, 222–226. [CrossRef] [PubMed]

48. Ulluwishewa, D.; Anderson, R.C.; McNabb, W.C.; Moughan, P.J.; Wells, J.M.; Roy, N.C. Regulation of tight junction permeability by intestinal bacteria and dietary components. *J. Nutr.* **2011**, *141*, 769–776. [CrossRef] [PubMed]

49. Gill, S.K.; Allerton, D.M.; Ansley-Robson, P.; Hemmings, K.; Cox, M.; Costa, R.J.S. Does short-term high dose probiotic supplementation containing *Lactobacillus casei* attenuate exertional-heat stress induced endotoxemia and cytokinaemia? *Int. J. Sport Nutr. Exerc. Metab.* **2016**, *26*, 268–275. [CrossRef] [PubMed]

50. Munford, R.S. Sensing gram-negative bacterial lipopolysaccharides: A human disease determinant? *Infect. Immun.* **2008**, *76*, 454–465. [CrossRef] [PubMed]

51. Mach, N.; Botella-Fuster, D. Endurance exercise and gut microbiota: A review. *J. Sports Health Sci.* **2016**, in press. [CrossRef]

52. Nakamura, Y.K.; Omaye, S.T. Metabolic disease and pro- and prebiotics: Mechanistic insights. *Nutr. Metab.* **2012**, *9*, 60. [CrossRef] [PubMed]

53. Lescheid, D.W. Probiotics as regulators of inflammation: A review. *Funct. Foods Health Dis.* **2014**, *4*, 299–311.

54. Pagnini, C.; Saeed, R.; Bamias, G.; Arseneau, K.O.; Pizarro, T.T.; Cominelli, F. Probiotics promote gut health through stimulation of epithelial innate immunity. *Proc. Natl. Acad. Sci. USA* **2010**, *107*, 454–459. [CrossRef] [PubMed]

55. Madden, J.A.J.; Plummer, S.F.; Tang, J.; Garaiova, I.; Plummer, N.T.; Herbison, M.; Hunter, J.O.; Shimada, T.; Cheng, L.; Shirakawa, T. Effects of probiotics on preventing disruption of the intestinal microflora following antibiotic therapy: A double-blind, placebo-controlled pilot study. *Int. Immunopharmacol.* **2005**, *5*, 1091–1097. [CrossRef] [PubMed]

56. Plummer, S.; Weaver, M.A.; Harris, J.C.; Dee, P.; Hunter, J. Clostridium difficile pilot study: Effects of probiotic supplementation on the incidence of *C. difficile* diarrhea. *Int. Microbiol.* **2004**, *7*, 59–62. [PubMed]

57. Dehghan, P.; Gargari, B.P.; Jafar-abadi, A.M. Oligofructose-enriched inulin improves some inflammatory markers and metabolic endotoxemia in women with type 2 diabetes mellitus: A randomized controlled clinical trial. *Nutrition* **2014**, *30*, 418–423. [CrossRef] [PubMed]

58. Rastall, R.A.; Gibson, G.R. Recent developments in prebiotics to selectively impact beneficial microbes and promote intestinal health. *Curr. Opin. Biotechnol.* **2015**, *32*, 42–46. [CrossRef] [PubMed]

59. Delzenne, N.M.; Neyrinck, A.M.; Cani, P.D. Gut microbiota and metabolic disorders: How prebiotic can work? *Br. J. Nutr.* **2013**, *109* (Suppl 2), S81–S85. [CrossRef] [PubMed]

60. Dewulf, E.M.; Cani, P.D.; Claus, S.P.; Fuentes, S.; Puylaert, P.G.B.; Neyrinck, A.M.; Bindels, L.B.; de Vos, W.M.; Gibson, G.R.; Thissen, J.-P.; et al. Insight into the prebiotic concept: Lessons from an exploratory, double-blind intervention study with inulin-type fructans in obese women. *Gut* **2013**, *62*, 1112–1121. [CrossRef] [PubMed]

61. Rajkumar, H.; Kumar, M.; Das, N.; Kumar, S.N.; Challa, H.R.; Nagpal, R. Effect of probiotic Lactobacillus salivarius UBL S22 and prebiotic fructo-oligosaccharide on serum lipids, inflammatory markers, insulin sensitivity, and gut bacteria in healthy young volunteers: A randomized controlled single-blind pilot study. *J. Cardiovasc. Pharmacol. Ther.* **2015**, *20*, 289–298. [CrossRef] [PubMed]

62. Lindsay, J.O.; Whelan, K.; Stagg, A.J.; Gobin, P.; Al-Hassi, H.O.; Rayment, N.; Kamm, M.A.; Knight, S.C.; Forbes, A. Clinical, microbiological, and immunological effects of fructo-oligosaccharide in patients with Crohn's disease. *Gut* **2006**, *55*, 348–355. [CrossRef] [PubMed]

63. Nova, E.; Viadel, B.; Warnberg, J.; Carreres, J.E.; Marcos, A. Beneficial effects of a synbiotic supplement on self-perceived gastrointestinal well-being and immunoinflammatory status of healthy adults. *J. Med. Food* **2011**, *14*, 79–85. [CrossRef] [PubMed]

64. Khanna, S.; Atalay, M.; Lakksonen, D.E.; Gul, M.; Roy, S.; Sen, C.L. α-lipoic acid supplementation: Tissue glutathione homeostasis at rest and after exercise. *J. Appl. Physiol.* **1999**, *86*, 1191–1196. [PubMed]

65. Shay, K.P.; Moreau, R.F.; Smith, E.J.; Smith, A.R.; Hagen, T.M. Alpha-lipoic acid as a dietary supplement: Molecular mechanisms and therapeutic potential. *Biochem. Biophys. Acta* **2009**, *1790*, 1149–1160. [CrossRef] [PubMed]

66. Heer, M.; Repond, F.; Hany, A.; Sulser, H.; Kehl, O.; Jager, K. Actue ischaemic colitis in a female long distance runner. *Gut* **1987**, *28*, 896–899. [CrossRef] [PubMed]

67. Buffinton, G.D.; Doe, W.F. Depleted mucosal antioxidant defences in inflammatory bowel disease. *Free Radic. Biol. Med.* **1995**, *19*, 911–918. [CrossRef]

68. Goraca, A.; Peichota, A.; Huk-Kolega, H. Effect of alpha-lipoic acid on LPS-induced oxidative stress in the heart. *J. Physiol. Pharmacol.* **2009**, *60*, 61–68. [PubMed]

69. Heibashy, M.I.A.; Mazen, G.M.A.; Shahin, M.I. The curative effects of some antioxidants on endotoxin induced with lipopolysaccharides in the liver of rats. *J. Am. Sci.* **2013**, *9*, 529–538.

70. Zhang, W.-J.; Wel, H.; Hagen, T.; Frel, B. α-lipoic acid attenuates LPS-induced inflammatory responses by activating the phosphoinositide 3-kinase/Akt signaling pathway. *Proc. Natl. Acad. Sci. USA* **2007**, *104*, 4077–4082. [CrossRef] [PubMed]

71. Kuennen, M.; Gillum, T.; Doklandy, K.; Bedrick, E.; Schneider, S.; Moseley, P. Thermotolerance and heat acclimcation may share a common mechanism in humans. *Am. J. Physiol. Regul. Integr. Comp. Physiol.* **2011**, *301*, R524–R533. [CrossRef] [PubMed]

72. Prado de Oliveira, E.; Jeukendrup, A. Nutritional recommendations to avoid gastrointestinal complaints during exercise. *Sports Sci. Exch.* **2013**, *26*, 1–4.

73. Pyne, D.B.; West, N.P.; Cox, A.J.; Cripps, A.W. Probitoics supplementation for athletes—Clinical and physiological effects. *Eur. J. Sport Sci.* **2015**, *15*, 63–72. [CrossRef] [PubMed]

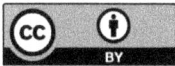

nutrients

MDPI

Case Report

Dietary Intake, Body Composition, and Menstrual Cycle Changes during Competition Preparation and Recovery in a Drug-Free Figure Competitor: A Case Study

Tanya M. Halliday [1,2,*], Jeremy P. Loenneke [3] and Brenda M. Davy [1]

[1]   Department of Human Nutrition, Foods, and Exercise, Virginia Tech, Blacksburg, VA 24060, USA;
       bdavy@vt.edu
[2]   Division of Endocrinology, Metabolism and Diabetes, School of Medicine,
       University of Colorado Anschutz Medical Campus, Aurora, CO 80045, USA
[3]   Kevser Ermin Applied Physiology Laboratory, Department of Health, Exercise Science and Recreation
       Management, University of Mississippi, University, MS 38677, USA; jploenne@olemiss.edu
*   Correspondence: tanyamh@vt.edu; Tel.: +1-540-231-8811

Received: 30 August 2016; Accepted: 16 November 2016; Published: 20 November 2016

Abstract: Physique competitions are events in which competitors are judged on muscular appearance and symmetry. The purpose of this retrospective case study was to describe changes in dietary intake, body mass/composition, and the menstrual cycle during the 20-week competition preparation (PREP) and 20-week post competition recovery (REC) periods of a drug-free amateur female figure competitor (age = 26–27, BMI = 19.5 kg/m^2). Dietary intake (via weighed food records) and body mass were assessed daily and averaged weekly. Body composition was estimated via Dual-energy X-ray absorptiometry (DXA) and 7-site skinfold measurements. Energy intake, body mass and composition, and energy availability decreased during the 20-week PREP period (changes of ~298 kcals, 5.1 kg, 6.5% body fat, and 5.4 kcal/kg fat free mass, respectively) and returned to baseline values by end of the 20-week REC period. Menstrual cycle irregularity was reported within the first month of PREP and the last menstruation was reported at week 11 of PREP. Given the potentially adverse health outcomes associated with caloric restriction, future, prospective cohort studies on the physiological response to PREP and REC are warranted in drug-free, female physique competitors.

Keywords: bodybuilders; physique athletes; competition preparation; competition recovery; dieting; energy availability; amenorrhea

1. Introduction

Physique competitions (bodybuilding, figure, and bikini) are unique athletic events in which competitors are judged on muscular appearance and symmetry rather than physical performance. In preparation for these contests competitors aim to decrease fat mass while maintaining lean mass through a combination of prolonged ($\geq$12 weeks) caloric restriction, resistance training, and aerobic exercise [1,2]. Currently, no evidence-based dietary guidelines exist for physique athletes to achieve body mass/composition goals for competition, or to re-gain appropriate levels of fat mass following competition, particularly in a manner that preserves (or at least minimizes risks to) overall health [1,3]. This may contribute to the large number of preparation strategies implemented by coaches and athletes, some of which may be dangerous (extremely low caloric intakes, reliance on un-tested supplements, extreme dehydration, etc.) [4–9]. Healthcare professionals working with these understudied athletes will need to understand the culture and associated constraints of the sport in order to assist competitors in developing nutrition strategies to support their training and competition goals.

Previous research on physique athletes is limited and has mainly focused on male competitors, female competitors using anabolic steroids, and/or the competition preparation (PREP) phase only [1,3,10–17]. Furthermore, the published literature on female physique competitors is limited by: (1) low methodological quality; (2) inadequate description of competition phase; and (3) being dated (e.g., published in the 1980s and 1990s when top-level competitors had lower body masses, and fewer competition categories existed [1,3]. Thus the data may be less applicable to current day physique competitors). Recent case studies of male physique competitors [11,18–20] have provided empirical evidence on the nutritional and exercise regimens, and the associated metabolic and physiological responses of these athletes. To our knowledge, no studies have provided a detailed account of both the PREP and competition recovery (REC) phases in drug-free female competitors. Given the potential health implications (e.g., female athlete triad) of obtaining a low level of fat mass through caloric restriction and exercise [21,22], evaluation of these athletes is warranted. To address gaps in the literature, the purpose of this case study was to describe changes in dietary intake, body mass and composition, and the menstrual cycle in a drug-free, female, figure competitor during both the PREP and REC periods.

2. Materials and Methods

This case study was considered exempt from Institutional Review Board review and approval. It was conducted and prepared in accordance with the Health Insurance Portability and Accountability Act.

2.1. Subject and Timeline Overview

The subject (26–27 years; BMI: 19.4 kg/m^2; body fat: 15%) was a Caucasian, drug-free, amateur figure competitor preparing for her first competition. The subject did not take any medications, including oral contraceptives, during the PREP or REC periods. The 20-week competition PREP and 20-week REC timeline for this competitor, including nutrition and exercise training programs were developed in collaboration with a contest preparation coach who is a certified personal trainer and professional male natural bodybuilder with 20 years of competition and coaching experience. Alterations to the program were determined based on body composition changes and subjective assessment of physique during posing practices. An overview of the timeline for study measurements is presented in Figure 1. In addition, the subject returned for assessment of body mass and composition (DXA) 32 weeks after the competition (i.e., 1 year since the initiation of PREP) and when menses resumed, 71 weeks post competition.

2.2. Dietary Intake

The subject electronically tracked dietary intake via weighed food records, using a commercially available digital food scale (Soehnle Optica$^\circledR$) to the nearest gram throughout PREP. Following the competition, the subject was less motivated to maintain a rigid diet and track intake as diligently. Thus, the 20-week REC period contains estimates of weekly macronutrient and caloric intake from a combination of weighed records and food diary estimates. Nutrient information was obtained from the USDA National Nutrient Database [23] or product-specific nutrition facts panels. Daily nutrient intake information (total kcals, macronutrient (g and %), and fiber (g)) was averaged each week.

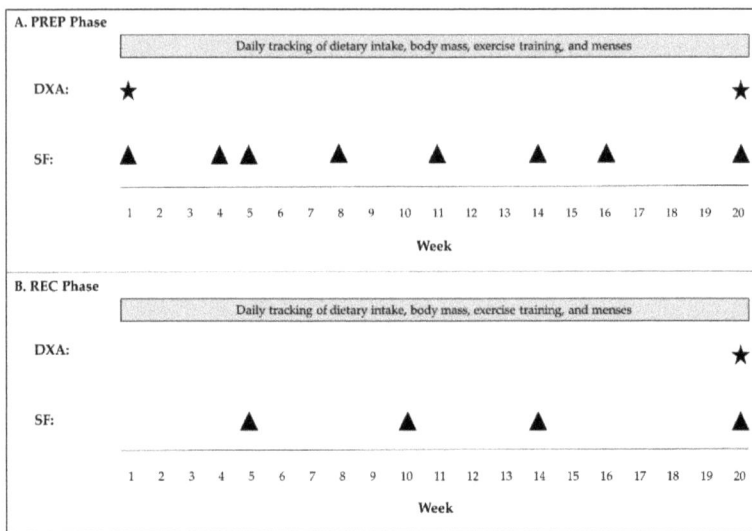

Figure 1. Timeline of Study Measurements (**A**) PREP and (**B**) REC phases. PREP: Competition preparation; REC: Competition recovery; DXA: Dual-energy X-ray absorptiometry; SF: Skinfolds.

2.3. Body Mass and Composition

The subject electronically tracked body mass daily on a commercially-available home scale (Health O Meter Professional®) throughout PREP and REC. Daily body masses were averaged each week. Body composition was assessed just before the PREP period began, the week of the competition (week 20 PREP), and at week 20 of the REC period via dual-energy X-ray absorptiometry (DXA; pre-PREP using Lunar Prodigy Advance, GE Medical Systems, software version 8.10e, Madison, WI, USA; and remainder of scans using Lunar iDXA, GE Medical Systems, software version enCORE 15, Madison, WI, USA model due to equipment upgrading in our laboratory) performed by a trained research technician licensed as a Radiologic Technologist-Limited in the state of Virginia. Skinfold thickness was measured 8 times during the 20-week PREP period and 4 times during the 20-week REC period via 7-site skinfold measurements according to ACSM guidelines [24] and using Jackson-Pollock generalized skinfold equation for body density [25] and the Siri equation for estimating body fat [24] by the subject's contest preparation coach.

2.4. Exercise Training

The subject recorded (paper/pen) exercise training daily for the duration of PREP and REC periods. Exercise Energy Expenditure (EEE) was estimated using the 2011 Compendium on Physical Activity [26].

2.5. Energy Availability

Before and at weeks, 1, 10, and 20 of PREP and weeks 10 and 20 of REC energy availability (EA) ((energy intake (kcals)-EEE (kcals))/fat-free mass (FFM) (kg)) [27] was calculated from the dietary intake record, exercise training record, and estimated FFM of the corresponding week. The established threshold of 30 kcal/kg was used as the reference level for comparing this subject's EA to the level below which adverse health outcomes have been detected [21].

2.6. Menstrual Cycle

Menses was tracked (paper/pen calendar) and reported by the subject for PREP and REC phases.

3. Results

3.1. Dietary Intake

The subject's diet during PREP and REC consisted of 2 days of high carbohydrate intake (~180–230 g/day), 3 days of moderate carbohydrate intake (~150–180 g/day), and 2 days of low carbohydrate intake (~100–150 g/day) each week. High carbohydrate intake days occurred on lower body resistance training days and low carbohydrate intake days occurred on off or low-intensity cardio training days. A sample daily weighed food record is presented in Table 1, representing typical food choices and portions consumed during both PREP and REC. Dietary supplement intake included: whey and casein protein powders, which were calculated into daily caloric and protein intake totals; and 5 g/day of creatine monohydrate from weeks 11 to 20 of PREP.

Table 1. Sample Weighed Food Record Representative of a Typical Day During both PREP and REC.

Food [1]	Preparation and/or Description	Weight (g) (Approximate Volume)
Breakfast:		
Oatmeal	With water	40 (dry)
		(1/2 cup, dry)
Whey Protein Isolate (De Novo Nutrition)	N/A	20
		(2/3 scoop)
Blueberries	Frozen, no sugar added	70
		(1/3 cup)
Peanut Butter	Natural, no added oil, sugar, or salt	15
		(1 Tbsp)
Morning Snacks:		
Greek Yogurt (Chobani)	Plain, non-fat	150
		(1 single-serve container)
Apple	Raw, with peel	180
		(1 medium, 3-inch diameter)
Almonds	Raw, unsalted	12
		(12 almonds)
Lunch:		
Broccoli	Steamed from fresh or frozen	142
		(1 small stalk)
Black Beans	Canned, drained and rinsed	120
		(1/2 cup)
Brown Rice, Jasmine	With water, no added oil or salt	98 (prepared)
		(1/2 cup, prepared)
Hummus (Sabra)	Classic flavor	28
		(2 Tbsp)
Whey Protein Isolate (De Novo Nutrition)	N/A	20
		(2/3 scoop)

Table 1. *Cont.*

Food [1]	Preparation and/or Description	Weight (g) (Approximate Volume)
Afternoon Snacks:		
Greek Yogurt (Chobani)	Plain, non-fat	150 (1 single-serve container)
Blueberries	Frozen, no sugar added	70 (1/3 cup)
Oatmeal	With water	40 (dry) (1/2 cup, dry)
Whey Protein Isolate (De Novo Nutrition)	N/A	20 (2/3 scoop)
Green Bell Pepper	Raw	164 (1 large, 3-inch diameter)
Dinner:		
Tilapia fillet	Baked, from frozen	114 (1.3 fillets)
Green Bell Pepper	Raw	164 (1 large, 3-inch diameter)
Kale	Raw	100 (6 cups, loosely packed)
Carrot	Raw	100 (0.9 cups, grated)
Red Cabbage	Raw	100 (1.1 cups, chopped)
Extra Virgin Olive Oil	Dressing for kale salad	10 (2 tsp)
Sesame Seed Oil	Dressing for kale salad	5 (1 tsp)
Rice Vinegar	Dressing for kale salad	15 (1 Tbsp)
Sesame Seeds	Whole, dry, dressing for kale salad	5 (1/2 Tbsp)
Brown Rice, Jasmine	With water, no added oil or salt	80 (prepared) (2/5 cup, prepared)
Evening Snacks:		
Almond Butter	Natural, no added oils, sugar, or salt	18 (1 Tbsp)
Beverage Intake [2]:		
Water	N/A	24–48 fl. oz.
Diet Soda	N/A	24–36 fl. oz.
Coffee/tea	Black, unsweetened	24–48 fl. oz.

PREP: Competition Preparation; REC: Competition recovery; Tbsp: Tablespoon. [1] Use of seasonings (e.g., salt) was not weighed or tracked; [2] Beverage intake was not weighed or rigidly tracked. It was reported by participant as typical consumption.

Changes in averaged weekly caloric intake are presented in Figure 2 for PREP and REC. Habitual energy and macronutrient intake at baseline (i.e., before PREP), weeks 1, 10, and 20 of PREP, and weeks 10 and 20 of REC are listed in Table 2.

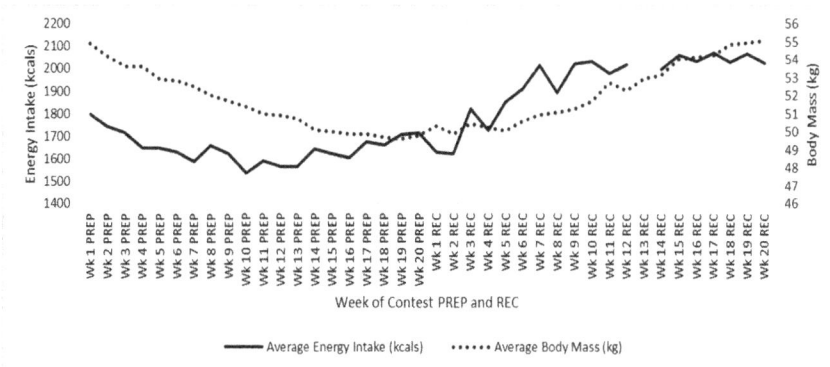

Figure 2. Changes in Energy Intake and Body Mass during Competition Preparation and Recovery. PREP: Competition preparation; REC: Competition recovery.

Table 2. Energy and Macronutrient Intake.

	Energy (kcals/Day)	CHO (g) (% Total kcals) (g/kg BM)	Protein (g) (% Total kcals) (g/kg BM)	Fat (g) (% Total kcals)	Fiber (g)
Baseline	2010	225 45% (4.1 g/kg)	120 24% (2.2 g/kg)	70 31%	48
Week 1 PREP	1798	187 42% (3.4 g/kg)	150 33% (2.7 g/kg)	50 25%	40
Week 10 PREP	1541	143 37% (2.7 g/kg)	150 39% (2.9 g/kg)	41 24%	24
Week 20 PREP	1712	188 44% (3.8 g/kg)	150 35% (3.0g/kg)	40 21%	34
Week 10 REC	2032	219 43% (4.2 g/kg)	146 29% (2.8 g/kg)	63 28%	49
Week 20 REC	2023	233 46% (4.2g/kg)	133 26% (2.4 g/kg)	62 28%	47

PREP: Competition preparation; REC: Competition recovery; CHO: carbohydrate; BM: body mass.

3.2. Body Mass and Composition

Changes in average weekly body mass are presented in Figure 2 for PREP and REC. Body mass decreased from 54.9 kg at Week 1 of PREP to 49.8 kg by Week 20 of PREP, and then increased to 55.1 kg by Week 20 REC. Body fat (assessed via DXA) decreased from 15.1% (8.3 kg) at baseline to 8.6% (4.3 kg) by Week 20 of PREP. Lean mass was maintained at 44.3 kg pre and post PREP (80.7% and 89% lean mass, respectively). By Week 20 REC, percent body fat had returned to baseline at 14.8%. By Week 32 of REC (e.g., 1 year since initiation of PREP), body mass had increased to 57.3 kg and body fat to 20%. By Week 71 REC (when menses resumed) body mass was 56.1 kg and body fat had been maintained at 20%.

Total and site-specific skinfold thickness changes during PREP and REC are presented in Figure 3. Total skinfold thickness decreased from 66.5 mm at Baseline to 30 mm by the week of competition

(Week 20 PREP) (corresponding to a decrease from 14.8% to 8.3% body fat, indicating concordance with the DXA results). Skinfold thickness steadily increased in the REC period and returned to baseline (64 mm) by Week 20 REC.

3.3. Exercise Training

Exercise training during PREP consisted of a high-volume resistance training program 4–5 days/ week (training all major muscle groups of the upper and lower body 2–3 days/week), brief (e.g., 10–30 min) high-intensity interval training 1–2 day(s)/week, and longer (e.g., 45–120 min) aerobic exercise session 1 day/week. This training regimen resulted in an EEE of 484, 459, and 440 kcal/day at weeks 1, 10, and 20 of PREP, respectively. Exercise training during REC consisted of a high-volume resistance training program 3–4 days/week, brief (10–30 min) high-intensity interval training 1–2 day(s)/week, and a longer (45–60 min) aerobic exercise session 1 day/week. This training regimen resulted in an EEE of 355 and 378 kcal/day at weeks 10 and 20 of REC, respectively.

3.4. Energy Availability and Menstrual Cycle

Prior to PREP and at weeks 1, 10, and 20 of PREP, EA was 32.7, 28.2, 23.2, and 27.3 kcal/kg FFM, respectively. At weeks 10 and 20 of REC, EA was estimated to have increased to 36.5 kcal/kg and 35.1 kcal/kg FFM, respectively. Our subject reported a habitual cycle length of ~42 days without use of hormonal birth control for several years prior to engaging in competition preparation. Menstrual cycle irregularity (spotting between typical menses) was reported within the first month of PREP and the last menstruation was reported at week 11 of PREP. Menses did not resume until 71 weeks following the competition.

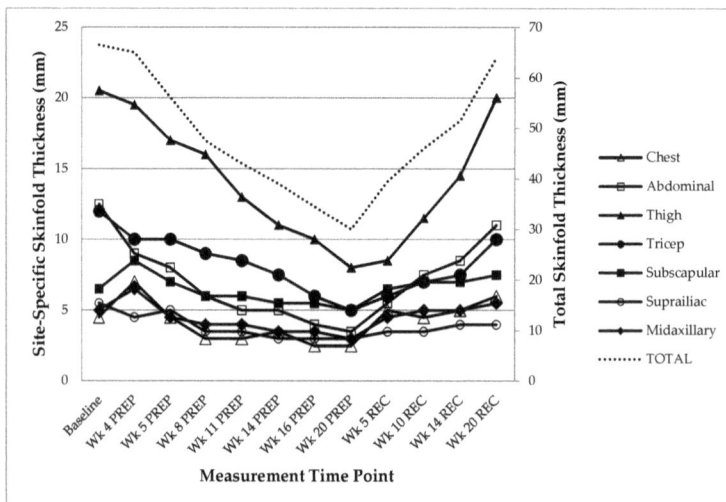

Figure 3. Total and Site-Specific Skinfold Thickness Changes. Wk: Week; PREP: Competition Preparation; REC: Competition recovery.

4. Discussion

This case study provides a detailed and comprehensive examination of the dietary and exercise habits, and the associated alterations in body mass, body composition, EA, and menses during both the PREP and REC phases for a drug free, female figure competitor. The major finding from this investigation was that caloric restriction, low EA, and decreased fat mass led to loss of menses early in the PREP phase. Despite a return to baseline levels of energy intake, EA, and fat mass during the

REC phase, resumption of menses was delayed. In addition, this investigation provides insight on the diet-related culture of the sport which is vital for healthcare professionals working with these clients to be familiar with.

4.1. Dietary Intake

4.1.1. Energy Intake

Competition PREP for our subject consisted of a gradual decrease in energy intake for the initial 10-weeks and then a gradual increase back to week 1 PREP energy intake by week 20 PREP (i.e., week of competition). Our subject's habitual (2010 kcals/day) and PREP energy intake (low of 1541 kcals/day at week 10) were greater than those previously reported in female physique competitors (average of 1636 and 1214 kcals/day, respectively) [1]. Energy intake at competition was similar for our subject and previous reports (1712 vs. 1739 kcals/day) [1]. However, prior investigations only monitored dietary intake for short periods of time, and many did not include information on dietary supplement use [1], thus limiting our ability to compare our more detailed analysis to previous reports.

Following the competition, our subject slowly increased energy intake. This was in an effort to limit a rapid increase in fat mass due to the known propensity for fat accumulation following energy restriction [28]. To our knowledge only one previous study assessed dietary intake following competition in female physique athletes. Walberg-Rankin et al. instructed female bodybuilders to keep 3-day food records the day of until 2 days following the competition and 19 to 21 days following the competition [14]. Compared with their participants' energy intakes in the 1 month prior to the competition (1536–1839 kcals/day), energy intake immediately post competition (3237 kcals) and 3 weeks post was significantly greater (2790 kcals). This was associated with a rapid increase in body mass that was 1.2 kg above their initially reported body mass 1 month before the competition. Our subject was more cautious in the REC period than the athletes previously studied by diligently increasing energy intake slowly and limiting days 'off' the diet.

4.1.2. Macronutrient Intake

During PREP, carbohydrate and fat intake decreased and protein intake increased compared to the subject's baseline dietary habits. Carbohydrate intake fell below the Acceptable Macronutrient Distribution Range (AMDR) of 45%–65% of total caloric intake and protein intake rose above the AMDR of 10%–35%. Our subject's macronutrient intake is consistent with previous reports in male and female physique competitors [1,11,14,20] which show carbohydrate intake below sports nutrition recommendations (e.g., 3–12 g/kg/day depending on training volume/intensity and body composition goals) [29] and protein intake above recommendations for strength training athletes (e.g., 1.2–2.0 g/kg/day) [29]. The elevated protein intake is presumably in an effort to maintain muscle mass (which our subject was successful at doing) during a period of weight loss, and is in line with recent findings demonstrating the efficacy of an increased protein intake during periods of energy restriction [30–32]. Following the competition, increases in energy intake were due to higher carbohydrate and fat intake. Protein intake decreased slightly, but still remained above 2.0 g/kg.

4.1.3. Fiber Intake

Fiber intake decreased during PREP, but remained above the Dietary Reference Intake of 14 g/1000 kcals [33], and increased during REC. This was due to a reliance on nutrient-dense, low-energy foods such as fruits and vegetables [34]. High intake of fibrous foods likely promoted feelings of fullness and enabled this competitor to adhere to the energy restriction [35–39]. In addition, high fruit and vegetable intake is beneficial in ensuring that micronutrient needs are met while energy intake is reduced, and therefore should be included in the development of nutrition recommendations for competition PREP [34,36]. Prior studies in physique competitors have not quantified fiber consumption or tracked dietary intake as accurately so it is unknown if this is typical practice amongst physique competitors.

4.2. Exercise Training and Body Mass and Composition

Exercise training consisted of a high-volume resistance training regimen and modest amounts of aerobic exercise. Contrary to previous reports from the 1990s [14,16,40], but in agreement with more recent data [1,11] alterations in body mass and composition occurred mainly by reduced energy intake and not increased aerobic exercise. This may be indicative of an overall shift in preparation strategy over time. However, anecdotally we have observed that some current day physique athletes do rely on high levels of aerobic exercise to decrease fat mass before competitions.

Unsurprisingly, 20-weeks of caloric restriction during PREP resulted in reduced body mass and fat mass, which was reversed when caloric intake increased during the 20-week REC phase. Lean mass was maintained during the PREP phase, likely due to a combination of high protein intake and the intensive resistance training program [30,31]. Our subject was lean (~15% body fat) at the start of competition preparation and achieved a body composition (~8%) similar to female bodybuilders previously studied [1,14,16]. While these reported body composition values are less than recommendations for essential fat for women [24], it is likely necessary in order to be competitive in this sport. As noted in the dietary intake section, the REC period has not been well studied in female physique competitors. Given the rapid increase in body mass (which overshot initial body mass) seen in the Walberg-Rankin et al. study [14], and an even more pronounced increase of 8.6 kg gain in body mass by 4 weeks post competition detected by Lamar-Hildebrand et al. in college-aged female bodybuilders [41] compared with the more controlled return to habitual body mass and composition in our subject, the REC period is deserving of additional investigation and likely requires unique dietary intake recommendations.

4.3. Energy Availability and Menstrual Cycle

The EA of our subject fell below recommended levels of 30 kcal/kg of FFM [27] upon initiation of PREP and remained below this level for the entire 20 weeks. In addition, disruption to normal menstruation was reported early and amenorrhea occurred by the end of PREP. Due to an increase in energy intake and a decline in exercise energy expenditure during REC, EA increased to >35 kcal/kg FFM by week 10 of REC. Despite the return of caloric intake and body composition and mass to baseline levels during the 20-week REC period, menses did not resume until 71 weeks following the competition. Interestingly, the subject had returned to our laboratory for assessment of body composition (via DXA) 32 weeks post competition (i.e., 1 year since the initiation of PREP) and at week 71 post competition when menses resumed. Body composition and mass at those two assessment time points (20% body fat, 57.3 kg and 20% body fat, 56.1 kg, respectively) were higher than the habitual body composition and mass (~15% body fat, 54.9 kg) our subject had maintained for years leading up to the competition.

This finding suggest that the reductions to EA and body composition which occur with preparation for physique competitions may have prolonged, detrimental effects on normal reproductive hormonal profiles. Resumption of menses may require that EA and body composition exceed baseline values for a prolonged period of time. Since our subject was concerned about the health implications of amenorrhea, she did not have plans to compete again. However, for competitors who plan to complete yearly, they may not have adequate time in between PREP cycles for menstrual cycle recovery. Prior investigations have noted that both resistance training and energy restriction are associated with alterations to reproductive hormones [14,42–44] leading to menstrual disruption (e.g., increases in estradiol and beta-endorphin which then reduce gonadotropin releasing hormone and luteinizing hormone pulsatility). Therefore, since physique athletes subject themselves to both intensive resistance training regimens and prolonged caloric restriction, they are at greater risk for menstrual disturbance and the associated insults to bone and metabolic health [21,22]. This has important ethical implications for the advice and treatment provided by coaches and health care professionals who work with these athletes.

Previous research on female athletes has established that those in lean build sports are more likely to have menstrual dysfunction than those in non-lean build sports [45]. However, while more common in this group of athletes than non-athletes, participation in physique competitions does not always lead to menstrual dysfunction [14,46]. Therefore, investigation of individual factors contributing to disruptions of normal menses, as well as analysis of alterations in reproductive hormones during PREP and REC warrant investigation in this at-risk group of athletes.

4.4. Strengths and Limitations

The current study has several strengths. Most notably this is the first to provide detailed, weighed dietary intake analysis over an extended time period (e.g., 40 weeks). This overcomes limitations of previous reports that rely solely on 1–3-day food records or food frequency questionnaires kept for a limited duration leading up to competitions [1]. Second, we accounted for intake of dietary supplementation, which has not been consistently reported in many earlier papers describing the dietary habits of physique competitors [1]. Third, we utilized DXA technology to evaluate changes in body composition. While we did rely on two separate DXA machines due to unavoidable equipment upgrades in our laboratory, the estimates tracked similarly with skinfold estimates, giving us greater confidence in our measurements. Fourth, this study is the first to estimate EA and track menses during PREP and REC. These are important considerations for the development of sports nutrition recommendations that will also support the long-term health of physique athletes. Finally, the case study approach is also a strength since longer-term, detailed information was obtained which would be challenging with a larger cohort [47]. These findings can be utilized to inform future studies in this athletic population.

Despite these strengths, we acknowledge limitations of this study. First, we did not collect biochemical or clinical data (aside from body composition). Future investigations should be done prospectively and plan to obtain blood and urine samples to evaluate alterations in hormonal and metabolite values related to weight loss/gain and menstrual function as well as relevant clinical outcomes (e.g., metabolic rate, blood pressure, heart rate, etc.). Second, we did not include psychological measures. Questionnaires related to dietary restraint, disinhibition, and disordered eating would be valuable to include in future longitudinal research on physique competitors. Third, our participant did not track timing of dietary intake and supplement use throughout the day, or in relation to workouts. While nutrient timing is an important and interesting sports nutrition consideration, this level of detail would likely be unrealistic in investigations of similar duration. Nonetheless, future trials and interventions focusing on this topic may provide important information on nutrient timing strategies to assist physique athletes in achieving their body composition and/or strength goals before and after competitions.

4.5. Future Directions

The popularity of physique competitions is increasing, with a greater number of organizations created and competitions held each year [48]. Therefore, research is needed in order to establish evidence-based nutrition and exercise recommendations related to improving performance, while minimizing potential adverse health outcomes of caloric restriction in these athletes. Randomized-controlled trials will likely be unfeasible in this population. Instead, long-term observational trials which track competitors during PREP and REC phases will be needed. Specific questions to answer include: What is the typical degree of caloric restriction competitors subject themselves to? What is the prevalence of the female athlete triad? What best predicts both performance and maintenance of health in these athletes (e.g., baseline caloric intake, degree of restriction employed, age, dietary composition, exercise energy expenditure, etc.)? What is the time course for recovery of physiological, metabolic, and menstrual responses to competition preparation? What is the long-term impact of several cycles of competition preparation and recovery on health outcomes? What are the psychological ramifications (e.g., eating attitudes, mood disturbance, and sleep habits) of physique competition participation? Overall, these competitors are a unique and understudied group of athletes whom much can be learned from in regards to the metabolic adaptations to caloric restriction during competition preparation and metabolic recovery during refeeding following competitions.

5. Conclusions

This case study provides the first long-term assessment of dietary intake, body mass/composition, and menstrual cycle changes associated with competition PREP and REC in a drug-free, female figure competitor. As expected caloric restriction and decreased EA led to a decline in fat and body mass and cessation of menses. Energy intake, body mass and fat mass returned to baseline levels by the end of the 20-week REC period. However, return of menstruation was delayed, not resuming until over a year following the competition. Our case study adds long-term, detailed information to the limited literature available on this population. Future studies should build upon this approach in order to lead to the creation of evidence-based dietary intake and exercise recommendations for physique competitors across the competitive cycle that aims to increase 'performance' (e.g., subjectively rated appearance) while maintaining the health of the competitors.

Author Contributions: T.M.H. and J.P.L. conceived and designed the study; T.M.H. collected the data and T.M.H., J.P.L. and B.M.D. analyzed and interpreted the data. T.M.H. was primarily responsible for writing the manuscript with input from J.P.L. and B.M.D. All authors read and approved the final manuscript.

Conflicts of Interest: The authors declare no conflict of interest.

References

1. Spendlove, J.; Mitchell, L.; Gifford, J.; Hackett, D.; Slater, G.; Cobley, S.; O'Connor, H. Dietary intake of competitive bodybuilders. *Sports Med.* **2015**, *45*, 1041–1063. [CrossRef] [PubMed]
2. Kennedy, R.H. *Encyclopedia of Bodybuilding: The Complete A–Z Book on Muscle Building*; Robert Kennedy Publishing: Toronto, ON, Canada, 2008.
3. Slater, G.; Phillips, S.M. Nutrition guidelines for strength sports: Sprinting, weightlifting, throwing events, and bodybuilding. *J. Sports Sci.* **2011**, *29* (Suppl. S1), S67–S77. [CrossRef] [PubMed]
4. Giampreti, A.; Lonati, D.; Locatelli, C.; Rocchi, L.; Campailla, M.T. Acute neurotoxicity after yohimbine ingestion by a body builder. *Clin. Toxicol.* **2009**, *47*, 827–829. [CrossRef] [PubMed]
5. Faber, M.; Benade, A.J. Nutrient intake and dietary supplementation in body-builders. *S. Afr. Med. J.* **1987**, *72*, 831–834. [PubMed]
6. Hackett, D.A.; Johnson, N.A.; Chow, C.M. Training practices and ergogenic aids used by male bodybuilders. *J. Strength Cond. Res./Natl. Strength Cond. Assoc.* **2013**, *27*, 1609–1617. [CrossRef] [PubMed]
7. Schafer, C.N.; Guldager, H.; Jorgensen, H.L. Multi-organ dysfunction in bodybuilding possibly caused by prolonged hypercalcemia due to multi-substance abuse: Case report and review of literature. *Int. J. Sports Med.* **2011**, *32*, 60–65. [CrossRef] [PubMed]
8. Andersen, R.E.; Barlett, S.J.; Morgan, G.D.; Brownell, K.D. Weight loss, psychological, and nutritional patterns in competitive male body builders. *Int. J. Eat. Disord.* **1995**, *18*, 49–57. [CrossRef]
9. Brill, J.B.; Keane, M.W. Supplementation patterns of competitive male and female bodybuilders. *Int. J. Sport Nutr.* **1994**, *4*, 398–412. [CrossRef] [PubMed]
10. Helms, E.R.; Aragon, A.A.; Fitschen, P.J. Evidence-based recommendations for natural bodybuilding contest preparation: Nutrition and supplementation. *J. Int. Soc. Sports Nutr.* **2014**, *11*. [CrossRef] [PubMed]
11. Rossow, L.M.; Fukuda, D.H.; Fahs, C.A.; Loenneke, J.P.; Stout, J.R. Natural bodybuilding competition preparation and recovery: A 12-month case study. *Int. J. Sports Physiol. Perform.* **2013**, *8*, 582–592. [CrossRef] [PubMed]
12. Bamman, M.M.; Hunter, G.R.; Newton, L.E.; Roney, R.K.; Khaled, M.A. Changes in body composition, diet, and strength of bodybuilders during the 12 weeks prior to competition. *J. Sports Med. Phys. Fit.* **1993**, *33*, 383–391.

13. Sandoval, W.M.; Heyward, V.H. Food selection patterns of bodybuilders. *Int. J. Sport Nutr.* **1991**, *1*, 61–68. [CrossRef] [PubMed]
14. Walberg-Rankin, J.; Edmonds, C.E.; Gwazdauskas, F.C. Diet and weight changes of female bodybuilders before and after competition. *Int. J. Sport Nutr.* **1993**, *3*, 87–102. [CrossRef] [PubMed]
15. Withers, R.T.; Noell, C.J.; Whittingham, N.O.; Chatterton, B.E.; Schultz, C.G.; Keeves, J.P. Body composition changes in elite male bodybuilders during preparation for competition. *Aust. J. Sci. Med. Sport* **1997**, *29*, 11–16. [CrossRef] [PubMed]
16. Van der Ploeg, G.E.; Brooks, A.G.; Withers, R.T.; Dollman, J.; Leaney, F.; Chatterton, B.E. Body composition changes in female bodybuilders during preparation for competition. *Eur. J. Clin. Nutr.* **2001**, *55*, 268–277. [CrossRef] [PubMed]
17. Lemon, P.W.; Tarnopolsky, M.A.; MacDougall, J.D.; Atkinson, S.A. Protein requirements and muscle mass/strength changes during intensive training in novice bodybuilders. *J. Appl. Physiol.* **1992**, *73*, 767–775. [PubMed]
18. Della Guardia, L.; Cavallaro, M.; Cena, H. The risks of self-made diets: The case of an amateur bodybuilder. *J. Int. Soc. Sports Nutr.* **2015**, *12*. [CrossRef] [PubMed]
19. Robinson, S.L.; Lambeth-Mansell, A.; Gillibrand, G.; Smith-Ryan, A.; Bannock, L. A nutrition and conditioning intervention for natural bodybuilding contest preparation: Case study. *J. Int. Soc. Sports Nutr.* **2015**, *12*. [CrossRef] [PubMed]
20. Kistler, B.M.; Fitschen, P.J.; Ranadive, S.M.; Fernhall, B.; Wilund, K.R. Case study: Natural bodybuilding contest preparation. *Int. J. Sport Nutr. Exerc. Metab.* **2014**, *24*, 694–700. [CrossRef] [PubMed]
21. Mountjoy, M.; Sundgot-Borgen, J.; Burke, L.; Carter, S.; Constantini, N.; Lebrun, C.; Meyer, N.; Sherman, R.; Steffen, K.; Budgett, R.; et al. The IOC consensus statement: Beyond the female athlete triad—Relative Energy Deficiency in Sport (RED-S). *Br. J. Sports Med.* **2014**, *48*, 491–497. [CrossRef] [PubMed]
22. De Souza, M.J.; Nattiv, A.; Joy, E.; Misra, M.; Williams, N.I.; Mallinson, R.J.; Gibbs, J.C.; Olmsted, M.; Goolsby, M.; Matheson, G. 2014 Female Athlete Triad Coalition Consensus Statement on Treatment and Return to Play of the Female Athlete Triad: 1st International Conference Held in San Francisco, California, May 2012 and 2nd International Conference Held in Indianapolis, Indiana, May 2013. *Br. J. Sports Med.* **2014**, *48*. [CrossRef]
23. National Nutrient Database for Standard Reference, Release 28. United Stated Department of Agriculture. Available online: http://www.ars.usda.gov/ba/bhnrc/ndl (accessed on 30 Septmeber 2015).
24. Pescatello, L.S.; American College of Sports Medicine. *Acsm's Guidelines for Exercise Testing and Prescription*; Wolters Kluwer/Lippincott Williams & Wilkins Health: Philadelphia, PA, USA, 2014.
25. Jackson, A.S.; Pollock, M.L.; Ward, A. Generalized equations for predicting body density of women. *Med. Sci. Sports Exerc.* **1980**, *12*, 175–181. [CrossRef] [PubMed]
26. Ainsworth, B.E.; Haskell, W.L.; Herrmann, S.D.; Meckes, N.; Bassett, D.R., Jr.; Tudor-Locke, C.; Greer, J.L.; Vezina, J.; Whitt-Glover, M.C.; Leon, A.S. 2011 compendium of physical activities: A second update of codes and met values. *Med. Sci. Sports Exerc.* **2011**, *43*, 1575–1581. [CrossRef] [PubMed]
27. Loucks, A.B.; Kiens, B.; Wright, H.H. Energy availability in athletes. *J. Sports Sci.* **2011**, *29* (Suppl. S1), S7–S15. [CrossRef] [PubMed]
28. Maclean, P.S.; Bergouignan, A.; Cornier, M.A.; Jackman, M.R. Biology's response to dieting: The impetus for weight regain. *Am. J. Physiol. Regul. Integr. Comp. Physiol.* **2011**, *301*, R581–R600. [CrossRef] [PubMed]
29. Thomas, D.T.; Erdman, K.A.; Burke, L.M. Position of the academy of nutrition and dietetics, dietitians of canada, and the american college of sports medicine: Nutrition and athletic performance. *J. Acad. Nutr. Diet.* **2016**, *116*, 501–528. [CrossRef] [PubMed]
30. Phillips, S.M.; van Loon, L.J. Dietary protein for athletes: From requirements to optimum adaptation. *J. Sports Sci.* **2011**, *29* (Suppl. S1), S29–S38. [CrossRef] [PubMed]
31. Longland, T.M.; Oikawa, S.Y.; Mitchell, C.J.; Devries, M.C.; Phillips, S.M. Higher compared with lower dietary protein during an energy deficit combined with intense exercise promotes greater lean mass gain and fat mass loss: A randomized trial. *Am. J. Clin. Nutr.* **2016**, *103*, 738–746. [CrossRef] [PubMed]
32. Mettler, S.; Mitchell, N.; Tipton, K.D. Increased protein intake reduces lean body mass loss during weight loss in athletes. *Med. Sci. Sports Exerc.* **2010**, *42*, 326–337. [CrossRef] [PubMed]
33. Institute of Medicine of the National Academies. *Dietary Reference Intakes for Energy, Carbohydrate, Fiber, Fat, Fatty Acids, Cholesterol, Protein, and Amino Acids*; National Academies Press: Washington, DC, USA, 2002.

34. Institute of Medicine of the National Academies. *Dietary Reference Intakes. Proposed Definition of Dietary Fiber;* National Academies Press: Washington, DC, USA, 2001.

35. Manore, M.M. Weight management for athletes and active individuals: A brief review. *Sports Med.* **2015**, *45* (Suppl. S1), S83–S92. [CrossRef] [PubMed]

36. Marlett, J.A.; McBurney, M.I.; Slavin, J.L. Position of the american dietetic association: Health implications of dietary fiber. *J. Am. Diet. Assoc.* **2002**, *102*, 993–1000. [CrossRef]

37. Harrold, J.; Breslin, L.; Walsh, J.; Halford, J.; Pelkman, C. Satiety effects of a whole-grain fibre composite ingredient: Reduced food intake and appetite ratings. *Food Funct.* **2014**, *5*, 2574–2581. [CrossRef] [PubMed]

38. Rolls, B.J. Dietary strategies for weight management. *Nestle Nutr. Inst. Workshop Ser.* **2012**, *73*, 37–48. [PubMed]

39. Slavin, J.L. Dietary fiber and body weight. *Nutrition* **2005**, *21*, 411–418. [CrossRef] [PubMed]

40. Kleiner, S.M.; Bazzarre, T.L.; Litchford, M.D. Metabolic profiles, diet, and health practices of championship male and female bodybuilders. *J. Am. Diet. Assoc.* **1990**, *90*, 962–967. [PubMed]

41. Lamar-Hildebrand, N.; Saldanha, L.; Endres, J. Dietary and exercise practices of college-aged female bodybuilders. *J. Am. Diet. Assoc.* **1989**, *89*, 1308–1310. [PubMed]

42. Walberg-Rankin, J.; Franke, W.D.; Gwazdauskas, F.C. Response of beta-endorphin and estradiol to resistance exercise in females during energy balance and energy restriction. *Int. J. Sports Med.* **1992**, *13*, 542–547. [CrossRef] [PubMed]

43. Cumming, D.C.; Wall, S.R.; Galbraith, M.A.; Belcastro, A.N. Reproductive hormone responses to resistance exercise. *Med. Sci. Sports Exerc.* **1987**, *19*, 234–238. [CrossRef] [PubMed]

44. Enea, C.; Boisseau, N.; Fargeas-Gluck, M.A.; Diaz, V.; Dugue, B. Circulating androgens in women: Exercise-induced changes. *Sports Med.* **2011**, *41*, 1–15. [CrossRef] [PubMed]

45. Beals, K.A.; Hill, A.K. The prevalence of disordered eating, menstrual dysfunction, and low bone mineral density among US collegiate athletes. *Int. J. Sport Nutr. Exerc. Metab.* **2006**, *16*, 1–23. [CrossRef] [PubMed]

46. Walberg, J.L.; Johnston, C.S. Menstrual function and eating behavior in female recreational weight lifters and competitive body builders. *Med. Sci. Sports Exerc.* **1991**, *23*, 30–36. [CrossRef] [PubMed]

47. Amerson, R. Making a case for the case study method. *J. Nurs. Educ.* **2011**, *50*, 427–428. [CrossRef] [PubMed]

48. History of Bodybuilding. Available online: http://historyofbodybuilding.org (accessed on 12 January 2016).

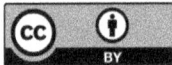

nutrients

MDPI

Article

Probiotic Supplements Beneficially Affect Tryptophan–Kynurenine Metabolism and Reduce the Incidence of Upper Respiratory Tract Infections in Trained Athletes: A Randomized, Double-Blinded, Placebo-Controlled Trial

Barbara Strasser [1,*], Daniela Geiger [2], Markus Schauer [2], Johanna M. Gostner [1], Hannes Gatterer [3], Martin Burtscher [3] and Dietmar Fuchs [2]

[1] Division of Medical Biochemistry, Biocenter, Medical University of Innsbruck, Innrain 80, 6020 Innsbruck, Austria; Johanna.Gostner@i-med.ac.at

[2] Division of Biological Chemistry, Biocenter, Medical University of Innsbruck, Innrain 80, 6020 Innsbruck, Austria; M.Sc.DanielaGeiger@gmail.com (D.G.); M.Schauer@hotmail.com (M.S.); Dietmar.Fuchs@i-med.ac.at (D.F.)

[3] Department of Sport Science, Medical Section, University of Innsbruck, Fuerstenweg 189, 6020 Innsbruck, Austria; Hannes.Gatterer@uibk.ac.at (H.G.); Martin.Burtscher@uibk.ac.at (M.B.)

* Correspondence: Barbara.Strasser@i-med.ac.at; Tel.: +43-512-9003 (ext. 70350)

Received: 12 July 2016; Accepted: 17 November 2016; Published: 23 November 2016

Abstract: Background: Prolonged intense exercise has been associated with transient suppression of immune function and an increased risk of infections. In this context, the catabolism of amino acid tryptophan via kynurenine may play an important role. The present study examined the effect of a probiotic supplement on the incidence of upper respiratory tract infections (URTI) and the metabolism of aromatic amino acids after exhaustive aerobic exercise in trained athletes during three months of winter training. Methods: Thirty-three highly trained individuals were randomly assigned to probiotic (PRO, $n = 17$) or placebo (PLA, $n = 16$) groups using double blind procedures, receiving either 1×10^{10} colony forming units (CFU) of a multi-species probiotic (*Bifidobacterium bifidum* W23, *Bifidobacterium lactis* W51, *Enterococcus faecium* W54, *Lactobacillus acidophilus* W22, *Lactobacillus brevis* W63, and *Lactococcus lactis* W58) or placebo once per day for 12 weeks. The serum concentrations of tryptophan, phenylalanine and their primary catabolites kynurenine and tyrosine, as well as the concentration of the immune activation marker neopterin were determined at baseline and after 12 weeks, both at rest and immediately after exercise. Participants completed a daily diary to identify any infectious symptoms. Results: After 12 weeks of treatment, post-exercise tryptophan levels were lowered by 11% (a significant change) in the PLA group compared to the concentrations measured before the intervention ($p = 0.02$), but remained unchanged in the PRO group. The ratio of subjects taking the placebo who experienced one or more URTI symptoms was increased 2.2-fold compared to those on probiotics (PLA 0.79, PRO 0.35; $p = 0.02$). Conclusion: Data indicate reduced exercise-induced tryptophan degradation rates in the PRO group. Daily supplementation with probiotics limited exercise-induced drops in tryptophan levels and reduced the incidence of URTI, however, did not benefit athletic performance.

Keywords: intense exercise; kynurenine; tryptophan; probiotics; upper respiratory tract infections

1. Introduction

Numerous studies have shown that prolonged intense physical exercise is associated with a transient depression of immune function in athletes. While moderate exercise beneficially influences the immune system [1], a heavy schedule of training and competition can lead to immune impairment associated with an increased risk of upper respiratory tract infections (URTIs) due to altered immune function [2,3]. It has been suggested that exhaustive exercise creates a potential 'open window' of decreased host protection, during which viruses and bacteria can gain a foothold, increasing the risk of developing an infection [4]. During major competitions of 2–3 weeks duration, typically about 7% of athletes experience at least one episode of illness and about half of these are respiratory [5]. Exercise immunological studies reported that infection episodes were preceded by declines in immunoglobulin A (IgA) in saliva [6–8]. Furthermore, results suggest a possible mechanism for the increased incidence of infection during intensified training via modulation of type 1/type 2 T lymphocyte distributions [9].

Physical exercise and sports influence immunoregulatory circuits which, as a primary response, involve the production of forward regulatory cytokines is followed by counter-regulation leading to an immunosuppressed state [3,10,11]. Downstream biochemical events include changes in tryptophan (Trp) metabolism when T helper cell type 1 (Th1-type) cytokine interferon-γ (IFN-γ) is released and induces tryptophan-degrading enzyme indoleamine 2,3-dioxygenase (IDO-1). In turn, blood concentrations of Trp become reduced, leading to various potential consequences [12]. The essential amino acid Trp is not only a precursor of the serotonin biosynthesis pathway but is also the key element for the formation of the energy carrier and coenzyme nicotinamide-adenine-dinucleotide NAD and its reduced form NADH via the so-called kynurenine (Kyn) pathway [13,14]. Recently, exhaustive aerobic exercise in athletes was reported to significantly impact on Trp–Kyn metabolism [15]. Results indicate an involvement of IDO-1 activation in enhanced Trp catabolism and Kyn production following demanding exercise [15]. The close association of Trp metabolites with neuropsychopharmacologically relevant metabolites may have special consequences for athletes since it influences immunosurveillance and the development of infections as well training adherence because of disturbed neurotransmitter biochemistry [16].

Trp is also an important target for the gut and brain interaction [17]. In addition to its resorption from dietary components, the composition of gut bacteria—the microbiome—is of enormous importance in the regulation of Trp. Available data suggest a role for the gut microbiota in actually modulating Trp and hence having control over serotonin levels in the host [18]. Recently, an inverse correlation of serum levels of Trp, tyrosine, and phenylalanine with concentration of fecal calprotectin, a marker for gut leakiness, has been reported in patients suffering from Alzheimer's disease, thus indicating a close relationship between the intestinal barrier function and aromatic amino acid concentration in the blood [19]. Furthermore, there is growing body of evidence indicating that the microbiota is sensitive to physiological changes associated with exercise [20,21]. For example, acute aerobic exercise reduces the expression of toll-like receptors (TLRs) in the monocyte cell-surface, contributing to post-exercise immunodepression, while over the long-term, a decrease in TLR expression may represent a beneficial effect because it decreases the inflammatory capacity of leukocytes, thus altering whole body chronic inflammation [22]. TLRs can activate dendritic cells, which are associated with the attenuation of immune activation and inflammation protection [20]. Notably, IDO-1 has been identified in mucosal Cluster of Differentiation 103 -expressing dendritic cells and has already been claimed to be a possible therapeutic target for gut disorders [23].

Dietary supplements containing probiotics can modify the population of the gut microflora and may provide a practical means of enhancing gut and systemic immune function, which was shown to be beneficial by reducing the infection frequency in sensible groups, e.g., elderly in group homes or children [24,25]. However, studies in these subject groups might not be reflective of athletes who have different gut microbiota [26]. Exercise and associated dietary extremes were shown to increase gut microbial diversity in comparison to sedentary people [27]. Some studies have established that probiotic intake can improve low-grade inflammation [28,29] and enhance resistance to URTI in athletes [30–32]. In a previous study, Lamprecht and colleagues found that adequate probiotic supplementation composed of six strains consisting of *Bifidobacterium bifidum* W23,

Bifidobacterium lactis W51, *Enterococcus faecium* W54, *Lactobacillus acidophilus* W22, *Lactobacillus brevis* W63, and *Lactococcus lactis* W58 could improve redox hemostasis and low-grade inflammation in men under sustained exercise stress [29]. The mechanisms behind these observations have not been widely investigated but may include direct interaction with gut microbiota, interaction with mucosal immune system and modulation of lung macrophage and T cell functions [33]. For example, one study observed that the IFN-γ response (a potent stimulus for IDO-1) was moderately higher with probiotic treatment than with placebo, associated with a significant reduction in the number of days of respiratory illness symptoms in highly trained distance runners [30]. Since Trp availability is primarily regulated via the Kyn pathway, the catabolism of amino acid Trp via Kyn may play an important role on the risk of developing an infection.

The aim of the present study was to examine the effect of a probiotic supplement on the incidence of URTI and Trp metabolism after exhaustive aerobic exercise in trained athletes during three months of winter training We hypothesized that daily supplementation with probiotics is beneficial in reducing the incidence of URTI in athletes during training periods in winter and is associated with modulation of the Trp—Kyn metabolic pathways.

2. Materials and Methods

2.1. Subjects

Thirty-three healthy and trained volunteer athletes (mean age 26.7 years; average body mass index 22 kg/m^2; average peak oxygen uptake 51.4 mL/kg/min) participated in this study that was conducted at the Department of Sport Science at the Leopold Franzens University of Innsbruck, Austria. Individuals were invited to participate if they were 20–35 years of age, non-smokers, had no previous history of muscle disorders and were free of heart, kidney, lung, neurologic, and psychiatric diseases. Athletes with a cardiorespiratory response and fitness of ≥150% of reference values during maximal exercise [34] were included. A questionnaire about medical history and previous training was filled out by each participant. In total, 33 individuals were enrolled with 29 participants (13 men 16 women) completing the study. Baseline characteristics of the subjects are presented in Table 1.

Table 1. Baseline characteristics, nutrition and performance data of the participants.

Variable	Unit	Probiotics (*n* = 14) Mean ± SD	Placebo (*n* = 15) Mean ± SD
Gender	male/female	8/6	5/10
Age	year	25.7 ± 3.5	26.6 ± 3.5
BMI	kg/m^2	22.2 ± 1.5	21.2 ± 2.7
Weight	kg	67.4 ± 9.6	62.9 ± 11.1
Body cell mass	kg	31.2 ± 6.6	28.7 ± 7.4
Total body fat	%	20.1 ± 5.7	19.5 ± 4.4
VO$_{2max}$	mL/kg/min	55.1 ± 6.4	47.5 ± 7.1 **
P$_{max}$	watt	325 ± 54.2	274 ± 51.6 *
P$_{rel}$	watt/kg	4.8 ± 0.3	4.3 ± 0.4 **
P$_{TT}$	watt	222 ± 41.9	181 ± 38.3 *
Energy intake	kcal/day	2821 ± 1374	2840 ± 1161
REE	kcal/day	1602 ± 206	1519 ± 2031
Protein	%	14.9 ± 3.3	15.0 ± 3.5
Carbohydrates	%	49.5 ± 12.4	49.3 ± 12.7
Fat	%	32.5 ± 10.8	33.0 ± 12.1
Fibers	g	33.0 ± 10.1	32.0 ± 14.2
Alcohol	g	11.1 ± 10.7	9.4 ± 9.5
Water	L	3.38 ± 0.58	3.37 ± 0.84

Values are means ± SD; Significant difference between the groups: * $p < 0.05$; ** $p < 0.01$; BMI: body mass index; VO$_{2max}$ = peak oxygen uptake; P$_{max}$ = peak power output; P$_{rel}$ = peak power output related to body weight; P$_{TT}$ = Time-trial power output; REE = resting energy expenditure.

Subjects who met the inclusion criteria of the study were randomly assigned to the treatment or placebo group. The randomization code was held by a third party and handed over for statistical analyses after collection of all data. All of the participants were informed of the risks and potential discomforts associated with the investigation and signed a written consent to participate. The study was approved by the Board for Ethical Questions in Science Ethics at the Leopold Franzens University of Innsbruck according to the principles expressed in the Declaration of Helsinki.

2.2. Study Intervention

Subjects randomized to probiotics (PRO, n = 17) received boxes with sachets containing multi-species probiotics composed of six strains consisting of *Bifidobacterium bifidum* W23, *Bifidobacterium lactis* W51, *Enterococcus faecium* W54, *Lactobacillus acidophilus* W22, *Lactobacillus brevis* W63, and *Lactococcus lactis* W58 (Ecologic® Performance, Winclove B.V., Amsterdam, The Netherlands). The total cell count was adjusted to 2.5×10^9 colony forming units (CFU) per gram. The candidate strains were selected upon their survival in the gastrointestinal tract, activity, intestinal barrier function, and anti-inflammatory properties and were used in a previous study on immune health in athletes [29]. The matrix consisting of cornstarch, maltodextrin, vegetable protein, $MgSO_4$, $MnSO_4$ and KCl. Subjects were instructed to take 1 sachet of 4 g per day, which is equivalent to 1×10^{10} CFU/day, with 100–125 mL of plain water, one hour prior to breakfast and throughout the 12 weeks. Those subjects assigned to the placebo group (PLA, n = 16) received identical boxes and sachets with the same instructions for use.

2.3. Study Protocol

During the three-month intervention period (January 2015 to March 2015) subjects were asked to maintain their normal diet and to continue with their normal training programs. In addition, participants agreed to avoid taking medicine including anti-inflammatory drugs (e.g., aspirin, ibuprofen, voltaren) and antibiotics, additional probiotics and dietary supplements such as fish oil, vitamins (vitamin C, vitamin E) and minerals (selenium). Consumption of alcohol (>10 and 20 g for women and men, respectively, per day), or any fermented dairy products (e.g., yoghurt) was not permitted during this period. During the first visit to the laboratory, measures of participants' weight and height were obtained using standardized methods and used to calculate body mass index (BMI, kg/m^2). Prior to and at the end of the study, all subjects were tested for body fat (in percent of body weight), body cell mass (kg), and resting energy expenditure (kcal/day) using the bioelectrical impedance analysis (BIA) method (BIA-2000-M, Data Input, Pöcking, Germany). Prior to the first blood draw and after 12 weeks of supplementation, participants were asked to complete a three-day food record to evaluate energy and nutrient intake. Diet records were analyzed for total calories, protein, carbohydrate, fat, alcohol, and water intake using "nut.s science" nutritional software (dato Denkwerkzeuge, Vienna, Austria). Weekly training (modality, frequency, intensity, volume) and illness (URTI symptoms and gastrointestinal GI complaints symptoms) logs were kept.

The illness symptoms listed on the self-constructed questionnaire, modified according to Gleeson et al. (2011) [31] were sore throat, runny nose, cough, fever, and weakness. Subjects were asked to rate the severity of their symptoms (very light, light, moderate, severe, very severe). The GI discomfort symptoms listed on the questionnaire were abdominal pain, diarrhea, loss of appetite, vomiting, and others. The incidence score relates to the number of participants who reported symptoms in each arm of the study. One or more symptoms on at least two consecutive days were defined as an episode of illness. Symptoms with an interval of only one day were counted as the same episode.

2.4. Exercise Tests

In the morning of the exercise test a standardized breakfast was provided 2 h prior to strenuous exercise tests (379 kcal; 88 energy percent carbohydrates, 11 energy percent proteins, and 1 energy percent fat). The composition of this standardized breakfast is shown in Table 2.

Table 2. Composition of the standardized breakfast 2 h prior to strenuous exercise tests.

Food	Energy (kcal)	Protein (g)	Carbohydrates (g)	Fat (g)
2 wheat rolls 100 g	260	8.70	52.7	0.90
Marmalade/jam 50 g	114	0.30	28.0	0.00
250 mL tea	5	0.75	0.25	0.25
250 mL water	-	-	-	-
Total	379	9.75	80.95	1.15
Meal energy (%)		11	88	1

For eligibility testing all subjects performed an incremental cycle ergometer exercise test until exhaustion. Cycle ergometry was performed on an electronically braked ergometer (Ergometrics 900, Ergoline, Germany) and started at a workload of 50/75 W (women/men) for 5 min (warm up) with a following increase in workload of 25 W per minute until exhaustion. Exhaustion was defined as the state when the pedaling rate dropped below 60 rpm. Heart rate and ventilatory parameters were monitored continuously (Oxycon mobile, Jaeger, Germany). Peak power output (P_{max}) was defined as the last completed workload rate plus the fraction of time spent in the final uncompleted work rate multiplied by 25 W [35]. Peak oxygen uptake (VO_{2max}) was defined as the highest 30-s average during the test.

After a 20 min resting period, athletes performed a 20-min maximal time-trial on a cycle ergometer (RBM Cyclus 2, Leipzig, Germany) as described by Faulhaber and colleagues [35]. Briefly, the cycle ergometer was shifted to a fixed pedal force in which power output was dependent on the pedaling rate. Pedal force for each participant was set so that pedaling at 100 rpm would produce about 70% (rounded to 5 W) of peak power output, which was determined by the incremental cycle ergometry. During the test, cyclists were strongly encouraged to choose a maximal pedaling rate that could be maintained for the respective test duration. The main outcome measurement was mean power output during the 20-min test, which was automatically calculated by the software of the ergometer. The participants were allowed to drink water ad libitum. Three months later this procedure was repeated on the same cycle ergometer and with the same investigator.

2.5. Blood Measurements

We conducted blood collections from the participants in the supine position from a medial cubital vein at baseline and after 12 weeks at rest and within 5 min after exercise (four blood draws per study participant). After centrifugation for 10 min cells were removed and plasma samples were frozen at $-20\,^{\circ}$C until analysis. Serum concentrations of Trp and Kyn as well as concentrations of phenylalanine (Phe) and tyrosine (Tyr) were determined by high-performance liquid chromatography (HPLC), as previously described [36,37]. The ratios of Kyn/Trp and Phe/Tyr were calculated as indexes of Trp degradation and phenylalanine 4-hydroxylase (PAH) activity, respectively. Pro-inflammatory cascades were found to be associated with disturbed PAH activity [37]. Serum neopterin concentrations were measured by ELISA (BRAHMS Diagnostics, Hennigsdorf, Germany) following the manufacturer's instructions [38].

2.6. Statistical Analysis

Per protocol analyses were performed using SPSS (IBM SPSS Statistics Version 22, IBM Corp., Armonk, NY, USA). Normality in the distribution of data was tested using the Kolmogorov-Smirnov's test and Boxplots. In the case of Gaussian distribution, baseline characteristics, performance data, nutrient and biological markers were compared by unpaired Student's *t*-test or Mann-Whitney-*U*-Test. Changes in variables during the study were analyzed by univariate analysis of variance (ANOVA) for parametric variables. The Wilcoxon-signed rank and Friedman test were applied to non-parametric data. Spearman's rank correlation was used to assess the association between two variables. Partial eta-squared values were calculated to estimate the effect of any statistically significant differences found. Using the guidelines of Cohen [39], 0.01 = small effect, 0.06 = moderate effect, and 0.14 = large effect. A *p*-value of less than 0.05 (two-tailed) was considered to indicate statistical significance. Data are presented as mean values ± standard deviation (SD) or by mean values ± standard error of the mean (SEM).

Sample size calculation was based on changes in exercise-induced Trp levels [40] from baseline to the end of the 12-week intervention between the PRO group and the control. We estimated between 10 and 12 subjects per group—depending on SD and effect size—to reach a probability of error (alpha/2) of 5% and 80% power. Allowing for a drop-out rate of 30%, 16 subjects per group were recruited.

3. Results

3.1. Study Population

Twenty-nine of the 33 randomized subjects completed the full program and entered statistical analyses. Three withdrew because of injury or persistent illness with antibiotic medications, one because of a longer training interruption. Returned sachet count after the treatment period revealed a compliance rate >95% in both groups (97.6% in the probiotics group, 98.8% in the control group). The lowest level of compliance for a subject was 86.9%. A CONSORT (Consolidated Standards of Reporting Trials) diagram outlining participant recruitment is depicted Figure 1.

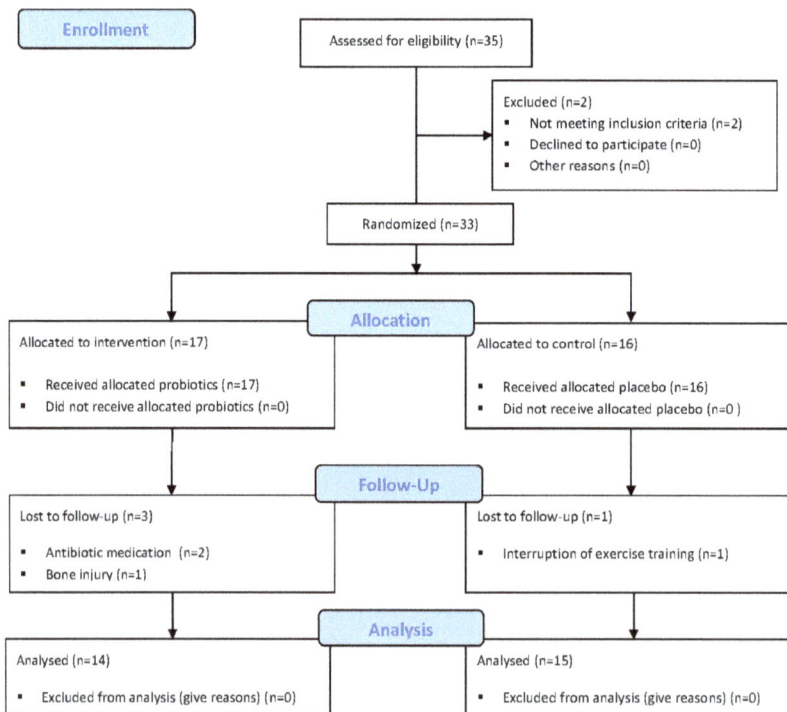

Figure 1. Flow of participations through each stage of the trial.

At baseline, a significant gender-dependent difference (females were overrepresented in the control group), VO_{2max} and Trp was observed between groups (*p* < 0.05). Females had a lower BMI, VO_{2max}, and mean power output during the 20-min test (P_{TT}) compared to male athletes, as Kyn levels were lower in females (*p* = 0.019). None of the other parameters were influenced by gender.

3.2. Training Loads

Analysis of training loads indicated that the weekly training of the aerobic system, mainly continuous endurance training at moderate intensity (60% to 80% VO_{2max}), varied significantly between the groups over the 12-week treatment period (Figure 2). The means were significantly higher in the probiotics group as compared to the placebo group: 8.0 ± 2.3 and 6.6 ± 4.3 h per week endurance training, respectively ($U = 2.597$, $p < 0.001$).

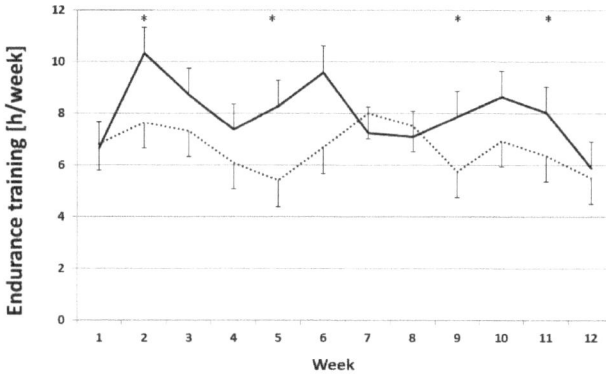

Figure 2. Training loads for endurance training (h/week) over the study period for the participants who completed the study. Graph shows mean ± standard error of the mean (SEM); * $p < 0.05$ (Mann-Whitney U test). Asterisks depict weeks with significant differences between PRO (—) and PLA (···) groups. PRO: probiotics-supplemented group; PLA: placebo group.

3.3. Body Composition, Nutrition, and Performance

After 12 weeks of treatment, there was no significant difference between probiotic supplementation groups and placebo groups in anthropometric characteristics, body composition, and food intake ($p > 0.05$). Performance (VO_{2max}) remained unchanged over time and still differed significantly between groups in week 12 ($p < 0.05$). Resting energy expenditure (REE, kcal/day) was significantly different between groups after 12-weeks of the study (mean ± SEM: 1617 ± 57 kcal/day and 1518 ± 56 kcal/day for PRO and PLA, respectively; $p < 0.05$, $\eta^2 = 0.13$; Figure 3).

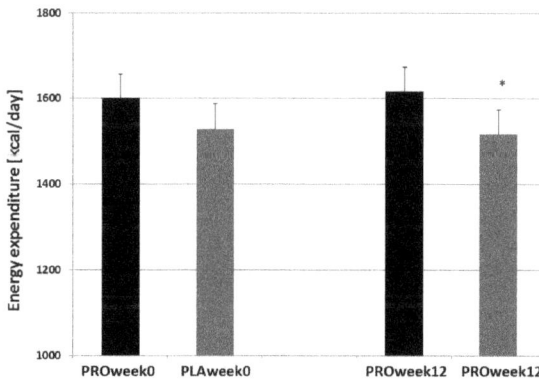

Figure 3. Resting energy expenditure (REE; (kcal/day)) in trained athletes before and after 12 weeks of treatment. PRO: probiotics-supplemented group ($n = 14$); PLA: placebo group ($n = 15$). Graph shows mean + SEM; * $p < 0.05$ (ANOVA).

3.4. Amino Acids

At the beginning of the study, exhaustive exercise induced a decrease in Trp levels in both the probiotic and the placebo group (Table 3). At the end of the experimental protocol, the exercise-induced Trp shift was comparable to the shift in week 0 in subjects who ingested probiotics but was more pronounced in in the placebo group (approximately 10% lower than in week 0, $p < 0.05$) (Figure 4).

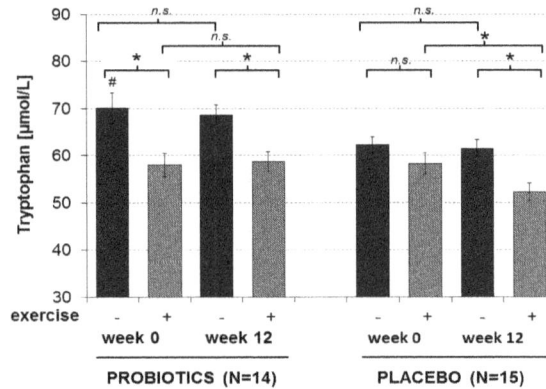

Figure 4. Tryptophan concentrations before and after exhaustive exercise in the probiotic ($n = 14$) and placebo ($n = 15$) group of trained athletes before and after 12 weeks of treatment (four blood draws per athlete). Graph shows mean $\pm$ SEM; * $p < 0.05$: Wilcoxon, # $p < 0.05$: week 0, before exercise placebo vs. probiotics: Mann-Whitney-U, n.s. = not statistically significant.

These data indicate reduced Trp degradation rates in subjects supplemented with probiotics, although this effect was not significant ($p = 0.13$, $\eta^2 = 0.08$). It should be mentioned that baseline Trp concentrations were slightly but significantly lower in the placebo group compared to the probiotics group, most probably due do the different percentage of female athletes in the groups. In parallel to Trp decrease, Kyn/Trp and neopterin levels were increased after exercise in both study groups at both time points.

Further, at the beginning of the study, VO$_{2max}$ correlated significantly with baseline concentrations of Trp ($rs = 0.562$, $p = 0.001$) and this relation remained significant after 12 weeks of treatment ($r = 0.497$, $p = 0.006$) but was no longer present after intense exercise.

Tyrosine levels significantly increased and Phe/Tyr significantly decreased with exhaustive exercise ($p = 0.018$ and $p < 0.001$, respectively), but there were no significant time-dependent differences between groups. Serum concentrations of Phe were not significantly affected, either by exercise or by supplementation (Table 3).

3.5. Immune System Biomarkers

Exhausting exercise was associated with a strong increase in neopterin levels up to +61% ($U = 4.420$, $p < 0.001$) and +63% of pre-exercise values ($U = 4.660$, $p < 0.001$), before and after 12 weeks of treatment, respectively, with no significant differences between and within groups over time. However, this increase was significantly influenced by endurance training volume with a strong inverse correlation between the athletes' training status and the concentrations of neopterin at exhaustion ($rs = -0.502$, $p < 0.01$).

Kyn concentrations were slightly increased with exercise by 7% ($U = 2.671$, $p < 0.01$) before and by 3% ($U = 0.923$, n.s.) after 12 weeks of intervention, contributing to the elevation of the Kyn/Trp ratios by 22% ($U = 4.544$, $p < 0.001$) and by 21% ($U = 4.433$, $p < 0.001$), respectively. Exercise induced a change in Kyn levels with time (ΔKyn), with a significant decline being overserved in the PLA group ($p = 0.04$), whereas an increase was seen in the PRO group, but this effect was not significant between groups ($p = 0.05$, $\eta^2 = 0.13$). At baseline, neopterin and Kyn/Trp ratios correlated significantly ($rs = 0.490$, $p < 0.01$), with the association even becoming slightly stronger upon exercise ($rs = 0.512$, $p < 0.01$). After 12 weeks there was no longer a significant relationship between pre-exercise neopterin and Kyn/Trp levels ($rs = 0.280$, n.s.), but it became again significant after exercise ($rs = 0.583$, $p = 0.001$). At the same time, higher neopterin levels correlated with lower Trp concentrations ($rs = -0.384$, $p < 0.05$).

Table 3. Amino acids and immune biomarkers in 29 athletes before and after 12 weeks of treatment either supplemented with probiotics or placebo measured before (PRE) and after exercise (POST).

Probiotics ($n = 14$)	Baseline PRE	Baseline POST	Week 12 PRE	Week 12 POST
Tryptophan (μmol/L)	70.07 ± 3.20 [a,e]	57.99 ± 2.47 [b]	68.64 ± 2.12 [c,k]	58.76 ± 2.11 [d]
Kynurenine (μmol/L)	1.98 ± 0.11	1.97 ± 0.07	1.83 ± 0.10	1.92 ± 0.11
Kyn/Trp (μmol/mmol)	28.35 ± 1.16 [f]	34.50 ± 1.46	26.94 ± 1.51 [l]	33.32 ± 2.19
Neopterin (nmol/L)	5.19 ± 0.23 [g]	8.43 ± 1.00	4.92 ± 0.31 [m]	7.74 ± 0.86
Tyrosine (μmol/L)	138.58 ± 29.96 [h]	145.06 ± 6.23	147.25 ± 24.01 [n]	149.22 ± 5.60
Phenylalanine (μmol/L)	69.59 ± 8.27 [i]	68.72 ± 2.06	72.16 ± 1.99 [o]	71.76 ± 1.90
Phe/Tyr (mol/mol)	0.52 ± 0.08 [j]	0.48 ± 0.01	0.50 ± 0.03 [p]	0.49 ± 0.02
Placebo ($n = 15$)	Baseline PRE	Baseline POST	Week 12 PRE	Week 12 POST
Tryptophan (μmol/L)	62.27 ± 1.72	58.27 ± 2.37	61.50 ± 1.84	52.26 ± 1.86
Kynurenine (μmol/L)	1.77 ± 0.13	2.02 ± 0.07	1.75 ± 0.08	1.77 ± 0.09
Kyn/Trp (μmol/mmol)	28.38 ± 1.81	34.49 ± 2.17	28.49 ± 1.03	34.03 ± 1.51
Neopterin (nmol/L)	6.63 ± 0.95	10.48 ± 1.56	5.65 ± 0.70	9.55 ± 2.06
Tyrosine (μmol/L)	131.15 ± 5.28	137.40 ± 5.42	126.41 ± 6.29	129.28 ± 5.76
Phenylalanine (μmol/L)	69.23 ± 2.45	68.55 ± 1.87	72.53 ± 1.67	70.09 ± 2.71
Phe/Tyr (mol/mol)	0.53 ± 0.02	0.50 ± 0.02	0.59 ± 0.03	0.55 ± 0.02

Values are means ± SEM. [a] $U = 2.095$, $p = 0.036$ (baseline PRE placebo vs. probiotics), [b] $U = 0.284$, $p = 0.777$ (baseline POST placebo vs. probiotics), [c] $U = 2.706$, $p = 0.007$ (week 12 PRE placebo vs. probiotics), [d] $U = 2.139$, $p = 0.032$ (week 12 POST placebo vs. probiotics), [e] $U = 3.384$, $p = 0.001$ (all athletes baseline PRE vs. POST), [f] $U = 4.660$, $p < 0.001$ (all athletes baseline PRE vs. POST), [g] $U = 4.420$, $p < 0.001$ (all athletes baseline PRE vs. POST), [h] $U = 2.011$, $p = 0.044$ (all athletes week 12 PRE vs. POST), [i] $U = 0.270$, $p = 0.787$ (all athletes week 12 PRE vs. post), [j] $U = 3.357$, $p = 0.001$ (all athletes week 12 PRE vs. post), [k] $U = 4.703$, $p < 0.001$ (all athletes week 12 PRE vs. POST), [l] $U = 4.433$, $p < 0.001$ (all athletes week 12 PRE vs. post), [m] $U = 4.544$, $p < 0.001$ (all athletes week 12 PRE vs. post), [n] $U = 0.443$, $p = 0.658$ (all athletes week 12 PRE vs. post), [o] $U = 0.660$, $p = 0.510$ (all athletes week 12 PRE vs. post), [p] $U = 1.208$, $p = 0.227$ (all athletes week 12 PRE vs. post).

3.6. Infection Incidence

Only one participant on the placebo experienced GI-discomfort symptoms during the study period. Analysis of the URTI-symptom questionnaires indicated that 55% (16 subjects) of the cohort experienced an URTI episode during the 12-week study period. Thirteen subjects did not experience any URTI episode during the study period. Before supplementation, 10 subjects on placebo and 12 subjects on probiotics experienced one or more URTI symptoms over the prior three months. After 12 weeks of treatment, 11 subjects on placebo and 5 subjects on probiotics experienced one or more URTI symptoms during the study period (Figure 5). The proportion of subjects who experienced one or more URTI symptoms during the study period was 2.2-fold higher in the placebo group than in the probiotics group (PLA 0.79, PRO 0.35; $p = 0.016$).

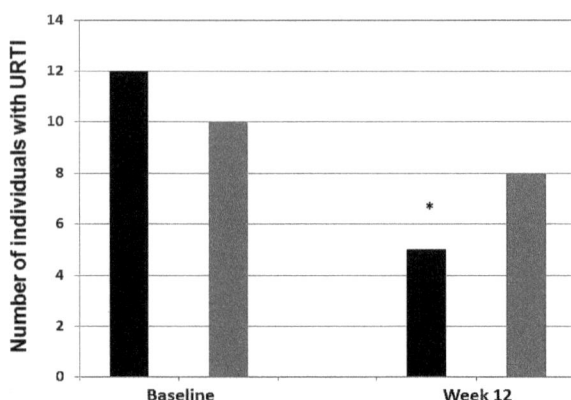

Figure 5. Incidence of upper respiratory tract infections (URTIs) in trained athletes before and after 12 weeks of treatment. The share of subjects on placebo (gray columns, 0.79) who experienced 1 or more URTI symptoms was 2.2-fold greater than those on probiotics (black columns, 0.35; * p = 0.016).

Individuals who developed URTI had higher degradation rates of Trp before exercise compared to those without URTI (Table 4). Additionally, a running nose, but not cough was associated with higher Kyn/Trp ratios compared to those individuals without such symptoms.

Table 4. Association between upper respiratory tract infection (URTI) incidence at week 12 and degree of tryptophan breakdown as indicated by Kyn/Trp (mean ± SEM). Bold text indicates a statistically significant correlation with a p-value less than 0.05.

URTI	Baseline PRE	Baseline POST	Week 12 PRE	Week 12 POST
yes	28.9 ± 1.7	34.9 ± 6.0	31.1 ± 5.1	38.9 ± 7.3
no	28.2 ± 6.5	34.4 ± 7.2	26.7 ± 4.3	32.0 ± 6.0
U/p-value	0.535/0.592	0.102/0.919	**2.039/0.041**	**2.090/0.037**

4. Discussion

This study illustrates a significant influence of probiotic supplementation on athletes who performed intense exercise. On the one hand, increased training load was measured and on the other hand, the rate of infectious complications was markedly reduced. However, whether this is based on the actual probiotic supplementation or due to other cofounding factors (baseline fitness, gender) is currently unknown. In addition, some of these influences appeared to be connected with alterations in Trp metabolism, e.g., Trp breakdown rates at the end of the study were significantly higher in individuals who developed infections as compared to those who did not. However, it was not determined whether higher Kyn/Trp ratios were observed, particularly in those individuals who experienced an infection close to the end of the study and it still remains to be elucidated whether there is a more direct association between probiotic supplementation and reduced Trp breakdown. Alternatively, different training loads between groups may have affected Trp metabolism, rather than the actions of the probiotic, since regular endurance exercise causes adaptations in Kyn metabolism [41].

4.1. Training Adherence

Supplementation with probiotics was associated with higher training loads vs. placebo. One explanation for these findings could be that probiotics may enable better performance capabilities and training adherence when the risk of URTI development is reduced, as individuals with fewer episodes of infections such as common colds and runny noses are able to train more often and harder than others. However, it could also be possible that existing URTI symptoms influenced training performance to a lesser extent in athletes on probiotics [31]. In any case, performance was not increased even with the higher training load in the probiotics group as compared to the placebo group, even if the training load was indeed an effect of the supplementation.

A potential role of Trp metabolism could be of relevance for the effects of probiotics on training adherence because individuals on probiotics showed higher serum Trp levels than those without such supplements. Higher serum Trp levels may improve the Trp transport into brain and support serotonin metabolism, which can influence an individual's sensation of fatigue and thus potentially affect training adherence and performance [42]. Interestingly, VO_{2max} correlated with pre-exercise Trp levels supporting a role of Trp metabolism in training performance. It could further relate to the recent findings of Kyn metabolism in skeletal muscle mediating resilience to stress-induced depression with endurance training, whereas less energetically demanding exercise protocols, such as high-force eccentric exercise, did not lead to adaptations in Kyn metabolism [41,43].

4.2. Tryptophan and the Gut Microbiome

Post exercise serum Trp levels declined but this was only true in the placebo group whereas serum Trp levels did not change but remained stable in individuals supplemented with probiotics. This difference could be due to an effect of probiotics on the microbiome composition in the gut, which may affect downstream immunoregulatory pathways. Alterations in the gut milieu influence Trp metabolism and the absorption and availability of the essential amino acids [17]. In addition, the altered composition of the microbiome may increase the biosynthesis of Trp by specific bacteria. Research in rats has shown that administration of the probiotic *Bifidobacteria infantis* attenuated pro-inflammatory immune responses following mitogen stimulation and, furthermore, there was a marked increase in plasma concentrations of Trp in the *Bifidobacteria*-treated rats when compared to controls [44], suggesting that bacteria can improve the available serotonin pool and ultimately elicit communication between the gut and the brain via serotonin [17,18]. In the present study, probiotics were able to selectively modulate Trp concentrations since no influence on the metabolism of Phe, another essential amino acid, was observed. Interestingly, no detectable effect of supplementation was found on concentrations of immune system biomarker neopterin and also Kyn/Trp ratios were not modulated. Further studies will be necessary to address these open questions.

4.3. Probiotics to Prevent URTIs

Some well-controlled studies in athletes have shown that daily probiotic ingestion results in fewer days of respiratory illness and lower severity of URTI symptoms [30–32]. A meta-analysis using data from both athlete and non-athlete studies concluded that there is a likely benefit of reducing URTI incidence [45]. The likely mechanisms of action for probiotics include direct interaction with the gut microbiota, interaction with the mucosal immune system and immune signaling to a variety of organs and systems [46]. A recent report by He and colleagues noted gender differences in the number and duration of respiratory-tract illness symptoms in endurance athletes during a winter training period indicating that females may be more susceptible to URTI than their male counterparts [5]. Furthermore, supplementation with *Lactobacillus fermentum* was associated with a reduction of the symptoms in clinical indices of URTI at high training loads in well-trained male cyclists but not in females, for whom there was some evidence of an increase in symptoms [47]. Thus, females may benefit from higher doses of probiotics. In the present study, females were overrepresented in the control group who experienced more than double the URTI symptoms, accompanied by higher Trp breakdown rates compared to those on probiotics. However, gender is not the basis for the observed effect on URTI incidence in this study. The interaction between gender and URTI was not statistically significant in either group before and after 12 weeks of treatment (Table 5). It remains unclear whether these findings are related to the influence of gender on Trp catabolism and further work is required to address this issue.

Table 5. Interaction between gender and illness symptoms in 29 athletes before and after 12 weeks of treatment either supplemented with probiotics (PRO) or placebo (PLA).

Illness Symptoms		Baseline U	p	Week 12 U	p
URTI	PRO	0.212	0.832	0.155	0.877
	PLA	0.748	0.454	0.399	0.690
Runny nose	PRO	0.212	0.832	0.329	0.742
	PLA	0	1	1.080	0.280
Cough	PRO	0.931	0.352	0.362	0.717
	PLA	1.497	0.134	1.497	0.134
Sore throat	PRO	1.041	0.298	0.866	0.386
	PLA	0.374	0.708	1.497	0.134
Fever	PRO	0.823	0.411	0	1
	PLA	0	1	0	1
Weakness	PRO	0.866	0.386	0	1
	PLA	0.519	0.604	0.519	0.604

Taken together, probiotic supplements on a daily basis enhance resistance to URTI in athletes and offer thus a potential intervention strategy during heavy exercise training periods, especially in the winter months. A prerequisite for robust immune function during intense exercise is, however, to avoid a long-term energy deficit, deficiencies of macronutrients and essential micronutrients, and to ingest carbohydrate during exercise [48].

4.4. Study Strengths and Limitations

This study has several strengths and limitations. A major strength was the randomized controlled, double-blinded, placebo-controlled study design and the use of an objective and standardized test for assessment of peak oxygen uptake and peak power output. The study was conducted with a multi-species probiotic consisting of *Bifidobacterium bifidum* W23, *Bifidobacterium lactis* W51, *Enterococcus faecium* W54, *Lactobacillus acidophilus* W22, *Lactobacillus brevis* W63, and *Lactococcus lactis* W58 at a total dose of 1 billion CFU. Total probiotic cell count varied between 11×10^9 CFU/g at the beginning of the study and 7×10^9 CFU/g at the end of the study. The individual amount of each strain is unknown. Returned sachet count after the treatment period revealed a high level of compliance in both groups (>95%). The 80% cutoff has been used for a majority of studies on medication adherence, especially for cardiovascular medications, since adherence based on this cutoff point has been associated with both intermediate and strong outcomes [49]. Although the 80% cutoff appears reasonable, the optimal level of adherence for dietary supplements may be higher than current cutoffs (e.g., 80% to 100%). Limitations of the study are the relatively small sample size and significant differences in gender composition of the subpopulations, which may have contributed to differences in illness symptoms and physiological parameters, e.g., VO_{2max} and weekly training logs between males and females. We did not randomize by body weight, performance, or any other variable that might have given us a better chance to catch differences in outcomes since women—overrepresented in the control group—generally show a lower VO_{2max}. Indeed, West et al. (2011) showed gender difference with probiotic supplementation in athletes with a significant reduction in respiratory infections (duration and severity) in males, but no effect in females [47]. Therefore, we analyzed the influence of gender on URTI. No significant effect of gender was observed for either group, before or after 12 weeks of treatment. However, Trp metabolism can be influenced to some extend by gender differences [50]. This aspect is mainly relevant for the results obtained at the baseline when Kyn levels were found to differ between groups. Another limitation of the study is that we were not able to calculate the severity of illness symptoms because of the high number of no replies. Furthermore, infections were only symptomatically monitored, but not serologically proven. It is assumed that

Nutrients **2016**, *8*, 752

common pathogens either of bacterial or viral origin have been involved in and could contribute to alterations of, e.g., Trp metabolism, which, because of its immunoregulatory influence, could increase the risk of such infections. Longitudinal research will be needed to clarify causal ordering.

5. Conclusions and Future Research

Daily supplementation with probiotics was found to be associated with a lower frequency of URTIs in athletes who underwent endurance training and seems to be beneficial in increasing training efficacy during training periods, however, no benefits to athletic performance were observed. Some of these effects appeared to be connected with alterations in Trp metabolism. Still, these findings are of a preliminary nature and warrant further investigation into the precise mechanisms involved. In addition, more research is required to clarify issues of strains, dose–response, mechanisms and best practice models for probiotic implementation in various sports disciplines. It should be further investigated as to whether regular exercise per se affects human microbiota characteristics, for how long and how much exercise is needed.

Acknowledgments: This study was sponsored by Winclove B.V., Amsterdam, The Netherlands, and Institute Allergosan GmbH, Graz, Austria. The Institute Allergosan GmbH, Graz, Austria covered the costs to publish in open access.

Author Contributions: B.S. and M.B. conceived and designed the experiments; D.G. and M.S. performed the experiments; J.M.G. and D.F. analyzed the data; H.G. contributed reagents/materials/analysis tools; B.S. and D.F. wrote the paper.

Conflicts of Interest: The authors declare no conflict of interest. The founding sponsors had no role in the design of the study; in the collection, analyses, or interpretation of data; in the writing of the manuscript, and in the decision to publish the results.

References

1. Nieman, D.C.; Henson, D.A.; Austin, M.D.; Sha, W. Upper respiratory tract infection is reduced in physically fit and active adults. *Br. J. Sports Med.* **2011**, *45*, 987–992. [CrossRef] [PubMed]
2. Gleeson, M.; Bishop, N.C. URI in athletes: Are mucosal immunity and cytokine responses key risk factors? *Exerc. Sport Sci. Rev.* **2013**, *41*, 148–153. [CrossRef] [PubMed]
3. Walsh, N.P.; Gleeson, M.; Shephard, R.J.; Gleeson, M.; Woods, J.A.; Bishop, N.C.; Fleshner, M.; Green, C.; Pedersen, B.K.; Hoffman-Goetz, L.; et al. Position statement. Part one: Immune function and exercise. *Exerc. Immunol. Rev.* **2011**, *17*, 6–63. [PubMed]
4. Nieman, D.C. Immune response to heavy exertion. *J. Appl. Physiol.* **1997**, *82*, 1385–1394. [PubMed]
5. He, C.S.; Bishop, N.C.; Handzlik, M.K.; Muhamad, A.S.; Gleeson, M. Sex differences in upper respiratory symptoms prevalence and oral-respiratory mucosal immunity in endurance athletes. *Exerc. Immunol. Rev.* **2014**, *20*, 8–22. [PubMed]
6. Fahlman, M.M.; Engels, H.J. Mucosal IgA and URTI in American college football players: A year longitudinal study. *Med. Sci. Sports Exerc.* **2005**, *37*, 374–380. [CrossRef] [PubMed]
7. Gleeson, M.; McDonald, W.A.; Pyne, D.B.; Cripps, A.W.; Francis, J.L.; Fricker, P.A.; Clancy, R.L. Salivary IgA levels and infection risk in elite swimmers. *Med. Sci. Sports Exerc.* **1999**, *31*, 67–73. [CrossRef] [PubMed]
8. Neville, V.; Gleeson, M.; Folland, J.P. Salivary IgA as a risk factor for upper respiratory infections in elite professional athletes. *Med. Sci. Sports Exerc.* **2008**, *40*, 1228–1236. [CrossRef] [PubMed]
9. Lancaster, G.I.; Halson, S.L.; Khan, Q.; Drysdale, P.; Wallace, F.; Jeukendrup, A.E.; Drayson, M.T.; Gleeson, M. Effects of acute exhaustive exercise and chronic exercise training on type 1 and type 2 T lymphocytes. *Exerc. Immunol. Rev.* **2004**, *10*, 91–106. [PubMed]
10. Sprenger, H.; Jacobs, C.; Nain, M.; Gressner, A.M.; Prinz, H.; Wesemann, W.; Gemsa, D. Enhanced release of cytokines, interleukin-2 receptors, and neopterin after long-distance running. *Clin. Immunol. Immunopathol.* **1992**, *63*, 188–195. [CrossRef]
11. Tilz, G.P.; Domej, W.; Diez-Ruiz, A.; Weiss, G.; Brezinschek, R.; Brezinschek, H.P.; Hüttl, E.; Pristautz, H.; Wachter, H.; Fuchs, D. Increased immune activation during and after physical exercise. *Immunobiology* **1993**, *188*, 194–202. [CrossRef]

12. Strasser, B.; Gostner, J.M.; Fuchs, D. Mood, food, and cognition: Role of tryptophan and serotonin. *Curr. Opin. Clin. Nutr. Metab. Care* **2016**, *19*, 55–61. [CrossRef] [PubMed]

13. Stone, T.W.; Perkins, M.N. Quinolinic acid: A potent endogenous excitant at amino acid receptors in CNS. *Eur. J. Pharmacol.* **1981**, *72*, 411–412. [CrossRef]

14. Chen, Y.; Guillemin, G.J. Kynurenine pathway metabolites in humans: Disease and healthy states. *Int. J. Tryptophan Res.* **2009**, *2*, 1–19. [PubMed]

15. Strasser, B.; Geiger, D.; Schauer, M.; Gatterer, H.; Burtscher, M.; Fuchs, D. Effects of exhaustive aerobic exercise on tryptophan-kynurenine metabolism in trained athletes. *PLoS ONE* **2016**, *11*, e0153617. [CrossRef] [PubMed]

16. Strasser, B.; Sperner-Unterweger, B.; Fuchs, D.; Gostner, J.M. Mechanisms of Inflammation-Associated Depression: Immune Influences on Tryptophan and Phenylalanine Metabolisms. *Curr. Top. Behav. Neurosci.* **2016**, in press.

17. Jenkins, T.A.; Nguyen, J.C.; Polglaze, K.E.; Bertrand, P.P. Influence of tryptophan and serotonin on mood and cognition with a possible role of the gut-brain axis. *Nutrients* **2016**, *8*. [CrossRef] [PubMed]

18. Evans, J.M.; Morris, L.S.; Marchesi, J.R. The gut microbiome: The role of a virtual organ in the endocrinology of the host. *J. Endocrinol.* **2013**, *218*, R37–R47. [CrossRef] [PubMed]

19. Leblhuber, F.; Geisler, S.; Steiner, K.; Fuchs, D.; Schütz, B. Elevated fecal calprotectin in patients with Alzheimer's dementia indicates leaky gut. *J. Neural Transm.* **2015**, *122*, 1319–1322. [CrossRef] [PubMed]

20. Bermon, S.; Petriz, B.; Kajėnienė, A.; Prestes, J.; Castell, L.; Franco, O.L. The microbiota: An exercise immunology perspective. *Exerc. Immunol. Rev.* **2015**, *21*, 70–79. [PubMed]

21. Cerdá, B.; Pérez, M.; Pérez-Santiago, J.D.; Tornero-Aguilera, J.F.; González-Soltero, R.; Larrosa, M. Gut Microbiota Modification: Another Piece in the Puzzle of the Benefits of Physical Exercise in Health? *Front. Physiol.* **2016**, *7*, 51. [CrossRef] [PubMed]

22. Gleeson, M.; McFarlin, B.; Flynn, M. Exercise and Toll-like receptors. *Exerc. Immunol. Rev.* **2006**, *12*, 34–53. [PubMed]

23. Matteoli, G.; Mazzini, E.; Iliev, I.D.; Mileti, E.; Fallarino, F.; Puccetti, P.; Chieppa, M.; Rescigno, M. Gut CD103+ dendritic cells express indoleamine 2,3-dioxygenase which influences T regulatory/T effector cell balance and oral tolerance induction. *Gut* **2010**, *59*, 595–604. [CrossRef] [PubMed]

24. Nagata, S.; Asahara, T.; Wang, C.; Suyama, Y.; Chonan, O.; Takano, K.; Daibou, M.; Takahashi, T.; Nomoto, K.; Yamashiro, Y. The Effectiveness of Lactobacillus Beverages in Controlling Infections among the Residents of an Aged Care Facility: A Randomized Placebo-Controlled Double-Blind Trial. *Ann. Nutr. Metab.* **2016**, *68*, 51–59. [CrossRef] [PubMed]

25. Wang, Y.; Li, X.; Ge, T.; Xiao, Y.; Liao, Y.; Cui, Y.; Zhang, Y.; Ho, W.; Yu, G.; Zhang, T. Probiotics for prevention and treatment of respiratory tract infections in children: A systematic review and meta-analysis of randomized controlled trials. *Medicine* **2016**, *95*, e4509. [CrossRef] [PubMed]

26. O'Sullivan, O.; Cronin, O.; Clarke, S.F.; Murphy, E.F.; Molloy, M.G.; Shanahan, F.; Cotter, P.D. Exercise and the microbiota. *Gut Microbes* **2015**, *6*, 131–136. [CrossRef] [PubMed]

27. Clarke, S.F.; Murphy, E.F.; O'Sullivan, O.; Lucey, A.J.; Humphreys, M.; Hogan, A.; Hayes, P.; O'Reilly, M.; Jeffery, I.B.; Wood-Martin, R.; et al. Exercise and associated dietary extremes impact on gut microbial diversity. *Gut* **2014**, *63*, 1913–1920. [CrossRef] [PubMed]

28. Jäger, R.; Purpura, M.; Stone, J.D.; Turner, S.M.; Anzalone, A.J.; Eimerbrink, M.J.; Pane, M.; Amoruso, A.; Rowlands, D.S.; Oliver, J.M. Probiotic *Streptococcus thermophilus* FP4 and Bifidobacterium breve BR03 Supplementation Attenuates Performance and Range-of-Motion Decrements Following Muscle Damaging Exercise. *Nutrients* **2016**, *8*, 642. [CrossRef] [PubMed]

29. Lamprecht, M.; Bogner, S.; Schippinger, G.; Steinbauer, K.; Fankhauser, F.; Hallstroem, S.; Schuetz, B.; Greilberger, J.F. Probiotic supplementation affects markers of intestinal barrier, oxidation, and inflammation in trained men; a randomized, double-blinded, placebo-controlled trial. *J. Int. Soc. Sports Nutr.* **2012**, *9*, 45. [CrossRef] [PubMed]

30. Cox, A.J.; Pyne, D.B.; Saunders, P.U.; Fricker, P.A. Oral administration of the probiotic Lactobacillus fermentum VRI-003 and mucosal immunity in endurance athletes. *Br. J. Sports Med.* **2010**, *44*, 222–226. [CrossRef] [PubMed]

31. Gleeson, M.; Bishop, N.C.; Oliveira, M.; Tauler, P. Daily probiotic's (*Lactobacillus casei* Shirota) reduction of infection incidence in athletes. *Int. J. Sport Nutr. Exerc. Metab.* **2011**, *21*, 55–64. [CrossRef] [PubMed]

32. Haywood, B.A.; Black, K.E.; Baker, D.; McGarvey, J.; Healey, P.; Brown, R.C. Probiotic supplementation reduces the duration and incidence of infections but not severity in elite rugby union players. *J. Sci. Med. Sport* **2014**, *17*, 356–360. [CrossRef] [PubMed]

33. West, N.P.; Pyne, D.B.; Peake, J.M.; Cripps, A.W. Probiotics, immunity and exercise: A review. *Exerc. Immunol. Rev.* **2009**, *15*, 107–126. [PubMed]

34. Edvardsen, E.; Scient, C.; Hansen, B.H.; Holme, I.M.; Dyrstad, S.M.; Anderssen, S.A. Reference values for cardiorespiratory response and fitness on the treadmill in a 20- to 85-year-old population. *Chest* **2013**, *144*, 241–248. [CrossRef] [PubMed]

35. Faulhaber, M.; Gatterer, H.; Haider, T.; Patterson, C.; Burtscher, M. Intermittent hypoxia does not affect endurance performance at moderate altitude in well-trained athletes. *J. Sports Sci.* **2010**, *28*, 513–519. [CrossRef] [PubMed]

36. Widner, B.; Werner, E.R.; Schennach, H.; Wachter, H.; Fuchs, D. Simultaneous measurement of serum tryptophan and kynurenine by HPLC. *Clin. Chem.* **1997**, *43*, 2424–2426. [PubMed]

37. Neurauter, G.; Scholl-Bürgi, S.; Haara, A.; Geisler, S.; Mayersbach, P.; Schennach, H.; Fuchs, D. Simultaneous measurement of phenylalanine and tyrosine by high performance liquid chromatography (HPLC) with fluorescence detection. *Clin. Biochem.* **2013**, *46*, 1848–1851. [CrossRef] [PubMed]

38. Geisler, S.; Mayersbach, P.; Becker, K.; Schennach, H.; Fuchs, D.; Gostner, J.M. Serum tryptophan, kynurenine, phenylalanine, tyrosine and neopterin concentrations in 100 healthy blood donors. *Pteridines* **2015**, *26*, 31–36. [CrossRef]

39. Cohen, J.W. *Statistical Power Analysis for the Behavioral Sciences*, 2nd ed.; Lawrence Erlbaum Associates Publishers: Mahwah, NJ, USA, 1988; pp. 284–287.

40. Areces, F.; González-Millán, C.; Salinero, J.J.; Abian-Vicen, J.; Lara, B.; Gallo-Salazar, C.; Ruiz-Vicente, D.; Del Coso, J. Changes in serum free amino acids and muscle fatigue experienced during a half-ironman triathlon. *PLoS ONE* **2015**, *10*, e0138376. [CrossRef] [PubMed]

41. Schlittler, M.; Goiny, M.; Agudelo, L.Z.; Venckunas, T.; Brazaitis, M.; Skurvydas, A.; Kamandulis, S.; Ruas, J.L.; Erhardt, S.; Westerblad, H.; et al. Endurance exercise increases skeletal muscle kynurenine aminotransferases and plasma kynurenic acid in humans. *Am. J. Physiol. Cell Physiol.* **2016**, *310*, C836–C840. [CrossRef] [PubMed]

42. Meeusen, R. Exercise, nutrition and the brain. *Sports Med.* **2014**, *44* (Suppl. 1), S47–S56. [CrossRef] [PubMed]

43. Agudelo, L.Z.; Femenía, T.; Orhan, F.; Porsmyr-Palmertz, M.; Goiny, M.; Martinez-Redondo, V.; Correia, J.C.; Izadi, M.; Bhat, M.; Schuppe-Koistinen, I.; et al. Skeletal muscle PGC-1α1 modulates kynurenine metabolism and mediates resilience to stress-induced depression. *Cell* **2014**, *159*, 33–45. [CrossRef] [PubMed]

44. Desbonnet, L.; Garrett, L.; Clarke, G.; Bienenstock, J.; Dinan, T.G. The probiotic *Bifidobacteria infantis*: An assessment of potential antidepressant properties in the rat. *J. Psychiatr. Res.* **2008**, *43*, 164–174. [CrossRef] [PubMed]

45. Hao, Q.; Dong, B.R.; Wu, T. Probiotics for preventing acute upper respiratory tract infections. *Cochrane Database Syst. Rev.* **2015**, *2*, CD006895.

46. Pyne, D.B.; West, N.P.; Cox, A.J.; Cripps, A.W. Probiotics supplementation for athletes—Clinical and physiological effects. *Eur. J. Sport Sci.* **2015**, *15*, 63–72. [CrossRef] [PubMed]

47. West, N.P.; Pyne, D.B.; Cripps, A.W.; Hopkins, W.G.; Eskesen, D.C.; Jairath, A.; Christophersen, C.T.; Conlon, M.A.; Fricker, P.A. *Lactobacillus fermentum* (PCC®) supplementation and gastrointestinal and respiratory-tract illness symptoms: A randomised control trial in athletes. *Nutr. J.* **2011**, *10*, 30. [CrossRef] [PubMed]

48. Gleeson, M. Nutritional support to maintain proper immune status during intense training. *Nestle Nutr. Inst. Workshop Ser.* **2013**, *75*, 85–97. [PubMed]

49. Ho, P.M.; Bryson, C.L.; Rumsfeld, J.S. Medication adherence: Its importance in cardiovascular outcomes. *Circulation* **2009**, *119*, 3028–3035. [CrossRef] [PubMed]

50. Carretti, N.; Florio, P.; Bertolin, A.; Costa, C.V.; Allegri, G.; Zilli, G. Serum fluctuations of total and free tryptophan levels during the menstrual cycle are related to gonadotrophins and reflect brain serotonin utilization. *Hum. Reprod.* **2005**, *20*, 1548–1553. [CrossRef] [PubMed]

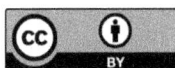

nutrients

MDPI

Article

Periodization of Carbohydrate Intake: Short-Term Effect on Performance

Laurie-Anne Marquet [1,2,*], Christophe Hausswirth [1], Odeline Molle [1], John A. Hawley [3,4], Louise M. Burke [3,5], Eve Tiollier [1] and Jeanick Brisswalter [2]

[1]   Laboratory of Sport, Expertise and Performance, French National Institute of Sport,
      Expertise and Performance (INSEP), 75012 Paris, France; hausswirthc@gmail.com (C.H.);
      odeline.molle@insep.fr (O.M.); eve.tiollier@insep.fr (E.T.)
[2]   Université Côte d'Azur, LAMHESS, 06205 Nice, France; brisswalter@unice.fr
[3]   Mary MacKillop Institute for Health Research, Centre for Exercise and Nutrition,
      Australian Catholic University, Melbourne, VIC 3065, Australia; John.Hawley@acu.edu.au (J.A.H.);
      louise.burke@ausport.gov.au (L.M.B.)
[4]   Research Institute for Sport and Exercise Sciences, Liverpool John Moores University, Liverpool L3 5UA, UK
[5]   Sports Nutrition, Australian Institute of Sport (AIS), Belconnen, ACT 2617, Australia
[*]   Correspondence: laurie-anne.marquet@insep.fr; Tel.: +33-141-744-138

Received: 15 September 2016; Accepted: 9 November 2016; Published: 25 November 2016

Abstract: Background: "Sleep-low" consists of a sequential periodization of carbohydrate (CHO) availability—low glycogen recovery after "train high" glycogen-depleting interval training, followed by an overnight-fast and light intensity training ("train low") the following day. This strategy leads to an upregulation of several exercise-responsive signaling proteins, but the chronic effect on performance has received less attention. We investigated the effects of short-term exposure to this strategy on endurance performance. Methods: Following training familiarization, 11 trained cyclists were divided into two groups for a one-week intervention—one group implemented three cycles of periodized CHO intake to achieve the sleep-low strategy over six training sessions (SL, CHO intake: 6 g·kg^{-1}·day^{-1}), whereas the control group consumed an even distribution of CHO over the day (CON). Tests were a 2 h submaximal ride and a 20 km time trial. Results: SL improved their performance (mean: +3.2%; $p < 0.05$) compared to CON. The improvement was associated with a change in pacing strategy with higher power output during the second part of the test. No change in substrate utilization was observed after the training period for either group. Conclusion: Implementing the "sleep-low" strategy for one week improved performance by the same magnitude previously seen in a three-week intervention, without any significant changes in selected markers of metabolism.

Keywords: carbohydrate; performance; training; cycling time trial; trained athletes; lipid oxidation; perception of effort

1. Introduction

Carbohydrate-based fuels (CHO) are the main substrates used by the brain and skeletal muscle during exercise. Thus, nutritional recommendations for competition performance promote strategies to achieve "high CHO availability", in the form of adequate pre-exercise glycogen concentrations and additional CHO intake during competition to meet the specific fuel needs of the event [1,2]. However, recent research has provided new insight into the interactions of exercise with "low CHO availability", whereby the adaptive responses to training or recovery are enhanced in an environment of low exogenous and endogenous CHO stores [3]. Within this framework, glycogen is not only considered as an energetic substrate, but more as a regulator of metabolic signaling responses [4].

The aim of training is to act as a chronic stimulus leading to physiological adaptations and an improvement in performance. The acute and chronic effect of endurance exercise on metabolic responses have already been widely described and include mitochondrial biogenesis, shifts in fiber composition toward type I fibers, and enhanced oxidative metabolism [5,6]. Substrate availability interacts with the contractile stimulus to modulate these physiological responses to training [7] Specifically, muscle glycogen content can modulate physiological adaptations induced by endurance training by upregulating transcription factors and regulators of gene expression such as *PGC-1α* [8] and *p53* [9]. Based on these observations, a growing interest in training under conditions of low glycogen availability and/or low exogenous glucose availability has developed [3].

Several studies have reported that commencing a training session with low glycogen availability enhances expression of genes involved in mitochondrial biogenesis and substrate metabolism [10–13]. However, these studies have typically failed to show improvements in performance, likely because the beneficial "molecular" effects are negated by a decreased ability to sustain high intensity exercise under the conditions of low CHO availability [12,13]. This has led to interest in a "periodized" approach to CHO availability in the training program, where sessions undertaken to promote adaptation are carefully integrated with others focused on high quality performance outcomes. The "sleep-low" (SL) strategy represents one such sequence of periodized CHO availability, which allows athletes to perform high intensity training sessions supported by high CHO availability while enhancing metabolic adaptation associated with low glycogen availability [14–17].

Specifically, this strategy consists of a cycling of (1) late afternoon scheduling of a high intensity training (HIT) session undertaken with high glycogen stores; (2) withholding of the ingestion of CHO after the session to maintain glycogen depletion during the overnight recovery period; and (3) a low–moderate intensity steady-state exercise session (LIT) in the following morning completed after an overnight fast. Previous studies have reported that this strategy leads to increased activity of several proteins with putative roles in training adaptation (AMPK, p38 MAPK, p53) [9,14] and higher rates of fat oxidation during submaximal exercise [14]. However, the effects on endurance performance are equivocal. Recently, we [15] reported that integrating SL strategy, three times a week, during a three-week training intervention (i.e., nine occurrences of the sequence) was associated with an improved endurance performance in well-trained subjects (+3% during a 10 km running trial), coupled with an increase in submaximal cycling efficiency. A control group, who undertook the same training program with a similar total intake of energy and CHO, but normally distributed over the day, failed to improve performance. Furthermore, the performance improvements achieved by the SL program were associated with a decrease in body fat (−1.05%) [15] without any negative impact on immune function or sleep quality [16]. The original concept underlying this strategy is the periodization of the CHO intake: instead of a chronically low CHO intake, which has been shown to alter glycogen metabolism [18], high-intensity training sessions are performed under conditions of high glycogen availability. The recovery period, which plays a central role in the development of training adaptation [19], is non optimal for prolonging the period of optimized response to the training stimulus [20]. Lower-intensity training (LIT) is performed while fasted to maximize cellular adaptations and enhance rates of lipid oxidation.

Although the intervention in our three-week study was successful in improving performance and body composition [15], we note challenges to the feasibility of free-living athletes achieving the required dietary manipulations and/or having the commitment to undertake the low CHO recovery and subsequent training [21]. It is therefore of interest to see if a shorter exposure to this CHO periodization strategy would be successful in inducing metabolic adaptations and performance improvement. Accordingly, the aim of the current study was to investigate the effect of an abbreviated program of the "sleep-low" strategy on endurance performance in well-trained athletes. We also examined whether any observed effects on performance are related to an enhancement of metabolic adaptations to training as previously suggested [3].

2. Materials and Methods

2.1. Study Population

Eleven endurance-trained male cyclists volunteered to participate in the study. They were healthy, aged between 18 and 40 years, and training at least 12 h/week, having at least 3 years of prior training. Their mean (±SD) age was 31.2 ± 7.1 years, their mean body mass was 71.1 ± 5.6 kg, their mean maximal oxygen consumption ($\dot{V}O_{2max}$) was 64.2 ± 6.0 mL·min^{-1}·kg^{-1}, and their mean maximal aerobic power (MAP, W) was 342 ± 38.3 W. Before entering the study, all participants were examined by a cardiologist to ensure they did not present with abnormal electrocardiograph pattern or contraindications to physical activity. The study's protocol was approved by local Ethic Committee 2015-AO1136-43 (Paris IDF X, France). After written and verbal explanation, all participants provided their written informed consent to participate.

2.2. Study Design

An overview of the study design is depicted in the Figure 1. Subjects were first assigned to a familiarization session to the testing protocol. Then, during the following two weeks, they trained according to their habitual training program. During the first week, they ate according to their usual dietary habits, documenting their food intake via a daily food diary. In the second week, they followed specific nutritional guidelines, which set their CHO intake at 6 g·kg^{-1}·day^{-1}, while continuing to keep their daily food diary. After the two weeks of habitual training load, subjects were assigned to the PRE test session. Then, they were randomly assigned to two different groups undertaking the same one-week training program but following different nutritional guidelines, according to the "sleep-low" strategy, previously described [14,15]. CHO intake was similar between groups (6 g·kg^{-1}·day^{-1}) but periodized differently over the day, according to the demands of the training sessions. Specifically, one group trained with a high CHO availability (control group, CON group, $n = 9$) with an even spread of CHO intake over the day and between training sessions. Meanwhile, the intervention group trained with a CHO intake that was periodized within the various days ("sleep-low" group, SL group, $n = 12$) such that no CHO was consumed between the high intensity interval training sessions (HIT) held late in the day and the end of the following morning's low–moderate intensity (LIT) training session. The protocol ended with a POST test session.

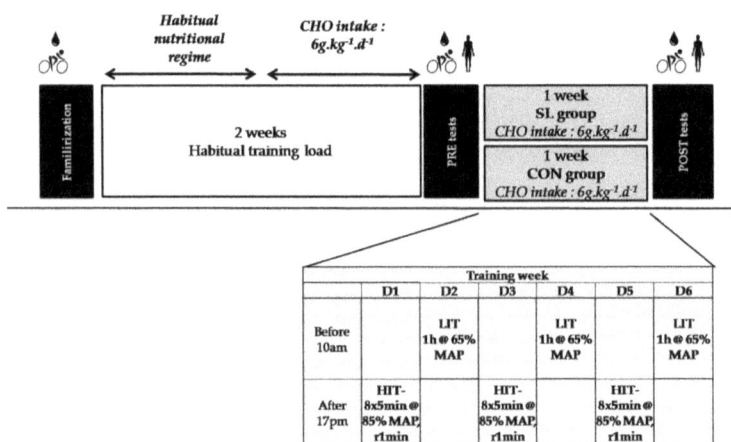

Figure 1. Overview of the experimental protocol; CHO: carbohydrates; HIT: high-intensity training session; LIT: light intensity training session; SL: Sleep-Low; CON: Control; MAP: Maximal aerobic power.

Since it was not possible to disguise the differences in dietary intake between the groups, this study could not be performed as a blinded intervention. In order to limit this bias, participants were not informed of the aim of the study (periodization of the CHO intake). They were neither aware of the number of groups in the study, the group to which they had been assigned, nor the program of the other group.

2.3. Preliminary Measurement of Maximal Oxygen Consumption

Before entering the study, all participants had to perform a $\dot{V}O_{2max}$ test, which was determined by an incremental test until exhaustion, on an electrically braked cycle ergometer (Excalibur Sport, Lode, Groningen, The Netherlands). Saddle and handlebar heights were set to match the usual positions used by participants, and these were standardized between sessions. The cycle ergometer was equipped with individual racing pedals, allowing participants to wear their own shoes. Subjects warmed up for 6 min at 100 W, then power output was increased by 25 W each successive 2 min until volitional exhaustion. Participants wore a face mask covering their mouth and nose to collect breath (Hans Rudolph, Kansas City, MO, USA). During the test, oxygen uptake ($\dot{V}O_2$), carbon dioxide uptake ($\dot{V}CO_2$), minute ventilation ($\dot{V}E$) and the respiratory exchange ratio (RER) were continuously recorded and monitored as breath-by-breath values (Quark, Cosmed, Rome, Italy). The gas and flow analyzers were calibrated prior to each test using ambient air, known-concentration gas ($O_2 = 16\%$, $CO_2 = 5\%$), and a 3 L syringe. The $\dot{V}O_{2max}$ was determined based on the highest 30 s average value. The MAP (W) was calculated as MAP = W completed + 25 × (t/120), where W is the last completed workload and t is the number of seconds in the last workload [22]. The MAP was used to adjust the workload in the testing session and the training program.

2.4. Training Protocol

The training program was divided in two phases. The first phase, lasting two weeks, was composed of the participants' habitual training programs. The second phase lasted one week and was similar for all participants, regardless of the nutritional group to which they were assigned. The training program (Figure 1) was based on our previous studies [15,16] and consisted of six training sessions over six consecutive days, including a HIT session in the afternoon (after 1700 h) and low–moderate intensity training session in the following morning (before 1000 h). The HIT session comprised a 10 min warm-up followed by eight repetitions lasting 5 min at 85% of MAP interspersed with 1 min of recovery (100 W). The cycling LIT sessions consisted of a steady-state 1 h session at 65% of MAP.

2.5. Nutritional Protocol

During the first week of the protocol of the habitual training load, participants were not assigned to specific nutritional guidelines. They were asked to complete a food diary in order to record their nutritional habits and examine how they differed from the nutritional interventions applied in the study. The second week of this first phase of the protocol, all participants were given dietary prescriptions, setting CHO intake at 6 g·kg^{-1}·day^{-1} in anticipation of the nutritional strategy of the second phase. Participants were given precise instructions for the weighed food allowances for each meal (breakfast, lunch, dinner, and during training) according to their body mass. During the week of modified training program, participants were separated into two groups: the CON group ($n = 9$) and the SL group ($n = 12$). They were instructed to ingest the same amount of CHO during the day (6 g·kg^{-1}) but spread differently over the day (Table 1). A full description of the dietary program can be found elsewhere [16]. Briefly, for the SL group, no CHO was consumed from the commencement of the HIT session on the evening of one day until after the completion of the LIT session on the following morning. Thereafter, CHO intake was resumed to meet daily targets. In this way, the HIT session was undertaken with high muscle glycogen concentrations ("train-high"), while recovery from this session and the completion of the LIT session was undertaken with low CHO availability due to depleted glycogen concentrations and an overnight fast ("sleep-low" and "train-low", respectively). Meanwhile, high glycogen availability was maintained in the CON group with regular intake of CHO at all meals throughout the day, and the intake of a sports drink (6% CHO, Gatorade, PepsiCo, Purchase, NY, USA) during training sessions. CHO was ingested at every meal. Each participant received written nutritional recommendations for each meal with quantities according to their group and weight. To prevent an unwanted loss of fat-free mass, a high-protein sugar-free drink (High Protein 15 g, UHS, Bruno, France) was prescribed before going to bed. To check compliance to the dietary protocols, participants were required to complete a daily food diary. They were instructed to give as many details as possible (food weights, pictures of dishes, descriptions of fat used to cook or flavor dishes, and the brand names of commercial food products). The diaries were inspected by the same researcher and analyzed using a self-made database of food composition.

Table 1. Total energy and macronutrient intake for sleep-low (SL) and control (CON) groups before starting the training program (BASELINE) and during the training/diet intervention (TRAINING) (mean ± SD).

		Total Energy Intake	Carbohydrate Intake	Lipid Intake	Protein Intake
		(kcal·Day^{-1})	(g·kg^{-1}·Day^{-1})	(g·kg^{-1}·Day^{-1})	(g·kg^{-1}·Day^{-1})
SL group	BASELINE	2658 ± 726	4.9 ± 1.3	1.2 ± 0.4	1.4 ± 0.4
$n = 12$	TRAINING	3079 ± 874	6.5 ± 2.2	0.9 ± 0.3	1.9 ± 0.2 *
CON group	BASELINE	2924 ± 967	5.2 ± 1.9	1.4 ± 0.5	1.4 ± 0.5
$n = 9$	TRAINING	2610 ± 488	5.0 ± 1.3	0.9 ± 0.3 *	1.6 ± 0.4

*: $p < 0.05$ as compared to PRE values.

Meals during the 24 h prior to the testing sessions (lunch, dinner, and breakfast) were identically prescribed for both groups to ensure that the same amount of CHO (total intake of 6 g·kg^{-1}·day^{-1}) was consumed.

2.6. Testing Protocol

Three sessions of testing were planned: familiarization, PRE, and POST tests. They were composed of two exercise sessions on the same day. The day after the last training session of the week, subjects reported to the laboratory at a standardized time. The first test was a 2 h submaximal cycling test at 60% of MAP at a self-selected cadence. The test started with 10 min at 100 W followed by 110 min at 60% of MAP. Participants wore a cardio belt to monitor heart rate (HR) constantly throughout the test, as well as a face mask to measure gas exchange. They wore the mask for the first 20 min and then the mask was removed for 10 min every 10 min, allowing the subjects to drink only water. Respiratory gases were collected and analyzed to assess cycling efficiency, substrate oxidation, and respiratory quotient. Specifically, whole body rates of CHO and fat oxidation (in g·min^{-1}) were calculated from $\dot{V}O_2$ and $\dot{V}CO_2$ values measured during the submaximal cycling test; calculations were made from gases collected during the last 60 s of each work interval of interest with nonprotein respiratory exchange ratio (RER) values being assessed according to standard equations [23]:

$$\text{CHO oxidation} = 4.210\dot{V}CO_2 - 2.962\dot{V}O_2 \tag{1}$$

$$\text{Fat oxidation} = 1.695\dot{V}O_2 - 1.701\dot{V}CO_2 \tag{2}$$

Three blood samples were collected during the submaximal test—immediately before, at 1 h, and at 2 h of the test—from a superficial forearm using venipuncture techniques. Four 33 mL samples of blood were collected into EDTA and Z Serum Clot Activator tubes (Greiner Bio-One, Frickenhausen, Germany).

The submaximal test was immediately followed by a 20 km time-trial (TT) performed on the participants' own bike mounted on a braked Cyclus2 ergometer (RBM GmbH, Leipzig, Germany). We tried to reproduce realistic conditions of a cycling race, within a laboratory environment. Ingestion of sports drink (6% CHO, Gatorade, PepsiCo, Purchase, NY, USA) was allowed during the time-trial, with the volume ingested during the familiarization being recorded and replicated during the ensuing testing sessions. No feedback was provided to the subjects during TT except for their gear ratio and the distance remaining. Rating perception of effort (RPE) was assessed verbally using the Borg 6–20 scale [24] every 5 km. Heart rate (HR) was continuously sampled every 5 s (Polar, Kempele, Finland) during the TT. The time, the mean power, and the mean speed were collected at the end of the TT. Pacing strategy was reported per kilometer during the TT. Participants were not informed of their results until the end of the study.

2.7. Blood Analysis

To avoid interassay variation, all blood samples were analyzed in a single batch at the end of the study. Blood samples were collected to measure plasma concentrations of markers of lipid metabolism (glycerol and free fatty acid) and markers of metabolic stress (adrenaline and noradrenaline). After collection, blood samples were immediately centrifuged at 4000 rev·min^{-1} for 10 min at 4 °C to separate plasma from red blood cells. Plasma was then stored in multiple aliquots (Eppendorf type, 1500 µL) at −80 °C until analysis. Catecholamine concentrations were determined with commercially available ELISA kits (Demeditec Diagnostics GmbH, Kiel, Germany). The assay for (adrenaline) had an intra-assay coefficient of variation (CV) of 24.7%–11.0% over a concentration range of 64.7–948 pg·mL^{-1} and an interassay CV of 14.5%–13.1% over a concentration range of 76.4–771 pg·mL^{-1}. The assay for noradrenaline had intra-assay CV of 12.8%–11.1% over a concentration range of 510–3363 pg·mL^{-1} and an interassay CV of 9.2%–9.2% over a concentration range of 445–3283 pg·mL^{-1}. All blood samples were analyzed in duplicate in respective wavelengths on a spectrophotometer Dynex MRXe (Legalla Biosciences, Chelmsford, MA, USA).

Plasma non-esterified fatty acids (NEFA) were determined with an enzymatic method (Wako Chemical, Neuss, Germany) and glycerol concentrations were measured with enzymatic colorimetric method Randox (Crumnil, Antrin, UK) on PENTRA 400 Horiba (ABX, Montpellier, France).

2.8. Body Composition

Measurement of whole body composition was undertaken on all subjects using dual-energy X-ray absorptiometry (Lunar IDXA, General Electric, Madison, WI, USA) at PRE and POST test sessions, the day after the performance tests. All measurements were taken early in the morning and in a fasted state [25].

2.9. Statistical Analysis

All statistical analyses were conducted using Statistica 7.1 software (StatSoft). All data are expressed as mean ± SD. Normality of data was tested using a Shapiro–Wilk normality test. Data which were not normally distributed were log-transformed. A repeated-measures analysis of variance (ANOVA) was used to calculate the effect of the dietary strategy (SL vs. CON) and the period (PRE and POST) on performance, blood parameters, and body composition. When a significant effect was found, post hoc tests were performed using Newman–Keuls procedures. Effect sizes for comparison were then calculated Cohen's d values. Values of 0.1, 0.3, and over 0.5 were respectively considered as small, medium, and large effect [26]. For all tests, the significance level was set at $p < 0.05$.

3. Results

3.1. Dietary Intervention

Analyses of food diaries revealed that participants complied with the nutritional guidelines of their prescribed diet (Table 1). There was no significant difference in the CHO intake between both groups before and after the training/diet intervention week, despite a slightly difference in the effective CHO intake. Total protein intake increased between the baseline training period and the training diet week (+36.3% and +20.4%, $p < 0.05$, d = 3.48 and d = 1.07, for SL and CON groups, respectively) but without any difference between groups. In both groups, there was also a reduction in reported intake of fat during the training/diet intervention period compared with baseline (−17.8% and −20.9%, $p < 0.01$, d = 2.13 and d = 2.81 for SL and CON groups, respectively).

3.2. Performance Tests

3.2.1. Twenty Kilometer Time-Trial Cycling Test Performance

Time to complete the 20 km cycling time-trial was reduced after the training period for all the subjects in SL (−3.23% ± 2.99%, $p < 0.05$, d = 1.58), whereas no change was recorded for CON (−1.04% ± 3.46%) (Figure 2). This improvement was due to a significantly higher mean power output (from 229 ± 36 to 250 ± 32 W, $p < 0.05$, d = 1.48) in SL.

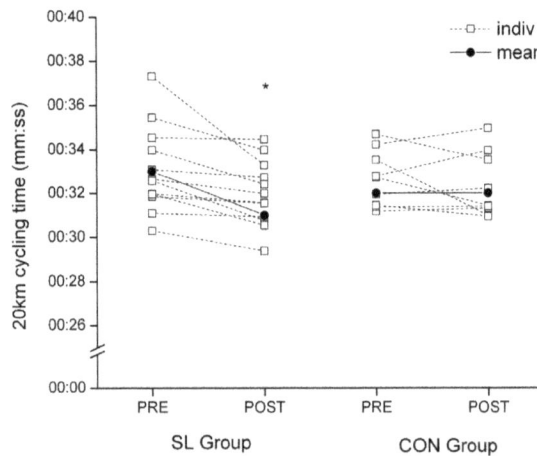

Figure 2. Individual 20 km cycling time-trial performance for SL and CON groups in PRE and POST tests. * Significantly different from PRE values, $p < 0.05$.

● Pacing strategy

The change in mean power over the duration of the time-trial is depicted in Figure 3. The SL strategy induced a significantly higher mean power at the 11th (+13.2% ± 15%, $p < 0.05$, d = 1.58), 13th (+18.1% ± 23.4%, $p < 0.01$, d = 1.95), 14th (+14.3% ± 14.6%, $p < 0.05$, d = 1.58), 15th (21.2% ± 12.8%, $p < 0.01$, d = 2.95), 16th (+11.8% ± 8.4%, $p < 0.05$, d = 1.92), and 17th kilometers (+12.4% ± 9.4%, $p < 0.05$, d = 1.74) (Figure 3a), whereas no change was observed after the training week for the CON group (Figure 3b). Both groups developed higher mean power at the 20th kilometer after the training week (+7.7% ± 14%, $p < 0.05$, d = 0.85 for SL group; +11.2% ± 20%, $p < 0.01$, d = 2.31 for CON group).

(a)

(b)

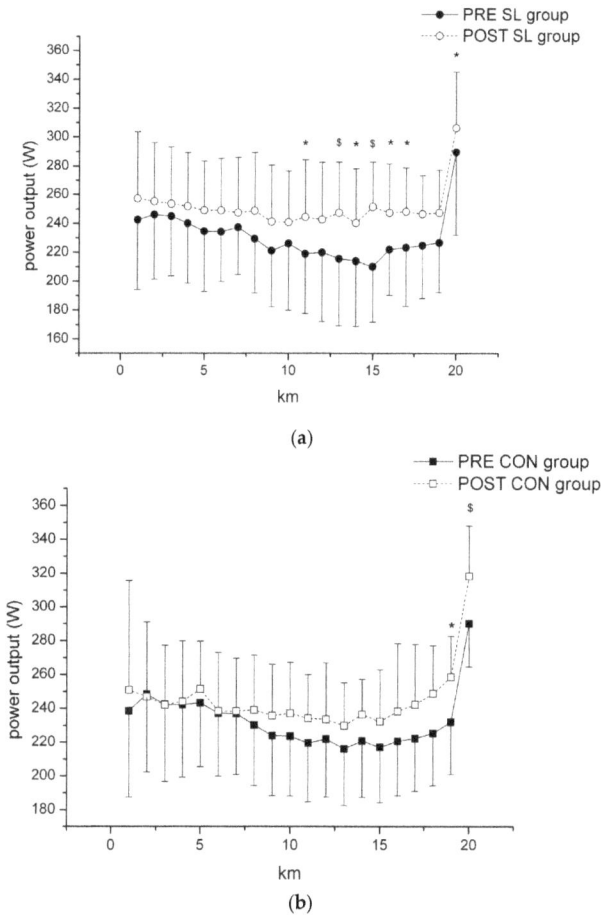

Figure 3. Pacing strategy (absolute change in power output per kilometer) during the 20 km cycling time-trial in PRE and POST tests for (a) SL group; and (b) CON group. * Significantly different from PRE values, $p < 0.05$. $ Significantly different from PRE values, $p < 0.01$.

- RPE

No difference in RPE values during the time trial was observed between PRE and POST tests for both groups (Table 2), despite the higher outputs of the SL group in the POST test trial

Table 2. Rating perception of effort (RPE) during the 20 km cycling time-trial every 5 km for SL and CON groups in PRE and POST tests.

		RPE				
		0	5 km	10 km	15 km	20 km
SL group	PRE	9 ± 1.2	14.7 ± 2.3	16.2 ± 1.6	17.3 ± 1.7	19 ± 1.2
	POST	10 ± 2.5	15 ± 2	16 ± 1.6	17.2 ± 1.3	19 ± 1
CON group	PRE	10.9 ± 2	14.7 ± 1.7	15.3 ± 2.3	16.2 ± 2	17.7 ± 1.9
	POST	13.1 ± 2.8	14.3 ± 1.7	15 ± 2.4	16 ± 1.7	18 ± 1.7

3.2.2. Submaximal Cycling Test

• Substrate oxidation

No significant differences between group and pre and post tests was observed for rates of CHO oxidation (mean values during the whole test: respectively for pre and post test for the SL group 2.0 ± 0.2 g·min^{-1} vs. 2.1 ± 0.2 g·min^{-1}; and for the CON group: 1.9 ± 0.5 g·min^{-1} vs. 2.1 ± 0.5 g·min^{-1}) or fat oxidation (respectively for pre and post test for the SL group 0.6 ± 0.3 g·min^{-1} vs. 0.9 ± 0.2 g·min^{-1}; and for the CON group: 0.7 ± 0.2 g·min^{-1} vs. 0.6 ± 0.2 g·min^{-1}).

• Blood analysis

Markers of lipid metabolism. Plasma concentrations of glycerol increased during the submaximal cycling test ($p < 0.001$) but differences between groups or between PRE and POST tests were not significant (Table 3). Similarly, there was an increase in plasma concentrations of free fatty acids during the test ($p < 0.001$) but without any difference between groups or between PRE and POST tests.

Markers of stress. Plasma catecholamine concentrations increased during the submaximal cycling test: the concentrations at 1 h and at 2 h were higher than resting concentrations for both groups ($p < 0.01$ for both markers). No significant difference in plasma catecholamine concentrations were observed before and after the training/diet intervention or between groups (Table 3).

Table 3. Blood analysis sampled before, during (at 1 h) and immediately after (at 2 h) the submaximal test for markers of lipid metabolism (glycerol, non-esterified fatty acid (NEFA)) and catecholamine concentrations.

		Glycerol (mmol·L^{-1})			NEFA (μmol·L^{-1})		
	Blood Sampling	Before	During	After	Before	During	After
SL group	PRE	0.02 ± 0.01	0.11 ± 0.06	0.25 ± 0.13	185 ± 115	308 ± 135	610 ± 209
	POST	0.02 ± 0.01	0.07 ± 0.04	0.22 ± 0.1	168 ± 79	229 ± 90	589 ± 213
CON group	PRE	0.03 ± 0.01	0.08 ± 0.03	0.21 ± 0.08	153 ± 60	241 ± 148	604 ± 284
	POST	0.03 ± 0.03	0.10 ± 0.05	0.22 ± 0.11	134 ± 59	341 ± 222	699 ± 457
		Adrenaline (ng·mL^{-1})			Noradrenaline (ng·mL^{-1})		
	Blood Sampling	Before	During	After	Before	During	After
SL group	PRE	0.10 ± 0.13	0.31 ± 0.25	1.1 ± 0.79	0.93 ± 0.92	4.17 ± 2.1 [$]	4.6 ± 3.8 [$]
	POST	0.07 ± 0.10	0.16 ± 0.17	0.73 ± 0.67 *	0.9 ± 0.6	3.8 ± 3.6 *	2.9 ± 2.2 *
CON group	PRE	0.18 ± 0.25	0.36 ± 0.1 [$]	0.27 ± 1.64 [$]	1.68 ± 1.0	4.13 ± 4.5	7.6 ± 4.4
	POST	0.04 ± 0.04	0.30 ± 0.13	0.48 ± 0.20	5.1 ± 7.2	10.1 ± 7.9	7.3 ± 6.9

[$] significantly different from PRE before values, $p < 0.01$; * significantly different from POST before values, $p < 0.05$.

3.3. Training Period

The perception of effort for the LIT training session during the intervention was significantly different between groups. Subjects who trained in a fasted state (SL group) perceived the LIT training sessions as harder (15.2 ± 1.9) than the subjects of the CON group (13.5 ± 2) ($p < 0.05$, d = 0.87).

3.4. Body Composition

There were no differences in body mass and fat-free mass for either group after the intervention week. However, there was a significant reduction in fat mass in the SL group only (-395 ± 491 g, $p < 0.05$, d = 0.34), whereas the change observed in the CON group was not significant (-151 ± 363 g).

4. Discussion

This study investigated the effect of a short-term exposure to a periodized "sleep-low" training/diet strategy on metabolism and performance of well-trained cyclists. The program involved exposure to three cycles of a sequence involving "train high, sleep low, and train low" based on periodizing CHO intake to achieve different levels of CHO availability for specific training sessions within a week of training. The main finding was a significant improvement in performance during a cycling time-trial after only one week of training under the "sleep-low" strategy (+3.2% ± 2.99%). This improvement is similar in magnitude to that observed previously after three weeks of SL training [15]. No significant effect was observed for any other physiological parameter. This enhanced performance was related to differences in pacing strategy, and higher levels of self-chosen power outputs in the athletes who undertook the periodized CHO intake protocol. These findings show the importance of pacing in the determination of performance, and suggest factors other than physiological or metabolic characteristics that have been previously reported in studies focusing on the effect of low glycogen availability during training [7].

Strategies that promote training adaptation with low CHO availability (overnight-fasted training, low-glycogen training, low glycogen recovery periods) are commonly observed among athletes, but are often implemented unintentionally or without strategy. The lack of efficacy of these protocols in some studies [12,13] suggests that unless they are implemented in a strategic way, the outcomes may not integrate with other aspects of the training program towards a clear performance improvement. A case study describing the real-life training program of three elite marathoners during a 16-week training program [21] illustrated a sophisticated approach to mixing and matching specific training sessions with varying CHO availability, with the frequency of low CHO training varying from 1.3 to 2.6 sessions/week of training at different times of the season. Our protocol involves a specific sequence of three different training/nutrient stimuli, and this study brings new information regarding how they might achieve benefits in a shorter period or be scheduled at a strategic time before competition [27], at least in athletes of this well-trained but sub-elite caliber.

The improvement in performance in the current study was associated with change in the pacing strategy. Among the participants in our group who undertook the "sleep-low" exposure, self-chosen power outputs in the second half of the time-trial (11th–17th kilometer) were higher despite the same perceived exertion. Factors affecting pacing strategies have been widely investigated during the last decade and several models have been proposed [28–31].

It has been suggested that endurance performance is centrally regulated by both intrinsic (cognitive, mental fatigue, physiological) and extrinsic (environmental) signals to preserve physiological limits [32]. In the psychobiological model of Marcora [31], pacing regulation could be explained using an effort-based decision-making model based on motivational intensity theory. This model states that the conscious regulation of pace is determined by five cognitive factors: (1) perception of effort; (2) potential motivation; (3) knowledge of the distance/time to cover; (4) knowledge of the distance/time remaining; and (5) previous experience of perception of effort during exercise of varying intensity and duration. In most of the cases, perception of effort is the key determinant of these models. In any event, the pacing strategy is adopted very rapidly, meaning that it is not only a function of metabolic changes [30].

One hypothesis to explain the impact of the periodization of CHO intake on the improvement of performance could reside in changes in resting muscle glycogen concentration. In a twice-daily training model in which the second session was undertaken with low glycogen availability, Hansen et al. and Yeo et al. [11,12] found a higher resting glycogen content in muscle that had received this exposure. It is possible that the participants in the SL group achieved an enhancement of glycogen storage leading to higher muscle glycogen concentration at the start of the 20 km time-trial. Muscle glycogen depletion, when the athlete is fed, is correlated to the development of fatigue [33]. The lower values of RPE after the training period can also be explained by higher muscle glycogen concentration. Rauch et al. [34] proposed that the power output developed is dependent on the brain, which anticipates the rate of muscle glycogen utilization leading to individual "critical" levels of endpoint muscle glycogen. In their study, eight subjects followed three days of carbohydrate loading or a normal diet with an exercise protocol in which they completed 2 h cycling at 65% of MAP interspersed with five 60 s sprints after 20, 40, 60, 80, and 100 min. This bout was followed immediately by a time-trial of 1 h. Although the power outputs developed in the trial following the normal diet were lower than those in the carbohydrate loading trial, endpoint muscle glycogen concentrations were similar in both conditions, despite different starting concentrations. Although we were unable to measure muscle glycogen in our study, it is possible that higher pre-exercise muscle glycogen concentrations in the SL group may "signal" to the brain to allow higher power output. Future studies should investigate this hypothesis.

One limitation of our study which could also explain the possibly higher muscular glycogen content is the trend for an increase in energy and CHO intake for the SL group between PRE and POST testing sessions, while it was slightly reduced for the CON group. We note that although we provided precise nutritional guidelines to participants, they were free-living and prepared their own meals. Therefore, slight deviations from the desired dietary control could have possibly induced a bias in the outcomes. It should be noted, however, that despite these trends in reported energy intake, the SL group reported a small decrease in fat mass over the intervention period.

Another interesting finding of our study is that the performance improvement seen in the SL group was not associated with the metabolic changes classically reported after training with low CHO availability [14]. No changes in fat oxidation were observed during the submaximal cycling bout in the SL participants, while blood analyses also failed to record any change in metabolites or catecholamine levels after one week of "sleep-low" training strategy. The lack of any effect of the SL strategy on substrate oxidation is similar to the findings of our first study using a three-week SL strategy [15], but contrasts with the observations from previous studies on training with low glycogen availability. Typically, these studies report higher activity of enzymes involved in fat metabolism [12,13], and changes in transcription for adaptive genes [14] or factors involved in mitochondrial biogenesis [17]. However, a difference between our study and others is that our performance tests were undertaken pre- and post- intervention with subjects following strategies of high CHO availability (i.e., high CHO diet in the preceding day, pre-exercise CHO intake, CHO intake during the exercise). Thus, previous studies reported the effect of exercise in fasted conditions [10,35] as well as the effect of training with low CHO availability. In terms of effects on catecholamine concentrations, the lack of changes in the current study are consistent with the findings of our longer study, in which an increase in resting catecholamine concentrations was observed in the second and the third week of the training/diet intervention. This indicates that a longer period of exposure is needed to achieve measurable modifications in plasma catecholamine concentration.

5. Conclusions

One week of training with sequential periodization of CHO availability for selected periods of training (recovery, light intensity training session) seems sufficient to improve performance in trained endurance athletes. This strategy could be implemented during the weeks preceding a competition before the taper period.

Acknowledgments: The author would like to thank Jocelyne Drai for her valuable help in the NEFA and glycerol analyses. No source of funding were use to conduct this research work or publish it in open access. The authors had no conflicts of interest that are directly relevant to this article.

Author Contributions: L.-A.M. has made substantial contributions to conception, design, acquisition of data, analysis and interpretation of data and has been involved in drafting the manuscript. C.H. has made substantial contributions to conception and design. O.M. has made substantial contributions to acquisition of data and analysis. J.A.H. has made substantial contributions to conception, design and has been involved in drafting the manuscript or revising it critically for important intellectual content. L.M.B. has made substantial contributions to conception, design and has been involved in drafting the manuscript or revising it critically for important intellectual content. E.T. has made substantial contributions to design and analysis. J.B. has made substantial contributions to conception, design, acquisition of data, analysis and interpretation of data and has been involved in drafting the manuscript.

Conflicts of Interest: The authors declare that they have no conflicts of interest.

References

1. Burke, L.M.; Hawley, J.A.; Wong, S.H.S.; Jeukendrup, A.E. Carbohydrates for training and competition. *J. Sports Sci.* **2011**, *29* (Suppl. 1), S17–S27. [CrossRef] [PubMed]
2. Thomas, D.T.; Erdman, K.A.; Burke, L.M. Position of the academy of nutrition and dietetics, dietitians of Canada, and the American college of sports medicine: Nutrition and athletic performance. *J. Acad. Nutr. Diet.* **2016**, *116*, 501–528. [CrossRef] [PubMed]
3. Hawley, J.A.; Morton, J.P. Ramping up the signal: Promoting endurance training adaptation in skeletal muscle by nutritional manipulation. *Clin. Exp. Pharmacol. Physiol.* **2014**, *41*, 608–613. [CrossRef] [PubMed]
4. Baar, K.; McGee, S. Optimizing training adaptations by manipulating glycogen. *Eur. J. Sport Sci.* **2008**, *8*, 97–106. [CrossRef]
5. Coffey, V.G.; Hawley, J.A. The molecular bases of training adaptation. *Sports Med.* **2007**, *37*, 737–763. [CrossRef] [PubMed]
6. Hawley, J.A. Adaptations of skeletal muscle to prolonged, intense endurance training. *Clin. Exp. Pharmacol. Physiol.* **2002**, *29*, 218–222. [CrossRef] [PubMed]
7. Hawley, J.A.; Gibala, M.J.; Bermon, S. International Association of Athletics Federations Innovations in athletic preparation: Role of substrate availability to modify training adaptation and performance. *J. Sports Sci.* **2007**, *25* (Suppl. 1), S115–S124. [CrossRef] [PubMed]
8. Psilander, N.; Frank, P.; Flockhart, M.; Sahlin, K. Exercise with low glycogen increases *PGC-1α* gene expression in human skeletal muscle. *Eur. J. Appl. Physiol.* **2013**, *113*, 951–963. [CrossRef] [PubMed]
9. Bartlett, J.D.; Louhelainen, J.; Iqbal, Z.; Cochran, A.J.; Gibala, M.J.; Gregson, W.; Close, G.L.; Drust, B.; Morton, J.P. Reduced carbohydrate availability enhances exercise-induced *p53* signaling in human skeletal muscle: Implications for mitochondrial biogenesis. *Am. J. Physiol. Regul. Integr. Comp. Physiol.* **2013**, *304*, R450–R458. [CrossRef] [PubMed]
10. Van Proeyen, K.; Szlufcik, K.; Nielens, H.; Ramaekers, M.; Hespel, P. Beneficial metabolic adaptations due to endurance exercise training in the fasted state. *J. Appl. Physiol.* **2011**, *110*, 236–245. [CrossRef] [PubMed]
11. Hansen, A.K.; Fischer, C.P.; Plomgaard, P.; Andersen, J.L.; Saltin, B.; Pedersen, B.K. Skeletal muscle adaptation: Training twice every second day vs. training once daily. *J. Appl. Physiol.* **2005**, *98*, 93–99. [CrossRef] [PubMed]
12. Yeo, W.K.; Paton, C.D.; Garnham, A.P.; Burke, L.M.; Carey, A.L.; Hawley, J.A. Skeletal muscle adaptation and performance responses to once a day versus twice every second day endurance training regimens. *J. Appl. Physiol.* **2008**, *105*, 1462–1470. [CrossRef] [PubMed]
13. Hulston, C.J.; Venables, M.C.; Mann, C.H.; Martin, C.; Philp, A.; Baar, K.; Jeukendrup, A.E. Training with low muscle glycogen enhances fat metabolism in well-trained cyclists. *Med. Sci. Sports Exerc.* **2010**, *42*, 2046–2055. [CrossRef] [PubMed]
14. Lane, S.C.; Camera, D.M.; Lassiter, D.G.; Areta, J.L.; Bird, S.R.; Yeo, W.K.; Jeacocke, N.A.; Krook, A.; Zierath, J.R.; Burke, L.M.; et al. Effects of sleeping with reduced carbohydrate availability on acute training responses. *J. Appl. Physiol.* **2015**, *119*, 643–655. [CrossRef] [PubMed]
15. Marquet, L.-A.; Brisswalter, J.; Louis, J.; Tiollier, E.; Burke, L.M.; Hawley, J.A.; Hausswirth, C. Enhanced endurance performance by periodization of carbohydrate intake: "Sleep Low" strategy. *Med. Sci. Sports Exerc.* **2016**, *48*, 663–672. [CrossRef] [PubMed]
16. Louis, J.; Marquet, L.-A.; Tiollier, E.; Bermon, S.; Hausswirth, C.; Brisswalter, J. The impact of sleeping with reduced glycogen stores on immunity and sleep in triathletes. *Eur. J. Appl. Physiol.* **2016**, *116*, 1–14. [CrossRef] [PubMed]
17. Impey, S.G.; Hammond, K.M.; Shepherd, S.O.; Sharples, A.P.; Stewart, C.; Limb, M.; Smith, K.; Philp, A.; Jeromson, S.; Hamilton, D.L.; et al. Fuel for the work required: A practical approach to amalgamating train-low paradigms for endurance athletes. *Physiol. Rep.* **2016**, *4*, e12803. [CrossRef] [PubMed]
18. Burke, L.M. Re-Examining high-fat diets for sports performance: Did we call the "Nail in the Coffin" too soon? *Sports Med.* **2015**, *5*, S33–S49. [CrossRef] [PubMed]

19. Pilegaard, H.; Ordway, G.A.; Saltin, B.; Neufer, P.D. Transcriptional regulation of gene expression in human skeletal muscle during recovery from exercise. *Am. J. Physiol. Endocrinol. Metab.* **2000**, *279*, E806–E814. [PubMed]

20. Pilegaard, H.; Osada, T.; Andersen, L.T.; Helge, J.W.; Saltin, B.; Neufer, P.D. Substrate availability and transcriptional regulation of metabolic genes in human skeletal muscle during recovery from exercise. *Metab. Clin. Exp.* **2005**, *54*, 1048–1055. [CrossRef] [PubMed]

21. Stellingwerf, T. Case study: Nutrition and training periodization in three elite marathon runners. *Int. J. Sport Nutr. Exerc. Metab.* **2012**, *22*, 392–400. [CrossRef] [PubMed]

22. Hawley, J.A.; Noakes, T.D. Peak power output predicts maximal oxygen uptake and performance time in trained cyclists. *Eur. J. Appl. Physiol. Occup. Physiol.* **1992**, *65*, 79–83. [CrossRef] [PubMed]

23. Jeukendrup, A.E.; Wallis, G.A. Measurement of substrate oxidation during exercise by means of gas exchange measurements. *Int. J. Sports Med.* **2005**, *26*, S28–S37. [CrossRef] [PubMed]

24. Borg, G. Perceived exertion as an indicator of somatic stress. *Scand. J. Rehabil. Med.* **1970**, *2*, 92–98. [PubMed]

25. Nana, A.; Slater, G.J.; Hopkins, W.G.; Halson, S.L.; Martin, D.T.; West, N.P.; Burke, L.M. Importance of standardized dxa protocol for assessing physique changes in athletes. *Int. J. Sport Nutr. Exerc. Metab.* **2014**, in press. [CrossRef] [PubMed]

26. Cohen, J. *Statistical Power Analysis for the Behavioral Sciences*; Lawrence Erlbaum Associates (LEA): Hillsdale, NJ, USA, 1988.

27. Issurin, V. Block periodization versus traditional training theory: A review. *J. Sports Med. Phys. Fit.* **2008**, *48*, 65–75.

28. Renfree, A.; Martin, L.; Micklewright, D.; Gibson, A.S.C. Application of decision-making theory to the regulation of muscular work rate during self-paced competitive endurance activity. *Sports Med.* **2013**, *44*, 147–158. [CrossRef] [PubMed]

29. Millet, G.Y. Can neuromuscular fatigue explain running strategies and performance in ultra-marathons? *Sports Med.* **2011**, *41*, 489–506. [CrossRef] [PubMed]

30. Noakes, T.D.; St Clair Gibson, A.; Lambert, E.V. From catastrophe to complexity: A novel model of integrative central neural regulation of effort and fatigue during exercise in humans: Summary and conclusions. *Br. J. Sports Med.* **2005**, *39*, 120–124. [CrossRef] [PubMed]

31. Marcora, S. Counterpoint: Afferent feedback from fatigued locomotor muscles is not an important determinant of endurance exercise performance. *J. Appl. Physiol.* **2010**, *108*, 454–456. [CrossRef] [PubMed]

32. Abbiss, C.R.; Laursen, P.B. Describing and understanding pacing strategies during athletic competition. *Sports Med.* **2008**, *38*, 239–252. [CrossRef] [PubMed]

33. Hermansen, L.; Hultman, E.; Saltin, B. Muscle glycogen during prolonged severe exercise. *Acta Physiol. Scand.* **1967**, *71*, 129–139. [CrossRef] [PubMed]

34. Rauch, H.G.L.; St Clair Gibson, A.; Lambert, E.V.; Noakes, T.D. A signalling role for muscle glycogen in the regulation of pace during prolonged exercise. *Br. J. Sports Med.* **2005**, *39*, 34–38. [CrossRef] [PubMed]

35. De Bock, K.; Richter, E.A.; Russell, A.P.; Eijnde, B.O.; Derave, W.; Ramaekers, M.; Koninckx, E.; Léger, B.; Verhaeghe, J.; Hespel, P. Exercise in the fasted state facilitates fibre type-specific intramyocellular lipid breakdown and stimulates glycogen resynthesis in humans. *J. Physiol. (Lond.)* **2005**, *564*, 649–660. [CrossRef] [PubMed]

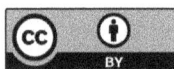

nutrients

MDPI

Review

Pre-Sleep Protein Ingestion to Improve the Skeletal Muscle Adaptive Response to Exercise Training

Jorn Trommelen and Luc J. C. van Loon *

NUTRIM School of Nutrition and Translational Research in Metabolism, Maastricht University Medical Centre+, P.O. Box 616, Maastricht 6200 MD, The Netherlands; jorn.trommelen@maastrichtuniversity.nl
* Correspondence: l.vanloon@maastrichtuniversity.nl; Tel.: +31-43-388-1397

Received: 14 September 2016; Accepted: 23 November 2016; Published: 28 November 2016

Abstract: Protein ingestion following resistance-type exercise stimulates muscle protein synthesis rates, and enhances the skeletal muscle adaptive response to prolonged resistance-type exercise training. As the adaptive response to a single bout of resistance exercise extends well beyond the first couple of hours of post-exercise recovery, recent studies have begun to investigate the impact of the timing and distribution of protein ingestion during more prolonged recovery periods. Recent work has shown that overnight muscle protein synthesis rates are restricted by the level of amino acid availability. Protein ingested prior to sleep is effectively digested and absorbed, and thereby stimulates muscle protein synthesis rates during overnight recovery. When applied during a prolonged period of resistance-type exercise training, protein supplementation prior to sleep can further augment gains in muscle mass and strength. Recent studies investigating the impact of pre-sleep protein ingestion suggest that at least 40 g of protein is required to display a robust increase in muscle protein synthesis rates throughout overnight sleep. Furthermore, prior exercise allows more of the pre-sleep protein-derived amino acids to be utilized for de novo muscle protein synthesis during sleep. In short, pre-sleep protein ingestion represents an effective dietary strategy to improve overnight muscle protein synthesis, thereby improving the skeletal muscle adaptive response to exercise training.

Keywords: sleep; recovery; exercise; hypertrophy; casein

1. Introduction

A single session of exercise stimulates muscle protein synthesis rates, and to a lesser extent, muscle protein breakdown rates [1,2]. However, the muscle protein net balance will remain negative in the absence of food intake [2]. Protein ingestion stimulates muscle protein synthesis and inhibits muscle protein breakdown rates, resulting in net muscle protein accretion during the acute stages of post-exercise recovery [3]. Therefore, post-exercise protein ingestion is widely applied as a strategy to augment post-exercise muscle protein synthesis rates and, as such, to facilitate the skeletal muscle adaptive response to exercise training. Various factors have been identified which can modulate the post-exercise muscle protein synthetic response to exercise including the amount [4,5], type [6,7], timing [8], and distribution [9] of protein ingestion.

Only few studies have investigated the dose-response relationship between protein ingestion and post-exercise muscle protein synthesis rates in young [4,5] and older adults [10–12]. Ingestion of 20 g egg or whey protein has been shown sufficient to maximize muscle protein synthesis rates during recovery from lower-body resistance-type exercise in young males [4,5]. More recent evidence indicates that this dose-response relationship may depend on the amount of muscle tissue that was recruited during exercise, with the ingestion of 40 g protein further increasing muscle protein synthesis rates during recovery from whole-body resistance-type exercise [13].

A large variety of dietary protein sources have been shown to stimulate post-exercise muscle protein synthesis rates, including egg protein [4], whey and casein protein [14], milk and beef protein [15], and soy protein [6]. However, dietary protein sources can differ in their capacity to stimulate muscle protein synthesis rates, which appears to be largely dependent on differences in protein digestion and absorption kinetics [14,16] and amino acid composition [6,17], with the leucine content being of particular relevance [18,19].

Besides the amount and type of ingested protein, the timing and distribution of protein ingestion throughout the day can modulate post-exercise muscle protein synthesis rates. An even distribution of total protein intake over the three main meals stimulates 24 h muscle protein synthesis rates more effectively than an unbalanced distribution in which the majority (>60%) of total daily protein intake is consumed at the evening meal [20]. During 12 h of post-exercise recovery, an intermediate pattern of protein ingestion (20 g every 3 h) seems to increase muscle protein synthesis rates to a greater extent than the same amount of protein provided in less frequent but larger amounts (40 g every 6 h), or in more frequent, smaller amounts (10 g every 6 h) [9]. Therefore, an effective pattern of daily protein intake distribution to support muscle protein synthesis is to provide at least 20 g of protein with each main meal with no more than 4–5 h between meals.

As overnight sleep is typically the longest post-absorptive period during the day, we have recently introduced the concept of protein ingestion prior to sleep as a means to augment post-exercise overnight muscle protein synthesis. The aim of this review is to discuss the current state of evidence regarding the efficacy of pre-sleep protein ingestion to stimulate overnight muscle reconditioning.

2. Overnight Protein Metabolism

In general, most studies assess the effects of food intake on the muscle protein synthetic response to exercise performed in an overnight fasted state. Such post-absorptive conditions differ from normal everyday practice in which recreational sports activities are often performed in the late afternoon or evening after a full day of habitual physical activity and food intake. Therefore, we evaluated the impact of exercise performed in a fed state in the evening and the efficacy of protein ingestion immediately after exercise on muscle protein synthesis during prolonged overnight recovery [21]. The ingestion of 20–25 g of protein during exercise increased muscle protein synthesis rates during exercise, but we observed no increase in muscle protein synthesis rates during the prolonged overnight recovery period. Muscle protein synthesis rates during overnight sleep were unexpectedly low, with values being even lower than those typically observed in the in the morning following an overnight fast. Thus, a day of habitual food intake and the ingestion of 20–25 g of protein during and/or immediately after an exercise bout performed in the evening does not suffice to augment overnight muscle protein reconditioning.

3. Does the Gut Function at Night?

As overnight muscle protein synthesis rates are surprisingly low [21], we questioned whether they are limited by overnight plasma amino acid availability. Therefore, we hypothesized that protein provision during sleep increases overnight plasma amino acid availability and stimulates overnight muscle protein synthesis rates. As human intestinal motility follows a circadian rhythm with reduced activity during the night [22], we first assessed whether dietary protein provision during sleep leads to proper dietary protein digestion and amino acid absorption. In a proof-of-principle study, we first administrated specifically produced intrinsically L-$[1-^{13}C]$-phenylalanine-labeled casein protein via a nasogastric tube while subjects were asleep and assessed the subsequent protein digestion and absorption kinetics [23]. We observed that administration of 40 g casein via a nasogastric tube during overnight sleep is followed by proper dietary protein digestion and absorption kinetics, thereby increasing overnight plasma amino acid availability and increasing muscle protein synthesis rates. Clearly, these data demonstrated that the gut functions properly at night and that protein provided during sleep strongly increases overnight muscle protein synthesis rates.

4. Pre-Sleep Protein Feeding as a Strategy to Increase Overnight Muscle Protein Synthesis

Our observation that protein administered during sleep is effectively digested and absorbed provided proof-of-principle that the gut functions properly during sleep [23]. However, nasogastric tube feeding does not represent a feasible feeding strategy for athletes. Therefore, our next step was to assess if protein ingestion prior to sleep would represent an effective dietary strategy to increase muscle protein synthesis rates during overnight post-exercise recovery [24]. Therefore, we studied recreational athletes during overnight recovery from a single bout of resistance-type exercise performed in the evening after a full day of dietary standardization. Immediately after exercise, all athletes ingested a recovery drink containing 20 g protein to maximize muscle protein synthesis rates during the acute stages of post-exercise recovery [4,24]. As explained above, this prescribed recovery strategy does not suffice to maintain elevated muscle protein synthesis rates during more prolonged overnight sleep [21]. Therefore, we provided subjects with either 40 g casein protein or a placebo drink immediately prior to sleep. In line with intragastric protein administration during sleep [23], the bolus of protein ingested prior to sleep was properly digested and absorbed throughout overnight sleep. The greater plasma amino acid availability following pre-sleep protein ingestion improved the overnight whole-body protein balance, allowing the net protein balance to become positive. In line, muscle protein synthesis rates were approximately 22% higher during overnight recovery when protein was ingested prior to sleep when compared to the placebo treatment. From these data we concluded that pre-sleep protein ingestion represents an effective dietary strategy to further augment the skeletal muscle adaptive response to resistance-type exercise training (Figure 1).

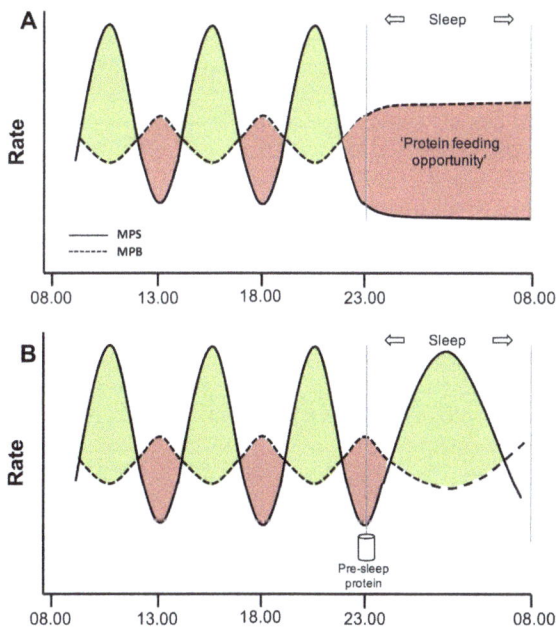

Figure 1. Schematic representation of the process of muscle protein synthesis (MPS) and muscle protein breakdown (MPB) throughout the day. Protein ingestion stimulates MPS rates and allows for net muscle protein accretion (green areas). During post-absorptive conditions, MPB rates exceed MPS rates, resulting in a net loss of muscle protein (red areas). Overnight sleep is the longest post-absorptive period of the day (**A**). Pre-sleep protein ingestion stimulates overnight muscle protein synthesis rates (**B**), thereby improving muscle reconditioning during overnight sleep.

To test this hypothesis, we assessed the impact of pre-sleep protein feeding to facilitate the skeletal muscle adaptive response to prolonged resistance-type exercise training [25]. Specifically, we selected healthy young men to participate in a 12-week resistance-type exercise training program (three exercise sessions per week) during which they ingested either 27.5 g of protein prior to sleep, or a non-caloric placebo. Muscle mass and strength increased to a greater extent in the group that ingested protein prior to sleep. These results indicate that protein supplementation prior to sleep represents an effective dietary strategy to augment the gains in muscle mass and strength during resistance-type exercise training. It remains to be established what dose and type of pre-sleep protein should be used to further optimize overnight muscle protein synthesis rates and, as such, can support greater gains in muscle mass and strength.

It should be noted that the ingestion of the pre-sleep protein supplement in both our acute and long-term studies was compared with a non-protein placebo, and not compared with protein supplementation provided at other time points. Therefore, we can only speculate on the surplus benefits of pre-sleep protein provision when compared to other time points. It can be speculated that the greater gains in muscle mass and strength are, at least partly, attributed to the pre-sleep timing of the protein supplement, as the vast majority of studies in which protein has been supplemented immediately before and/or after exercise do not show an increase in muscle mass gains when compared to a placebo [26]. However, it has been suggested that protein supplementation increases muscle mass gains mainly as a function of increased total protein intake, rather than the specific timing of a protein supplement [27,28]. As a meta-analysis was required to demonstrate that additional protein intake augments training-induced muscle hypertrophy [26], it seems unlikely that a possible positive effect of protein timing (i.e., protein supplementation at a time point compared to protein supplementation at different time point) on muscle mass gains can be detected in a longitudinal study. While it is currently unclear whether pre-sleep protein ingestion is superior to protein ingestion at a different time point, we propose that a more relevant question is whether pre-sleep protein ingestion is additive to protein intake earlier in the day. We suggest that athletes should aim to ingest sufficient protein intake at every meal to maximize muscle protein synthesis until the next meal. We have recently shown that the ingestion of large amounts of protein in the early post-exercise recovery phase does not compromise the muscle protein synthetic response to protein ingestion at a later stage [29]. This suggests that every meal moment represents a unique opportunity to stimulate muscle protein synthesis and that the muscle protein synthetic response to each meal may be additive. In addition, we have recently shown that athletes typically consume well above 1.2 g protein/kg/day, with the majority of protein consumed during the three main meals, and only a small amount of protein eaten as an evening snack (~7 g) [30]. As such, additional pre-sleep protein ingestion represents a practical strategy to increase the total daily protein intake, add another meal moment, and increase the overnight muscle protein synthesis rates; this effect is likely additive to muscle protein synthesis rates observed throughout the day.

5. Pre-Sleep Protein Feeding Characteristics

While we have identified the overnight sleeping period as a new window of opportunity to augment post-exercise training adaptations, it remains to be established how we can maximize the impact of pre-sleep protein feeding on overnight muscle protein synthesis rates. Previously we have shown that the ingestion of 40 g protein prior to sleep stimulates overnight muscle protein rates [24], which is considerably more than the 20 g of protein that is supposed to maximize muscle protein synthesis rates during the first few hours of post-exercise recovery [4,5]. Therefore, we questioned if a more moderate amount of protein would suffice to augment overnight muscle protein synthesis rates. To address this issue, we performed a follow-up study similar in design to our previous pre-sleep protein work, with the main difference that we provided 30 g of highly enriched intrinsically labeled protein prior to sleep, with or without an additional 2 g of free leucine. In contrast to our previous findings with 40 g protein, the ingestion of 30 g protein prior to sleep did not significantly increase overnight muscle protein synthesis rates (preliminary observations). This suggests that a pre-sleep protein dose-response relationship exists, which differs from the immediate post-exercise recovery period during which the ingestion of merely 20 g protein seems to maximize post-exercise muscle protein synthesis rates in young adults.

The ingestion of highly enriched, intrinsically L-[1-^{13}C]-phenylalanine-labeled protein allowed us to also directly assess the metabolic fate of the pre-sleep dietary protein-derived amino acids. Pre-sleep protein-derived L-[1-^{13}C]-phenylalanine was incorporated in de novo muscle protein as evidenced by the increase in muscle protein–bound L-[1-^{13}C]-phenylalanine following overnight recovery, demonstrating that the pre-sleep protein provided amino acids as precursors for de novo myofibrillar protein accretion during overnight sleep. This provides mechanistic evidence to support our observation that the ingestion of 30 g protein prior to sleep augments muscle mass during three months of resistance-type exercise training [25]. However, our data suggest that at least 40 g of pre-sleep protein is required to induce a more substantial, detectable increase in muscle protein synthesis rates when assessed acutely over a 7.5 h overnight period.

As we anticipated that 30 g of pre-sleep protein might not be sufficient to adequately increase overnight muscle protein synthesis rates, we included a third treatment in which 2 g crystalline leucine was added to the 30 g bolus of protein. The addition of supplemental free leucine to a suboptimal amount of protein has been shown to enhance post-exercise muscle protein synthesis rates [18,19,31,32]. Despite these previous observations, co-ingesting free leucine with 30 g of casein prior to sleep did not augment the overnight muscle protein synthetic response. Given the extended duration of overnight sleep compared to a typical postprandial period (8 vs. 4–5 h), it is tempting to speculate that larger amounts of protein ($\geq$40 g) are required to maximize muscle protein synthesis rates during overnight sleep.

6. Prior Exercise

It has been well established that the muscle protein synthetic response to protein ingestion is enhanced following exercise when exercise is performed in the morning following an overnight fast [12,33]. Recently, we evaluated the effect of resistance-type exercise performed in the evening on the muscle protein synthetic response to pre-sleep protein ingestion [34]. Postprandial overnight muscle protein synthesis rates were higher when exercise had been performed earlier that evening and more of the ingested protein-derived amino acids were directed towards de novo myofibrillar protein synthesis during overnight sleep. Therefore, protein ingestion prior to sleep represents an effective strategy to enhance overnight muscle reconditioning and is likely of even more relevance on exercise training days. In line, we have shown that physical activity performed in the evening increases the overnight muscle protein synthetic response to pre-sleep protein ingestion in older adults [35]. Clearly, combing pre-sleep protein ingestion with resistance-type exercise represents a more effective strategy to further enhance overnight skeletal muscle protein synthesis rates and increases the efficiency by which dietary protein is used for muscle protein accretion (Figure 2).

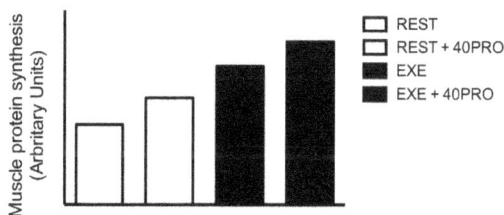

Figure 2. Conceptual framework of the overnight muscle protein synthetic response to 40 g of pre-sleep protein feeding at rest or following prior exercise.

7. Type of Pre-Sleep Protein

As protein sources differ in their capacity to stimulate muscle protein synthesis, the type of protein ingested prior to sleep may modulate the overnight muscle protein synthetic response. So far, all studies assessing the efficacy of pre-sleep protein ingestion on exercise reconditioning have provided casein protein. Casein is a more slowly digestible protein source, allowing a more moderate but prolonged rise in plasma amino acid concentrations [17]. Given the extended nature of overnight sleep, it could be speculated that such a more sustained postprandial aminoacidemia during overnight sleep is preferred as it will provide precursors to support muscle protein synthesis rates throughout the entire night. In contrast, whey protein is a more rapidly digestible protein, resulting in a pronounced but transient rise in plasma amino acid concentrations [17]. Ingestion of a single bolus of whey protein has been shown to stimulate muscle protein synthesis rates to a greater degree than casein protein when assessed over periods up to 6 h [6,17,36]. This has been attributed to the more rapid protein digestion and amino acid absorption kinetics as well as the higher leucine content in whey versus casein protein, resulting in a more rapid rise in postprandial plasma leucine concentrations [37]. It remains to be established if whey is superior to casein protein when ingested prior to sleep and muscle protein synthesis rates are assessed over a more prolonged overnight period of 7.5 h. The plasma levels of leucine do not seem to be the only factor in this regard, as we recently did not observe any differences in overnight muscle protein synthesis rates following the ingestion of 30 g casein with or without 2 g crystalline leucine (preliminary observations). Snijders et al. [25] provided a casein protein supplement that consisted of 50% micellar casein and 50% casein hydrolysate. When casein protein is hydrolyzed, its digestion and absorption properties resemble a more rapid digestible protein [38]. Therefore, pre-sleep ingestion of a mixture of a slow and more rapidly digestible protein source appears to be effective to augment muscle mass and strength gains during a prolonged resistance-type exercise program. We speculate that a variety of high-quality animal-based protein sources can augment overnight muscle protein synthesis rates when provided in sufficient amounts ($\geq$40 g; Table 1), with relatively minor differences in efficacy between sources.

Table 1. Quantity of protein sources to provide 40 g pre-sleep protein.

Food Item	Quantity
Cooked eggs	7 eggs
Low fat milk	5 cups (1025 mL)
Low fat yogurt	5 cups (1176 mL)
Chicken breast	2 breasts (176 g)
Steak	2 steaks (168 g)
Protein concentrate in water	3 scoops (60 g)
Protein concentrate in low-fat milk	2 scoops in 300 mL

8. Applications

Overnight sleep has emerged as a novel window of opportunity to modulate muscle protein metabolism. Pre-sleep protein ingestion represents an effective dietary strategy to stimulate both the acute and long-term skeletal muscle adaptive response to resistance-type exercise training [24,25]. There are numerous other potential applications of protein ingestion prior to sleep. Protein ingestion prior to sleep may also enhance exercise training adaptations to other exercise modalities. However, research on the impact of protein supplementation on other modes of exercise such as concurrent training [39] or endurance-type exercise training [40] is surprisingly scarce. While protein ingested immediately after endurance-type exercise does not appear to further augment mitochondrial protein synthesis rates [40], amino acid administration at rest stimulates mitochondrial protein synthesis rates [41]. It remains to be established if pre-sleep protein can augment the adaptive response to endurance-type exercise training with greater increases in skeletal muscle oxidative capacity, vascular density and/or endurance performance capacity.

Protein administration during sleep has been shown to stimulate overnight muscle protein synthesis rates in older adults [23]. Consequently, pre-sleep protein feeding may also represent an effective interventional strategy to support muscle mass maintenance in the older population or possibly even in patients in more clinically compromised conditions characterized by accelerated muscle loss such as acute sickness, systematic inflammation, and muscle disuse [42,43].

9. Conclusions

Muscle protein synthesis rates are particularly low during sleep, even when 20 g protein is ingested immediately after exercise performed in the evening. Protein ingested immediately prior to sleep is effectively digested and absorbed, thereby increasing amino acid availability during overnight sleep. Greater amino acid availability during sleep stimulates muscle protein synthesis rates and improves whole-body protein net balance during overnight recovery. At least 40 g of dietary protein should be ingested prior to sleep to elicit a robust stimulation of muscle protein synthesis rates throughout the night. Resistance-type exercise performed during the day augments the overnight muscle protein synthetic response to pre-sleep protein ingestion and allows more of the protein-derived amino acids to be used as precursors for de novo muscle protein synthesis. When applied during prolonged resistance-type exercise, pre-sleep protein supplementation can be used effectively to further increase gains in muscle mass and strength.

Author Contributions: Jorn Trommelen wrote the draft manuscript, Luc J. C. van Loon revised the manuscript.

Conflicts of Interest: The authors declare no conflict of interest.

References

1. Biolo, G.; Maggi, S.P.; Williams, B.D.; Tipton, K.D.; Wolfe, R.R. Increased rates of muscle protein turnover and amino acid transport after resistance exercise in humans. *Am. J. Physiol.* **1995**, *268*, E514–E520. [PubMed]
2. Phillips, S.M.; Tipton, K.D.; Aarsland, A.; Wolf, S.E.; Wolfe, R.R. Mixed muscle protein synthesis and breakdown after resistance exercise in humans. *Am. J. Physiol.* **1997**, *273*, E99–E107. [PubMed]
3. Tipton, K.D.; Ferrando, A.A.; Phillips, S.M.; Doyle, D.J.; Wolfe, R.R. Postexercise net protein synthesis in human muscle from orally administered amino acids. *Am. J. Physiol.* **1999**, *276*, E628–E634. [PubMed]
4. Moore, D.R.; Robinson, M.J.; Fry, J.L.; Tang, J.E.; Glover, E.I.; Wilkinson, S.B.; Prior, T.; Tarnopolsky, M.A.; Phillips, S.M. Ingested protein dose response of muscle and albumin protein synthesis after resistance exercise in young men. *Am. J. Clin. Nutr.* **2009**, *89*, 161–168. [CrossRef] [PubMed]
5. Witard, O.C.; Jackman, S.R.; Breen, L.; Smith, K.; Selby, A.; Tipton, K.D. Myofibrillar muscle protein synthesis rates subsequent to a meal in response to increasing doses of whey protein at rest and after resistance exercise. *Am. J. Clin. Nutr.* **2013**, *99*, 86–95. [CrossRef] [PubMed]
6. Tang, J.E.; Moore, D.R.; Kujbida, G.W.; Tarnopolsky, M.A.; Phillips, S.M. Ingestion of whey hydrolysate, casein, or soy protein isolate: Effects on mixed muscle protein synthesis at rest and following resistance exercise in young men. *J. Appl. Physiol.* **2009**, *107*, 987–992. [CrossRef] [PubMed]
7. Wilkinson, S.B.; Tarnopolsky, M.A.; Macdonald, M.J.; Macdonald, J.R.; Armstrong, D.; Phillips, S.M. Consumption of fluid skim milk promotes greater muscle protein accretion after resistance exercise than does consumption of an isonitrogenous and isoenergetic soy-protein beverage. *Am. J. Clin. Nutr.* **2007**, *85*, 1031–1040. [PubMed]
8. Levenhagen, D.K.; Gresham, J.D.; Carlson, M.G.; Maron, D.J.; Borel, M.J.; Flakoll, P.J. Postexercise nutrient intake timing in humans is critical to recovery of leg glucose and protein homeostasis. *Am. J. Physiol. Endocrinol. Metab.* **2001**, *280*, E982–E993. [PubMed]
9. Areta, J.L.; Burke, L.M.; Ross, M.L.; Camera, D.M.; West, D.W.D.; Broad, E.M.; Jeacocke, N.A.; Moore, D.R.; Stellingwerff, T.; Phillips, S.M.; et al. Timing and distribution of protein ingestion during prolonged recovery from resistance exercise alters myofibrillar protein synthesis. *J. Physiol.* **2013**, *591*, 2319–2331. [CrossRef] [PubMed]

10. Yang, Y.; Breen, L.; Burd, N.A.; Hector, A.J.; Churchward-Venne, T.A.; Josse, A.R.; Tarnopolsky, M.A.; Phillips, S.M. Resistance exercise enhances myofibrillar protein synthesis with graded intakes of whey protein in older men. *Br. J. Nutr.* **2012**, *108*, 1780–1788. [CrossRef] [PubMed]

11. Yang, Y.; Churchward-Venne, T.A.; Burd, N.A.; Breen, L.; Tarnopolsky, M.A.; Phillips, S.M. Myofibrillar protein synthesis following ingestion of soy protein isolate at rest and after resistance exercise in elderly men. *Nutr. Metab.* **2012**, *9*, 57. [CrossRef] [PubMed]

12. Robinson, M.J.; Burd, N.A.; Breen, L.; Rerecich, T.; Yang, Y.; Hector, A.J.; Baker, S.K.; Phillips, S.M. Dose-dependent responses of myofibrillar protein synthesis with beef ingestion are enhanced with resistance exercise in middle-aged men. *Appl. Physiol. Nutr. Metab.* **2013**, *38*, 120–125. [CrossRef] [PubMed]

13. Macnaughton, L.S.; Wardle, S.L.; Witard, O.C.; McGlory, C.; Hamilton, D.L.; Jeromson, S.; Lawrence, C.E.; Wallis, G.A.; Tipton, K.D. The response of muscle protein synthesis following whole-body resistance exercise is greater following 40 g than 20 g of ingested whey protein. *Physiol. Rep.* **2016**, *4*, e12893. [CrossRef] [PubMed]

14. Tipton, K.D.; Elliott, T.A.; Cree, M.G.; Wolf, S.E.; Sanford, A.P.; Wolfe, R.R. Ingestion of casein and whey proteins result in muscle anabolism after resistance exercise. *Med. Sci. Sports Exerc.* **2004**, *36*, 2073–2081. [CrossRef] [PubMed]

15. Burd, N.A.; Gorissen, S.H.; van Vliet, S.; Snijders, T.; van Loon, L.J. Differences in postprandial protein handling after beef compared with milk ingestion during postexercise recovery: A randomized controlled trial. *Am. J. Clin. Nutr.* **2015**, *102*, 828–836. [CrossRef] [PubMed]

16. West, D.W.D.; Burd, N.A.; Coffey, V.G.; Baker, S.K.; Burke, L.M.; Hawley, J.A.; Moore, D.R.; Stellingwerff, T.; Phillips, S.M. Rapid aminoacidemia enhances myofibrillar protein synthesis and anabolic intramuscular signaling responses after resistance exercise. *Am. J. Clin. Nutr.* **2011**, *94*, 795–803. [CrossRef] [PubMed]

17. Pennings, B.; Boirie, Y.; Senden, J.M.G.; Gijsen, A.P.; Kuipers, H.; van Loon, L.J.C. Whey protein stimulates postprandial muscle protein accretion more effectively than do casein and casein hydrolysate in older men. *Am. J. Clin. Nutr.* **2011**, *93*, 997–1005. [CrossRef] [PubMed]

18. Churchward-Venne, T.A.; Breen, L.; Di Donato, D.M.; Hector, A.J.; Mitchell, C.J.; Moore, D.R.; Stellingwerff, T.; Breuille, D.; Offord, E.A.; Baker, S.K.; et al. Leucine supplementation of a low-protein mixed macronutrient beverage enhances myofibrillar protein synthesis in young men: A double-blind, randomized trial. *Am. J. Clin. Nutr.* **2014**, *99*, 276–286. [CrossRef] [PubMed]

19. Wall, B.T.; Hamer, H.M.; de Lange, A.; Kiskini, A.; Groen, B.B.L.; Senden, J.M.G.; Gijsen, A.P.; Verdijk, L.B.; van Loon, L.J.C. Leucine co-ingestion improves post-prandial muscle protein accretion in elderly men. *Clin. Nutr.* **2013**, *32*, 412–419. [CrossRef] [PubMed]

20. Mamerow, M.M.; Mettler, J.A.; English, K.L.; Casperson, S.L.; Arentson-Lantz, E.; Sheffield-Moore, M.; Layman, D.K.; Paddon-Jones, D. Dietary protein distribution positively influences 24-h muscle protein synthesis in healthy adults. *J. Nutr.* **2014**, *144*, 876–880. [CrossRef] [PubMed]

21. Beelen, M.; Tieland, M.; Gijsen, A.P.; Vandereyt, H.; Kies, A.K.; Kuipers, H.; Saris, W.H.M.; Koopman, R.; van Loon, L.J.C. Coingestion of carbohydrate and protein hydrolysate stimulates muscle protein synthesis during exercise in young men, with no further increase during subsequent overnight recovery. *J. Nutr.* **2008**, *138*, 2198–2204. [CrossRef] [PubMed]

22. Furukawa, Y.; Cook, I.J.; Panagopoulos, V.; McEvoy, R.D.; Sharp, D.J.; Simula, M. Relationship between sleep patterns and human colonic motor patterns. *Gastroenterology* **1994**, *107*, 1372–1381. [CrossRef]

23. Groen, B.B.L.; Res, P.T.; Pennings, B.; Hertle, E.; Senden, J.M.G.; Saris, W.H.M.; van Loon, L.J.C. Intragastric protein administration stimulates overnight muscle protein synthesis in elderly men. *Am. J. Physiol. Endocrinol. Metab.* **2012**, *302*, E52–E60. [CrossRef] [PubMed]

24. Res, P.T.; Groen, B.; Pennings, B.; Beelen, M.; Wallis, G.A.; Gijsen, A.P.; Senden, J.M.G.; van Loon, L.J.C. Protein ingestion before sleep improves postexercise overnight recovery. *Med. Sci. Sports Exerc.* **2012**, *44*, 1560–1569. [CrossRef] [PubMed]

25. Snijders, T.; Res, P.T.; Smeets, J.S.J.; van Vliet, S.; van Kranenburg, J.; Maase, K.; Kies, A.K.; Verdijk, L.B.; van Loon, L.J.C. Protein ingestion before sleep increases muscle mass and strength gains during prolonged resistance-type exercise training in healthy young men. *J. Nutr.* **2015**, *145*, 1178–1184. [CrossRef] [PubMed]

26. Cermak, N.M.; Res, P.T.; de Groot, L.C.; Saris, W.H.; van Loon, L.J. Protein supplementation augments the adaptive response of skeletal muscle to resistance-type exercise training: A meta-analysis. *Am. J. Clin. Nutr.* **2012**, *96*, 1454–1464. [CrossRef] [PubMed]

27. Reidy, P.T.; Rasmussen, B.B. Role of ingested amino acids and protein in the promotion of resistance exercise-induced muscle protein anabolism. *J. Nutr.* **2016**, *146*, 155–183. [CrossRef] [PubMed]
28. Schoenfeld, B.J.; Aragon, A.A.; Krieger, J.W. The effect of protein timing on muscle strength and hypertrophy: A meta-analysis. *J. Int. Soc. Sports Nutr.* **2013**, *10*, 53. [CrossRef] [PubMed]
29. Wall, B.T.; Burd, N.A.; Franssen, R.; Gorissen, S.H.; Snijders, T.; Senden, J.M.; Gijsen, A.P.; van Loon, L.J.C. Pre-sleep protein ingestion does not compromise the muscle protein synthetic response to protein ingested the following morning. *Am. J. Physiol. Endocrinol. Metab.* **2016**. [CrossRef] [PubMed]
30. Gillen, J.B.; Trommelen, J.; Wardenaar, F.C.; Brinkmans, N.Y.J.; Versteegen, J.J.; Jonvik, K.L.; Kapp, C.; de Vries, J.; van den Borne, J.J.G.C.; Gibala, M.J.; et al. Dietary protein intake and distribution patterns of well-trained dutch athletes. *Int. J. Sport Nutr. Exerc. Metab.* **2016**. [CrossRef] [PubMed]
31. Katsanos, C.S.; Kobayashi, H.; Sheffield-Moore, M.; Aarsland, A.; Wolfe, R.R. A high proportion of leucine is required for optimal stimulation of the rate of muscle protein synthesis by essential amino acids in the elderly. *Am. J. Physiol. Endocrinol. Metab.* **2006**, *291*, E381–E387. [CrossRef] [PubMed]
32. Rieu, I.; Balage, M.; Sornet, C.; Giraudet, C.; Pujos, E.; Grizard, J.; Mosoni, L.; Dardevet, D. Leucine supplementation improves muscle protein synthesis in elderly men independently of hyperaminoacidaemia. *J. Physiol.* **2006**, *575*, 305–315. [CrossRef] [PubMed]
33. Pennings, B.; Koopman, R.; Beelen, M.; Senden, J.M.G.; Saris, W.H.M.; van Loon, L.J.C. Exercising before protein intake allows for greater use of dietary protein-derived amino acids for de novo muscle protein synthesis in both young and elderly men. *Am. J. Clin. Nutr.* **2011**, *93*, 322–331. [CrossRef] [PubMed]
34. Trommelen, J.; Holwerda, A.M.; Kouw, I.W.K.; Langer, H.; Halson, S.L.; Rollo, I.; Verdijk, L.B.; van Loon, L.J.C. Resistance exercise augments postprandial overnight muscle protein synthesis rates. *Med. Sci. Sports Exerc.* **2016**, *48*, 2517–2525. [CrossRef] [PubMed]
35. Holwerda, A.M.; Kouw, I.W. K.; Trommelen, J.; Halson, S.L.; Wodzig, W.K.; Verdijk, L.B.; van Loon, L.J. Physical activity performed in the evening increases the overnight muscle protein synthetic response to presleep protein ingestion in older men. *J. Nutr.* **2016**, *146*, 1307–1314. [CrossRef] [PubMed]
36. Burd, N.A.; Yang, Y.; Moore, D.R.; Tang, J.E.; Tarnopolsky, M.A.; Phillips, S.M. Greater stimulation of myofibrillar protein synthesis with ingestion of whey protein isolate v. micellar casein at rest and after resistance exercise in elderly men. *Br. J. Nutr.* **2012**, *108*, 958–962. [CrossRef] [PubMed]
37. Devries, M.C.; Phillips, S.M. Supplemental protein in support of muscle mass and health: Advantage whey. *J. Food Sci.* **2015**, *80*, A8–A15. [CrossRef] [PubMed]
38. Koopman, R.; Crombach, N.; Gijsen, A.P.; Walrand, S.; Fauquant, J.; Kies, A.K.; Lemosquet, S.; Saris, W.H.M.; Boirie, Y.; van Loon, L.J.C. Ingestion of a protein hydrolysate is accompanied by an accelerated in vivo digestion and absorption rate when compared with its intact protein. *Am. J. Clin. Nutr.* **2009**, *90*, 106–115. [CrossRef] [PubMed]
39. Perez-Schindler, J.; Hamilton, D.L.; Moore, D.R.; Baar, K.; Philp, A. Nutritional strategies to support concurrent training. *Eur. J. Sport Sci.* **2015**, *15*, 41–52. [CrossRef] [PubMed]
40. Moore, D.R.; Camera, D.M.; Areta, J.L.; Hawley, J.A. Beyond muscle hypertrophy: Why dietary protein is important for endurance athletes 1. *Appl. Physiol. Nutr. Metab.* **2014**, *39*, 987–997. [CrossRef] [PubMed]
41. Bohe, J.; Low, A.; Wolfe, R.R.; Rennie, M.J. Human muscle protein synthesis is modulated by extracellular, not intramuscular amino acid availability: A dose-response study. *J. Physiol.* **2003**, *552*, 315–324. [CrossRef] [PubMed]
42. Kortebein, P.; Ferrando, A.; Lombeida, J.; Wolfe, R.; Evans, W.J. Effect of 10 days of bed rest on skeletal muscle in healthy older adults. *JAMA* **2007**, *297*, 1772–1774. [CrossRef] [PubMed]
43. Klaude, M.; Mori, M.; Tjader, I.; Gustafsson, T.; Wernerman, J.; Rooyackers, O. Protein metabolism and gene expression in skeletal muscle of critically ill patients with sepsis. *Clin. Sci.* **2012**, *122*, 133–142. [CrossRef] [PubMed]

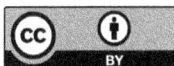

nutrients

MDPI

Article

Vitamin D and Weight Cycling: Impact on Injury, Illness, and Inflammation in Collegiate Wrestlers

Jacqueline N. Barcal [1,2], Joi T. Thomas [2], Bruce W. Hollis [3], Kathy J. Austin [4], Brenda M. Alexander [4] and D. Enette Larson-Meyer [1,*]

[1] Department of Family and Consumer Sciences, University of Wyoming, 1000 E. University Avenue, Laramie, WY 82071, USA; jbarcal@uwyo.edu
[2] Department of Athletics, University of Wyoming, 1000 E. University Avenue, Laramie, WY 82071, USA; thomasjj@uwyo.edu
[3] Dr. Bruce Hollis' Laboratory at the Medical University of South Carolina, Charleston, SC 29425, USA; hollisb@musc.edu
[4] Department of Animal Sciences; University of Wyoming, 1000 E. University Avenue, Laramie, WY 82071, USA; KathyAus@uwyo.edu (K.J.A.); BAlex@uwyo.edu (B.M.A.)
* Correspondence: enette@uwyo.edu; Tel.: +1-307-766-4378; Fax: +1-307-766-5686

Received: 28 August 2016; Accepted: 18 November 2016; Published: 30 November 2016

Abstract: This study explored the link between vitamin D status and frequency of skin infections, inflammation, and injury in college wrestlers during an academic year. Methods: Serum 25-hydroxyvitamin D (25(OH)D) (n = 19), plasma cytokine (TNF-α, IL-6, IL-10) (n = 18) concentrations, and body weight/composition were measured and injury/illness/skin infection data were collected in fall, winter, and spring. Results: In the fall, 74% of wrestlers had vitamin D concentrations <32 ng/mL which increased to 94% in winter and spring. Wrestlers lost an average of 3.4 ± 3.9 kg (p < 0.001) during the season with corresponding decreases in fat mass and increases in lean mass (p < 0.01). An inverse association between 25(OH)D concentrations and total body mass and body fat percentage was observed at all-time points (p < 0.01). Concentrations of cytokines were highly variable among individuals and did not change across time (p > 0.05). Correlations between vitamin D status, cytokines, or frequency of illness, injury, or skin infections were not observed. Conclusions: A high prevalence of vitamin D insufficiency (<32 ng/mL) and deficiency (<20 ng/mL) was observed in wrestlers and was associated with higher adiposity. It remains unclear if higher vitamin D status would reduce injury, illness, and skin infection risk.

Keywords: vitamin D; wrestling; exercise; athletes; inflammation

1. Introduction

Increasing evidence has linked low vitamin D status to a variety of health conditions including osteoporosis, cardiovascular disease, diabetes, depression, multiple sclerosis, rheumatoid arthritis and certain types of cancer [1–3]. Research has also observed a link between low vitamin D status and increased susceptibility of upper respiratory tract infections (URTI) [4] including influenza and the common cold [4,5]. Even though vitamin D is considered a vitamin, it is unique in that it both acts as a hormone, assisting in regulation of serum calcium, and may be obtained from dietary and endogenously synthesized sources. Endogenous synthesis occurs in the skin with exposure to sufficient ultra violet B (UVB) light [1,6] during peak hours (10 a.m. to 2 p.m.). Vitamin D cannot be made in the winter months at distances greater than 37 degrees north or south [2]. Natural or fortified dietary sources include fatty fish, whole milk, and some brands of yogurt, margarine, fruit juice, and ready-to-eat cereals [2]. Although vitamin D deficiency has been considered a nutritional problem of the past, it has re-emerged as a public health concern. In fact, some researchers believe it is an unrecognized epidemic in adults lacking exposure to adequate sunlight [1].

In athletic populations, vitamin D may be important for optimal health and performance. Vitamin D deficiency has been associated with reduced strength [7], prolonged recovery from surgery [8], altered inflammatory markers [9,10], and increased risk for injury and illness [11–13] in both athletes and non-athletes. In athletes, the prevalence of vitamin D deficiency and insufficiency varies by sport, training location, skin color [13], adequate sunlight exposure between 10 a.m. and 2 p.m., is more prevalent among athletes who train indoors versus outdoors [11,14,15], and who have higher body fat percentages [16]. A summary of vitamin D status documented in athletes and active individuals is outlined in Table S1. Vitamin D status is generally lower in the winter and among athletes who train predominantly indoors versus outdoors and who live at higher latitudes (i.e., >37 degrees North or South). In addition, serum concentrations tend to decline between fall and spring, and supplementation may or may not be effective for reaching optimum concentrations depending on dosage [17]. Current studies are inconsistent as to whether or not having higher vitamin D status translates to improved performance measures [18].

Wrestlers, particularly at the college level, are at risk for skin infections from mat and skin-to-skin contact and may be more prone to both compromised immune function and poor vitamin D status due to nutrient restriction from cutting weight [19–21], indoor training, and competing during a season of limited sun exposure (October-March) when URTI risk is elevated [11,22]. Although the vitamin D status of collegiate athletes has previously been evaluated, little is known about the status of wrestlers who may be at increased risk for deficiency/insufficiency due to indoor training and chronic dietary restriction and weight cycling. Therefore, the purpose of this study was to assess vitamin D status of male college wrestlers during the academic year and determine if low vitamin D status (i.e., low circulating concentrations of 25-hydroxy vitamin D) was associated with documented incidence of acute illness, including skin infections, and with circulating pro-inflammatory cytokines interleukin-6 (IL-6) and tumor necrosis factor-alpha (TNF-α) and the anti-inflammatory cytokine interleukin-10 (IL-10). A secondary purpose was to explore whether weight and body composition changes further impacted seasonal changes in vitamin D concentration and cytokine concentrations. We hypothesized that wrestlers with suboptimal vitamin D status (25(OH)D <32 ng/mL) would have a higher incidence of acute illness including URTI and skin infections, higher pro-inflammatory markers, and lower anti-inflammatory markers compared to wrestlers with optimal vitamin D status (25(OH)D >40 ng/mL).

2. Materials and Methods

2.1. Study Design

This study took place during the 2014–2015 college academic year. All University of Wyoming (UW) athletes ≥18 years on UW's National Collegiate Athletic Association (NCAA) Division I wrestling team ($n = 25$) were invited to participate. Participation, however, was not required and the coaching staff received no information on which wrestlers participated in the study so as to avoid potential bias during training or competition. The study was approved by the UW Institutional Review Board (approval code #20140703JB00477, 3 July 2014) with written, informed consent obtained prior to participation.

2.2. Study Overview

Blood was drawn three times during the academic year (September, January, and April) in accordance with seasonal training and typically occurred in the morning after an overnight fast. Athletes were instructed to avoid exercise for at least 12 h prior to the draw. Height and weight were measured and a short questionnaire, administered at these same time points was used to assess vitamin D intake and lifestyle factors which may impact vitamin D status (i.e., estimated time spent outdoors, sunscreen use, use of tanning beds, etc.) [11]. The vitamin D questionnaire was administered in a private setting and took approximately 10 min to complete [11]. Body composition was analyzed by dual energy X-ray absorptiometry (DXA) and occurred no more than 7 days away from the blood draw. Selected information contained within the athletes' medical charts, including illness and infection history (i.e., upper respiratory tract infections, gastritis, skin infection, etc.), illness progression, prescribed medications, and supplement use was obtained from medical records documented by the Sports Medicine staff as part of routine care.

2.3. Blood Analysis

Blood samples were appropriately post-processed and kept frozen at −20 degrees Celsius until analysis. 25(OH)D concentration was evaluated by Diasorin 25(OH)D radioimmunoassay (Bruce Hollis' Laboratory, the Medical University of South Carolina, Charleston, SC, USA). Inflammatory markers (TNF-α, IL-6, IL-10) were analyzed via enzyme-linked immunosorbent assay (ELISA) (QIAGEN, Santa Clarita, CA, USA) according to manufacturer's instructions. For cytokine analysis, plasma samples were thawed immediately before being assayed and vortexed for approximately 5 s to ensure adequate mixing. Absorbance was read at 450 nm using a standard ELISA microplate reader. Standards were diluted using a 1:2 dilution series. The eight standards of known cytokine concentrations included in each assay ranged from 15–2000 pg/mL. All samples were analyzed in duplicate. A log transformation was used to generate a regression equation to predict cytokine concentrations, reported as pg/mL.

2.4. Body Composition

Body composition was assessed via DXA. Subjects were instructed to avoid food and exercise at least two hours prior to testing. When possible, testing was done first thing in the morning (6:00–9:00 a.m.) after an overnight fast and abstaining from training for at least 12 h. Body mass (kg), fat mass (kg), fat free mass (kg), and body fat percentage were utilized for statistical analysis.

2.5. Weight Collection

Weekly weights were obtained from coaching staff from 3 September to 28 February. Wrestlers were weighed on the same scale, with minimal clothing, in their locker room prior to afternoon practice on each Monday by one of the wrestling coaches. In order to calculate the amount of weight lost each week to "make weight" for competition, each athlete's weight class was subtracted from his recorded Monday weight with the assumption that he would have to lose that amount in order to compete at the end of the week (Friday/Saturday). Because heavyweights are less likely to partake in traditional weight cutting practices, heavyweights were omitted from statistical analyses addressing weekly and seasonal weight changes. These weights were also utilized to calculate average weekly weight changes (Monday to Monday).

2.6. Injury, Illness, and Skin Infection

As part of routine medical care, injury, illness, and skin infection data were collected by the team physician and documented in student-athlete medical charts. In addition to documentation done by the physician, a certified athletic trainer (ATC) assigned to the sport performed daily skin checks and was present at each training session. The daily skin check allowed wrestlers to report any unusual formations on the skin.

2.7. Statistical Procedures

A sample size calculation for a descriptive study of a continuous variable (i.e., 25(OH)D concentration) was conducted using the average standard deviation for college athletes participating in indoor sports during the fall (8.2 ng/mL) and winter (5.6 ng/mL) from pervious data [11].

Using a 95% confidence interval (CI), an $n = 19$ to 41 was estimated for a total desired CI width of 5 and a sample of 10 to 21 was needed for a total CI width of 7 [23]. Correlation sample calculations for previously identified associations between 25(OH)D and fat mass ($r = -0.42$) [16], frequency of URTI ($r = -0.40$) [11] and TNF-α concentration ($r = -0.63$) [24] using previous coefficients as the expected correlation coefficient (one-tailed $\alpha = 0.05$ and $\beta = 0.20$) estimated that a sample size of $n = 14$ to 37 would be needed to determine whether correlation coefficients differed from zero. Given these calculations, efforts were placed on recruitment and longitudinal retention of as many of our total population of wrestlers of $n = 25$.

Data were analyzed using IBM SPSS Statistics 23 software. Repeated measures analysis of variance (ANOVA) was utilized to assess the change in body weight/body composition, serum 25(OH)D, and plasma cytokine concentrations over time. Correlation coefficients (Pearson's) were used to evaluate the associations among 25(OH)D and body weight/adiposity, weight change during the season, dietary and supplemental vitamin D intake (including vitamin D and calcium), frequency of infection and illness, and cytokine concentrations. Additional multilinear regression modeling was used to evaluate the association between vitamin D status and body weight/body composition adjusting for weight cycling pattern, weight class, age, athletic eligibility year, and other significant predictors (based on analysis of simple correlation coefficients). Spearman's rank correlations were used to identify intra-cytokine association and association with vitamin D, body composition, illness, injury, and skin infection prevalence.

3. Results

Twenty male wrestlers initially volunteered to participate in the study; nineteen wrestlers reported to baseline testing. All 19 initial participants completed baseline vitamin D testing (September), but body composition data could not be obtained on one athlete due to scheduling conflicts. Baseline characteristics for the 18 wrestlers for which body composition was available are summarized in Table 1.

Table 1. Baseline characteristics of 18 male wrestlers [1].

Age (years)	Height (cm)	Weight (kg)	BMI (kg/m^2)	Body Fat (%)
20.9 ± 2.0	171.8 ± 15.3	87.4 ± 18.6	27.3 ± 4.0	19.0 ± 7.0
19–23	162.6–193.0	62.0–121.7	22.6–35.4	12.5–37.7

[1] Data reported as mean $\pm$ SD with range listed beneath; Caucasian ($n = 15$); Spanish Italian ($n = 1$); Asian ($n = 2$). Abbreviations: BMI, body mass index.

By the winter data collection point (January), three participants discontinued participation for undisclosed reasons. Complete longitudinal data for vitamin D was therefore available on 16 wrestlers for winter and spring collection and logitudinal body composition and cytokine data were only available on 15 due to difficulty with a blood draw in the fall ($n = 1$) and scheduling conflicts with the DXA measurement ($n = 1$).

During the 2014–2015 academic season, the team as a whole participated in 5 tournaments, 15 dual meets, and six wrestlers competed in the NCAA Division I Wrestling Championships. Starters wrestled an average of 31 matches. Among the athletes who completed the study, there was representation from each of the ten weight classes and each class weight class included a conference dual starter with the exception of the 141 lb weight class in which only fall data was available.

3.1. Vitamin D Status

As shown in Figure 1 below, serum 25(OH)D changed across time ($p < 0.001$) and was highest in the fall and lowest in the winter. In the fall ($n = 19$), five athletes (26.3%) had sufficient vitamin D status whereas twelve (63.2%) and two (10.5%) presented with insufficient (20–32 ng/mL) and deficient status (<20 ng/mL), respectively. In the winter and spring ($n = 16$), one athlete (6%) had sufficient status, and eleven (69%) and four (25%) had insufficient and deficient status, respectively. None of the athletes experienced optimal 25(OH)D status (>40 ng/mL) [5,11] at any time point across the season.

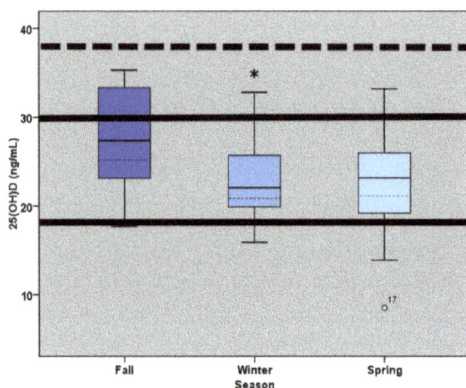

Figure 1. Box plots illustrating the distribution of 25(OH)D concentration (ng/mL) in the fall (n = 19), winter (n = 16), and spring (n = 16). Box extents indicate the 25th and 75th percentile, with the median indicated by a solid dark line and the mean indicated by a dashed line. Central vertical lines (whiskers) extend up to 1.5 interquartile ranges from the end of the box. A circle marks individual points outside of the whiskers indicating a value between 1.5 and 3.0 interquartile ranges of the box. 25(OH)D concentrations <20 ng/mL are considered deficient, concentrations between 20 and 32 ng/mL are considered insufficient (solid horizontal lines), and concentrations >40 ng/mL are considered optimal. * Significant decrease in 25(OH)D observed between fall and winter (p < 0.001), reported as mean ± SD.

3.2. Body Weight and Body Composition

Body weight changes over the course of the training season/academic year (September–May) ranged from −12.0 kg to +4.5 kg with an average season weight change of −3.4 ± 3.8 kg (n = 16, p = 0.003). Most of the weight loss, averaging 4.1 ± 2.4 kg (−1.0 kg to −9.5 kg), occurred between the fall and winter. This was followed by an average weight gain of 0.21 ± 2.4 kg (−6.0 ± 4.1 kg) per wrestler in between winter and spring. The trend for weight gain between winter and spring remained when omitting the four heavy weight wrestlers in the group (0.06 ± 0.12 kg), but was not apparent when accounting for the nine conference season starters (0.003 ± 0.171 kg). Among the entire group for which weekly weight changes were available (n = 19), mean week-to-week weight change (Monday to Monday) averaged −0.19 ± 0.10 kg (−0.37 kg to −0.06) over the course of the study. This minimal change in weekly weight became even smaller when accounting for season starters only (n = 10) and also when omitting heavyweights (n = 15). Despite minimal changes in weight between team weekly weigh-ins, the amount of weight lost each week to make competition weight, not including heavy weights (n = 15), averaged 4.6 ± 1.0 kg (6.3% ± 1.5%). Similar results were observed when accounting for starters. Average weekly weight change did not change across any time point (fall to winter, winter to spring, or fall to spring, p > 0.05).

As summarized in Table 2, body composition changed across the training season/academic year (n = 15, p < 0.01) despite the minimal week-to-week variability in body weight. Absolute total body mass, body mass index (BMI), fat mass, and body fat percentage decreased whereas lean body mass and bone mineral density (BMD) increased.

3.3. Cytokine Concentrations and Inter-Cytokine Relationship

As shown in Table 3, there was considerable variability in the concentrations of the various cytokines among individuals and across the academic year (n = 15). Concentrations of IL-6 and TNF-α were numerically higher in the fall and spring and lowest in winter whereas concentrations of IL-10 demonstrated the opposite pattern. These slight alterations, however, were not different across time ($p > 0.05$).

Table 2. Body composition across the academic year [1].

Measurement	Fall	Winter	Spring	Sig. (p) [2]
Weight (kg)	90.6 ± 18.0	86.5 ± 17.0	86.7 ± 16.0	<0.001
BMI (kg/m^2)	27.6 ± 3.9	26.4 ± 3.6	26.7 ± 3.4	0.001
Lean Mass (kg)	69.0 ± 10.4	70.8 ± 9.8	70.5 ± 9.8	0.003
Fat Mass (kg)	17.6 ± 10.2	11.8 ± 9.4	12.1 ± 9.1	<0.001
Body Fat (%)	19.4 ± 7.1	13.2 ± 7.4	12.8 ± 5.0	<0.001
BMD (g/cm^2)	1.42 ± 0.1	1.45 ± 0.1	1.47 ± 0.1	0.001

[1] Data reported as mean $\pm$ SD; [2] Repeated measures ANOVA of body composition changes across time ($n = 15$) (statistic $\times$ time effect).

Table 3. Cytokine concentrations across the academic year [1].

Cytokine	Fall	Winter	Spring	Sig. (p) [2]
IL-6 (pg/dL)	110 ± 229	73 ± 144	120 ± 306	0.335
IL-10 (pg/dL)	254 ± 469	362 ± 938	246 ± 559	0.270
TNF-α (pg/dL)	1549 ± 2361	886 ± 1117	1293 ± 2197	0.287

[1] Data reported as mean $\pm$ SD. [2] Repeated measures ANOVA of body composition changes across time ($n = 15$) (statistic $\times$ time effect).

In addition, cytokine concentrations were highly inter-correlated at all time points (Pearson's). IL-6 was positively correlated with both IL-10 and TNF-α during the fall ($n = 18$), winter ($n = 15$), and spring ($n = 15$) (IL-10: $r = 0.924$, $r = 0.856$, and $r = 0.846$, $p < 0.001$, respectively; TNF-α: $r = 0.950$, $r = 0.837$, and $r = 0.945$, $p < 0.001$, respectively). IL-10 also positively correlated with TNF-α at all time points ($r = 0.897$, $r = 0.767$, and $r = 0.969$, $p < 0.001$, respectively).

3.4. Illness, Injury, and Skin Infection

Skin infection occurrence over the course of the season (September–May) averaged 1.8 ± 1.3 per participant with fifteen (79%) subjects experiencing at least one skin infection by the end of fall with four (11%) new infections being documented between winter and spring. A total of 35 skin infections were reported over the course of the season with a majority ($n = 31$, 89%) being reported between the fall and winter. Herpes ($n = 19$), ringworm ($n = 4$), and impetigo ($n = 2$) were the most common diagnoses between fall and winter while only herpes ($n = 4$) was reported between the winter and spring. The forehead was the most common skin infection site ($n = 8$) followed by the ear, back, arm/wrist, and lip being the second most frequent location ($n = 4$).

Eight subjects experienced a documented illness over the course of the study with one subject contracting two illnesses. Six of these were reported between the fall and winter and three were reported between winter and spring. The primary diagnosis was URTI ($n = 8$) which included cough, congestion, and sinus infection.

There were a total of nine injuries reported in seven different athletes over the year with an average of 0.5 ± 0.7 injuries per wrestler. Collectively, there were 50 total skin infections, illnesses, and injuries reported over the year averaging 2.6 ± 1.5 per wrestler ($n = 19$).

3.5. Vitamin D

3.5.1. Vitamin D Intake and Relation to Vitamin D Status

Intake of vitamin D from food alone or food plus supplements is summarized in Table 4. Athletes did not meet the recommended dietary allowance (RDA) for vitamin D intake from food alone (600 IU) at any time point during the year. When supplements were included, seven athletes met the RDA in the fall, five in the winter, and four in the spring. There were no significant changes in dietary vitamin D intake from food alone or food plus supplements across time ($n = 16$, $p = 0.25$ and $p = 0.707$, respectively).

Table 4. Vitamin D intake from food and supplements across the academic year [1].

Vitamin D Source	Fall	Winter	Spring
Dietary Intake	257 ± 212	211 ± 135	250 ± 191
Intake from Supplements	443 ± 996	370 ± 569	296 ± 758
Combined Vitamin D Intake	1549 ± 2361	886 ± 1117	1293 ± 2197

[1] Reported as International Units (IU), mean $\pm$ SD ($n = 16$).

Vitamin D intake from food alone or food plus supplements was not associated with serum 25(OH)D concentrations at any time point ($p \geq 0.05$). However, in the spring there was a positive association between both total vitamin D intake and vitamin D intake from supplements and vitamin D category (i.e., deficient, insufficient, etc.) such that those with higher overall vitamin D intake had higher categorical status ($n = 16$, $r = 0.563$, $p = 0.02$ and $r = 0.556$, $p = 0.02$, respectively).

3.5.2. Relation between Vitamin D Status and Body Composition

25(OH)D was negatively correlated with body fat percentage in the fall ($n = 18$, $r = -0.481$, $p = 0.043$), winter ($n = 16$, $r = -0.521$, $p = 0.038$), and spring ($n = 16$, $r = -0.565$, $p = 0.18$). 25(OH)D was correlated with fat mass in the spring only ($n = 16$, $r = -0.652$, $p = 0.005$) as shown in Figure 2, with a trend for a similar association in the winter ($n = 16$, $r = -0.446$, $p = 0.083$), but not the fall ($n = 18$, $r = -0.385$, $p = 0.115$). 25(OH)D, however, was not associated with total body mass, lean mass, or BMI at any time point ($p > 0.05$). There was an interaction with vitamin D category (sufficient, insufficient, and deficient) and total body mass ($p = 0.012$), fat mass ($p = 0.001$), and body fat percentage ($p = 0.001$) such that those with higher weight and adiposity had lower status. The change in vitamin D status from fall to winter and from winter to spring, however, did not appear to be associated with the change in total body mass or fat mass over these same time points ($p > 0.05$). However, average weekly weight fluctuations (Monday to Monday) from fall to spring positively correlated with spring 25(OH)D ($n = 16$, $r = 0.663$, $p = 0.005$,) such that those with larger average weekly weight changes had higher vitamin D status in the spring.

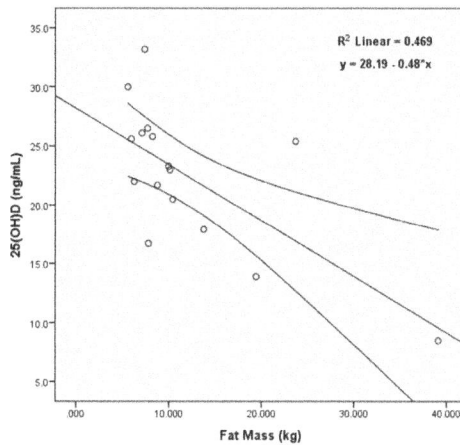

Figure 2. Linear regression model illustrating the association between 25(OH)D and fat mass (kg) in the spring ($n = 16$). Negative associations between these two variables were also observed in the fall and winter.

3.5.3. Relation between Vitamin D Status and Cytokines

Neither 25(OH)D or vitamin D category (sufficient, insufficient, and deficient) correlated with IL-6, IL-10, or TNF-α at any time point ($n = 15$, $p > 0.05$, Pearson's correlation).

3.5.4. Relation between Vitamin D Status and Illness, Injury, and Skin Infections

Neither 25(OH)D or vitamin D category (sufficient, insufficient, and deficient) was associated with number of illnesses or skin infections at any time point or over the course of the academic year ($n = 15$, $p > 0.05$), however, winter vitamin D category was positively associated with number of injuries incurred from fall to winter such that those with higher status experienced more injuries ($r = 0.550$, $p = 0.020$).

3.6. Cytokines

3.6.1. Relation between Body Composition and Cytokines

At no time point did body composition (total body mass, body fat percentage, fat mass, lean mass, or BMD) influence IL-6, IL-10, or TNF-α over time ($p > 0.05$). Fall and winter fat mass influenced the change in TNF-α over time that approached statistical significance ($n = 15$, $p = 0.62 \times$ time effect, $p = 0.73 \times$ time effect).

3.6.2. Relation between Weight Loss and Cytokines

Average weekly weight fluctuations over the course of the year (fall to spring) and cytokine concentrations were not correlated at any time point ($p > 0.05$). Significant correlations were found between weight change from fall to winter and winter cytokine concentrations ($n = 15$, Table 5).

Table 5. Association between cytokine concentrations in the winter and total body mass change between fall and winter (*n* = 15).

Spearman's Rank	Correlation (r)	Sig. (p)
IL-6	0.497	0.060
IL-10	0.561	0.029
TNF-α	0.540	0.038

3.6.3. Relation between Cytokine Concentrations and Prevalence of Illness, Injury, and Skin Infection

Cytokine concentrations were not associated with the prevalence of illness, injury, or skin infections at any time point during the study (*n* = 15, *p* > 0.05).

4. Discussion

This study evaluated the vitamin D status of male collegiate wrestlers over the course of an academic year and aimed to determine whether vitamin D status was influenced by vitamin D intake and body composition. We also aimed to determine whether vitamin D status influenced cytokine concentrations, injury, illness, and skin infection incidence. Furthermore, it was evaluated whether wrestlers who "cut" more weight over the course of the season, experienced greater season-induced changes in vitamin D status and/or cytokine concentrations. We found a high prevalence of vitamin D insufficiency and deficiency in wrestlers throughout the academic year, which ranged from 74% in the fall to 94% in the winter and spring, that was inversely associated with body fat percentage and was influenced by week-to-week weight fluctuations, but was not impacted by intake or overall weight loss throughout the season. An association between serum 25(OH)D concentration and risk of injury, infection or illness was not observed.

Despite an initially high prevalence of vitamin D insufficiency and deficiency in the fall, the status of college wrestlers declined significantly across the academic year as has been previously shown in other athlete groups [11,25–30]. The majority of the decline occurred between the fall (September) and winter (January) with the incidence of insufficiency/deficiency reaching 94% in the winter and spring. The overall prevalence of suboptimal status was higher than previously reported in our laboratory in college athletes from mixed sports [11,24] and those of other indoor athletes [26,27] and sportsmen training near the equator where suspected sun avoidance was the culture [31]. Although it was not surprising that wrestlers had low vitamin D status in the winter and spring due to their exclusive indoor training regimen, it was somewhat surprising that status was so low in the fall when wrestlers engaged in close to eight weeks of outdoor training typically between 2:00 and 5:00 p.m. in mostly sunny conditions at an elevation of between ~7200 and 8400 feet [25]. The higher than expected prevalence of insufficiency and deficiency may be a combination of late afternoon training, which misses peak hours of 10:00 a.m.–2:00 p.m., clothing worn, or the higher body fat percentage of some of the athletes [16] when weekly weigh-ins are not required. In agreement with previous studies in both athletes and non-athletes [16,30,32–34], body adiposity was negatively associated with serum 25(OH)D concentration across the academic year. Although the specific mechanism for this association is not fully understood, the lipophilic properties of vitamin D are thought to allow sequestration in adipose tissue, which thereby decreases circulating 25(OH)D concentrations [30,35].

The overall low vitamin D intake may have also contributed to low status. Vitamin D intake was, on average, less than 50% of the RDA across the season, which is consistent with research in other athletic populations [11,25,26,36]. Vitamin D supplementation was also low. For instance, depending on the time of the year, only two to three wrestlers reported taking a vitamin D supplement and only five to six reported taking a multi-vitamin. In agreement with previous studies [11,32], vitamin D intake from food or supplements was not directly associated with vitamin D status. Ironically, in the current study the wrestler with the lowest serum 25(OH)D concentration had the highest body mass, the third highest body fat percentage, and reported taking a vitamin D supplement during the entire academic year. He also experienced a significant decline in body fat percentage (37.7% in the fall to 19.6% in the spring). This suggests that the supplemental dose taken (not reported) was not sufficient to counteract the negative influence of adiposity on status across the season despite a significant reduction in body adiposity.

Unique to this study was our evaluation of whether vitamin D status impacted cytokine concentrations over the course of the year. Our initial hypothesis was that athletes with lower vitamin D status would have higher pro-inflammatory cytokines and lower anti-inflammatory cytokines than those with higher status. Our lack of an association between serum 25(OH)D and cytokine concentrations during the season, however, may be explained by the overall low vitamin D status of our wrestlers and/or the high variability in cytokine concentrations throughout the year. Although all blood cytokine concentrations were obtained after at least 12 h of physical inactivity, approximately eight weeks (August–September) of conditioning (6 days/week) and strength training (3 days/week) occurred before the initial data collection in September. Thus, preseason training may have elevated cytokines in some or all athletes. It is not well established how a single bout of exercise or regular training influences cytokine concentrations, or how long athletes should refrain from exercise to reveal cytokine samples reflective of overall health. For example, some research has shown that after a single bout of intense physical activity, cytokine concentrations return to baseline within 2–3 h after exercise terminates [9,37] while others suggest that cytokines remain elevated even 24 h following exercise [38,39].

In the present study, IL-6 and TNF-α concentrations decreased between fall and winter. This was followed by an increase back toward the fall baseline between winter and spring. IL-10 concentration, in contrast, increased between the fall and winter also returning toward baseline in the spring. The decrease in TNF-α concentration between the fall and winter was somewhat unexpected due to intense practices and weight training sessions 5–6 days per week, which would be expected to induce a low level inflammatory response. Perhaps, TNF-α was not elevated due to a concurrent rise in IL-10 concentrations. IL-10 is a potent anti-inflammatory cytokine that has been shown to assist in the down-regulation of TNF-α during exercise [37,40]. In agreement with our findings, previous research has also shown a lack of correlation between 25(OH)D and TNF-α [32,41–45]. Our lack of a relationship between vitamin D status and TNF-α concentration, however, is contradictory to Willis et al. [24], and others who have found a significant inverse relationship between 25(OH)D and TNF-α concentrations in both humans and mice [45–48].

In the current study, the majority of skin infections were reported between the fall and winter ($n = 31$) as compared to between winter to spring ($n = 4$). This was somewhat expected, as wrestlers transition from summer conditioning and strength training to training in the wrestling room where skin-to-skin and skin-to-mat contact are more frequent. This time period also coincides with the suspected reduction in cutaneous vitamin D synthesis (from limited sun exposure and reduced synthesis capacity) and frequent dietary restriction as wrestlers work to maintain competition weight on a week-to-week basis. As previously noted, the majority of the decrease in serum 25(OH)D concentration occurred between fall and winter (28.2 ± 5.2 vs. 22.8 ± 4.6 ng/mL), however, vitamin D intake remained unchanged despite the suspected intentional energy restriction, at least in some wrestlers. We had hypothesized, however, that the increased skin infection risk would be associated with low serum 25(OH)D. The hormonally active form of vitamin D, $1,25(OH)_2D_3$, has been shown to up-regulate expression of anti-microbial peptides (AMP's) and assist in the defense against bacterial infection [49]. Our lack of association between vitamin D status and frequency of both skin and other documented illnesses, nevertheless, may be due to the overall high frequency of vitamin D insufficiency and deficiency. This precluded maintenance of 25(OH)D concentrations in a range not high enough to experience a beneficial effect. For example, when Halliday et al. evaluated the relationship between vitamin D status and illness in collegiate athletes from our same university, athletes with higher 25(OH)D concentration in the winter and spring were found to experience fewer illnesses over the course of the year [11]. Reduction in illness frequency, however, was not apparent until serum 25(OH)D concentrations approached approximately 40 ng/mL [11]. In the current study, only one wrestler maintained vitamin D status in the sufficient category (>32 ng/mL) in both winter and spring and none maintained 25(OH)D concentration greater than 40 ng/mL. Future research should include a vitamin D supplementation trial that elevates concentrations of 25(OH)D above 40 ng/mL to allow for a better analysis of the impact of maintaining optimal vitamin D status on inflammation, illness, and skin infection in wrestlers.

The present study did not reveal a consistent relationship between vitamin D status and number of injuries sustained. This may be partially explained by our low injury rate, injury underreporting, or small sample size. In the present study, our injury frequency averaged approximately 0.5 injuries per wrestler which was lower than previous reports in male ballet dancers (1.9 injuries/dancer) [50], Taiwanese elite wrestlers (4.2 injuries/wrestler) [51], and high school wrestlers (5.2 injuries/wrestler) [52]. With the identification of vitamin D receptors in skeletal muscle cells [53], it is not surprising that several previous studies have found associations between higher vitamin D status and fewer incidences of injuries, including in professional American football athletes [54,55]. Furthermore, vitamin D supplementation in ballet dancers has been shown to reduce injuries over a 4-month period when compared to no supplementation [7]. Other research has indicated that while maintaining higher vitamin D concentrations may not prevent injury, it may assist in expediting recovery [56]. One unexpected result of the current study was the positive correlation between vitamin D status in the winter and the number of injuries that occurred between the fall and winter. It is likely that this association is coincidental due to the small number of injuries and small sample size. Overuse, over-training, and/or poor wrestling technique may also confound our findings. Unfortunately, duration of injury or injury rehabilitation response was not evaluated in the present study.

Collectively, the reported total number of skin infections, illnesses, and injuries averaged 2.7 ± 1.5 per wrestler ($n = 20$), however, actual rates may be higher due to underreporting by the athlete to avoid restrictions from practice and/or competition. The five injuries that occurred in the four wrestlers between fall and winter included a concussion, wrist fracture, meniscus tear, foot sprain, and a shoulder pain complaint due to surgery that occurred at the beginning of the semester.

We found that fat mass at all three time points (fall, winter, and spring) influenced the change in TNF-α across time. This finding is in agreement with previous reports indicating a positive association between adiposity and inflammation [36]. This may warrant special attention to those athletes with higher adiposity, as they may be more prone to injury and illness. Interestingly, a non-significant inverse relationship between all winter cytokine concentrations and the total number of illnesses, injuries, and skin infections was observed, implying that between September and January, a period when training is at its peak, lower cytokine concentrations were associated with increased risk for illness, skin infection or injury.

In the current study it is important to note that over the course of the season wrestlers lost an average of 3.5 kg (−12.0 to +4.5 kg), which is lower than the 7.9 ± 0.8 kg loss reported by Melby et al. [57]. On average, wrestlers started the training week (Monday) 4.6 ± 1.0 kg ($6.3\% \pm 1.5\%$) over their weight class suggesting an approximate 5 kg weight loss each week (Monday–Friday) to "make weight" for competition. The weight loss observed in this study is on the lower end of the previously reported weekly loss of 5.0–9.1 kg reported by Steen and Brownell [19], but higher than the 2.3 and 3.4 kg deficits observed by Lakin, Steen, and Oppliger [20] and Lingor and Olson [21], respectively. Furthermore, average weekly weight loss, Monday to Monday, averaged <0.5 kg which is significantly lower than the suggested weight loss between Monday to Friday and lower than any of the aforementioned studies [19–21]. No significant differences in average weekly weight loss between starters and non-starters were observed. This may be due to non-starters competing in non-conference dual meets on the weekends requiring them to engage in similar weight management behaviors as starters. Culturally, coaches also implemented a "maximum weight over" policy that prohibited wrestlers from participating in normal practice activities if they reported to Monday training more than 4.6 kg over their weight class. The positive association between average weekly weight change (Monday to Monday) over the course of the season and spring 25(OH)D concentration and status implies that those who had larger weekly weight fluctuations tended to have higher vitamin D by the spring, which is in contrast to our hypothesis. While unexpected, this observation may reflect a release of vitamin D from adipose tissue by those wrestlers who lost more weight each week.

Limitations

Although our study captured a unique group of athletes potentially at increased risk for poor vitamin D status, it has several limitations. This includes the small sample size, limited racial differences, and the limited variability in 25(OH)D among individual wrestlers at all-time points. For example, a majority of wrestlers in fall, winter, and spring had serum 25 (OH)D concentrations in the deficient and insufficient range with only a few athletes ($n = 5$ in the fall and $n = 1$ in the winter) with concentrations in the sufficient range and none in the optimal range. This precludes comparisons between those with deficient/insufficient status and those sufficient or optimal status, and also limits statistical power. In addition, participants in the current study were closely monitored by a registered dietitian (J.N.B.) which may have positively influenced dietary habits (resulting in better fueling choices, healthier weight loss practices, and lowered post-exercise cytokine responses). The "maximum weight over" policy established by the sport coaches to prevent wrestlers from reporting to Monday practice more than 4.6 kg over their weight class, may have reduced week-to-week weight fluctuations. The low number of skin infections, illnesses, and injuries reported in the current study between the winter and spring may be the result of under-reporting, under-recording, or season-to-season variability of which made detection of relations with vitamin D status difficult. In addition, data collection, particularly for cytokine concentrations, began after approximately eight weeks of fall conditioning (August-September) which may have altered the true picture of how vitamin D status influences such concentrations during training and competition, however, they are a reality for the in-season college athletes. Finally, vitamin D binding protein (VDBP) and gene polymorphisms were not addressed in this study which may have influenced 25(OH)D concentrations [58,59].

5. Conclusions

This study is the first, to our knowledge, to directly analyze the relationship between vitamin D status' and weight cycling's impact on inflammation, skin infection, illness, and injury in wrestlers. Overall, there was a lack of association between vitamin D and prevalence of illness, injury, and skin infection which was in partial contrast to our hypothesis and supports the need for further research in wrestlers. Future research should attempt to analyze a larger sample size, include a supplementation group, and also include wrestlers from varying latitudes. Although we were not able to shed light on the ability of vitamin D to influence cytokines or reduce risk of illness, injury, or infection, our study revealed that despite the stereotypical extreme weight making practices of wrestlers, this group experienced minimal weekly weight fluctuations to reach their goal weight and this likely contributed to their ability to maintain or gain lean body mass while decreasing body fat over the course of the year. Although most of the wrestlers did not utilize vitamin D supplements, exploring the potential benefits of vitamin D supplementation for reducing frequency of illness, injury, and skin infections should be explored in future research especially in a group that appears to have a high prevalence of insufficiency and deficiency.

Supplementary Materials: The following are available online at http://www.mdpi.com/2072-6643/8/12/775/s1, Table S1: Summary of Vitamin D Status in Athletes and Active Individuals.

Acknowledgments: This study was partially funded by a $2,500 graduate research grant provided by the Sports Cardiovascular and Wellness Nutrition (SCAN) dietetic practice group of the Academy of Nutrition and Dietetics (AND). The authors would like to extend a special thank you to the University of Wyoming athletics and sports medicine departments as well as the university's wrestling program for their support and participation in this study.

Author Contributions: J.N.B. and E.L.M. conceived and designed the research protocol, collected the data, performed statistical analysis and data interpretation and wrote and edited the manuscript; B.W.H. performed the blood analysis for 25(OH)D concentrations and provided input on results analysis, J.N.B. and E.L.M. ran the statistical analysis; QIAGEN© contributed reagents and materials for cytokine analysis, K.J.A. and the Department of Animal Science provided the lab equipment for analysis; J.N.B. wrote the paper.

Conflicts of Interest: The authors declare no conflict of interest. The founding sponsors had no role in the design of the study; in the collection, analyses, or interpretation of data; in the writing of the manuscript, and in the decision to publish the results.

References

1. Holick, M.F. Evolution and function of vitamin D. *Recent Results Cancer Res.* **2003**, *164*, 3–28. [PubMed]
2. Holick, M.F. Sunlight and vitamin D for bone health and prevention of autoimmune diseases, cancers, and cardiovascular disease. *Am. J. Clin. Nutr.* **2004**, *80*, 1678S–1688S. [PubMed]
3. Chiu, K.C.; Chu, A.; Go, V.L.; Saad, M.F. Hypovitaminosis D is associated with insulin resistance and beta cell dysfunction. *Am. J. Clin. Nutr.* **2004**, *79*, 820–825. [PubMed]
4. Laaksi, I.; Ruohola, J.P.; Tuohimaa, P.; Auvinen, A.; Haataja, R.; Pihlajamaki, H.; Ylikomi, T. An association of serum vitamin D concentrations <40 nmol/L with acute respiratory tract infection in young Finnish men. *Am. J. Clin. Nutr.* **2007**, *86*, 714–717. [PubMed]
5. Cannell, J.J.; Vieth, R.; Umhau, J.C.; Holick, M.F.; Grant, W.B.; Madronich, S.; Garland, C.F.; Giovannucci, E. Epidemic influenza and vitamin D. *Epidemiol. Infect.* **2006**, *134*, 1129–1140. [CrossRef] [PubMed]
6. Iwamoto, J.; Yeh, J.K.; Takeda, T.; Sato, Y. Effects of vitamin D supplementation on calcium balance and bone growth in young rats fed normal or low calcium diet. *Horm. Res.* **2004**, *61*, 293–299. [CrossRef] [PubMed]
7. Wyon, M.A.; Koutedakis, Y.; Wolman, R.; Nevill, A.M.; Allen, N. The influence of winter vitamin D supplementation on muscle function and injury occurrence in elite ballet dancers: A controlled study. *J. Sci. Med. Sport* **2014**, *17*, 8–12. [CrossRef] [PubMed]
8. Barker, T.; Martins, T.B.; Hill, H.R.; Kjeldsberg, C.R.; Trawick, R.H.; Weaver, L.K.; Traber, M.G. Low Vitamin D Impairs Strength Recovery After Anterior Cruciate Ligament Surgery. *J. Evid. Based Complement. Altern. Med.* **2011**, *16*, 201–209. [CrossRef]
9. Barker, T.; Martins, T.B.; Hill, H.R.; Kjeldsberg, C.R.; Dixon, B.M.; Schneider, E.D.; Henriksen, V.T.; Weaver, L.K. Vitamin D sufficiency associates with an increase in anti-inflammatory cytokines after intense exercise in humans. *Cytokine* **2014**, *65*, 134–137. [CrossRef] [PubMed]
10. Plunkett, B.A.; Callister, R.; Watson, T.A.; Garg, M.L. Dietary antioxidant restriction affects the inflammatory response in athletes. *Br. J. Nutr.* **2010**, *103*, 1179–1184. [CrossRef] [PubMed]
11. Halliday, T.; Peterson, N.; Thomas, J.; Kleppinger, K.; Hollis, B.; Larson-Meyer, D. Vitamin D Status Relative to Diet, Lifestyle, Injury and Illness in College Athletes. *Med. Sci. Sports Exerc.* **2011**, *42*, 335–343. [CrossRef] [PubMed]
12. Umeda, T.; Nakaji, S.; Shimoyama, T.; Kojima, A.; Yamamoto, Y.; Sugawara, K. Adverse effects of energy restriction on changes in immunoglobulins and complements during weight reduction in judoists. *J. Sports Med. Phys. Fit.* **2004**, *44*, 328–334.
13. He, C.-S. Influence of vitamin D status on respiratory infection incidence and immune function during 4 months of winter training in endurance sport athletes. *Exerc. Immunol. Rev.* **2013**, *19*, 1077–5552.
14. Larson-Meyer, D.E.; Willis, K.S. Vitamin D and athletes. *Curr. Sports Med. Rep.* **2010**, *9*, 220–226. [CrossRef] [PubMed]
15. Farrokhyar, F.; Tabasinejad, R.; Dao, D.; Peterson, D.; Ayeni, O.R.; Hadioonzadeh, R.; Bhandari, M. Prevalence of vitamin D inadequacy in athletes: A systematic-review and meta-analysis. *Sports Med.* **2015**, *45*, 365–378. [CrossRef] [PubMed]
16. Heller, J.E.; Thomas, J.J.; Hollis, B.W.; Larson-Meyer, D.E. Relation between vitamin D status and body composition in collegiate athletes. *Int. J. Sport Nutr. Exerc. Metab.* **2015**, *25*, 128–135. [CrossRef] [PubMed]
17. Barger-Lux, M.J.; Heaney, R.P.; Dowell, S.; Chen, T.C.; Holick, M.F. Vitamin D and its major metabolites: Serum levels after graded oral dosing in healthy men. *Osteoporos. Int.* **1998**, *8*, 222–230. [CrossRef] [PubMed]
18. Chiang, C.M.; Ismaeel, A.; Griffis, R.B.; Weems, S. Effects of Vitamin D Supplementation on Muscle Strength in Athletes: A Systematic Review. *J. Strength Cond. Res.* **2016**, in press. [CrossRef] [PubMed]

19. Steen, S.N.; Brownell, K.D. Patterns of weight loss and regain in wrestlers: Has the tradition changed? *Med. Sci. Sports Exerc.* **1990**, *22*, 762–768. [CrossRef] [PubMed]
20. Lakin, J.A.; Steen, S.N.; Oppliger, R.A. Eating behaviors, weight loss methods, and nutrition practices among high school wrestlers. *J. Community Health Nurs.* **1990**, *7*, 223–234. [CrossRef] [PubMed]
21. Lingor, R.J.; Olson, A. Fluid and diet patterns associated with weight cycling and changes in body composition assessed by continuous monitoring throughout a college wrestling season. *J. Strength Cond. Res.* **2010**, *24*, 1763–1772. [CrossRef] [PubMed]
22. Willis, K.S.; Peterson, N.J.; Larson-Meyer, D.E. Should we be concerned about the vitamin D status of athletes? *Int. J. Sport Nutr. Exerc. Metab.* **2008**, *18*, 204–224. [CrossRef] [PubMed]
23. Hulley, S.B.; Cummings, S.R.; Browner, W.S.; Grady, D.; Newman, T.B. *Designing Clinical Research: An Epidemiologic Approach*, 4th ed.; Lippincott Williams & Wilkins: Philadelphia, PA, USA, 2013; Appendix 6D; p. 80.
24. Willis, K.S.; Smith, D.T.; Broughton, K.S.; Larson-Meyer, D.E. Vitamin D status and biomarkers of inflammation in runners. *Open Access J. Sports Med.* **2012**, *3*, 35–42. [PubMed]
25. Storlie, D.M.; Pritchett, K.; Pritchett, R.; Cashman, L. 12-Week Vitamin D Supplementation Trial Does Not Significantly Influence Seasonal 25(OH)D Status in Male Collegiate Athletes. *Int. J. Health Nutr.* **2011**, *2*, 8–13.
26. Bescos Garcia, R.; Rodriguez Guisado, F.A. Low levels of vitamin D in professional basketball players after wintertime: Relationship with dietary intake of vitamin D and calcium. *Nutr. Hosp.* **2011**, *26*, 945–951. [PubMed]
27. Wolman, R.; Wyon, M.A.; Koutedakis, Y.; Nevill, A.M.; Eastell, R.; Allen, N. Vitamin D status in professional ballet dancers: Winter vs. summer. *J. Sci. Med. Sport* **2013**, *16*, 388–391. [CrossRef] [PubMed]
28. Villacis, D.; Yi, A.; Jahn, R.; Kephart, C.J.; Charlton, T.; Gamradt, S.C.; Romano, R.; Tibone, J.E.; Hatch, G.F., 3rd. Prevalence of Abnormal Vitamin D Levels Among Division I NCAA Athletes. *Sports Health* **2014**, *6*, 340–347. [CrossRef] [PubMed]
29. Kopec, A.; Solarz, K.; Majda, F.; Slowinska-Lisowska, M.; Medras, M. An evaluation of the levels of vitamin D and bone turnover markers after the summer and winter periods in polish professional soccer players. *J. Hum. Kinet.* **2013**, *38*, 135–140. [CrossRef] [PubMed]
30. Holick, M.F. Vitamin D deficiency. *N. Engl. J. Med.* **2007**, *357*, 266–281. [CrossRef] [PubMed]
31. Hamilton, B.; Grantham, J.; Racinais, S.; Chalabi, H. Vitamin D deficiency is endemic in Middle Eastern sportsmen. *Public Health Nutr.* **2010**, *13*, 1528–1534. [CrossRef] [PubMed]
32. Lewis, R.M.; Redzic, M.; Thomas, D.T. The effects of season-long vitamin D supplementation on collegiate swimmers and divers. *Int. J. Sport Nutr. Exerc. Metab.* **2013**, *23*, 431–440. [CrossRef] [PubMed]
33. Looker, A.C. Do body fat and exercise modulate vitamin D status? Vitamin D and Cancer: Current Dilemmas and Future Needs. National Institutes of Health, Bethesda, Maryland, USA, May 7–8, 2007. *Nutr. Rev.* **2007**, *65*, S124–S126. [CrossRef] [PubMed]
34. Wortsman, J.; Matsuoka, L.Y.; Chen, T.C.; Lu, Z.; Holick, M.F. Decreased bioavailability of vitamin D in obesity. *Am. J. Clin. Nutr.* **2000**, *72*, 690–693. [PubMed]
35. Mutt, S.J.; Hypponen, E.; Saarnio, J.; Jarvelin, M.R.; Herzig, K.H. Vitamin D and adipose tissue-more than storage. *Front. Physiol.* **2014**, *5*, 228. [CrossRef] [PubMed]
36. Gibson, J.C.; Stuart-Hill, L.; Martin, S.; Gaul, C. Nutrition status of junior elite Canadian female soccer athletes. *Int. J. Sport Nutr. Exerc. Metab.* **2011**, *21*, 507–514. [CrossRef] [PubMed]
37. Ostrowski, K.; Rohde, T.; Asp, S.; Schjerling, P.; Pedersen, B.K. Pro- and anti-inflammatory cytokine balance in strenuous exercise in humans. *J. Physiol.* **1999**, *515*, 287–291. [CrossRef] [PubMed]
38. Louis, E.; Raue, U.; Yifan, Y.; Jemiolo, B.; Trappe, S. Time course of proteolytic, cytokine, and myostatin gene expression after acute exercise in human skeletal muscle. *J. Appl. Physiol.* **2007**, *103*, 1744–1751. [CrossRef] [PubMed]
39. Ostapiuk-Karolczuk, J.; Zembron-Lacny, A.; Naczk, M.; Gajewski, M.; Kasperska, A.; Dziewiecka, H.; Szyszka, K. Cytokines and cellular inflammatory sequence in non-athletes after prolonged exercise. *J. Sports Med. Phys. Fit.* **2012**, *52*, 563–568.
40. Chernoff, A.E.; Granowitz, E.V.; Shapiro, L.; Vannier, E.; Lonnemann, G.; Angel, J.B.; Kennedy, J.S.; Rabson, A.R.; Wolff, S.M.; Dinarello, C.A. A randomized, controlled trial of IL-10 in humans. Inhibition of inflammatory cytokine production and immune responses. *J. Immunol.* **1995**, *154*, 5492–5499. [PubMed]

41. Gannage-Yared, M.H.; Azoury, M.; Mansour, I.; Baddoura, R.; Halaby, G.; Naaman, R. Effects of a short-term calcium and vitamin D treatment on serum cytokines, bone markers, insulin and lipid concentrations in healthy post-menopausal women. *J. Endocrinol. Investig* **2003**, *26*, 748–753. [CrossRef] [PubMed]

42. Yusupov, E.; Li-Ng, M.; Pollack, S.; Yeh, J.K.; Mikhail, M.; Aloia, J.F. Vitamin D and serum cytokines in a randomized clinical trial. *Int. J. Endocrinol.* **2010**, *2010*, 305054. [CrossRef] [PubMed]

43. Barnes, M.S.; Horigan, G.; Cashman, K.D.; Hill, T.R.; Forsythe, L.K.; Lucey, A.J.; McSorley, E.M.; Kiely, M.; Bonham, M.P.; Magee, P.J.; et al. Maintenance of wintertime vitamin D status with cholecalciferol supplementation is not associated with alterations in serum cytokine concentrations among apparently healthy younger or older adults. *J. Nutr.* **2011**, *141*, 476–481. [CrossRef] [PubMed]

44. Beilfuss, J.; Berg, V.; Sneve, M.; Jorde, R.; Kamycheva, E. Effects of a 1-year supplementation with cholecalciferol on interleukin-6, tumor necrosis factor-alpha and insulin resistance in overweight and obese subjects. *Cytokine* **2012**, *60*, 870–874. [CrossRef] [PubMed]

45. Carrillo, A.E.; Flynn, M.G.; Pinkston, C.; Markofski, M.M.; Jiang, Y.; Donkin, S.S.; Teegarden, D. Vitamin D supplementation during exercise training does not alter inflammatory biomarkers in overweight and obese subjects. *Eur. J. Appl. Physiol.* **2012**, *112*, 3045–3052. [CrossRef] [PubMed]

46. Peterson, C.A.; Heffernan, M.E. Serum tumor necrosis factor-alpha concentrations are negatively correlated with serum 25(OH)D concentrations in healthy women. *J. Inflamm. (Lond.)* **2008**, *5*, 10. [CrossRef] [PubMed]

47. Zhu, Y.; Mahon, B.D.; Froicu, M.; Cantorna, M.T. Calcium and 1 alpha,25-dihydroxyvitamin D3 target the TNF-alpha pathway to suppress experimental inflammatory bowel disease. *Eur. J. Immunol.* **2005**, *35*, 217–224. [CrossRef] [PubMed]

48. Choi, M.; Park, H.; Cho, S.; Lee, M. Vitamin D3 supplementation modulates inflammatory responses from the muscle damage induced by high-intensity exercise in SD rats. *Cytokine* **2013**, *63*, 27–35. [CrossRef] [PubMed]

49. Liu, P.T.; Stenger, S.; Li, H.; Wenzel, L.; Tan, B.H.; Krutzik, S.R.; Ochoa, M.T.; Schauber, J.; Wu, K.; Meinken, C.; et al. Toll-like receptor triggering of a vitamin D-mediated human antimicrobial response. *Science* **2006**, *311*, 1770–1773. [CrossRef] [PubMed]

50. Ducher, G.; Kukuljan, S.; Hill, B.; Garnham, A.P.; Nowson, C.A.; Kimlin, M.G.; Cook, J. Vitamin D status and musculoskeletal health in adolescent male ballet dancers a pilot study. *J. Dance Med. Sci.* **2011**, *15*, 99–107. [PubMed]

51. Lin, Z.P.; Chen, Y.H.; Chia, F.; Wu, H.J.; Lan, L.W.; Lin, J.G. Episodes of injuries and frequent usage of traditional Chinese medicine for Taiwanese elite wrestling athletes. *Am. J. Chin. Med.* **2011**, *39*, 233–241. [CrossRef] [PubMed]

52. Pasque, C.B.; Hewett, T.E. A prospective study of high school wrestling injuries. *Am. J. Sports Med.* **2000**, *28*, 509–515. [PubMed]

53. Bischoff-Ferrari, H.A.; Borchers, M.; Gudat, F.; Durmuller, U.; Stahelin, H.B.; Dick, W. Vitamin D receptor expression in human muscle tissue decreases with age. *J. Bone Miner. Res.* **2004**, *19*, 265–269. [CrossRef] [PubMed]

54. Maroon, J.C.; Mathyssek, C.M.; Bost, J.W.; Amos, A.; Winkelman, R.; Yates, A.P.; Duca, M.A.; Norwig, J.A. Vitamin D profile in National Football League players. *Am. J. Sports Med.* **2015**, *43*, 1241–1245. [CrossRef] [PubMed]

55. Shindle, M.K.; Voos, J.E.; Gulotta, L. Vitamin D status in a professional American Football team. In Proceedings of the AOSSM Annual Meeting, San Diego, CA, USA, 7–10 July 2011.

56. Barker, T.; Henriksen, V.T.; Martins, T.B.; Hill, H.R.; Kjeldsberg, C.R.; Schneider, E.D.; Dixon, B.M.; Weaver, L.K. Higher serum 25-hydroxyvitamin D concentrations associate with a faster recovery of skeletal muscle strength after muscular injury. *Nutrients* **2013**, *5*, 1253–1275. [CrossRef] [PubMed]

57. Melby, C.L.; Schmidt, W.D.; Corrigan, D. Resting metabolic rate in weight-cycling collegiate wrestlers compared with physically active, noncycling control subjects. *Am. J. Clin. Nutr.* **1990**, *52*, 409–414. [PubMed]

58. Elkum, N.; Alkayal, F.; Noronha, F.; Ali, M.M.; Melhem, M.; Al-Arouj, M.; Bennakhi, A.; Behbehani, K.; Alsmadi, O.; Abubaker, J. Vitamin D Insufficiency in Arabs and South Asians Positively Associates with Polymorphisms in GC and CYP2R1 Genes. *PLoS ONE* **2014**, *9*, e113102. [CrossRef] [PubMed]
59. Malik, S.; Fu, L.; Juras, D.J.; Karmali, M.; Wong, B.Y.L.; Gozdzik, A.; Cole, D.E.C. Common variants of the vitamin D binding protein gene and adverse health outcomes. *Crit. Rev. Clin. Lab. Sci.* **2013**, *50*, 1–22. [CrossRef] [PubMed]

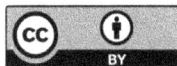

nutrients

MDPI

Article

Comparison of Site-Specific Bone Mineral Densities between Endurance Runners and Sprinters in Adolescent Women

Aoi Ikedo [1], Aya Ishibashi [1,2], Saori Matsumiya [1,3], Aya Kaizaki [4], Kumiko Ebi [1] and Satoshi Fujita [1,*]

[1]   Graduate School of Sport and Health Science, Ritsumeikan University, Kusatsu 525-8577, Japan; gr0167si@ed.ritsumei.ac.jp (A.I.), gr0167kx@ed.ritsumei.ac.jp (A.I.), saori.m0824@gmail.com (S.M.), ab@fc.ritsumei.ac.jp (K.E.)
[2]   Department of Sports Science, Japan Institute of Sports Science, Nishigaoka, Kitaku, Tokyo 115-0056, Japan
[3]   Department of Food Science and Nutrition, Mukogawa Women's University, Nishinomiya 663-8558, Japan
[4]   Research Organization of Science and Technology, Ritsumeikan University, Kusatsu 525-8577, Japan; kaizaki@fc.ritsumei.ac.jp
*   Correspondence: safujita@fc.ritsumei.ac.jp; Tel.: +81-077-561-5229

Received: 31 August 2016; Accepted: 21 November 2016; Published: 30 November 2016

Abstract: We aimed to compare site-specific bone mineral densities (BMDs) between adolescent endurance runners and sprinters and examine the relationship of fat-free mass (FFM) and nutrient intake on BMD. In this cross-sectional study, 37 adolescent female endurance runners and sprinters (16.1 ± 0.8 years) were recruited. BMD and FFM were assessed by dual-energy X-ray absorptiometry. Nutrient intake and menstrual state were evaluated by questionnaires. After adjusting for covariates, spine and total bone less head (TBLH) BMDs were significantly higher in sprinters than endurance runners (TBLH, 1.02 ± 0.05 vs. 0.98 ± 0.06 g/cm^2; spine, 0.99 ± 0.06 vs. 0.94 ± 0.06 g/cm^2; $p < 0.05$). There was no significant difference between groups in other sites. The rate of menstrual abnormality was higher in endurance runners compared with sprinters (56.3% vs. 23.8%; $p < 0.05$). FFM was a significant covariate for BMD on all sites except the spine ($p < 0.05$). Dietary intake of vitamin D was identified as a significant covariate only for pelvic BMD ($p < 0.05$). The BMDs of different sites among endurance runners and sprinters were strongly related to FFM. However, the association of FFM with spine BMD cannot be explained by FFM alone. Other factors, including nutrition and/or mechanical loading, may affect the spine BMD.

Keywords: adolescent; sprinters; endurance runners; bone mineral density; fat-free mass; nutrition

1. Introduction

Weight-bearing exercise has positive effects on bone metabolism across the age spectrum [1]. Adolescence is a critical time for bone mineral accrual [2]. Exercises that generate relatively high intensity loading forces enhance bone mineral accretion in adolescents [1]. Thus, adolescent athletes typically have higher bone mass compared with their nonathletic peers [3].

Endurance running has been associated with reduced risks for hypertension, hyperlipidemia, and diabetes [4]. Furthermore, regular running has been reported to reduce proportions of all-cause mortality and disability [5]. However, a subset of adolescent athletes may have impaired bone health [6,7]. Although endurance running is weight-bearing exercise, it has been associated with negative effects on bone in some populations, as indicated by reduced spine bone mineral density (BMD) in endurance runners [8,9]. In contrast, although both sprinters and endurance runners mainly use the lower limbs during exercise, sprinters demonstrate a higher BMD than endurance runners.

The reason for a lower BMD in adolescent female endurance runners may be that this subject group has a greater running distance to cover, higher rate of menstrual irregularities, lower body mass index (BMI), and lower lean tissue mass [6] than sprinters of the same age group. Kusy et al. reported that sprinters in the masters age category have a higher BMD as well as bone mineral content (BMC) at the leg, hip, lumbar spine, and trunk than endurance athletes [10], whereas Bennell et al. reported that differences in the BMD between sprinters and endurance runners (17–26 years) exist only in the lumbar spine [11].

So far, the effect of the ground reaction force has been considered the most significant contributing factor for bone formation [11,12]. However, based on previous studies [10,11], the differences in BMD between sprinters and endurance runners could not be explained solely by the effect of the ground reaction force. Furthermore, although generally higher muscle mass and optimal nutrition is related with increased BMD, the effects of muscle mass and nutrition on BMD among endurance runners and sprinters have not been explored. Recent studies have only focused on BMD in endurance runners [6–9,13]. Clarifying the differences in site-specific BMDs between sprinters and endurance runners may reveal specific factors contributing to BMD gain in sprinters and endurance runners.

The aim of the present study was to compare site-specific BMDs between female adolescent endurance runners and sprinters, and to examine the relationship of fat-free mass (FFM) and nutrient intake with the BMD of different sites.

2. Materials and Methods

2.1. Study Design and Recruitment

In this cross-sectional study, we recruited 37 high school track and field female athletes (16.1 ± 0.8 years old; competition history of 3.4 ± 1.9 years), including endurance runners (>800 m, $n = 16$) and sprinters (100–400 m, $n = 21$). Study investigators recruited participants from five high schools in the Kansai district of Japan. The study protocol was approved by the Ethics Committee for Human Experiments at Ritsumeikan University (BKC-IRB-2013-031), and was conducted in accordance with the Declaration of Helsinki. All subjects and legal guardians of subjects provided informed consent for participation in this study.

2.2. BMD and Body Composition

We measured the height, body weight, and BMI of each subject. The body mass, fat mass, percent body fat, FFM, and bone mass were evaluated by a dual-energy X-ray absorptiometry (DXA, Lunar Prodigy; GE Healthcare, Tokyo, Japan). During DXA measurements, subjects maintained a supine position. From total body scans, we used enCORE version 15 software (GE Medical Systems Lunar, Madison, WI, USA), which automated measurements of FFM and fat mass (arms, legs, torso, gynoid (gluteal area), and total body), BMD (total bone less head (TBLH), arms, spine, pelvis, and legs), and percent body fat. For screening of at-risk athletes at younger than 20 years for low BMD, TBLH BMD measurement is recommended [14].

2.3. Menstrual State and Stress Fracture History

Menstrual state and stress fracture history were evaluated using questionnaires. For the menstrual state, the age of menarche and characteristics of the menstrual cycle were evaluated. Cycle lengths longer than 45 or shorter than 21 days were considered abnormal [15]. Stress fracture history was defined as having received a diagnosis of stress fracture in a medical institution.

2.4. Food Frequency Questionnaire

A food frequency questionnaire based on the food group (FFQg) was used to estimate usual energy and nutrient intake in athletes. The FFQg estimated nutrient intake from the ingestion frequency and food intake during one week from the most recent 1–2 months [16].

2.5. Physical Activity and Running Distance

Physical activity was estimated from three-day physical activity records. Subjects were instructed to estimate the practice time in minutes.

Running distance was estimated as the mean running distance per one-week from two-week running distance records. Physical activity and running distance were analyzed from the recovered questionnaires (33/37 questionnaires were recovered).

2.6. Statistical Analysis

Statistical analyses were performed with SPSS software version 19.0 (IBM, Tokyo, Japan). All values are expressed as mean ± SD. The independent *t*-test was used to determine differences in physical characteristics, FFM, and BMD between endurance runners and sprinters. An analysis of covariance (ANCOVA) was performed to compare BMD between endurance runners and sprinters, adjusted for age, height, FFM, and fat mass (of total body, arms, torso, gynoid (the gluteal area), and legs), menstrual abnormality, menarche, stress fracture history, and nutrient intake. Those variables that have been reported as important determinant of BMD in previous studies were selected as independent variables [3,6,17,18]. In addition, in a previous study, calcium and vitamin D were chosen as nutrients important for bone health [3]. Of those two nutrients, vitamin D was chosen as covariate, since there was a significant correlation with BMD in the current study. A *p* value < 0.05 was considered statistically significant.

3. Results

3.1. Subject Characteristics

Table 1 shows the subject characteristics. Endurance runners had a significantly higher running volume than sprinters ($p < 0.01$). Endurance runners also demonstrated a higher incidence of menstrual abnormality ($p < 0.01$) than sprinters. Table 2 shows the physical activities of subjects. Duration of practice was not different between two groups. However, running distance was significantly higher in endurance runners compared with sprinters. Table 3 shows the daily energy and nutrient intake. There was no significant difference between any parameters among the two groups.

Table 1. Subjects characteristics.

	Endurance Runners (*n* = 16)	Sprinters (*n* = 21)
Age	16.3 ± 0.8	16.0 ± 0.7
Menstrual abnormality (%)	56.3	23.8 **
Height (cm)	156.7 ±3.7	158.8 ± 4.5
Weight (kg)	47.6 ± 4.6	50.7 ± 5.3
BMI (kg/m^2)	19.4 ± 1.5	20.1 ± 1.9
Fat mass (%)	19.9 ±4.6	19.5 ± 4.4

All values are mean ± SD; **: $p < 0.01$ vs. endurance runners.

Table 2. Physical activity.

	Endurance Runners (*n* = 14)	Sprinters (*n* = 21)
Practice time (min/day)	99.6 ± 38.7	109.7 ± 33.1
Running distance (km/week)	58.5 ± 27.1	10.4 ± 5.3 **

All values are mean ± SD; **: $p < 0.01$ vs. endurance runners.

Table 3. Energy and nutrient intake.

	Endurance Runners (*n* = 16)	Sprinters (*n* = 21)
Energy (kcal/day)	1927 ± 336	2099 ± 625
Protein (g/day)	70.0 ± 15.1	70.2 ± 20.5
Fat (g/day)	65.1 ± 18.1	78.1 ± 30.3
Carbohydrate (g/day)	258.5 ± 55.6	271.8 ± 78.8
Calcium (mg/day)	582 ± 205	595 ± 270
Magnesium (mg/day)	242 ± 52	232 ± 92
Phosphorus (mg/day)	1052 ± 251	1059 ± 345
Iron (mg/day)	7.5 ± 1.6	7.4 ± 3.1
Vitamin A (µg/day)	578 ± 161	553 ± 210
Vitamin D (µg/day)	6.4 ± 2.9	5.2 ± 2.9
Vitamin K (µg/day)	216 ± 65	182 ± 84
Vitamin B_1 (mg/day)	0.97 ± 0.21	1.00 ± 0.35
Vitamin B_2 (mg/day)	1.14 ± 0.32	1.21 ± 0.41
Vitamin B_6 (mg/day)	1.09 ± 0.22	1.03 ± 0.40
Vitamin B_{12} (µg/day)	6.0 ± 2.3	5.4 ± 2.6
Vitamin C (mg/day)	104 ± 25	88 ± 43

All values are mean ± SD.

3.2. Comparison between Endurance Runners and Sprinters

Table 4 shows subject FFM and BMD values. Endurance runners had a significantly lower FFM in all sites—except for the torso—compared to sprinters. Endurance runners had significantly lower arm, pelvic, spine, and TBLH BMDs than sprinters. However, the leg BMD was not significantly different between endurance runners and sprinters.

In ANCOVA with adjustment for covariates such as age, height, FFM, fat mass, menstrual abnormality, menarche, stress fracture history, and vitamin D intake, the spine and TBLH BMDs remained significantly higher in sprinters than endurance runners ($p < 0.05$) (Figure 1). In contrast, there were no significant between-group differences in other sites.

Table 4. FFM and BMD value among endurance runners and sprinters.

		Endurance Runners (*n* = 16)	Sprinters (*n* = 21)
FFM	Arms (kg)	3.2 ± 0.3	3.6 ± 0.4 **
	Legs (kg)	12.5 ± 1.3	13.7 ± 1.1 **
	Torso (kg)	17.0 ± 1.7	17.8 ± 1.3
	Gynoid (kg)	5.4 ± 0.5	5.9 ± 0.5 **
	Total body (kg)	36.0 ± 3.2	38.3 ± 2.6 *
BMD	Arms (g/cm^2)	0.767 ± 0.039	0.805 ± 0.038 **
	Legs (g/cm^2)	1.211 ± 0.091	1.262 ± 0.077
	Pelvic (g/cm^2)	1.097 ± 0.086	1.163 ± 0.099 *
	Spine (g/cm^2)	0.942 ± 0.064	0.985 ± 0.062 *
	TBLH (g/cm^2)	0.981 ± 0.061	1.023 ± 0.050 *

All values are mean ± SD; FFM: fat-free mass, BMD: bone mineral density, Gynoid: the gluteal area, TBLH: Total Bone Less Head; **: $p < 0.01$, *: $p < 0.05$ vs. endurance runners.

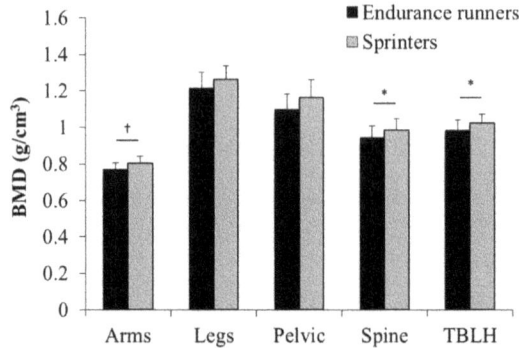

Figure 1. Comparison of adjusted BMD between endurance runners and sprinters. Endurance runners vs. sprinters; Spine: 0.94 ± 0.06 vs. 0.98 ± 0.06 g/cm^2, TBLH: 0.98 ± 0.06 vs. 1.02 ± 0.05; *: $p < 0.05$, †: $p = 0.06$.

3.3. Effect of Covariates on the BMD of Different Sites

In ANCOVA, FFM was a significant covariate for arms ($p < 0.01$), legs ($p < 0.05$), and pelvic ($p < 0.05$) BMD, and tended to be a covariate for TBLH BMD ($p = 0.05$) (Table 5). Additionally, vitamin D intake was identified as a significant covariate for arms ($p < 0.05$), pelvic ($p < 0.01$), and spine ($p < 0.05$) BMD, and tended to be a covariate for TBLH BMD ($p = 0.05$). Moreover, menarche was a significant covariate for arms BMD ($p < 0.05$).

Table 5. Multivariable linear regression model on BMD of all subjects.

	Arms	Legs	Pelvic	Spine	TBLH
Age	0.48	1.74	2.61	0.06	0.48
Height	0.34	0.06	0.01	0.00	0.06
FFM (each site)	11.37 **	4.83 *	7.49 *	0.05	4.13 †
Fat-mass (each site)	0.86	0.10	3.45	0.21	0.25
Menstrual abnormality	0.40	2.05	0.14	1.31	0.86
Menarche	6.13 *	1.78	0.17	1.04	1.61
Stress fracture history	2.00	0.97	0.18	0.88	1.29
Vitamin D intake	4.82 *	1.49	8.08 **	4.31 *	4.04 †

All values are *F* values; **: $p < 0.01$, *: $p < 0.05$, †: $p = 0.05$.

4. Discussion

The purpose of this cross-sectional study was to compare BMDs of various sites and examine the association with different factors on the BMD among female high school track and field athletes. The main finding of our results was that endurance runners had significantly lower BMD in spine and TBLH as compared with sprinters, even after adjusting for covariates. In addition, vitamin D intake seems to have a site-specific association with arms, pelvic, and spine BMD. Furthermore, FFM was a significant covariate for most BMDs, with the exception of the spine.

4.1. The Difference between the BMD of Sprinters and Endurance Runners

When comparing the BMD of sprinters and endurance runners using a *t*-test, the BMDs of the arms, pelvis, spine, and TBLH in sprinters were significantly higher than those in endurance runners. However, after adjusting for covariates, between-group differences remained significant only for spine and TBLH BMDs.

In a previous study, ground reaction force with foot-strike during running was reported to be 1–2 times the body weight for low intensity forms of running (e.g., endurance) while it becomes 2–4 times the body weight for high intensity forms of running (e.g., sprint) [19]. According to the mechanostat theory, an increase in the bone mass is caused by larger bone deformation (e.g., high ground reaction force) which exceeds the normal strain for modeling [20]. However, the ground reaction force decreases as it is transmitted upward to the pelvis and spine from legs [13]. Since endurance runners experience smaller ground reaction force than sprinters, endurance runners may have less loading and deformation to spine bone when compared with sprinters with higher ground reaction forces. Additionally, in a previous study, weekly running volume was inversely correlated with lumbar spine BMD [21,22]. Greater running distance results in large energy expenditures, and one possible explanation for its effect on bone is via a potential catabolism when energy intake was insufficient, leading to low energy availability. Low energy availability has been shown to increase bone resorption and decrease bone formation, potentially mediated by reduced levels of insulin-like growth factor 1 or estradiol, resulting in low BMD [23,24]. Trabecular bone such as spine has been shown to be easily influenced by low energy availability [13]. Average running volumes of previously reported studies were 68.4 ± 12.1 km/week [21] and 32 ± 8 km/week [22] for endurance runners. Our current study participants exercised 58.5 ± 27.1 km/week among endurance runners and only 10.4 ± 5.3 km/week among sprinters, while their energy intake was identical between groups. Therefore, the low BMD of endurance runners may have been caused by both smaller mechanical loading as well as less energy availability as compared with sprinters.

Previous studies comparing the BMD of endurance runners and sprinters have often shown a difference in the leg BMD between the two groups [11,25]. However, this difference was not observed in the present study. The reason for this difference may be related to the subjects' age and competition history. In a previous study, the subjects were over 17 years of age, and they had a competition history of over a decade [25]. In addition, in a previous study comparing the BMD of 13- to 18-year-old runners and non-runners, when separated by age, runners had significantly lower total body BMD compared with non-runners in the 17- to 18-year-old age group, but no difference was observed among groups of 13- to 16-years old [13]. The subjects in the present study had a mean age of 16.1 ± 0.8 years and mean competition history of 3.4 ± 1.9 years. Therefore, the lack of observed difference in leg BMD among long distance runners and sprinters may be caused by their age (bones being still in the growth stage) and relatively short competition history.

4.2. Relationship between Muscle Mass and BMD

After adjusting for age, height, FFM, fat-mass, menstrual abnormality, menarche, stress fracture history, and vitamin D intake, there were no significant group differences in the BMDs of the arms, legs, and pelvis. Among these confounding factors, FFM had the greater F value at each site. Thus, the FFM could have a strong influence on the BMDs among all sites. However, FFM was not found to be a significant covariate for spine BMD, while vitamin D intake was a significant covariate. Therefore, these results suggest that the spine might be more affected by nutrient factors such as vitamin D

The close relationship between muscle mass and bone mass has been known for a long time [26]. In a previous study, sprinters were shown to have a higher FFM than endurance runners. Kusy and Zielinski [10] demonstrated that greater skeletal size allows exertion of larger muscle forces, supporting engagement in sprint disciplines, or forces exerted during sprinting induce skeletal adaptation and augment BMD. In addition, in a longitudinal study of 68 children (8 to 14 years), the maximal increase in lean body mass (LBM) occurred a several months before the maximal increase in BMC, indicating a close relationship between muscle and bone development [27]. These findings suggest that among adolescent female track and field athletes in their growth period, sprinters may have higher FFM and exercise intensity than endurance runners. Thus, in accordance with mechanostat theory, sprinters demonstrate higher BMDs than endurance runners.

4.3. Effect of Site-Specificity in Vitamin D

Vitamin D intake seems to have a site-specific relationship with arms ($p < 0.01$), pelvis ($p < 0.05$), and spine ($p < 0.05$) BMDs. A previous study using a vitamin D analogue indicated that the effect with vitamin D differs between cortical and trabecular bone. Takahashi et al. [28] concluded that vitamin D compounds might suppress receptor activator of nuclear factor-kappa B ligand (RANKL) activity in superficial osteoblastic cells of the trabecular bone. RANKL is an essential cytokine for activating osteoclast (increase in bone resorption). Therefore, habitual high vitamin D intake has a potential positive effect on pelvic and spine BMDs of trabecular bone. On the other hand, vitamin D intake was identified as a significant covariate for arms BMD. The bone of the arms consists mostly of cortical bone, since it is long bone. Thus, the aforementioned explanation for vitamin D and trabecular bone may seem inconsistent. However, FFM and menarche were demonstrated as significant covariates for arms. Since running puts minimal mechanical stress on arms, other variables such as FFM and nutrients may have had a larger influence. In the present study, the strongest covariate for arms BMD was FFM ($F = 11.37$, $p < 0.01$). However, since the results of the present study cannot explain the causal relationship, further study is warranted.

4.4. Study Limitations

This study included a relatively small sample size. Furthermore, the causal relationship cannot be determined by the current cross-sectional study without an inactive control group. Several parameters were not evaluated, such as bone metabolism markers, sex hormones (e.g., estrogen and progesterone), and reproductive maturation (such as tanner breast stage). Moreover, a previous study reported that subclinical ovulatory disturbance provides negative effect on bone [29]; however, the present study did not assess that. Low-dose oral contraceptives may impair the attainment of peak bone mass [30]. It should be noted, however, that the subjects of the present study were not taking oral contraceptives. In addition, FFQs for dietary assessment have been validated on collegiate woman, and not with the same age group of subjects in the current study. Accordingly, the dietitians used food samples to demonstrate the correct portion of specific foods. Future prospective studies are needed in other populations to determine variations, and intervention studies are warranted to determine the effects of FFM and vitamin D on site-specific BMDs.

5. Conclusions

We conclude that differences in the BMDs of different sites among endurance runners and sprinters were strongly affected by FFM. Furthermore, vitamin D intake also seems to have site-specific associations with BMDs. However, the relationship of FFM on spine BMD cannot be explained by FFM alone. Other variables, including nutrition (e.g., vitamin D) and/or mechanical loading may have been associated with spine BMD.

Acknowledgments: This work was supported by the Ritsumeikan Global Innovation Research Organization.

Author Contributions: Aoi Ikedo, Kumiko Ebi and Satoshi Fujita conceived and designed the experiments; Aoi Ikedo, Aya Ishibashi, Saori Matsumiya and Aya Kaizaki performed the experiments; Aoi Ikedo analyzed the data; Aoi Ikedo, Aya Ishibashi, Saori Matsumiya, Aya Kaizaki contributed reagents/materials/analysis tools; Aoi Ikedo and Satoshi Fujita wrote the paper.

Conflicts of Interest: The authors declare no conflict of interest.

References

1. Kohrt, W.M.; Bloomfield, S.A.; Little, K.D.; Nelson, M.E.; Yingling, V.R. American College of Sports Medicine Position Stand: Physical activity and bone health. *Med. Sci. Sports Exerc.* **2004**, *36*, 1985–1996. [CrossRef] [PubMed]
2. Gibbs, J.C.; Williams, N.I.; de Souza, M.J. Prevalence of individual and combined components of the female athlete triad. *Med. Sci. Sports Exerc.* **2013**, *45*, 985–996. [CrossRef] [PubMed]

3. Mountjoy, M.; Sundgot-Borgen, J.; Burke, L.; Carter, S.; Constantini, N.; Lebrun, C.; Meyer, N.; Sherman, R.; Steffen, K.; Budgett, R.; et al. The IOC consensus statement: Beyond the Female Athlete Triad—Relative Energy Deficiency in Sport (RED-S). *Br. J. Sports Med.* **2014**, *48*, 491–497. [CrossRef] [PubMed]

4. Williams, P.T. Lower prevalence of hypertension, hypercholesterolemia, and diabetes in marathoners. *Med. Sci. Sports Exerc.* **2009**, *41*, 523–529. [CrossRef] [PubMed]

5. Chakravarty, E.F.; Hubert, H.B.; Lingala, V.B.; Fries, J.F. Reduced disability and mortality among aging runners: A 21-year longitudinal study. *Arch. Intern. Med.* **2008**, *168*, 1638–1646. [CrossRef] [PubMed]

6. Barrack, M.T.; Rauh, M.J.; Nichols, J.F. Prevalence of and traits associated with low BMD among female adolescent runners. *Med. Sci. Sports Exerc.* **2008**, *40*, 2015–2021. [CrossRef] [PubMed]

7. Tenforde, A.S.; Fredericson, M.; Sayres, L.C.; Cutti, P.; Sainani, K.L. Identifying sex-specific risk factors for low bone mineral density in adolescent runners. *Am. J. Sports Med.* **2015**, *43*, 1494–1504. [CrossRef] [PubMed]

8. Bilanin, J.E.; Blanchard, M.S.; Russek-Cohen, E. Lower vertebral bone density in male long distance runners. *Med. Sci. Sports Exerc.* **1989**, *21*, 66–70. [CrossRef] [PubMed]

9. Hind, K.; Truscott, J.G.; Evans, J.A. Low lumbar spine bone mineral density in both male and female endurance runners. *Bone* **2006**, *39*, 880–885. [CrossRef] [PubMed]

10. Kusy, K.; Zielinski, J. Sprinters versus long-distance runners: how to grow old healthy. *Exerc. Sport Sci. Rev.* **2015**, *43*, 57–64. [CrossRef] [PubMed]

11. Bennell, K.L.; Malcolm, S.A.; Khan, K.M.; Thomas, S.A.; Reid, S.J.; Brukner, P.D.; Ebeling, P.R.; Wark, J.D. Bone mass and bone turnover in power athletes, endurance athletes, and controls: A 12-month longitudinal study. *Bone* **1997**, *20*, 477–484. [CrossRef]

12. Wosk, J.; Voloshin, A. Wave attenuation in skeletons of young healthy persons. *J. Biomech.* **1981**, *14*, 261–267. [CrossRef]

13. Barrack, M.T.; Rauh, M.J.; Nichols, J.F. Cross-sectional evidence of suppressed bone mineral accrual among female adolescent runners. *J. Bone Miner. Res.* **2010**, *25*, 1850–1857. [CrossRef] [PubMed]

14. Gordon, C.M.; Bachrach, L.K.; Carpenter, T.O.; Crabtree, N.; El-Hajj Fuleihan, G.; Kutilek, S.; Lorenc, R.S.; Tosi, L.L.; Ward, K.A.; Ward, L.M.; et al. Dual energy X-ray absorptiometry interpretation and reporting in children and adolescents: The 2007 ISCD Pediatric Official Positions. *J. Clin. Densitom.* **2008**, *11*, 43–58. [CrossRef] [PubMed]

15. The American Congress of Obstetricians and Gynecologists (ACOG). Menstruation in girls and adolescents: Using the menstrual cycle as a vital sign. *Obstet. Gynecol.* **2006**, *108*, 1323–1328.

16. Takahashi, K.; Yoshiyama, Y.; Kaimoto, T.; Kunii, D.; Komatsu, T.; Yamamoto, S. Validation of a food frequency questionair based on food groups for estimating individual nutrient intake. *Jpn. J. Nutr. Diet.* **2001**, *59*, 221–232. [CrossRef]

17. Valimaki, V.V.; Alfthan, H.; Lehmuskallio, E.; Loyttyniemi, E.; Sahi, T.; Suominen, H.; Valimaki, M.J. Risk factors for clinical stress fractures in male military recruits: A prospective cohort study. *Bone* **2005**, *37*, 267–273. [CrossRef] [PubMed]

18. Heaney, R.P.; Abrams, S.; Dawson-Hughes, B.; Looker, A.; Marcus, R.; Matkovic, V.; Weaver, C. Peak bone mass. *Osteoporos. Int.* **2000**, *11*, 985–1009. [CrossRef] [PubMed]

19. Groothausen, J.; Siemer, H.; Kemper, H.C.G.; Twisk, J.; Welten, D.C. Influence of peak strain on lumbar bone mineral density: An analysis of 15-year physical activity in young males and females. *Pediatr. Exerc. Sci.* **1997**, *9*, 159–173. [CrossRef]

20. Frost, H.M. Why do marathon runners have less bone than weight lifters? A vital-biomechanical view and explanation. *Bone* **1997**, *20*, 183–189. [CrossRef]

21. Winters, K.M.; Adams, W.C.; Meredith, C.N.; Loan, M.D.; Lasley, B.L. Bone density and cyclic ovarian function in trained runners and active controls. *Med. Sci. Sports Exerc.* **1996**, *28*, 776–785. [CrossRef] [PubMed]

22. Burrows, M.; Nevill, A.M.; Bird, S.; Simpson, D. Physiological factors associated with low bone mineral density in female endurance runners. *Br. J. Sports Med.* **2003**, *37*, 67–71. [CrossRef] [PubMed]

23. Ackerman, K.E.; Nazem, T.; Chapko, D.; Russell, M.; Mendes, N.; Taylor, A.P.; Bouxsein, M.L.; Misra, M. Bone microarchitecture is impaired in adolescent amenorrheic athletes compared with eumenorrheic athletes and nonathletic controls. *J. Clin. Endocrinol. Metab.* **2011**, *96*, 3123–3133. [CrossRef] [PubMed]

24. Grinspoon, S.; Baum, H.; Lee, K.; Anderson, E.; Herzog, D.; Klibanski, A. Effects of short-term recombinant human insulin-like growth factor I administration on bone turnover in osteopenic women with anorexia nervosa. *J. Clin. Endocrinol. Metab.* **1996**, *81*, 3864–3870. [PubMed]
25. Magkos, F.; Yannakoulia, M.; Kavouras, S.A.; Sidossis, L.S. The type and intensity of exercise have independent and additive effects on bone mineral density. *Int. J. Sports Med.* **2007**, *28*, 773–779. [CrossRef] [PubMed]
26. Doyle, F.; Brown, J.; Lachance, C. Relation between bone mass and muscle weight. *Lancet* **1970**, *1*, 391–393. [CrossRef]
27. Rauch, F.; Bailey, D.A.; Baxter-Jones, A.; Mirwald, R.; Faulkner, R. The 'muscle-bone unit' during the pubertal growth spurt. *Bone* **2004**, *34*, 771–775. [CrossRef] [PubMed]
28. Takahashi, N.; Udagawa, N.; Suda, T. Vitamin D endocrine system and osteoclasts. *BoneKEy Rep.* **2014**, *3*, 495. [CrossRef] [PubMed]
29. Li, D.; Hitchcock, C.L.; Barr, S.I.; Yu, T.; Prior, J.C. Negative spinal bone mineral density changes and subclinical ovulatory disturbances—Prospective data in healthy premenopausal women with regular menstrual cycles. *Epidemiol. Rev.* **2014**, *36*, 137–147. [CrossRef] [PubMed]
30. Hartard, M.; Kleinmond, C.; Wiseman, M.; Weissenbacher, E.R.; Felsenberg, D.; Erben, R.G. Detrimental effect of oral contraceptives on parameters of bone mass and geometry in a cohort of 248 young women. *Bone* **2007**, *40*, 444–450. [CrossRef] [PubMed]

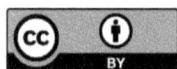

nutrients

MDPI

Article

Nutrition Assessment of B-Vitamins in Highly Active and Sedentary Women

Kathleen Woolf [1,*], Nicole L. Hahn [2], Megan M. Christensen [3], Amanda Carlson-Phillips [4] and Christine M. Hansen [5]

1   Department of Nutrition and Food Studies, Steinhardt School of Culture, Education,
    and Human Development, New York University, 411 Lafayette, 5th Floor, New York, NY 10003, USA
2   Department of Culinary and Nutrition Services, Banner Boswell Medical Center,
    10401 W. Thunderbird Boulevard, Sun City, AZ 85351, USA; nicole.hahn@bannerhealth.com
3   Department of Nutrition and Food Services, VA Salt Lake City Health Care System, 500 Foothill Drive,
    Salt Lake City, UT 84148, USA; megan.christensen@va.gov
4   Department of Performance Innovation, Exos, 2629 E. Rose Garden Lane, Phoenix, AZ 85050, USA;
    acarlson@teamexos.com
5   Nutrition Consultant, PO Box 184, Veneta, OR 97487, USA; veggiedoc@gmail.com
*   Correspondence: kathleen.woolf@nyu.edu; Tel.: +1-212-992-7898

Received: 1 September 2016; Accepted: 20 March 2017; Published: 26 March 2017

Abstract: Background: Female athletes and active women require adequate nutrition for optimal health and performance. Nutrition assessments are needed to identify potential nutrients of concern. Folate, vitamin B6, and vitamin B12 function in important pathways used during physical activity and female athletes may be at risk for poor status of these micronutrients. This cross-sectional study described a comprehensive nutrition assessment of the B-vitamins (folate, vitamin B6, and vitamin B12) using both dietary (food and dietary supplements) and biochemical assessments among highly active and sedentary women. Methods: Highly active (n = 29; age 20 ± 2 years; body mass index (BMI) 23.8 ± 3.5 kg/m^2) and sedentary (n = 29; age 24 ± 3 years; BMI 22.6 ± 3.0 kg/m^2) women were recruited for this study. Participants completed 7-day weighed food records and a fasting blood draw. Results: Although the highly active women reported higher intakes of energy ($p < 0.01$), folate ($p < 0.01$), vitamin B6 ($p < 0.01$), and vitamin B12 ($p < 0.01$), no significant differences were found between the groups for biomarkers of folate, vitamin B6, and vitamin B12. All of the highly active women had biomarkers within the desired reference ranges, suggesting good status. In general, most participants were able to meet the 1998 Recommended Daily Allowance (RDA) from food alone. For the women that reported using dietary supplements, micronutrient intakes met the 1998 RDA and in some cases, exceeded the Tolerable Upper Intake Level. Conclusion: This nutrition assessment documented good status for folate, vitamin B6, and vitamin B12 in the highly active women. Similar assessment approaches (food, dietary supplements, and biomarkers) should to completed with other nutrients of concern for the female athlete.

Keywords: B-vitamins; folate; vitamin B6; vitamin B12; female athlete

1. Introduction

Female athletes and active women require adequate nutrition to stay healthy and perform optimally. Comprehensive nutrition assessments, including dietary, biochemical, anthropometric, clinical, and environmental components, are needed to identify specific nutrition-related problems that may impact overall health and performance. For example, the B-vitamins play important roles in maintaining the health of female athletes and active women, serving as coenzymes in pathways critical for physical activity [1–6]. Folate functions as a coenzyme in reactions of deoxyribonucleic acid (DNA) synthesis, red blood cell synthesis, and amino acid metabolism, including the conversion of homocysteine to methionine [4,7]. Pyridoxal 5′-phosphate (PLP), the biologically active form of vitamin B6 in the human body, serves as a coenzyme in transamination and deamination reactions of amino acid metabolism and activates the rate-limiting step of glycogen breakdown [4,8,9]. Vitamin B12 functions as a coenzyme in methyl transfer reactions (i.e., homocysteine to methionine) and helps recycle folate [4,10]. Vitamin B12 also assists with the breakdown of odd-numbered fatty acid chains, DNA synthesis, and the production of red blood cells. Because folate, vitamin B6, and vitamin B12 assist with the metabolism of homocysteine, plasma homocysteine concentrations increase without adequate supplies of folate, vitamin B6, and vitamin B12, leading to an increased risk of cardiovascular disease [11]. Thus, these B-vitamins aid in the utilization of energy, metabolism of amino acids, maintenance of red blood cells, and regeneration of tissue. Comprehensive nutrition assessment of these key micronutrients is crucial to an athlete's success.

Unfortunately, many athletes, females in particular, may be at risk of poor dietary intakes for folate, vitamin B6, and vitamin B12 [12]. For instance, female athletes may not compensate for the energy expenditure associated with increased physical activity [13]. This behavior puts them at risk of low energy availability and many macronutrient and micronutrient deficits. In many sports, success is associated with a thin physique, thus encouraging excessive training and/or suboptimal dietary intakes [14,15]. Unfortunately, inadequate dietary intakes can impair an athlete's performance and lead to fatigue, injury, and/or altered concentration [12]. Additionally, female athletes and active women may have less folate, vitamin B6, and vitamin B12 available for metabolism of homocysteine, potentially leading to elevated plasma homocysteine concentrations compared to their physically inactive peers.

Dietary assessment has been utilized to assess dietary intakes for folate, vitamin B6, and vitamin B12 and determine adequacy. Recent dietary intakes for the United States (US) adult population have been well summarized from the National Health and Examination Surveys (NHANES) [16]. For female athletes and active women, reported dietary intakes for these micronutrients tend to come from older studies and are challenging to interpret due to changes in the reference ranges used to define nutrient adequacy. When completing dietary assessment for folate, time of data collection should also be considered to account for the 1996 US mandatory fortification of enriched grain products with folic acid [17]. In 1998, the latest reference values for these micronutrients were published as part of the Dietary Reference Intakes (DRIs) [18]. The DRIs express nutrient adequacy as the Estimated Average Requirement (EAR) (representing 50% of the population's requirement) and the Recommended Dietary Allowance (RDA) (representing 97.5% of the population's requirement). However, the EAR may not be sufficient for a physically active adult, adding to the difficulty to make generalizations about nutrient adequacy. Notwithstanding these concerns, some studies report mean dietary intakes for folate in female athletes less than the 1998 EAR (320 μg/day DFE) [19–24]. However, more recent studies report higher dietary intakes for folate among female athletes [25,26], which may be a reflection of folic acid fortification. For vitamin B6, most studies in female athletes document adequate intakes when compared to the 1998 RDA (1.3 mg/day) and EAR (1.1 mg/day) [21,22,25,26]. Studies comparing dietary intakes of vitamin B6 to the 1980 RDA (2 mg/day for adult females) or 1989 RDA (1.6 mg/day for adult females), values much higher than the 1998 RDA, typically report inadequate mean intakes for female athletes [4,19,22,27]. Because vitamin B6 plays a major role in the metabolic pathways required during exercise (i.e., amino acid metabolism, gluconeogenesis, glycogenolysis), some research suggests that female athletes may require two to three times the 1998 RDA of vitamin B6 due to their increased physical activity patterns and protein requirements [4,8]. For vitamin B12, some studies report adequate dietary intakes in female athletes [19–21,25,26], while other studies report inadequate intakes [13,23].

Because of the risk of inadequate dietary intakes of folate, vitamin B6, and vitamin B12 in female athletes, some research has included biochemical assessment in the evaluation of nutrient status. Unfortunately, the results are quite mixed. For example, Matter et al. examined folate status in non-supplementing female marathon runners and reported that 33% had poor status evidenced by low serum folate concentrations [28]. However, Beals and Manore examined serum folate concentrations in female athletes and reported only 4% with poor folate status [29]. Approximately 50% of the female athletes in this study reported taking a dietary supplement. Other research has reported good folate status in female recreational athletes [26,30], runners [31], and endurance athletes [32]. Research has also examined vitamin B6 status in both male and female athletes, with equally mixed outcomes. For instance, Raczynski and Szczepanska assessed vitamin B6 status of elite male and female Polish athletes over 6 years using the erythrocyte alanine aminotransaminase activity coefficient, a functional measure of vitamin B6, and reported poor status in 9% of the athletes [33]. In this study, endurance athletes had the highest prevalence of poor status of vitamin B6 (13%). Poor vitamin B6 status was highest in the pre-Olympic years (16%) and lowest in Olympic years (3%), when athletes may have focused more on dietary intakes and dietary supplementation. More recently, Joubert and Manore reported good status in a study of 64 recreationally active athletes (38 female) using plasma PLP [26]. Most studies of vitamin B12 status in female athletes suggest the risk of poor status is low, when adequate energy and animal products are consumed. Although the research is much more limited, good vitamin B12 status has been reported in female ultra-marathoners [34] and recreationally active adults [26].

More research should include comprehensive nutrition assessments to examine B-vitamin status in female athletes, especially for folate, vitamin B6, and vitamin B12. When completing dietary assessments, previous research has not included the contribution of natural sources and synthetic sources (fortified foods, dietary supplements) to dietary intakes. To determine nutrient status, biochemical assessment should also be included. Unfortunately, mixed gender studies have included more male participants than female participants, limiting information on the B-vitamin status of the female athlete. Thus, the purpose of this study was to describe the approach and results of a comprehensive nutrition assessment for B-vitamins (folate, vitamin B6, and vitamin B12), including dietary (food and dietary supplements) and biochemical assessments, among highly active and sedentary women.

2. Methods

2.1. Participant Recruitment and Study Design

This cross-sectional study completed a nutrition assessment of the B-vitamins (folate, vitamin B6, and vitamin B12) among highly active and sedentary women. This study was approved by the Institutional Review Board (IRB) at Arizona State University (IRB #0511000343; initial approval date 15 December 2005) and the University Committee on Activities Involving Human Subjects at New York University (IRB #11-8778; initial approval date 9 January 2012) and was conducted according to these guidelines.

Highly active and sedentary women between 18 and 35 years of age were recruited as the research participants for this study. Recruitment flyers were posted at university and college campuses, athletic training facilities, community centers, libraries, and throughout the local community. The study investigators also sent recruitment flyers to collegiate teams. The recruitment flyers briefly described the study and invited women to contact the study investigators for more information.

The study investigators determined eligibility over the telephone based on the following criteria: age (between 18 and 35 years), weight stable (<10% weight loss or gain within the past 6 months), no pregnancy or breastfeeding within the past year, nonsmoker or limited social smoker (quit smoking at least 6 months prior to study entry or smoke a few cigarettes socially on one occasion and then not smoke again for several days or weeks), and activity (highly active group defined as engaging in ≥12 h per week of programmed physical activity; sedentary group defined as engaging in <2 h of programmed physical activity per week). These activity levels must have been maintained for at least a year prior to study participation. Women who met the study criteria were invited to schedule a study appointment.

2.2. Procedures

The study participants completed two study visits. During the first visit, participants received detailed information about the study and signed an informed consent form. Height and weight were measured and body mass index (BMI) was calculated for each study participant. Participants were interviewed about the use of medications (prescription and over-the-counter) and dietary supplements (i.e., protein, energy, carbohydrate, meal replacement, vitamin, mineral, or herbal) and completed a health history questionnaire. Participants were asked to keep a 7-day weighed food record, noting all foods, beverages, and dietary supplements consumed. The study investigators provided participants with a food scale (Metrokane Gourmet Weigh Scale, Metrokane, New York, NY, USA) and showed them how to weigh foods. Participants were encouraged to include food labels for packaged items and provide measurements in teaspoons, tablespoons, or cups for foods not able to be weighed.

A second study visit was scheduled after the participants completed the food records. At this visit, participants completed an eight-hour fasting blood draw to determine blood biomarkers of folate, vitamin B6, and vitamin B12. The food records and study questionnaires were reviewed for completeness and study supplies were retrieved.

2.3. Anthropometric Assessment

Height was determined using a portable stadiometer (Invicta Plastics Limited, Oadby, Leicester, UK) to the nearest 0.1 centimeter without shoes. A Seca Bella 840 electronic flat scale (Seca North America, Chino, CA, USA) obtained each participant's weight to the nearest 0.1 kilogram.

2.4. Dietary and Physical Activity Assessment

Participants completed a 7-day weighed food record to examine dietary intake of energy, folate, vitamin B6, and vitamin B12. At the end of each day, participants recorded the type and duration of any programmed physical activity completed. The food records were analyzed using Food Processor, version 8.5 (Esha Research, Salem, OR, USA) and the United States Department of Agriculture (USDA) National Nutrient Database for Standard Reference, Release 20. The USDA database provided additional micronutrient information for commercial products. Folate intakes included assessments of dietary food folate (natural), synthetic folic acid added to fortified foods, and dietary folate equivalents (DFE) ((synthetic folic acid × 1.7) + food folate (natural)). The intake total included both natural and synthetic forms of vitamin B12. For vitamin B6, the intake total included vitamin B6 from food. Dietary intakes over the 7-days were averaged to determine the reported daily intake.

Micronutrient intakes (folic acid, vitamin B6, and vitamin B12) from supplements were added to the totals from food for those participants that reported using dietary supplements. The amount of folic acid from supplements was multiplied by 1.7 before adding to the total from food. Intakes from dietary supplements were summarized to reflect reported average daily intakes, considering dosage and usage patterns (days/week or days/month).

The estimated energy requirement (EER) was calculated for each participant using the appropriate age and gender equation [35]. For the active women, the "very active" physical activity coefficient was used in the equation. For the sedentary women, the "sedentary" physical activity coefficient was used. Energy intake/EER was determined for each participant.

2.5. Biochemical Assessment

Participants completed an eight-hour fasting blood draw to determine concentrations of plasma folate, red blood cell folate, plasma vitamin B6, vitamin B12, transcobalamin II, and homocysteine. Blood samples were immediately placed on ice and centrifuged within 30 min at 3000× g for 10 min at 4 °C. After centrifugation, the blood was separated and the plasma samples stored at −44 °C until analysis. Sonora Quest (Phoenix, AZ, USA), an independent laboratory, determined mean cell volume, hemoglobin, hematocrit, and high sensitivity C-reactive protein (CRP) concentrations.

For the analysis of red blood cell folate, a whole blood dilution (1:21) was prepared by combining 100 µL of well-suspended blood to 2 mL of newly made 0.2% ascorbic acid solution. The diluted samples were wrapped in foil to prevent light penetration and stored at −44 °C until the time of analysis. Plasma folate and red blood cell concentrations were analyzed using the Becton Dickinson SimulTRAC®-S Solid Phase Radioassay Kit (Becton, Dickinson and Company, Franklin Lakes, NJ, USA) for Vitamin B12 (^{57}Co) and Folate (^{125}I).

High performance liquid chromatography (HPLC) was used to determine vitamin B6 status of the participants using PLP as the biomarker [36]. HPLC utilizes reverse-phase ion pairing to separate B6 vitamers, which are chromatographically measured at an excitation wavelength of 330 nm and fluorescent emission of 400 nm.

Vitamin B12 status was assessed using plasma vitamin B12 and holotranscobalamin II (transcobalamin II) concentrations [37]. Transcobalamin II represents newly absorbed vitamin B12 enroute to the hematopoietic system and proliferating cells and is a more sensitive indicator of vitamin B12 status than plasma vitamin B12. Transcobalamin II was assessed by first preparing a slurry that contained 3 g synthetic amorphous precipitated silica in 20 mL of deionized water [38,39]. Transcobalamin II was absorbed from the samples by adding 100 µL of the prepared slurry to 500 µL of plasma and letting the samples sit at room temperature for 10 min. The samples were then centrifuged at 5000× g for 10 min. The supernatant was retained for further analysis. The Becton Dickinson SimulTRAC®-S Solid Phase Radioassay Kit (Becton, Dickinson and Company, Franklin Lakes, NJ, USA) for Vitamin B12 (^{57}Co) and Folate (^{125}I) was used to measure plasma vitamin B12 and holo-haptocorrin concentrations. Transcolbalamin II concentrations were determined by subtracting the holo-haptocorrin concentrations from the total plasma vitamin B12 concentration.

Fasting plasma homocysteine, a functional biomarker of folate, vitamin B6, and vitamin B12 status, was also measured by HPLC with fluorescence [40,41].

2.6. Statistical Analysis

Power calculations were completed using the reported vitamin B6 and folate dietary intakes for athletes and sedentary individuals from the research literature [42,43]. Using a difference of 0.2 mg, a sample size of 15 women per group would be sufficient to detect a difference in reported vitamin B6 intake between groups with a power of 0.80 and α = 0.05. However, a sample size of 57 women per group would be required to detect a difference in reported folate intake (using a difference of 50 µg) between groups with a power of 0.80 and α = 0.05, beyond the reach of this pilot study. Thus, we aimed to have 30 women per group and recruited additional women to allow for attrition. Prior to the statistical analysis, the data were tested for normality. Histograms of the study outcome measures visually assessed the distribution of the data. The Kolmogorov-Smirnov statistic was also used to assess normality of the distribution scores. Descriptive statistics (mean and standard deviation) were determined for the demographic data for the two groups of women. Independent sample *t*-tests compared the outcome measures between groups for the normally distributed variables. Because CRP did not have a normal distribution, the Mann-Whitney U test was used to examine the differences between groups. The median and interquartile range were used to summarize these values. Data were analyzed using IBM Statistical Package for the Social Sciences (SPSS) Statistics for Windows, version 22.0 (IBM Corporation, Armonk, NY, USA) version 14.0 and determined to be significant if $p < 0.05$.

3. Results

3.1. Descriptive Characteristics

Seventy-five participants signed consent forms (41 highly active women and 34 sedentary women). However, 11 highly active and 3 sedentary women decided not to finish the study. One highly active woman was eliminated because she was not as active as previously reported. Two sedentary women were eliminated; one had a blood disorder, and one had an activity level that was greater than 2 h per day. The present analysis includes 29 highly active women and 29 sedentary women.

Table 1 summarizes the descriptive characteristics for the 58 participants. The sedentary women were older than the highly active women ($p < 0.01$). Although the highly active women were heavier than the sedentary women, height and BMI were not significantly different between the two groups of women. The majority of participants in both groups, 69% of the highly active women and 82% percent of the sedentary women, reported their race/ethnicity as Caucasian (not of Hispanic origin). The highly active women reported consuming more total energy ($p < 0.01$) and relative energy (kcal/kg body weight) ($p = 0.01$) than the sedentary women. Although EER was significantly greater in the highly active women compared to the sedentary women ($p < 0.01$), there were no differences between groups for percent energy intake/EER.

Table 1. Descriptive characteristics of highly active and sedentary women [a].

Characteristics	Activity Level		*p*-Value
	Highly Active	Sedentary	
	n = 29	*n* = 29	
Descriptives			
Age (years)	20 ± 2	24 ± 3	<0.01 **
Height (cm)	169 ± 7	166 ± 8	0.11
Weight (kg)	68 ± 9	62 ± 10	0.03 *
Body mass index (kg/m^2)	23.8 ± 3.5	22.6 ± 3.0	0.17
Programmed physical activity (min/day)	169 ± 241	6 ± 8	
Energy intake			
Total energy (kcal/day)	2373 ± 616	1820 ± 403	<0.01 **
Relative energy (kcal/kg body weight)	35.2 ± 8.9	29.6 ± 7.2	0.01 *
Energy expenditure			
Estimated energy requirement (EER) (kcal)	2350 ± 168	1972 ± 132	<0.01 **
Energy intake/EER (%)	101 ± 25	92 ± 19	0.15
Race/ethnicity [b]			
African American (*n* (%))	0 (0)	0 (0)	
Asian/Pacific Islander (*n* (%))	1 (3)	0 (0)	
Native American (*n* (%))	0 (0)	1 (4)	
Caucasian (not of Hispanic origin) (*n* (%))	20 (69)	23 (82)	
Hispanic (*n* (%))	8 (28)	4 (14)	
Sport			
Basketball (*n* (%))	1 (3)		
Cross country/Long distance running (*n* (%))	3 (10)		
Gymnastics (*n* (%))	1 (3)		
Ice hockey (*n* (%))	1 (3)		
Softball (*n* (%))	3 (10)		
Swimming (*n* (%))	11 (38)		
Tennis (*n* (%))	4 (11)		
Volleyball (*n* (%))	5 (17)		

[a] Values are reported as mean ± standard deviation, except where noted; [b] One sedentary participant did not provide this information; * $p < 0.05$; ** $p < 0.01$.

Table 1 also describes the highly active women by their sport. The highly active women consisted of student athletes from Division I, Division II, and community college athletic teams.

3.2. Dietary Assessment

Tables 2–6 summarize the reported micronutrient intake of the 58 highly active and sedentary women. Folate intakes from food (natural sources, fortified foods) and dietary supplements are summarized in Table 2. The highly active women reported a greater intake of natural folate (μg/day) ($p < 0.01$), folic acid from fortified foods (μg/day) ($p = 0.03$), and folate (natural + fortified foods) (μg/day dietary folate equivalents (DFE)) ($p < 0.01$) than the sedentary women. There were no differences between the two groups of women for folate density (μg/day DFE/1000 kcal). For those participants that reported dietary supplement use (highly active = 9; sedentary = 12), the sedentary women consumed more folic acid from dietary supplements (μg/day) ($p = 0.04$) than the active women. However, there were no additional differences in folate intakes between the groups for participants that reported using dietary supplements.

Table 2. Folate intakes (food and dietary supplements) in highly active and sedentary women [a].

	Activity Level		
Intake Variable [b]	**Highly Active**	**Sedentary**	*p*-**Value**
	n = 29	*n* = 29	
Folate intake from food			
Folate (natural) (μg/day)	284 ± 119 256 (175)	190 ± 75 190 (116)	<0.01 **
Folic acid (fortified foods) (μg/day)	345 ± 213 302 (272)	238 ± 140 197 (155)	0.03 *
Folate (natural + fortified foods) (μg/day DFE) [c,d]	867 ± 391 777 (520)	595 ± 250 537 (344)	<0.01 **
Folate density (μg DFE/1000 kcal) [c,e]	364 ± 135 325 (205)	336 ± 154 288 (132)	0.47
Supplement contribution for those that reported supplement use			
Participants that reported folate dietary supplement use (*n* (%))	9 (31)	12 (41)	
Folic acid (dietary supplements) (μg/day)	564 ± 272 588 (364)	935 ± 438 680 (595)	0.04 *
Folate (natural) + folic acid (fortified foods + dietary supplements) (μg/day DFE) [c,d]	1470 ± 672 1232 (941)	1468 ± 473 1447 (670)	0.99
Folate (natural) + folic acid (fortified foods + dietary supplements) density (μg DFE/1000 kcal) [c,e]	621 ± 299 509 (358)	904 ± 365 775 (508)	0.07

[a] Values expressed as mean ± standard deviation and median (interquartile range), except where noted. [b] Intake variable determined by 7-day weighed food records analyzed using the United States Department of Agriculture (USDA) National Nutrient Database for Standard Reference, Release 20. [c] μg/day of DFE (Dietary Folate Equivalents) = (folic acid × 1.7) + natural food folate. [d] Folate Recommended Dietary Allowance (RDA) for women ages 14–18 = 400 μg/day of DFE. Folate RDA for women ages 19–50 = 400 μg/day of DFE. [e] Recommended value for DFE density: 250 μg of DFE/1000 kcals [44]. * $p < 0.05$. ** $p < 0.01$.

Table 3. Vitamin B6 intakes (food and dietary supplements) in highly active and sedentary women [a].

Intake Variable [b]	Activity Level		p-Value
	Highly Active n = 29	Sedentary n = 29	
Vitamin B6 intake from food			
Vitamin B6 (mg/day) [c]	3.5 ± 2.2 2.8 (1.9)	1.8 ± 0.7 1.6 (0.8)	<0.01 **
Vitamin B6 density (mg/1000 kcal) [d]	1.6 ± 1.2 1.1 (0.8)	1.0 ± 0.4 0.9 (0.5)	0.03 *
Supplement contribution for those that reported supplement use			
Participants that reported vitamin B6 dietary supplement use (n (%))	8 (28)	12 (41)	
Vitamin B6 (dietary supplements) (mg/day)	7.6 ± 9.2 2.7 (14.0)	14.0 ± 29.4 2.3 (3.0)	0.56
Vitamin B6 (food) + vitamin B6 (dietary supplements) (mg/day) [c]	11.5 ± 9.8 7.6 (15.4)	15.8 ± 29.3 4.4 (3.2)	0.70
Vitamin B6 (food) + vitamin B6 (dietary supplements) density (mg/1000 kcal) [d]	5.0 ± 4.1 3.4 (7.9)	9.0 ± 15.3 2.5 (3.6)	0.49

[a] Values expressed as mean ± standard deviation and median (interquartile range), except where noted. [b] Intake variable determined by 7-day weighed food records analyzed using the United States Department of Agriculture (USDA) National Nutrient Database for Standard Reference, Release 20. [c] RDA for vitamin B6 for girls ages 14–18 = 1.2 mg/day. RDA for vitamin B6 for women ages 19–50 = 1.3 mg/day. [d] Recommended value for vitamin B6 density: 1 mg/1000 kcals [44]. * $p < 0.05$. ** $p < 0.01$.

Table 4. Vitamin B12 intakes (food and dietary supplements) in highly active and sedentary women [a].

Intake Variable [b]	Activity Level		p-Value
	Highly Active n = 29	Sedentary n = 29	
Vitamin B12 intake from food			
Synthetic vitamin B12 (µg/day)	3.8 ± 5.8 2.7 (1.6)	1.6 ± 2.2 0.7 (1.8)	0.05
Vitamin B12 (µg/day) [c]	8.1 ± 6.3 6.1 (5.4)	4.7 ± 2.4 4.3 (2.0)	<0.01 **
Vitamin B12 density (µg/1000 kcal) [d]	3.6 ± 3.7 2.9 (1.3)	2.7 ± 1.5 2.2 (1.5)	0.21
Supplement contribution for those that reported supplement use			
Participants that reported vitamin B12 dietary supplement use (n(%))	9 (31)	12 (41)	
Vitamin B12 (dietary supplements) (µg/day)	34.8 ± 63.5 10.3 (33.0)	36.4 ± 73.8 7.0 (21.0)	0.96
Vitamin B12 (food) + vitamin B12 (dietary supplements) (µg/day) [c]	38.3 ± 66.0 10.4 (35.6)	37.6 ± 74.0 9.1 (21.6)	0.98
Vitamin B12 (food) + vitamin B12 (dietary supplements) density (µg/1000 kcal) [d]	15.9 ± 25.6 6.5 (16.2)	23.7 ± 48.4 5.6 (15.8)	0.66

[a] Values expressed as mean ± standard deviation and median (interquartile range), except where noted. [b] Intake variable determined by 7-day weighed food records analyzed using the United States Department of Agriculture (USDA) National Nutrient Database for Standard Reference, Release 20. [c] RDA for vitamin B12 for girls ages 14–18 = 2.4 µg/day. RDA for vitamin B12 for women ages 19–50 = 2.4 µg/day. Values include natural vitamin B12 and synthetic vitamin B12 added to food. [d] Recommended value for vitamin B12 density: 1.5 µg/1000 kcals [44]. * $p < 0.05$. ** $p < 0.01$.

Table 5. Evaluation of nutrient adequacy from food using DRI [a] recommendations of highly active and sedentary women.

Nutrient/DRI Factors	Activity Level		Reference Values: Girls 14–18 years [b]	Reference Values: Women 19–50 years [b]
	Highly Active	Sedentary		
	n = 29	*n* = 29		
Folate				
Met EAR (*n* (%)) [c]	28 (96)	26 (90)	330 µg/day	320 µg/day
Met RDA (*n* (%)) [d]	26 (90)	23 (79)	400 µg/day	400 µg/day
Exceeded UL (*n* (%)) [e,f]	4 (14)	1 (3)	800 µg/day	1000 µg/day
Vitamin B6				
Met EAR (*n* (%)) [c]	29 (100)	26 (90)	1.0 mg/day	1.1 mg/day
Met RDA (*n* (%)) [d]	27 (93)	25 (86)	1.2 mg/day	1.3 mg/day
Exceeded UL (*n* (%)) [e]	0 (0)	0 (0)	80 mg/day	100 mg/day
Vitamin B12				
Met EAR (*n* (%)) [c]	29 (100)	29 (100)	2.0 µg/day	2.0 µg/day
Met RDA (*n* (%)) [d]	29 (100)	27 (93)	2.4 µg/day	2.4 µg/day
Exceeded UL (*n* (%)) [e,g]	–	–	–	–

[a] DRI = Dietary Reference Intakes. [b] Reference value from Food and Nutrition Board, Institute of Medicine [18]. [c] EAR = Estimated Average Requirement. [d] RDA = Recommended Daily Allowance. [e] UL = Tolerable Upper Intake Level. [f] Because the UL for folate applies to synthetic forms (fortified foods, dietary supplements), this assessment only includes the contribution from fortified foods. [g] A UL for vitamin B12 has not been established.

Table 6. Evaluation of nutrient adequacy from food and supplements using the DRI [a] recommendations for the highly active and sedentary women that reported dietary supplement use.

Nutrient/DRI Factors	Activity Level		Reference Values: Girls 14–18 Yeras [b]	Reference Values: Women 19–50 Years [b]
	Highly Active	Sedentary		
Folate				
Participants that reported folate dietary supplement use	*n* = 9	*n* = 12		
Met EAR (*n* (%)) [c]	9 (100)	12 (100)	330 µg/day	320 µg/day
Met RDA (*n* (%)) [d]	9 (100)	12 (100)	400 µg/day	400 µg/day
Exceeded UL (*n* (%)) [e,f]	5 (56)	8 (67)	800 µg/day	1000 µg/day
Vitamin B6				
Participants that reported vitamin B6 dietary supplement use	*n* = 8	*n* = 12		
Met EAR (*n* (%)) [c]	8 (100)	12 (100)	1.0 mg/day	1.1 mg/day
Met RDA (*n* (%)) [d]	8 (100)	12 (100)	1.2 mg/day	1.3 mg/day
Exceeded UL (*n* (%)) [e]	0 (0)	1 (8)	80 mg/day	100 mg/day
Vitamin B12				
Participants that reported vitamin B12 dietary supplement use	*n* = 9	*n* = 12		
Met EAR (*n* (%)) [c]	9 (100)	12 (100)	2.0 µg/day	2.0 µg/day
Met RDA (*n* (%)) [d]	9 (100)	12 (100)	2.4 µg/day	2.4 µg/day
Exceeded UL (*n* (%)) [e,g]	–	–	–	–

[a] DRI—Dietary Reference Intakes. [b] Reference value from Food and Nutrition Board, Institute of Medicine [18]. [c] EAR—Estimated Average Requirement. [d] RDA—Recommended Daily Allowance. [e] UL—Tolerable Upper Intake Level. [f] Because the UL for folate applies to synthetic forms (fortified foods, dietary supplements), this assessment only includes the contribution from fortified foods and dietary supplements. [g] A UL for vitamin B12 has not been established.

Table 3 outlines the vitamin B6 intake from food and dietary supplements for the 58 highly active and sedentary women. Significant differences between groups were found in vitamin B6 intake from food (mg/day) ($p < 0.01$) and vitamin B6 density from food (mg/1000 kcal) ($p = 0.03$). Eight highly active and 12 sedentary women reported the use of supplements containing vitamin B6. However, there were no significant differences between groups for vitamin B6 intakes for those participants that used dietary supplements.

Dietary and supplemental intake of vitamin B12 is summarized in Table 4. The highly active women reported a significantly higher intake of vitamin B12 from food (μg/day) ($p < 0.01$) than the sedentary women. No significant differences were found between groups for synthetic vitamin B12 added to food (μg/day) and vitamin B12 density (μg/1000 kcal) from food. Nine highly active women reported the use of supplements containing vitamin B12 compared to 12 sedentary participants. However, there were no significant differences between groups for vitamin B12 intakes for those participants that reported using dietary supplements.

Table 5 describes the adequacy of dietary micronutrient intake as set by the DRI recommendations for folate, vitamin B6, and vitamin B12. Ninety-six percent of the highly active women and 90% of the sedentary participants met the EAR for folate. Ninety percent of the highly active women and 79% of the sedentary women met the RDA for folate. Fourteen percent of the highly active women and 3% of the sedentary women exceeded the UL (Tolerable Upper Intake Level) for folate, a guideline that only applies to synthetic forms of the nutrient (i.e., fortified foods, dietary supplements). Thus, folic acid from fortified foods was the form of folate used in this estimation. For vitamin B6, 100% of the highly active women and 90% of the sedentary women met the EAR. Ninety-three percent of the highly active women and 86% of the sedentary women met the RDA for vitamin B6. The UL was not exceeded by either group of women for vitamin B6. For vitamin B12, 100% of the highly active women met the EAR and RDA. One hundred percent of the sedentary women met the EAR for vitamin B12 and 93% of the sedentary women met the RDA. Currently, a UL for vitamin B12 has not been established.

Table 6 describes the adequacy of dietary micronutrient intake from food and dietary supplements as set by the DRI recommendations for folate, vitamin B6, and vitamin B12 for those participants reporting dietary supplement use. All of the highly active and sedentary participants met the EAR and RDA for folate, vitamin B6, and vitamin B12 when including both food and dietary supplements. However, 5 of the highly active (56% of those reporting dietary supplement use) and 8 of the sedentary women (67% of reporting dietary supplement use) exceeded the UL for folate, a guideline referring to synthetic folate sources (i.e., fortified foods, dietary supplements). None of the highly active woman exceeded the UL for vitamin B6, whereas 1 sedentary woman did.

3.3. Blood Biochemical Assessment

Table 7 summarizes biomarkers of B-vitamin status for the two groups of women. No differences were found between groups for any of the biomarkers for folate, vitamin B6, and vitamin B12. None of the participants had a plasma folate, red blood cell folate, or plasma vitamin B12 concentration below the reference range. However, two (7%) of the sedentary participants had plasma transcobalamin II concentrations below the reference range. Two (7%) of the highly active women and two (7%) of the sedentary participants had plasma transcobalamin II concentrations above the reference range. Additionally, two (7%) of the sedentary participants had PLP concentrations below the reference range.

Table 7 also describes the hematological data for the study participants. One athlete had a mean corpuscular volume (MCV), hemoglobin, and hematocrit values below the reference range. No participant was found to have an MCV value above the reference range. However, there were no significant differences between groups for these three hematological markers and CRP. Thirty-four percent of the athletes and 28% of the sedentary participants had CRP values above the reference value.

Table 7. Biochemical markers of highly active and sedentary women [a,b].

Blood Parameter	Reference Range	Activity Level		p-Value
		Highly Active	Sedentary	
		n = 29	n = 29	
Folate [c]	>3 ng/mL	11 ± 4	11 ± 4	0.91
Number below reference range (n (%))		0 (0)	0 (0)	
Red blood cell folate [c]	>140 ng/mL	444 ± 83	436 ± 122	0.79
Number below reference range (n (%))		0 (0)	0 (0)	
Vitamin B12 [c]	>170 pg/mL	647 ± 267	552 ± 168	0.11
Number below reference range (n (%))		0 (0)	0 (0)	
Transcobalamin II [d]	13–244 pg/mL	148 ± 115	146 ± 82	0.92
Number below reference range (n (%))		0 (0)	2 (7)	
Number above reference range (n (%))		2 (7)	2 (7)	
Pyridoxal 5'-phosphate [c]	>20 nmol/L	53 ± 34	45 ± 26	0.33
Number below reference range (n (%))		0 (0)	2 (7)	
Homocysteine [c]	<14 µmol/L	6 ± 2	6 ± 2	0.93
Number above reference range (n (%))		0 (0)	0 (0)	
Mean corpuscular volume [e]	78–100 fL	89 ± 6	89 ± 3	0.91
Participants below the reference range (n (%))		1 (3)	0 (0)	
Hemoglobin [e]	11.5–16.0 g/dL	13.5 ± 1.1	13.8 ± 0.7	0.23
Participants below the reference range (n (%))		1 (3)	0 (0)	
Hematocrit [e]	35%–48%	40 ± 3	40 ± 2	0.78
Participants below the reference range (n (%))		1 (3)	0 (0)	
High sensitivity C-reactive protein [e] median (interquartile range)	<1.0 mg/L	0.5 (3.2)	0.4 (1.0)	0.55
Participants above the reference range (n (%))		10 (34)	8 (28)	

[a] Mean ± standard deviation, except where noted. [b] Independent sample t-tests used to examine differences for all parameters except C-reactive protein (Mann Whitney U test). [c] Reference value from Food and Nutrition Board, Institute of Medicine [18]. [d] Reference value from Herzlich and Herbert [37]. [e] Reference value from Sonora Quest Laboratories. * $p < 0.05$.

4. Discussion

This study is one of few that summarizes a comprehensive nutrition assessment of the B-vitamins using dietary (food and dietary supplements) and biochemical assessments in highly active women compared to a control group of sedentary women. As part of the dietary assessment, food records were collected over 7 days (longer than other studies in the research literature) to determine nutrient adequacy using the DRIs for folate, vitamin B6, and vitamin B12. The average micronutrient intake of the highly active and sedentary participants not only met the 1998 DRIs, but were much higher than the dietary intakes reported in previous studies. Additionally, four highly active women and one sedentary participant exceeded the UL for folate with the consumption of fortified foods. Information was collected on dietary supplement use as part of the dietary assessment. The participants that used dietary supplements met the 1998 RDA for folate, vitamin B6, and vitamin B12. Furthermore, five highly active and eight sedentary women exceeded the UL for folate when the intake included both food and supplements. Dietary supplement use has not always been reported or included in previous studies. As part of the biochemical assessment, biomarkers for folate, vitamin B6, and vitamin B12 were determined. The mean values for the biomarkers were not significantly different between the two groups of women. All of the highly active women had biomarkers for folate, vitamin B6, and vitamin B12 within the reference ranges, suggesting good status. However, two sedentary women had low transcobalamin II concentrations, suggesting poor status of vitamin B12, and two different sedentary women had low PLP concentrations, suggesting poor status of vitamin B6.

4.1. Dietary Assessment

Folate, vitamin B6, and vitamin B12 intakes from food were significantly higher in the highly active women compared to the sedentary women. This finding may be related to the significantly higher energy intake by the highly active women. Only vitamin B6 was significantly different between groups for nutrient density, with a higher density in the highly active women; however, nutrient density recommendations were met for all three nutrients by both groups. Thus, the highly active women were not necessarily consuming more nutrient dense foods, especially for folate and vitamin B12. Athletes with lower energy requirements may benefit from nutrition education to help them select more nutritious foods in the diet. The average dietary intake of vitamin B6, folate, and vitamin B12 for the women in our study exceeded the 1998 RDAs for folate (400 µg/day of DFE), vitamin B6 (1.2 mg/day for girls 14–18 years; 1.3 mg/day for women 19–50 years), and vitamin B12 (2.4 µg/day). The reported dietary intakes from this study are also much higher than the intakes reported in recent NHANES data (i.e., women 20–29 years of age: vitamin B6 = 1.91 mg, folate = 471 µg DFE, vitamin B12 = 4.23 µg) [16].

In our study, the dietary intakes for folate are higher than those reported by female athletes in previous studies conducted after the mandatory folic acid fortification [13,14,23,26]. For example, 25 synchronized figure skaters reported average intakes for folate of 65% of the 1998 RDA [14]. In another study, pre- and post-season intakes for folate were examined in 13 intercollegiate female soccer players [13]. Pre-season intakes were 271 ± 130 µg/day, while the post-season intake was reported as 186 ± 113 µg/day. Similarly, Leydon and Wall examined dietary intakes among female jockeys and reported average dietary intakes of only 132 ± 52 µg/day [23]. Among female recreational athletes, Joubert and Manore reported higher dietary intakes for folate of 428 ± 125 µg/day for female athletes participating primarily in low intensity activities and 511 ± 105 µg/day for female athletes participating in high intensity activities [26].

Similarly, the reported vitamin B6 intakes in our study are higher than those reported by female athletes in the research literature [13,14,23,26]. Among female soccer players, the mean pre-season vitamin B6 intake met the 1998 RDA, but the mean post-season intake did not [13]. The post-season overall energy intake was less than the pre-season intake and could account for a decreased vitamin B6 intake. Ziegler et al. examined the vitamin B6 intake of female synchronized figure skaters utilizing 3-day food records of 123 athletes and reported results by age [14]. The mean values for all participants and the girls aged 14–18 years did not meet the 1998 RDA for vitamin B6. The lower intakes reported in this study may be due to lower energy intakes as figure skating is seen as a weight conscious sport. For female jockeys, another weight conscious sport, the average vitamin B6 intakes were 0.90 ± 0.49 mg/day, less than the 1998 RDA and EAR [23]. However, other research has reported adequate vitamin B6 intakes. For instance, Joubert and Manore reported mean vitamin B6 intakes from 2.2 ± 1.6 to 2.4 ± 0.7 mg/day in recreational athletes, above the current RDA of 1.3 mg/day for women 19–50 years of age [26].

In the research literature, the mean intakes of vitamin B12 for female athletes are lower than those found in our study [13,14,23,26]. For example, the average pre- and post-season vitamin B12 intakes of female soccer players were 4.5 ± 1.9 µg/day and 2.1 ± 1.7 µg/day, respectively [13]. The pre-season intake was also higher in dietary protein, which possibly influenced the average vitamin B12 intake. The post-season average intake did not meet the 1998 RDA, but was adequate when compared to the EAR, a guideline that may not be appropriate for an athlete. In female synchronized figure skaters, the average intake met the 1998 RDA [14]. However, younger skaters (14–18 years) had average intakes of 2.2 µg/day for vitamin B12, less than the RDA. Leydon and Wall reported dietary intakes of vitamin B12 less than the RDA among female jockeys (2.15 ± 1.07 µg/day) [23]. Joubert and Manore reported dietary intakes for vitamin B12 that exceeded the RDA among female recreational athletes (5.3 ± 2.5 to 5.3 ± 4.8 µg/day) [26]. Our highly active women reported much higher vitamin B12 intakes (active = 8.1 ± 6.3 µg/day; sedentary = 4.7 ± 2.4 µg/day), which may be attributed to a more complete dietary assessment, utilizing a dietary software database that also included synthetic food sources of vitamin B12.

The current study reported higher intakes of vitamin B6, folate, and vitamin B12 than most other studies. Several factors may have contributed to this finding. First, when the dietary software program was missing micronutrient information for the B vitamins, we used the USDA nutrient database to reanalyze the food records. The USDA nutrient database was more complete in regards to B-vitamin content, including synthetic forms of folate and vitamin B12. Other studies may have used software with similar missing data, thus, leading to an underestimation of dietary intakes. Second, our participants reported average intakes of 867 ± 391 µg/day (active) and 595 ± 250 µg/day (sedentary) DFE for folate. Food records showed large quantities of ready-to-eat breakfast cereals consumed by both groups of women. Some participants consumed >3 cups per sitting with multiple sittings per day. Four (14%) of the highly-active and one (3%) of the sedentary women had folate intakes that exceeded the UL of 1000 µg/day. Among US adults, Yang et al. reported that 2.7% of adults consumed more than the UL of folic acid, a percentage similar to the sedentary women in our study [45]. Thus, the consumption of ready-to-eat cereal was most likely associated with the higher dietary intakes of folic acid.

Two studies in female athletes also included dietary supplements when completing a dietary assessment of B-vitamins [25,34]. Singh et al. examined dietary intakes of ultra-marathon runners and found the average intake of vitamin B6 from food was 2.6 ± 0.3 mg/day for the usual diet and 2.3 ± 0.3 mg/day for the pre-race diet [34]. Vitamin B6 intake jumped to 7.3 ± 2.2 mg/day (usual diet) and 7.0 ± 2.4 mg/day (pre-race diet) when food and supplement intakes were combined. Average dietary folate intakes of the ultra-marathon runners were 391 µg/day, which only met the 1998 EAR of 320 µg/day of DFE [34]. When supplemental folic acid was included, average intakes of dietary folate increased (629 ±102 µg/day for usual intake and 513 ± 92 µg/day for pre-race intake). Singh et al. reported the average intake of vitamin B12 from food as 6.1 µg/day for the usual diet and 4.5 µg/day for the pre-race diet from food. Inclusion of supplemental vitamin B12 intake increased the total intake to 51.3 µg/day (usual diet) and 51.8 µg/day (pre-race diet), well above the 1998 RDA. Beshgetoor and Nichols also described the food and supplement intake of 25 female master cyclists and runners [25]. The mean intake of vitamin B6 for the supplementing athletes (SA) and the non-supplementing athletes (NSA) was 15 ± 5 mg/day and 3 ± 1 mg/day, respectively. Both groups met the 1998 RDA. The mean intake of folate for the SA and NSA was 486 ± 55 and 402 ± 115 µg/day DFE, respectively. The mean vitamin B12 intake for the SA and NSA was 18 ± 5 and 6 ± 2 µg/day, respectively, well above the EAR and RDA. Similarly, our study also documented higher consumption of folate, vitamin B6, and vitamin B12 for the highly active and sedentary women when both food and dietary supplements were included in the nutrient totals as part of the dietary assessment.

4.2. Biochemical Assessment

As part of the biochemical assessment, we examined biomarkers for folate, vitamin B6, and vitamin B12 in highly active and sedentary women. There were no significant differences between groups for any of the B-vitamin biomarkers. All of the highly active women had biomarkers within the reference ranges for plasma folate, RBC folate, plasma vitamin B6, vitamin B12, and homocysteine. Two sedentary women had transcobalamin II concentrations below the reference range of 13–244 pg/mL, suggesting poor vitamin B12 status from the biochemical assessment. When examining their dietary assessment data, neither participant reported using dietary supplements and one reported a vitamin B12 intake much lower than the group mean (2.8 µg/day). Two of the sedentary women had PLP concentrations <20 nmol/L, suggesting poor status of vitamin B6. Upon further examination of their dietary assessment data, one was non-supplementing and reported an average vitamin B6 intake of 1.35 mg/day. The other sedentary participant reported using a dietary supplement containing vitamin B6 (2 mg/day) and was consuming on average 1.54 mg/day of vitamin B6 from food. Ten of the highly active women had elevated CRP concentrations, which may be a sign of inflammation due to over training [46–48]. Eight of the sedentary women had elevated CRP levels as well, which may be related to environmental factors, such as stress at home or work, pollution, illness, or other factors. The more than adequate dietary intakes of folate, vitamin B6, and vitamin B12 certainly impacted the nutrient biomarkers.

Plasma homocysteine concentrations, a functional biomarker of B-vitamin status, were within the normal range in our highly active and sedentary women and there were no differences between the groups of women. The amount of training performed by our participants did not impact plasma homocysteine concentrations. Similarly, the adequate dietary intakes for folate, vitamin B6, and vitamin B12 may have influenced plasma homocysteine concentrations. Some studies have documented acute increases in homocysteine after exercise, but then a return to baseline after a recovery or resting period. For instance, Wright et al. reported homocysteine concentrations in men increased immediately after a 30 minute bicycle ride, but began to decrease within 30 min after exercise [49]. In another study involving winter athletes, plasma homocysteine concentrations were higher during training and competition compared to baseline [50]. Dehydration and decreased blood volume after strenuous exercise may be a factor in these study results. Similarly, Gelecek and colleagues reported increases in homocysteine concentrations from baseline after one exercise session and a 6 week exercise training program [51]. These results can also be a factor of dehydration. Our study documented biomarkers for folate, vitamin B6, and vitamin B12 within the reference range for the highly active women, but we did not examine the effect of acute physical activity on these parameters.

4.3. Limitations

The first limitation is related to the self-reported food and activity logs. Participants were instructed how to complete the forms and provided written information to use as a guide. However, many food records needed clarification of contents, amounts consumed, and preparation. Participants may have omitted some of their dietary intake to make it look as though they consumed less. Examples include omitting "unhealthy" foods and reporting intake of more socially desirable foods. The second limitation is that the results of this study are not applicable to all female athletes as we did not have representatives from every sport discipline. Due to the small sample sizes included in our study (basketball, $n = 1$; cross country/long-distance running, $n = 3$; gymnastics, $n = 1$; ice hockey, $n = 1$; softball, $n = 3$; swimming, $n = 11$; tennis, $n = 4$; volleyball, $n = 5$), our results may not be generalizable to female athletes participating in these same sports. A third limitation is the classification of activity level using self-report of programmed physical activity. For instance, the sedentary women could have reported engaging in <2 h of programmed physical activity but have jobs that require them to stand, walk, and complete physical movement throughout the day (i.e., childcare, retail sales, landscaping), thus confounding the results. Fourth, due to limited research, power calculations were not computed for reported vitamin B12 dietary intakes and B-vitamin biomarkers. The study was not powered to detect differences between the active and sedentary women in reported dietary folate intakes and may not have been sufficiently powered to detect differences in the other study outcome measures. This low statistical power reduces the chance of detecting any true differences between the study groups and increases the likelihood of making a type II error. Thus, the study results should be interpreted with caution and may not be generalizable to other groups of highly active and sedentary women. Fifth, selection bias may have influenced the study results. Because the participants volunteered for this nutrition study, they may be more interested in health and nutrition than their peers and may not appropriately represent other highly active and sedentary young women. Another limitation is whether the participants followed the parameters of the fasting blood draw (8-h fasting). Participants were asked the time when food/meal was consumed before the blood draw. There is also the possibility the participants did not refrain from physical activity or smoking (if they reported social smoking) for 48 h prior to the blood draw. Acute bouts of strenuous exercise may have an impact on CRP levels and smoking may alter folate status and CRP concentrations [46–48,52].

4.4. Future Studies

This study is one of few to comprehensively assess B-vitamin status (folate, vitamin B6, and vitamin B12) using both dietary (food, dietary supplements) and biochemical assessments in highly active and sedentary women. We did not report losses of the B-vitamins or complete a clinical exam looking for physical signs and symptoms related to B-vitamin status. Additional biomarkers (both static and functional) could further describe B-vitamin status of highly active women. Future studies should also incorporate larger sample sizes representing athletes from varied sports.

5. Conclusions

This study described a comprehensive nutrition assessment of the B-vitamins in highly active and sedentary women. Although the highly active women had significantly higher dietary intakes of energy, folate, vitamin B6, and vitamin B12, there were no significant differences between groups for the biomarkers of B-vitamin status. The dietary intakes reported by the women in this study were much higher than the dietary intakes reported in the research literature. Additionally, 5 women (4 highly active, 1 sedentary) exceeded the UL for folate with the consumption of fortified foods. In this study, all of the women that used dietary supplements met the 1998 RDA for folate, vitamin B6, and vitamin B12. However, the UL for folate was exceeded by 5 highly active and 8 sedentary women when the intake included both food and supplements. Furthermore, all of the highly active women had biomarkers of B-vitamin status within the reference ranges, reflecting the adequate dietary intakes (food, dietary supplements) for folate, vitamin B6, and vitamin B12.

Acknowledgments: The authors and co-authors did not receive any funding to conduct this study.

Author Contributions: The study was designed by K.W., N.H., M.M.C., and A.C.-P.; data were collected and analyzed by K.W., N.H., M.M.C., A.C.-P., and C.H.; data interpretation and manuscript preparation were undertaken by K.W. and N.H. All authors approved the final version of the manuscript.

Conflicts of Interest: The authors declare no conflict of interest.

References

1. Lukaski, H.C.L. Vitamin and mineral status. Effects on physical performance. *Nutrition* **2004**, *20*, 632–644. [CrossRef] [PubMed]
2. Maughan, R.J. Role of micronutrients in sport and physical activity. *Br. Med. Bull.* **1999**, *55*, 683–690. [CrossRef] [PubMed]
3. Volpe, S.L. Micronutrient requirements for athletes. *Clin. Sports Med.* **2007**, *26*, 119–130. [CrossRef] [PubMed]
4. Woolf, K.; LoBuono, D.L.; Manore, M.M. B-vitamins and the female athlete. In *Nutrition and the Female Athlete. From Research to Practice*; Beals, K.A., Ed.; CRC Press: Boca Raton, FL, USA, 2013; pp. 139–180.
5. Woolf, K.; Manore, M.M. B-vitamins and exercise: Does exercise alter requirements. *Int. J. Sport Nutr. Exerc. Metab.* **2006**, *16*, 453–484. [CrossRef] [PubMed]
6. Woolf, K.; Manore, M.M. Micronutrients important for exercise. In *Advances in Sport and Exercise Science Series: Nutrition and Sport*; Spurway, N., MacLaren, D., Eds.; Elsevier: Philadelphia, PA, USA, 2007; pp. 119–136.
7. Stover, P.J. Folic Acid. In *Modern Nutrition in Health and Disease*, 11th ed.; Ross, A.C., Caballero, B., Cousins, R.J., Tucker, K.L., Ziegler, T.R., Eds.; Lippincott Williams & Wilkins: Philadelphia, PA, USA, 2014; pp. 325–330.
8. Hansen, C.M.; Manore, M.M. Vitamin B6. In *Sports Nutrition: Vitamins and Trace Elements*; Driskell, J.A., Wolinsky, I., Eds.; CRC Press: Boca Raton, FL, USA, 2005; pp. 81–91.
9. Da Silva, V.R.; Mackey, A.D.; Davis, S.R.; Gregory, J.F., III. Vitamin B6. In *Modern Nutrition in Health and Disease*, 11th ed.; Ross, A.C., Caballero, B., Cousins, R.J., Tucker, K.L., Ziegler, T.R., Eds.; Lippincott Williams & Wilkins: Philadelphia, PA, USA, 2014; pp. 341–350.
10. Carmel, R. Cobalamin (Vitamin B12). In *Modern Nutrition in Health and Disease*, 11th ed.; Ross, A.C., Caballero, B., Cousins, R.J., Tucker, K.L., Ziegler, T.R., Eds.; Lippincott Williams & Wilkins: Philadelphia, PA, USA, 2014; pp. 369–389.
11. Debreceni, B.; Debreceni, L. The role of homocysteine-lowering B-vitamins in the primary prevention of cardiovascular disease. *Cardiovasc Ther.* **2014**, *32*, 130–138. [CrossRef] [PubMed]
12. Thomas, D.T.; Erdman, K.A.; Burke, L.M. Position of the Academy of Nutrition and Dietetics, Dietitians of Canada, and the American College of Sports Medicine: Nutrition and athletic performance. *J. Acad. Nutr. Diet.* **2016**, *116*, 501–528. [CrossRef] [PubMed]
13. Clark, M.; Reed, D.B.; Crouse, S.F.; Armstrong, R.B. Pre- and post-season dietary intake, body composition, and performance indices of NCAA division I female soccer players. *Int. J. Sport Nutr. Exerc. Metab.* **2003**, *13*, 303–319. [CrossRef] [PubMed]

14. Ziegler, P.J.; Kannan, S.; Jonnalagadda, S.S.; Krishnakumar, A.; Taksali, S.E.; Nelson, J.A. Dietary intake, body image perceptions, and weight concerns of female US international synchronized figure skating teams. *Int. J. Sport Nutr. Exerc. Metab.* **2005**, *15*, 550–566. [CrossRef] [PubMed]

15. Brownell, K.D. Dieting and the search for the perfect body: Where physiology and culture collide. *Behav. Ther.* **1991**, *22*, 1–12. [CrossRef]

16. US Department of Agriculture, Agricultural Research Service, Beltsville Human Nutrition Research Center, Food Surveys Research Group (Beltsville, MD) and US Department of Health and Human Services, Centers for Disease Control and Prevention, National Center for Health Statistics (Hyattsville, MD). What we eat in America, NHANES 2013–2014. Data: Nutrient Intakes from Food and Beverages. Available online: http://www.ars.usda.gov/northeast-area/beltsville-human-nutrition-research-center/food-surveys-research-group/docs/wweianhanes-overview/ (accessed on 10 November 2016).

17. Food and Drug Administration. Food Standards: Amendment of Standards of Identity for Enriched Grain Products to Require Addition of Folic Acid. Final Rule; Federal Register: Washington, DC, USA, 1996; Volume 61, pp. 8781–8797.

18. Food and Nutrition Board, Institute of Medicine. *Dietary Reference Intakes for Thiamin, Riboflavin, Niacin, Vitamin B6, Folate, Vitamin B12, Pantothenic Acid, Biotin, and Choline*; National Academy Press: Washington, DC, USA, 1998.

19. Keith, R.E.; O'Keeffe, K.A.; Alt, L.A.; Young, K.L. Dietary status of trained female cyclists. *J. Am. Diet. Assoc.* **1989**, *89*, 1620–1623. [PubMed]

20. Manore, M.M.; Besenfelder, P.D.; Wells, C.L.; Carroll, S.S.; Hooker, S.P. Nutrient intakes and iron status in female long-distance runners during training. *J. Am. Diet. Assoc.* **1989**, *89*, 257–259. [PubMed]

21. Nieman, D.C.; Butler, J.V.; Pollett, L.M.; Dietrich, S.J.; Lutz, R.D. Nutrient intake of marathon runners. *J. Am. Diet. Assoc.* **1989**, *89*, 1273–1278. [PubMed]

22. Faber, M.; Benade, A.J. Mineral and vitamin intake in field athletes (discus-, hammer-, javelin-throwers and shotputters). *Int. J. Sports Med.* **1991**, *12*, 324–327. [CrossRef] [PubMed]

23. Leydon, M.A.; Wall, C. New Zealands jockeys' dietary habits and their potential impact on health. *Int. J. Sport Nutr. Exerc. Metab.* **2002**, *12*, 220–237. [CrossRef] [PubMed]

24. Worme, J.D.; Doubt, T.J.; Singh, A.; Ryan, C.J.; Moses, F.M.; Deuster, P.A. Dietary patterns, gastrointestinal complaints, and nutrition knowledge of recreational triathletes. *Am. J. Clin. Nutr.* **1990**, *51*, 690–697. [PubMed]

25. Beshgetoor, D.; Nichols, J.F. Dietary intake and supplement use in female master cyclists and runners. *Int. J. Sport Nutr. Exerc. Metab.* **2003**, *13*, 166–172. [CrossRef] [PubMed]

26. Joubert, L.M.; Manore, M.M. The role of physical activity level and B-vitamin status on blood homocysteine levels. *Med. Sci. Sports Exerc.* **2008**, *40*, 1923–1931. [CrossRef] [PubMed]

27. Steen, S.N.; Mayer, K.; Brownell, K.D.; Wadden, T.A. Dietary intake of female collegiate heavyweight rowers. *Int. J. Sport Nutr.* **1995**, *5*, 225–231. [CrossRef] [PubMed]

28. Matter, M.; Stittfall, T.; Graves, J.; Myburgh, K.; Adams, B.; Jacobs, P.; Noakes, T.D. The effect of iron and folate therapy on maximal exercise performance in female marathon runners with iron and folate deficiency. *Clin. Sci.* **1987**, *72*, 415–422. [CrossRef] [PubMed]

29. Beals, K.A.; Manore, M.M. Nutritional status of female athletes with subclinical eating disorders. *J. Am. Diet. Asssoc.* **1998**, *98*, 419–425. [CrossRef]

30. Di Santolo, M.; Banfi, G.; Stel, G.; Cauci, S. Association of recreational physical activity with homocysteine, folate and lipid markers in young women. *Eur. J. Appl. Physiol.* **2009**, *105*, 111–118. [CrossRef] [PubMed]

31. Hoch, A.Z.; Lynch, S.L.; Jurva, J.W.; Schimke, J.E.; Gutterman, D.D. Folic acid supplementation improves vascular function in amenorrheic runners. *Clinl. J. Sports Med.* **2010**, *20*, 205–210. [CrossRef] [PubMed]

32. Herrmann, M.; Obeid, R.; Scharhag, J.; Kindermann, W.; Herrmann, W. Altered vitamin B-12 status in recreational endurance athletes. *Int. J. Sports Nutr. Exerc. Metab.* **2005**, *15*, 433–441. [CrossRef]

33. Raczynski, G.; Szczepanska, B. Longitudinal studies on vitamin B-1 and B-6 status in Polish elite athletes. *Biol. Sport* **1993**, *10*, 189–194.

34. Singh, A.; Evans, P.; Gallagher, K.L.; Deuster, P.A. Dietary intakes and biochemical profiles of nutritional status of ultra marathoners. *Med. Sci. Sports Exerc.* **1992**, *25*, 328–334.

35. Food and Nutrition Board, Institute of Medicine. Dietary Reference Intakes for Energy, Carbohydrate, Fiber, Fat, Fatty Acids, Cholesterol, Protein, and Amino Acids. National Academy Press: Washington, DC, USA, 2002.

36. Sampson, D.A.; O'Connor, D.K. Response of B-6 vitamers in plasma, erythrocytes and tissues to vitamin B6 depletion and repletion in the rat. *J. Nutr.* **1989**, *119*, 1940–1948. [PubMed]

37. Herzlich, B.; Herbert, V. Depletion of serum holotranscobalamin II. An early sign of negative vitamin B12 balance. *Lab. Investig.* **1998**, *58*, 332–337.

38. Das, K.C.; Manusselis, C.; Herbert, V. Determination of Vitamin B12 (cobalamin) in serum and erythrocytes by radioassay, and of holotranscobalamin II (holo-TC II) and holo-haptocorrin (holo-TC I and III) in serum by absorbing holo-TC II on microfine silica. *J. Nutr. Biochem* **1991**, *2*, 455–464. [CrossRef]

39. Wickramasinghe, S.N.; Fida, S. Correlations between holo transcobalamin II, holo-haptocorrin, and total B12 in serum samples from healthy subjects and patients. *J. Clin. Pathol.* **1993**, *46*, 537–539. [CrossRef] [PubMed]

40. Durand, P.; Fortin, L.J.; Lussier-Cacan, S.; Davignon, J.; Blache, D. Hyperhomocysteinemia induced by folic acid deficiency and methionine load–applications of a modified HPLC method. *Clin. Chim. Acta* **1996**, *252*, 83–93. [CrossRef]

41. Jacobsen, D.W.; Gatautis, V.J.; Green, R.; Robinson, K.; Savon, S.R.; Secic, M.J.J.; Otto, J.M.; Taylor, L.M., Jr. Rapid HPLC determination of total homocysteine and other thiols in serum and plasma: Sex differences and correlation with cobalamin and folate concentrations in healthy subjects. *Clin. Chem.* **1994**, *40*, 873–881. [PubMed]

42. Guilland, J.C.; Penaranda, T.; Gallet, C.; Boggio, V.; Fuchs, F.; Klepping, J. Vitamin status of young athletes incluind the effects of supplementation. *Med. Sci. Sports Exerc.* **1989**, *21*, 441–449. [CrossRef] [PubMed]

43. Rankinen, T.L.S.; Vanninen, E.; Pentilla, R.; Rauramaa, R.; Uusitupa, M. Nutritional status of the Finnish elite ski jumpers. *Med. Sci. Sports Exerc.* **1998**, *30*, 1592–1597. [CrossRef] [PubMed]

44. Hansen, R.G.; Wyse, B.W. Expression of nutrient allowances per 1000 kilocalories. *J. Am. Diet. Assoc.* **1980**, *76*, 223–227. [PubMed]

45. Yang, Q.; Cogswell, M.E.; Hamner, H.C.; Carriquiry, A.; Bailey, L.B.; Pfeiffer, C.M.; Berry, R.J. Folic acid source, usual intake, and folate and vitamin B12 status in US adults: National Health and Nutrition Examination Survey (NHANES) 2003–2006. *Am. J. Clin. Nutr.* **2010**, *91*, 64–72. [CrossRef] [PubMed]

46. Taylor, C.; Rogers, G.; Goodman, C.; Baynes, R.D.; Bothwell, T.H.; Bezwoda, W.R.; Kramer, F.; Hattingh, J. Hematologic, iron-related, and acute-phase protein responses to sustained strenuous exercise. *J. Appl. Physiol.* **1987**, *62*, 464–469. [PubMed]

47. Weight, L.M.; Alexander, D.; Jacobs, P. Strenuous exercise: Analogous to the acute-phase response. *Clin. Sci.* **1991**, *81*, 677–683. [CrossRef] [PubMed]

48. Kasapis, C.; Thompson, P.D. The effects of physical activity on serum C-reactive protein and inflammatory markers: A systemic review. *J. Am. Coll. Cardiol.* **2005**, *45*, 1563–1569. [CrossRef] [PubMed]

49. Wright, M.; Francis, K.; Cornwell, P. Effect of acute exercise on plasma homocysteine. *J. Sports Med. Phys. Fit.* **1998**, *38*, 262–265.

50. Borrione, P.; Pigozzi, F.; Massazza, G.; Schonhuber, H.; Viberti, G.; Paccotti, P.; Angeli, A. Hyperhomocysteinemia in winter elite athletes: A longitudinal study. *J. Endocrinol. Investig.* **2007**, *30*, 367–375. [CrossRef] [PubMed]

51. Gelecek, N.; Teoman, N.; Ozdirenc, M.; Pinar, L.; Akan, P.; Bediz, C.; Kozan, O. Influences of acute and chronic aerobic exercise on the plasma homocysteine level. *Ann. Nutr. Metab.* **2007**, *51*, 53–58. [CrossRef] [PubMed]

52. McPhillips, J.B.; Eaton, C.B.; Gans, K.M.; Derby, C.A.; Lasater, T.M.; McKenney, J.L.; Carleton, R.A. Dietary differences in smokers and nonsmokers from two southeastern New England communities. *J. Am. Diet. Assoc.* **1994**, *94*, 287–292. [CrossRef]

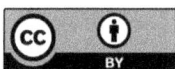

nutrients

MDPI

Concept Paper

"Eat as If You Could Save the Planet and Win!" Sustainability Integration into Nutrition for Exercise and Sport

Nanna Meyer [1,*] and Alba Reguant-Closa [2]

[1]   Health Sciences Department, University of Colorado, Colorado Springs, CO 80918, USA
[2]   International Doctoral School, University of Andorra, Principality of Andorra, Sant Julià de Lòria AD600, Andorra; albareguantclosa@gmail.com
*   Correspondence: nmeyer2@uccs.edu; Tel.: +1-(719)-255-3760

Received: 31 December 2016; Accepted: 14 April 2017; Published: 21 April 2017

Abstract: Today's industrial food production contributes significantly to environmental degradation. Meat production accounts for the largest impact, including greenhouse gas emissions, land and water use. While food production and consumption are important aspects when addressing climate change, this article focuses predominantly on dietary change that promotes both health for planet and people with focus on athletes. Healthy, sustainable eating recommendations begin to appear in various governmental guidelines. However, there remains resistance to the suggested reductions in meat consumption. While food citizens are likely to choose what is good for them and the planet, others may not, unless healthy eating initiatives integrate creative food literacy approaches with experiential learning as a potential vehicle for change. This concept paper is organized in three sections: (1) Environmental impact of food; (2) health and sustainability connections; and (3) application in sports and exercise. For active individuals, this article focuses on the quantity of protein, highlighting meat and dairy, and quality of food, with topics such as organic production and biodiversity. Finally, the timing of when to integrate sustainability principles in sport nutrition is discussed, followed by practical applications for education and inclusion in team, institutional, and event operations.

Keywords: sustainability; food; environment; sports nutrition; athlete; health; sustainable diet; food literacy

1. Introduction

There is an urgent need to reduce the degradation of natural resources and limit global warming, while providing healthy and sustainably produced food to a growing population. Agriculture contributes greatly to climate change and resource extraction, with animal-based foods playing a major role in greenhouse gas (GhG) emissions, loss of land, water, and biodiversity [1–4] Further, current dietary patterns contribute to chronic disease through inadequate intakes of plant-based foods and high consumption of red and processed meat [5,6]. In addition, climate change itself will negatively affect food production should temperatures continue to rise, resulting in reduced yields [7,8]—possibly as much as 30–40% loss by the turn of the century [9]. Adding to this, the consequential sea level rise due to ice melt in the Arctic, displacing not only people but also valuable agricultural land [10], and thus, indicating that food security will likely become the major threat to humans on earth. While agriculture itself must assume more sustainable practices, despite the continued need for intensification [11], strategies for adopting diets with lower environmental impact that are healthy, economically viable, and socially and culturally acceptable are also needed. Thus, for the first time in the history of dietary guidance, food and climate change are crossing paths, and promoting a sustainable, healthful diet, also fit for the athlete, is now more than ever arising as an urgent public and planetary message.

This concept paper is organized in three sections: (1) Environmental impact of food; (2) health and sustainability connections; and (3) application in sports and exercise. For active individuals, this article focuses on the quantity of protein, highlighting meat and dairy, and the quality of food, with topics such as organic production and biodiversity. Finally, the timing of when to integrate sustainability principles in sport nutrition is discussed, followed by practical applications for education and inclusion in team, institutional, and event operations.

1.1. Environmental Impact of Food

The environmental impact of food production affects both terrestrial and marine environments. Agriculture uses about one third of arable land, almost three fourths of global water resources, and one fifth of energy. Thus, agriculture is a major contributor to resource depletion [12]. Agriculture also emits large quantities of GhGs. Agriculture accounts for 30% of total GhG emissions from pre-production, production, to post-production [7,13,14], with direct emissions from agriculture contributing the most [7].

Greenhouse gas emissions are quantified in terms of carbon dioxide equivalents (CO_2eq), collectively also known as global warming potential. Carbon dioxide (CO_2) is the most prominent anthropogenic GhG with a global warming potential of 1. Nitrous oxide (N_2O) and methane (CH_4) are the other two major GhGs, with global warming potential of over 300 and 25 times that of CO_2, respectively, expressed over a 100-year lifespan [15]. Thus, these GhGs contribute significantly to global warming, and therefore, are at least as important to mitigate as CO_2.

Direct emissions from agriculture account for the largest fraction in agriculture-related GhG emissions, by generating CO_2, N_2O, and CH_4 directly on the farm [7]. Nitrous oxide arises from fertilizer applied to soil, as part of the denitrification process. Agriculture produces 65% of all N_2O [16,17]. Methane is generated in large quantities from enteric fermentation and manure from ruminants [1,17–19] and, to a smaller extent, from rice production [14]. Further direct, on-farm emissions originate from fossil fuel dependence to run tractors and machinery, which release CO_2 [7,20]. Adding to this the high demand for animal feed, such as corn and soy, from agriculture, animal agriculture (especially ruminant) plays the biggest role in food-generated GhG emissions and global warming potential [19], exceeding the production of vegetables, grains, and legumes [21,22]. While direct emissions from agriculture contribute the greatest in global warming potential, pre-production processes also include resource-intensive fertilizer, pesticide and herbicide production, which emit GhGs [14]. Climate change mitigation, especially from direct emissions, is critical, as estimates indicate an additional 35–60% rise in CH_4 and N_2O already by 2030 [23]. Table 1 shows GhG emissions per kilogram of various foods.

Food production requires arable land, but there are not unlimited resources. About 33% of Earth's ice-free surface is used for agriculture [12]. Animal agriculture requires large amounts of land—approximately half of all of agriculture—not only for the animals, but also to produce their feed [1,19,24]. Agriculture has negatively affected the land, with excessive chemical input, causing poor soil health and pollution, with potential adverse human health effects [25–32]. While meat production has become industrial and inexpensive, its impact on animals and people have been largely neglected [19,33,34]. To meet a rising demand for food, especially meat, ecosystems continue to be compromised to clear more land [1,7]. This land clearing is also called deforestation and is an indirect but large contributor to agriculture's impact on the environment, including the loss of biodiversity [1,2,4].

Table 1. Greenhouse gas (GhGs) emissions in food.

Low GhGs	Medium GhGs	High GhGs
<1 kg CO_2 eq/kg edible weight	1–4 kg CO_2 eq/kg edible weight	>4 kg CO_2 eq/kg edible weight
Potatoes	Chicken	* Beef
Pasta	Milk, butter, yogurt	* Lamb
Bread	Eggs	Pork
Oats and other grain	Rice	Turkey
Vegetables (e.g., onions, peas, carrots, corn, brassica)	Breakfast cereals	Fish
Fruits (e.g., apples, pears, citrus, plums, grapes)	Spreads	Cheese
Beans/lentils	Nuts/Seeds	
Confectionary	Biscuits, cakes, dessert	
Savory Snacks	Fruit (e.g., berries, banana, melons, salad)	
	Vegetables (e.g., salad, mushrooms, green beans, cauliflower, broccoli, squash)	

* May be as high as 20–50 kg CO_2 eq/kg edible weight. Average CO_2 emissions for driving car are 0.186 kg CO_2 eq/km driven. Adapted from [35] (with permission).

Post-production GhG emissions include emissions from food storage, packaging, distribution, transport, and end-consumer effects (e.g., waste). Compared to agriculture's direct emissions, post-production GhG emissions are considered small [14,36]. Taken together, direct (on farm) and indirect (deforestation) effects of agriculture contribute the largest part of all food-related GhG emissions and land use.

Although not always counted in environmental food studies, post-production includes waste. Globally, about one third of food produced is discarded per year [36] with enormous global warming potential [37]. Food loss can occur along the entire supply chain, from harvest to consumer-level discards. The amount of food waste is generally higher in developed countries, although developing nations also show food loss, especially during production and harvest [38]. In developed nations, consumer-level food waste (e.g., households) is significant [39]. In the US, food waste from households has increased by 50% since the 1970s [40]. On average, 40% of food in the US is wasted each year [41]. This amounts to 9 kg of food wasted per person per month or 200 kg of food per 4-person household per year. This has been estimated to cost the American family at least $589 and the entire country $165 billion per year [42]. Food waste is a significant contributor to resource depletion, considering energy, water, and land are needed for production, distribution, and storage of the food that goes uneaten. Moreover, discarding the food adds a further burden to the environment, accounting for 25% of landfill-generated CH_4 [41]. Thus, besides the energy-costly inputs and GhG emissions from food produced that is unconsumed, wasting it contributes to environmental degradation.

Finally, a significant impact of agriculture on the environment is also its water use. About 70% of all surface and ground water goes to agriculture, with many aquifers showing diminishing reserves [43]. As water resources are becoming equally scarce as land, it is important to consider the significantly greater water footprint of beef production as compared with alternative meat and plant sources [19,21, 44], although there are some exceptions [13].

Studies that focus on food and the environment use Life Cycle Assessment (LCA) to quantify global warming potential of the entire food supply chain—from cradle to grave, including all resources used and all emissions to air, soil, and water. While GhG emissions specific to agriculture are commonly reported, comprehensive LCA studies also include land and water use, toxicity to ecosystems and human health, biodiversity loss, eutrophication, and ocean acidification [45]. Although beyond the scope of this paper, the reader is encouraged to consult further literature on this topic [7,13,14,46,47].

1.2. Dietary Change to Reduce Environmental Impact

Studies have shown that dietary change can play a significant role in reducing the impact of agriculture on global warming potential, land and water use. Recently, scientists have also linked environmental impact, nutrition, and health in the discourse of dietary change [13,48–50]. When considering dietary change as a realistic pathway for the reduction in GhG emissions, land and water use, one of the simplest approaches is to follow healthy dietary guidelines, including a reduction in calories [50,51]. This should not be underestimated since reducing calories, especially if achieved by increasing fruit, vegetables, and dietary fiber at the expense of meat, would result in weight loss and improved health, with enormous impacts on society, including health care cost [51–55].

Animal agriculture is the most costly for the environment [19,21,52]. Eshel et al. 2014 have demonstrated that ruminant (beef) production requires 28 and 11 times more land and water and emits 5 times more GhG, compared with the production of non-ruminant protein sources (e.g., chicken, pork, eggs). Converted to food and protein, beef has a 35:1 feed-to-food caloric ratio compared with a 10:1 ratio for other animal proteins and an 800:1 ratio for feed calories-to-protein ratio, which is almost 10 times lower for other animal protein sources [19]. Thus, eating less beef is becoming an important dietary message worldwide [56]. However, there can be even greater reductions by lowering meat consumption in general [19], and replacing meat, and especially ruminant meat, with plant-based alternatives, which reduces land, energy, and water use, while lowering GhG emissions and waste [21]. While dairy is more efficient than beef, emitting less GhGs, dairy production exceeds egg, poultry, and pork production in land and water use [19,53,57]. Thus, dairy production also contributes to the expansion of cropland and resource extraction which, together with beef production, eventually exceeds the Earth's safe operating space [58].

Reducing beef consumption and replacing some with plant-based sources, chicken, pork, or eggs could decrease GhG emissions by up to 35% from the food sector [35]; however, a moderate reduction and replacing beef with dairy has a negligible effect [50]. Replacing beef with fish may provide some benefit but this largely depends on the type of fish, its production system, and fish feed used in aquacultures [3]. Eating less beef can reduce land use by 50% to 70% (see reviews by Hallström et al., 2015 and Aleksandrowicz et al., 2016 [50,59]). Thus, consuming less beef (and dairy) could slow land clearing for feed production and some of this land could be repurposed to grow food for human consumption [53].

Eating less animal and more plant protein in general is also in line with governmental dietary guidelines [56], since most developed nations exceed protein, and especially meat, recommendations [3]. A recent article entitled "Protein production: planet, profit, plus people?" recommends people eat one third less protein overall, replace one further third of their protein intake by plants such as beans, nuts, and grains, and choose the final third from free-range animals [60]. Based on annual per capita intake data [61], if this rule were applied to meat intake, this would still give the average American 80–100 grams (3–4 ounces, oz) per day.

Considering dietary change that could contribute to climate change mitigation, shifting from a typical Western diet to a more environmentally sustainable diet with less meat and more plants would work [59]. Being vegetarian or vegan would be better, with over 30% and up to 70% reduction potential in GhG emissions and land use [21,59,62] and 50% less water use [59]. However, vegetarian or vegan lifestyles may not be preferred for many people [63]. In addition, recent advances also point toward beneficial roles of well-managed, sustainable grazing practices that promote carbon sequestration on rangelands [64], and some areas in the world are less suited for crop production but still provide a great place for livestock, including ruminants. Adding more value to the consumption of meat is necessary [60], however. Thus, in the above example by Aiking (2014), the last third of what used to make up a meat-based dish, should contain a source that can be traced back to its origin, showing a healthy environment where animals are part of an intact ecosystem, given a good life and an end with dignity [60].

2. Dietary Guidelines and Sustainability

It is quite clear that eating less meat (especially less red and processed meat), besides eating less overall and more whole and plant-based foods (i.e., vegetables, fruit, nuts, beans, grains), would be one of the most important dietary strategies for both planet and people. These recommendations are also grounded in the dietary guidelines of many countries, some of which have integrated sustainability [56].

In recent years, governmental dietary recommendations from various countries have begun to integrate sustainability. According to a recent report by the Food and Agriculture Organization (FAO) [56], of 83 countries that have official dietary guidelines, there are 4 reported countries that reference environmental factors in their dietary guidelines. These include Sweden, Germany, Brazil, and Qatar. Table 2 highlights sustainability commitments beyond those generally targeted to health (e.g., increase plant foods).

Table 2. Sustainability commitments in Germany, Brazil, Sweden, and Qatar.

	Germany	Brazil	Sweden	Qatar
Sustainability Highlights	Eat meat in moderation. Use fresh ingredients. Take your time and enjoy eating. Eat fish once or twice a week.	Choose seasonally and locally grown produce. Try to restrict the amount of red meat. Limit the amount of processed foods. Eat in company. Develop, exercise and share cooking skills. Plan your time and make food and eating important in your life.	Eat less red and processed meat (no more than 500 g of cooked meat per week). Choose eco-labelled seafood. Try to maintain energy balance by eating just the right amount.	Limit red meat to 500 g per week. Avoid processed meat. Eat less fast foods and processed foods. Build and model healthy patterns for your family. Eat at least one meal together daily with family.

The first country world-wide to awaken awareness regarding sustainability and food consumption was Sweden in 2009, calling for a reduction in meat in consumers [65], with a cohort of countries today advising to reduce overall meat consumption to 500 g per week (16–17 oz) [56]. Current meat intake in the US is almost 4 kg (9 pounds, lbs) of trimmed, boneless meat per week, with an annual per capita consumption of almost 90 kg (195 lbs) [66]. However, the US is not alone, as many European and South American countries, along with Australia are also high, but not quite as high. Calculating the yearly per capita consumption per sustainability guidelines, with 500 g per week or a total of 26 kg annually, this equates to about one third of the current US consumption pattern.

While inclusion of sustainability into the US Dietary Guidelines would have been highly significant, considering (1) the high calorie and meat consumption in the US and (2) the potential global impact of US dietary guidelines [67], it remained invisible in the official guidelines [68]. Although not part of national dietary advice, several countries have published scientific papers that focus on mathematical modeling to derive a regional, sustainable and healthy diet alternative to what is considered the norm. The New Nordic Diet and the Low Lands Diet are two such examples. Both studies focused on less meat, more (Nordic Diet) or less (Low Lands Diet) fish, and local, traditional foods, and both used the Mediterranean diet as benchmark to link health and sustainability [69,70]. Further, there are several quasi-official guidelines, from government agencies or government-funded entities that also include sustainability [56]. Most recently, the Netherlands published an update through the Netherlands Nutrition Centre, calling its citizens to action to reduce red meat intake to less than 300 g per week, while the UK's governmental agency, encompassing England, Wales, Scotland, and Ireland also added a 7% reduction of dairy products [71].

2.1. Are People Willing to Change Diets to Protect the Environment?

When dietary guidelines promote a change, press releases are often the next step, communicating the governmental messages to the public. However, it is well known that dietary guidelines are only marginally followed [72] and that eating behaviors are difficult to change [63], especially if guidelines remain a verbal or written recommendation without the practical skill building required to put the guidelines into practice [73]. In addition, simply telling people what they should eat without communicating the reason behind this recommendation or focusing too much on diet and health may not work either. For example, Hekler and colleagues (2010) showed that a college course on society, ethics, and food changed eating practices more favorably than in students taking courses in health with a focus on biology, obesity, psychology, or community [74]. However, what about sustainability and the environment? Do people (1) understand the link between eating less meat and climate change and (2) would they make the change if it were both good for health and good for the planet?

"Eat as if there is no tomorrow" [63] studied a sample of Scottish people living in rural and urban areas using focus groups and interviews. The purpose of the study was to examine the perceptions of people toward eating less meat. The authors identified the following common themes, using a qualitative analysis: there was (1) a general lack of awareness related to the link between climate change and meat consumption and (2) little understanding that personal choice regarding meat consumption had anything to do with climate change. Finally, the study also showed that those interviewed were generally resistant to reducing meat intake.

Meat is a traditional menu ingredient in many cultures—meat is often the center piece of the plate. It should be apparent that dietary behavior change will only occur if people begin to understand how best to reduce meat intake. This requires innovative menu design, similar to what has been proposed by the Culinary Institute of America (CIA) and Harvard School of Public Health with the Menus of Change initiative [75], in addition to public campaigns such as Meatless Mondays [76]. This was also the synthesis of a recent study [73], proposing that besides policy change, innovative culinary training through reskilling to cook more balanced vegetarian meals would be necessary. In other words, food literacy training will be needed to bring these ideas closer to consumers.

Regardless of approach taken, promoting meat reduction for personal and planetary health, may continue to be challenging, as was shown by de Boer, de Witt, and Aiking, 2016. These authors studied people's perceptions as to the extent to which personal dietary change could mitigate climate change [55]. Few recognized eating less meat as an effective way to mitigate climate change, but those who did, showed greater willingness to eat less meat. When asked to rate personal preference of (1) eating less meat; (2) eating more organic food; and (3) eating more local/seasonal food as a vehicle to mitigate climate change, eating more locally/seasonally grown food appealed to more individuals than the other two, including the message of eating less meat [55].

2.2. Duality of Sustainability and Health

As we begin to imagine how to integrate sustainability into healthy and athletic lifestyles through the food we chose, we must define what constitutes sustainable food. Sustainability means that "humanity has the ability to make development sustainable—to ensure that it meets the needs of the present without compromising the ability of future generations to meet their own needs" [77] (p. 5). The three pillars of sustainability which include equity, environment, and economics often focus on what is currently unsustainable, for example in food production, but also tend not to challenge the consumer in moving to sustainable development. Sustainability is a moving target, dynamic and ever changing, as the planet is changing. Thus, adapting with the goal to mitigate climate change is needed in all sectors of production, distribution, consumption, and resource recovery, globally as well as locally. While there are numerous examples of sustainable agricultural advances, including organic production [78] and perennial polycultures [79], promoting greater social equity for farmers and welfare for animals and focusing on sustainable consumption patterns are also important. So, what is a sustainable diet? "A sustainable diet is a diet with low environmental impacts which contributes to food and nutrition security and to a healthy life for present and future generations. A sustainable food system is protective and respectful of biodiversity and ecosystems, culturally acceptable, accessible, economically fair and affordable, nutritionally adequate, safe and healthy, while optimizing natural and human resources" [80] (p. 111).

In 2014, Kjærgård and colleagues published a framework on how to link sustainability and health and by doing so, dual benefits could be observed [81]. These authors referred to their concept as a duality between sustainability and health. Considering sustainable food choices, a sustainable diet would also be a healthy diet. To understand this duality concept a bit deeper, the example of meat shows the duality of sustainability and health quite well. In general, livestock production, especially beef production, is associated with resource depletion and pollution [4] and contributes significantly to GhG emissions, biodiversity loss, and high health care costs [2]. Excessive red meat consumption has been associated with poor health outcomes, such as cardiovascular disease, obesity, diabetes, and cancer [5,7,82,83]. In addition, how animals are raised in some countries, in confined animal feeding operations (CAFOs), is also of concern regarding animal and worker welfare in the context of community prosperity, health, and quality of life near CAFOs, and human antibiotic resistance from non-therapeutic use of antibiotics in such production systems [84]. The duality of health and sustainability shows that addressing the "eat less meat" message has co-benefits for both sustainability and health. From the consumer side, dietary approaches that promote high protein intakes, such as the westernized diets and those recently termed "the diets of the healthy and wealthy" [85] fail to consider this duality approach, and thus, slow the shift urgently needed to promote both sustainable and healthful eating. There are other examples that provide insight into the intertwined synergies between sustainability and health, such as the ecosystem and health services arising from urban farms and community gardens [86] as well as reducing food waste [87].

Taken together, the inclusion of sustainability in nutrition and health is critical for current and future generations. The science of nutrition must embrace environmental considerations similar to the time when public health nutrition emerged from the science of nutrition for individuals and expanded its reach to communities [54]. "The nutrition of individuals and communities can only be maintained within an environmentally sustainable context, which is currently under serious threat." [54] (p. 817). Thus, we are in the center of a difficult reality—a sustainable food system needs the support of an intact ecosystem, but the way we currently eat contributes directly to its degradation [54].

3. Eat as If You Could Save the Planet and Win!

Whether the intention is health, fitness, and/or sports performance, integrating environmental consciousness when making dietary choices, seems no longer an option but rather a necessity. And while global warming and climate change are often overwhelming topics, dreaming the alternative fires up the imagination of young people, as so beautifully described in the Future of Health by Hanlon and colleagues [88]. Thus, to end a long discourse on the unsustainability of the current food system and its apparent lack to teach us anything about good food and healthy communities or environmental conservation, while the alternative does, the next section will focus on how to integrate these ideas into the daily eating practices of those who train to win.

3.1. Ecological Footprint: This Gets us Thinking

To understand one's own impact on the environment, it is always a good exercise to calculate the ecological footprint [89]. This is especially true with respect to dietary choices, as most people do not make the connection between their own eating and climate change [63]. However, there are also tradeoffs. Some might travel a lot by plane, which increases one's footprint significantly. A good tradeoff would be to make sustainable dietary choices to contribute to environmental protection.

3.2. Sustainability in Sports Nutrition?

The integration of environmental nutrition concepts might not be as intuitive in sports nutrition but there are many entry points. One might also argue that due to high energy intakes to meet energy demand, enormous use of packaged foods and bottled beverages, equipment, materials, and heavy travel schedules athletes and their teams should integrate sustainable practices whenever possible.

From a health perspective, athletes lead a more sustainable lifestyle than most of society. Athletes rarely burden the health care system due to chronic disease such as obesity and diabetes. And participating in sports should play a substantial role in making sustainable healthy lifestyle choices. Athletes are also great icons for kids to pick up sports. Athletes are role models for society at large and are generally represented by values of good sportsmanship [90]. Athletes are also great spokespeople, sharing their lessons learned through sports (e.g., time management, discipline to work hard, the importance of rituals, discerning the meaning of failure or injuries). While still dormant, athletes could become a strong voice for planetary health, and begin to realize that success in sport depends, in part, on an intact food system. Athlete or non-athlete, all young people should receive sustainability literacy training, and a covert approach to nutrition education may work best, using experiential learning through taste education, farm visits, cooking and eating together. The conversation around the digital-free table can further the understanding of contemporary food topics and build knowledge surrounding the current issues of the food system and what the sustainable, tasty alternative is all about.

Finally, the sustainable diet is not only the athlete's responsibility. As we see with other big topics in sport nutrition such as eating disorders [91,92], if coaches, service providers, and administrators are supporting the underlying rationale of a refreshed approach to nutrition education, using sustainability principles, it will enable change. Athletes, coaches, service providers, and administrators all serve as role models for societal change, thus, the adoption of sustainability principles, while coming from the bottom up in our examples, are best diffused if top to bottom is committed and understands the rationale behind the effort. True sport needs true food!

Therefore, let's get athletes on board in saving the planet and winning! Because sport nutrition is often focused on quantity, quality, and timing of food intake relative to training and competition, below we list sustainability actions for these overall themes, add a section about food literacy and food citizenship for athletes, and consider some final thoughts regarding the integration of sustainable practices for teams, institutions, and international events, such as the Olympic Games.

We will focus on several areas that may apply to exercisers and fitness enthusiasts in general, but athletes in particular, making small steps toward a more sustainable diet as the overarching goal, and this begins with the work of the sport nutrition professional.

3.3. Quantity of Food

3.3.1. Eat Less and Better Meat

Athletes' diets are generally high enough in protein [93,94], if not excessive [95,96]. Current protein recommendations have increased for athletes [97], ranging from 1.2–2 g/kg body weight (BW)/day, especially if the goal is muscle protein accretion [98]. Recently, these recommendations were translated into practical strategies to help athletes maintain protein consumption at intervals throughout the day in the amounts of 0.25–0.3 g/kg BW [99] or about 20 g [100] per meal, given several eating occasions (best every 4 h) [101] per day and before sleeping [102]. This has also been summarized in the recently released position paper on Nutrition and Athletic Performance [97]. That athletes follow guidelines for protein intake is shown in the most recent dietary study on a sample of well-trained Dutch athletes, with mean daily protein intakes of 108 ± 33 g (1.5 ± 04 g/kg BW/day) and 90 ± 24 g (1.4 ± 0.4 g/kg BW/day) in men and women, respectively [94].

There have also been recent trends for even higher protein recommendations to promote health [103], support weight loss strategies [104], to preserve lean body mass (LBM) under hypocaloric situations [105], in resistance-type sports such as bodybuilding [106], and corporate sports performance programs [107]. That athletes, especially in strength and power sports, accomplish higher protein intakes has also been shown [108], with recent reports also highlighting the issue of extremely high protein intakes in some athletes [96,109]. Even though data are limited, practitioners should be well aware of excessive protein intakes in some athletes, aligning with current sport nutrition trends, including the paleo diet. Finally, practitioners may inadvertently promote high protein intakes, considering educational tools and strategies or athletes may simply get too much by eating a lot, since protein is a function of energy intake [110]. However, what are the concerns besides the fact that some athletes may overdo it without proper guidance?

Because this paper is about sustainable diets, the question arises if current protein recommendations for athletes and actual intakes are going to align with global recommendations to reduce rather than increase protein intake in developed countries. Meeting protein recommendations in athletes per se may not necessarily be the issue. The issue is that the continued emphasis on higher protein needs will likely increase the demand for animal protein, including meat, dairy, and eggs. Considering the 50% rise in the world's population since 2000 and society's insatiable hunger for meat, the world meat and cheese demand will double by 2050, further burdening the planet [4]. Animal proteins are already consumed in greater quantities than plant proteins, in both the general [66,111] and athletic population [94], and the US considerably exceeds European countries in daily animal protein consumption [112].

Table 3 shows hypothetical amounts of meat (in this case beef) in reference to the (1) non-athlete recommended daily allowance (RDA) for protein [113]; (2) current athlete protein recommendation (~1.5 g/kg BW/day [97]); and (3) recently suggested athlete protein recommendations under energy restriction for weight loss (~2.5 g/kg BW/day [104,105]). It is assumed under this example, that 50% of dietary protein is supplied by meat. This is a rather conservative estimate based on total animal protein intakes typically exceeding 65% in the general population [111].

Table 3. Daily protein recommendations using estimated daily meat contributions for athletes and non-athletes.

Example	Units	Non-Athlete PRO RDA	Athlete's Standard PRO	Athlete's Hypocaloric PRO
60 kg female	PRO (g/day)	48	90	150
	Cooked Meat Contribution as 50% of total PRO (g/day) *	92	172	288
80 kg male	PRO (g/day)	64	120	200
	Cooked Meat Contribution as 50% of total PRO (g/day) *	123	230	387

* meat contribution at 50% of total protein recommendation, calculated for cooked ground lean beef (15% fat); 100 g edible portion equals 26 g of protein (similar for chicken, pork, lamb). Athlete's standard diet calculated at protein recommendation of 1.5 g/kg/day [97]. Athlete's hypocaloric diet calculated at protein recommendation of 2.5 g/kg/day [104,105]. PRO = Protein. Most sustainable and healthy dietary recommendations target 300 g of red meat or 500 g of total meat per week [56]. RDA = Recommended Daily Allowance. Table shows how easily athletes may exceed these weekly meat recommendations if they ate 50% meat of the total protein recommended per day.

From Table 3, we can see that meat consumption may easily exceed what is currently considered sustainable, as a total of 500 grams (17.6 oz) of meat per week (~70 grams per day; 2.5 oz) and less or equal to 300 grams (10.6 oz) of red meat per week (~45 grams per day; 1.6 oz/day) would be the upper limit per person. These are also the upper limits for meat consumption of most countries' dietary guidelines [56], including those for Americans, to promote health [68].

If the recommendation by Aiking (2014) could be implemented it would mean to cut 1/3 of the protein (in this case we would focus on meat, especially red meat), replace 1/3 with plant protein (beans including soy, grain, nuts, seeds), and to choose grass-fed or pasture-raised animal protein sources to obtain higher quality meat with greater omega 3 fatty acids and antioxidants, [114], not to mention less agricultural chemicals and antibiotic residues [60].

Let's look at an example integrating the recommendation by Aiking (2014) from above [60] but with focus on meat, especially red meat. If an 80-kg heavy male athlete eats 120 grams of protein of which 50% comes from meat, it equals approximately 240 grams of cooked meat per day. This is more than 3 times the 70-gram daily benchmark. Thus, if the athlete follows the recommendation for an environmentally friendly protein intake by Aiking (2014), they would first reduce this amount by 80 grams of meat which equals approximately 20 grams of protein [60]. Second, the athlete would creatively adapt protein intake, according to the Protein Flip Initiative (see Table 4), and replace another 80 grams (or 20 grams of protein) by plant sources (See Table 5). The question that will arise is whether the athlete should replace the first third of meat that was cut out, and if so, how would this be done within sustainable boundaries? The answer may be substituting red meat with chicken, pork, or eggs, or choosing a greater proportion of plant-based proteins (e.g., beans, peas, nuts, seeds, and/or grains). However, plant protein may lack essential amino acids (EAA), and thus, may be required in greater amounts to meet the RDA. A recent study compared the land use change and GhG emissions of various animal and plant sources in amounts corresponding to the RDA for EAA [115]. Interestingly, environmental impacts were no longer as discriminatory for animal versus plant proteins, with exception of soy, which showed the lowest GhG emissions and land use. However, we should be cautious when interpreting these data, because people eat a variety of foods in variable amounts to meet daily protein and EAA needs. According to the American Academy of Nutrition and Dietetics Position Paper on Vegetarian Nutrition [116], it is not necessary to get all EAA at one meal, and especially not from one plant or animal. Rather, EAA are accumulated over the course of a day from various foods, and it is not uncommon to find vegetarian meals enhanced with small amounts of animal protein (e.g., dairy, eggs), while vegan meals may include various protein-rich plant foods. Thus, the key message for omnivores is to reduce total amount of animal sources of protein, while for vegans, the message may be to ensure diets meet daily EAA needs by eating sufficient amounts of food, along with a combination of protein-rich, plant-based sources. Working toward a more balanced approach between animal and plant proteins should be the primary goal for both planetary and personal health. Considering the higher protein needs in athletes [97], bugs may be the most suited protein to make up the difference from non-athletic controls, however, at substantially lower environmental cost.

3.3.2. Insects

Insects may well be the next protein source with which excessive meat may need to be replaced. Insects are nutritious, with similar amounts of protein compared to livestock and high levels of vitamins and minerals. Insects can also be a good source of essential fatty acids. Insects emit much lower GhG due to their highly efficient feed-to-protein conversion rates and insects have very low water requirement [117]. Insect powder may become a viable option for post-exercise recovery nutrition in liquid or solid food products, some of which are already on the market. In addition, plant-protein alternatives, such as pea (*pisum sativum*) protein powder, may also present a carbon-friendly source for athletes [118]. Obviously, much more research is needed to compare various plant protein alternatives and insects to the well-researched and popularly used dairy proteins post-exercise. So, what about dairy?

3.3.3. Dairy

Milk, yogurt, Greek yogurt, and cheese all add up quickly, and most Americans, including athletes, may indeed meet the US dietary guidelines, recommending 700 mL of dairy products per day [61]. While milk consumption has gradually decreased over the past decades, cheese, yogurt, and whey intakes have dramatically increased [61]. It is estimated that milk production contributes 2.7% to total GhG emissions [119], although there is great variability based on farming systems [119], with industrial systems generally showing lower GhG emissions due to higher feed digestibility and milk productivity per unit of product, compared to extensive farming systems. However, if other components of environmental degradation (e.g., pollution of waterways and biodiversity), increased energy demand, and human and animal welfare—basically the sustainability of dairy production—are questioned [120], the impact of intensification may well be greater [119].

Nutrients **2017**, *9*, 412

Table 4. Examples for protein flip menus and burgers.

Meal	Actual	PRO g	Protein Flip	PRO g	Comments
Grilled Beef with Quinoa and Veggies United States Olympic Committee Colorado Springs	4 oz beef	26	2 oz 100% grassfed beef	13	Rename to Southwest Anasazi Bean and Beef Bowl.
	4 oz kale and quinoa	4	4 oz kale and quinoa	4	Launch educational campaign on protein flip.
	4 oz broccoli	3	2 oz Anasazi beans	10	Add history of Colorado beans and quinoa.
	1/2 stuffed portobello	5	4 oz broccoli	4	
			1/2 stuffed portobello	5	
	total	38	total	36	
Pork loin with Poblano Chili and Rice United States Olympic Committee Colorado Springs	4 oz pork loin	26	2 oz organic pork loin	13	Rename to Ancient Grains with Poblano Chili Pork.
	4 oz poblano chili	3	4 oz poblano chili	3	Launch educational campaign on protein flip.
	4 oz white rice with veg	4	6 oz farro, beans, veggies	12	Integrate nutritional benefits of ancient grains.
					Add history of emmer and biodiversity of grains.
	total	33	total	30	
SWELL Burger University of Colorado Colorado Springs	4 oz beef burger	22	2 oz 100% grassfed beef	10	This meal is served at UCCS Food Next Door.
	white bun	5	1.75 tsp black beans	2	SWELL Burger uses the protein flip approach.
	1 cup dinner salad	1	1.75 tsp quinoa	1	Launch educational campaign on protein flip.
			1.75 tsp hemp	3	Integrate sustainable food literacy.
			1 T peppers, carrots, leeks, chard	1	Highlight nutritional benefits of grassfed beef.
			garlic, chili, cumin, chives		Include social justice issues regarding CAFO.
			1 slice socca (chick pea flatbread)	4	Highlight Slow Meat and Menus of Change ideas.
			SWELL kale salad with roasted veg	2	
			pumpkin seeds	2	
	total	28	total	25	

SWELL: Sustainability, Wellness, & Learning; UCCS: University of Colorado, Colorado Springs; PRO: Protein; CAFO: Confined Animal Feeding Operation; ounces (oz; 1 oz = 28.4 g); tsp: teaspoon; T: tablespoon.

Table 5. Cooked amounts of plant and animal-based foods delivering 20 g of protein.

Food	Grams	Ounces	Cups	T	Calories	Limiting Amino Acids	Leucine (g)
Anasazi Beans	322	11.4	1.4	23	426	Sulfur containing AA	1.2
Black Beans	295	10.4	1.3	21	295	Sulfur containing AA	1.3
Chickpeas	284	10	1.3	20	336	Sulfur containing AA	1
Soybeans	204	7.2	1	14	268	Complete plant protein	2.3
Lentils	250	8.8	1.1	18	253	Sulfur containing AA	1.3
Tofu	284	10	1.3	20	189	Complete plant protein	1.3
Tempeh	306	10.8	1.4	22	265	Complete plant protein	2.4
Edamame	318	11.2	1.4	22	265	Complete plant protein	1.2
Seitan	408	14.4	1.8	29	270	Complete plant protein	no data
Buckwheat	755	26.6	3.3	53	516	Complete plant protein	0.4
Quinoa	567	20	2.5	40	555	Complete plant protein	0.5
Millet	748	26.4	3.3	53	683	Lysine, threonine	0.8
Amaranth	500	17.6	2.2	35	552	Complete plant protein	no data
Einkorn	145	5.1	0.6	10	218	no data	no data
Emmer	227	8	1	16	200	Lysine	0.3
Spelt	411	14.5	1.8	29	445	No data	no data
Kamut	411	14.5	1.8	29	454	Lysine	0.8
Almonds	227	8	1	16	575	Methionine, Cysteine	2.1
Peanut butter	68	2.4	0.3	5	470	Methionine, Cysteine	3.9
Hemp seeds	57	2	0.3	4	160	Lysine	0.7
Pumpkin seeds	132	4.6	0.6	9	433	Complete plant protein	3
Beef 15% fat	73	2.4	0.3	5	157	Complete protein	1.7
Chicken	91	3.2	0.4	6	100	Complete protein	3.3
Pork	73	2.4	0.3	5	152	Complete protein	1.9
Milk 2% fat	567	20.0	2.5	40	284	Complete protein	0.8
Eggs	188	6.4	0.8	13	291	Complete protein	2
Fish (tuna)	141	4.8	0.6	10	179	Complete protein	3.2

T: tablespoon. Combining protein-rich, plant-based foods will be the best strategy in obtaining all amino acids if partially or fully replacing animal-based foods.

Globally, about 45%, 20%, and 35% of milk is processed into cheese, milk powders, and fresh or fermented dairy products, respectively [119]. In the US, 50% of raw milk is generally processed into cheese [121]. Milk production generates about 1 kg of CO_2 eq/kg of milk (or 2.4 CO_2 eq/kg ready to consume milk) at farm gate [119]. Additional processing, transport, and distribution for dairy products, such as cheese, whey and yogurt increase GhG emissions [119]. Finished products, such as cheese and yogurt, show greater emissions due to the fact they need more milk per unit produced (see Table 1).

Depending on current dairy intake, a climate friendly start could be to reduce dairy products in general, and cheese in particular, due to greater GhG emissions [35]. The UK [122] currently suggests a 7% decrease in dairy, among reductions in meat, for all citizens to participate in consumer-driven climate change mitigation. This is world-wide the only guideline that targets reductions in dairy. Athletes may want to focus on milk, rich in whey, in the recovery period after an important workout, since this is an effective protocol to promote post-exercise protein synthesis [97] and is palatable. Whether environmental differences exist among milk-derived protein depends on what functional unit is used to express GhG emissions. A Canadian study shows that per gram of protein, GhG emissions are similar or slightly less for cheese and yogurt compared with milk. However, per kg product, milk ranks significantly lower in GhG emissions than cheese and yogurt [123]. Should an athlete need to focus on extra weight/muscle gain, casein-rich Greek yogurts appear popular before going to bed to promote protein synthesis at night [102]; however, Greek yogurt emits more GhGs than regular yogurt, because its production requires more milk [121].

While sweetened yogurts are often loaded with sugar and unrecognizable ingredients, a good choice is the least processed type that contains naturally occurring beneficial bacteria from fermentation. These bacteria are generally known as probiotics and are thought to boost gut health [124]. Thus, for both the environment and health, less processing in yogurts may be the way to go. Because most of the sport nutrition research has been conducted using dairy products, future studies are needed on more environmentally conscious plant protein alternatives and insect protein. This is especially important for athletes who, by default, likely exceed animal protein recommendations from meat and dairy (including whey), currently deemed unsuitable to protect the environment.

3.3.4. Reinventing the Athlete's Plate

To make the message of meat (and dairy) reduction palatable, practically engaging initiatives are needed. Choosing less and better meat is Slow Food's global strategy [125] for developed nations, where meat intake is generally very high. Flipping protein on the plate and making meat the topping or side dish is a strategy promoted through the Culinary Institute of America's Protein Flip initiative [75,126], which originated from the Menus of Change collaborative between the CIA and Harvard School of Public Health. Recreating the plate using meat as a garnish and complementing this dish with whole grain pasta, potatoes, vegetables, and protein-rich grain, legumes, nuts, and seeds is also an easy and creative way to rebuild an athlete's plate. This is the current topic of ongoing research at the United States Olympic Committee's (USOC) Food and Nutrition Services, as the Athlete's Plate [127] was shown to promote more protein than recommended for easy, moderate, and hard training days [128]. Further analysis indicates that the protein dished up on the plates by trained professionals was mostly of animal origin (more than 70%) with marginal amounts of plant protein [129]. It is expected, as was previously shown [73], that food service organization and restaurants may lack the experience with meat-reduced, vegan and vegetarian cuisine. Thus, while flipping proteins of animal-based plates is becoming more popular, taking a closer look at vegan and vegetarian menus and their composition will also help promote plant-based meals for omnivores. Once culinary professionals, students, and nutrition professionals tackle such menus, calculating nutrient profiles could be helpful [130,131], as the outcome of a protein flip menu should not compromise nutrient density—in fact, it should improve it. Most athletes consume sufficient calories to meet micronutrient needs and the majority also takes dietary supplements [132] and eats fortified foods (e.g., cereals, bars), which makes the integration of plant-based eating less concerning. Our preliminary work with the USOC Food and Nutrition Services shows hypothetically that (1) protein flip menus (with less meat) and (2) improved vegetarian menus, increase rather than compromise nutrients, while protein remains at moderate yet recommended levels for athletes [133]. The University of Colorado, Colorado Springs, having transitioned from a corporate to a self-operated dining and hospitality system, recently adopted the CIA's Menus of Change initiative and serves a very popular protein flip burger at its local food station called "Food Next Door" [134] (see Table 4 for examples).

Protein flip and vegetarian menus provide greater amounts of carbohydrate and fiber [116]. While extra carbohydrates are performance-enhancing, there may be concerns that phytates from fiber may inhibit iron absorption, thus, making the iron from meat less available. One strategy to assist with improving bioavailability of these changed menus is through iron enhancers, including fermented foods. Lactic fermentation is one of the oldest methods for food preservation [135]. Research shows that lactic fermentation of vegetables, corn, and soybeans can drastically reduce phytate content [136], thereby reducing its effect on nutrient absorption. For iron absorption, the mechanism is thought to be through the increase in ferric iron (Fe^{3+}), enhancing iron bioavailability [135]. It has also been shown that fermented sauerkraut improves iron absorption [137] and that fermented foods contribute to enhanced nutrient bioavailability in Asian cultures [138].

3.3.5. An Omnivore's Choice to Eat Vegan

While vegan diets may need more caution to ensure protein quantity, quality, and complementarity as well as achieving athletes' energy availability, it is generally accepted that these diets do not present with adverse health [116] or performance effects [139–142]. In fact, most data show that plant-based diets are not only great for the environment [13,50], but also human health [13,116,142], and they may promote performance enhancement [123,143]. While some athletes may use vegan diets to mask an eating disorder, there is no evidence that vegan or vegetarian diets cause eating disorders [144]. Considering that a reduction in meat, using more plant-based approaches, is effective in decreasing environmental impact does not mean that athletes must turn vegan. However, integrating meat-less meals and days in omnivorous athletes is not only fun and healthful but it is also educational. Making tasty and nutritionally-balanced vegan meals can also mean a new challenge for those in the kitchen. If proper screening and assessment of individual athlete risk precedes the introduction of plant-based dietary approaches, and education is provided about the rationale for such an approach, there should be no concern.

The best start into an environmentally friendlier diet for athletes is to start right here. As sport nutrition professionals, we need to understand the impact diet has on the environment. Athletes can simply consider the total animal and plant protein contributions in their diet and aim to reduce (not eliminate) red meat first, followed by integration of more plant-based protein choices. A closer look at dairy protein may also be warranted. If everyone in the United States ate no meat just one day per week, it would account for the carbon equivalents of driving 91 billion miles less or taking 7.6 million cars off the road [145]. Reducing meat consumption, in general, can have significant savings overall in food-related GhG emissions and land-use change, exceeding what can be achieved from the transportation sector [50]. Recent research also highlights the individuality of diets and that reductions in environmental impact can be achieved using various approaches, not necessarily compromising personal, cultural, or economic factors [146]. While animal protein reductions in athletes should be of primary importance considering environmental conservation, overall protein intake, nutritional status and the athlete's cultural background will determine if this is the best approach to take. However, we should not forget to highlight athletes who have been using vegan and vegetarian approaches and athletes who stand up for a healthier environment and restorative farming practices [147].

3.4. Quality of Food

3.4.1. Plant Biodiversity—Diet Diversity

In the last 100 years, three quarters of plant and animal species globally have been lost, and the majority of the world's food supply comes from a dozen plant and a handful of animal species [80]. At the same time, food processing has increased in a way that creates an artificial diversity and a false sense of food security, when browsing through endless aisles in a grocery store. Perhaps it is this level of agricultural simplification that has made the broad field of nutrition oblivious to the topic of biodiversity. Balanced nutrition depends not only on a variety of foods in the diet. The human diet also depends on the diversity within a food crop [148]. While largely understudied and under-documented, fragmented data show vast differences in nutrients within the same species; for example, in potatoes, rice, mangoes, bananas [149,150], and tomatoes [151], but also indigenous corn grown in the American Southwest [152]. Perhaps one of the most striking results in nutrient density comes from the potato, a staple of many countries, and often marginalized as a processed fast food not tolerated on healthy plates. Potato biodiversity is still broad, with over 5000 known varieties remaining and vastly differing nutrient content [150], particularly for sugar, protein, potassium and vitamin C. Similarly, wild plants, still contributing significantly to the health-promoting properties of the Mediterranean regions, have higher amounts of vitamins A, C, and those of the B-complex compared to their cultivated counterparts [153]. Interestingly, wild and local foods are increasingly being recognized as an integral part of contemporary nutrition, as countries are redefining their dietary guidelines, linking sustainable and healthful eating in a traditional context [154,155]. Unfortunately, crop biodiversity and its role in nutrition is generally neglected and this may be due to the field's professionals [149]. Perhaps a visual comparison as shown in a recent New York Times article [156] brings the message home. We simply assume that a tomato is a tomato and that nutrient density will remain the same despite significant differences [151]. It is true that nutrition education appears to be almost blind to biodiversity [80], although resources are available [157]. Diet biodiversity is becoming a rapidly emerging field but has remained understudied, especially in the nutrition sciences. However, with the return to the farm, scientists are recognizing that agricultural biodiversity can support food and diet diversity, thereby improving nutrition and health [158]. Research is also emerging that agricultural intensification, characteristic of high yield outputs, is associated with the loss of rare plant species [159], but shifting to more sustainable systems, biodiversity may be conserved and ecological functions secured [11]. Losing biodiversity means loss of diet quality, which can lead to micronutrient deficiencies, food insecurity, more pests on farms, fragile ecosystems, and the loss of culture and tradition. Thus, biodiversity should not only be recognized as an important player in sustainable agriculture, but also as a necessary contributor to a healthy diet [160].

3.4.2. Nutrient Composition and Nutrient Density

Dietary choice from the farm or factory gate produces variable foods with variable consequences. Meat and dairy from cows grazing on pastures all their lives provide a nutritionally superior [114], healthier, and safer product [25,52,84], especially considering antibiotic use in CAFOs [161,162]. However, grassfed beef is generally more expensive and considered less sustainable because more land is needed for animals to graze, with greater GhG emissions per kg of beef produced [18]. Unfortunately, animal welfare is not yet part of LCA studies, thus, intensive, as opposed to extensive farming systems, usually fare better in both GhG emissions and land use [18].

Considering the topic of fish, omega-3 fatty acids, especially eicosapentaenoic acid (EPA) and docosahexaenoic acid (DHA) found variably in fish, wild and farmed, have significant health benefits [163] recognized by health organizations world-wide [164]. Fish oils are also popular in athletes [165]. However, fish has been a topic of much debate, not only because of variable omega 3 fatty acid content but also environmental contaminants. Whether farmed fish contains lower, comparable, or greater amounts of EPA and DHA than a wild-caught counterpart continues to be an equivocal topic [166–169]. The type of feed (plant vs. fish-based) used in farmed fish is one important consideration [170]. Recent trends of vegetable oils in salmon feed have shown to increase the proportion of omega 6 fatty acids, while omega 3 fatty acids decrease [171], potentially impacting negatively on both fish and human health [172]. Although wild fish supply is diminishing fast, if people were to eat the wild fish that are seasonally available rather than the wild fish they desire (e.g., salmon), there would continue to be some level of access—at least for a little while [173]. However, wild fish supplies will not be able to meet the rising demand of a growing world population [3], nor will wild fish necessarily be free of pollutants [168]. Already to date, more than 50% of all fish consumed globally come from aquacultures [3]. Aquacultures generally emit lower GhG compared to wild fisheries, although concerns exist about the feed used in aquacultures [18]. While disconnecting marine resources from fish farming is recognized as an invaluable progress for protecting marine ecosystems, it does not come without increasing challenges about the feed used in aquacultures, especially if produced terrestrially [174]. Perhaps plant alternatives (e.g., microalgae) will be able to provide sustainable solutions in the future, so humans can continue to benefit from fish-derived EPA and DHA.

What about conventional versus organic production? Organic milk provides a superior nutritional profile than conventional milk, with organic milk containing more protein and omega 3 fatty acids [175], and raw milk may provide potential protection against allergies, although there is a greater risk of pathogens [176,177]. On a crop-level, nutrient composition in food has suffered in the last sixty years, with nutrient losses of up to 30%, most likely due to depletion of soil nutrient quality [178]. Conventional agriculture may produce food more economically and in higher quantities. However, research is gradually emerging, showing ecological and human health repercussions of such systems [19–21,25,26,29]. Organically grown soybeans show significantly higher nutrient composition, including amino acids, total protein and several micronutrients, compared to conventional and genetically modified (GM) soybeans. While the debate continues whether organic vs. conventional produce is superior in nutrients [78,179], organic foods contain significantly less herbicides, pesticides, toxins, and antibiotic residues [179,180] compared with conventionally produced food. Organic systems can also be more energy-efficient, may thrive in drought conditions, tend not to pollute waterways with synthetic pesticides and nitrate, and typically protect ecosystem services, such as biodiversity (see Reganold and Wachter, 2016, for an excellent review [78]). Finally, while largely understudied considering nutrient content, local food systems provide the most direct pathway from farm to table, with potential for greater nutrient density due to seasonality and reduced transit time from farm to consumer [181].

Taken together, from animals to plants, we must begin to pay attention to the quality of food. In addition, people must understand that dietary choices have the power to either protect or degrade ecosystem and health services. This knowledge may be difficult to teach in a classroom, and it is not nearly as fun as going to the farm. Farm field trips may be especially health-promoting for young, active children, as recent studies show the immune benefit of growing up on the farm [182].

3.4.3. The Grain Chain

The discourse on better food for health of both planet and people, however, is not complete without a discussion on grains. In addition, grains remain the world's most important staple [80] and may be a key strategy of the Menus of Change initiative. And yet, there has not been more controversy regarding issues of modern wheat [183], including its higher amounts of triggering gluten proteins [184]. Gluten-free eating has seen a tremendous popularity. In athletes, studies show that over 40% of athletes adhere to a gluten-free diet even if they do not have to [185], and despite the fact such diets do not improve performance [186]. However, are all grains as evil as they sound?

First, whole grains are packed with fiber, protein, carbohydrate, and B-vitamins and studies show whole grains reduce all-cause mortality and morbidity, with lower risk for cardiovascular disease, cancer, and diabetes [187]. When wheat is grown organically it has been shown to contain superior nutritional profiles compared to conventional wheat [188].

Wheat's nutritional profile has significantly decreased since the 1960s [189–191], while the number of new gluten proteins has increased [192], and this is reportedly not due to changes in soil, but changes in wheat hybridization. On the other hand, ancient wheat such as einkorn, emmer, kamut, durum, and spelt, celebrating a recent comeback, exceed nutrient composition (e.g., protein, lipids, minerals and elements, antioxidants such as lutein) compared to modern wheat [190,193–195]. A recent study on khorosan, also known by the name Kamut, shows greater anti-inflammatory effects through antioxidants, blood minerals, and reduced metabolic (e.g., lipids, glucose) and oxidative stress markers in healthy subjects consuming khorosan in bread, pasta, and crackers for 8 weeks, compared to consuming these products made with a semi whole-wheat product [196]. Thus, these older cultivars may contribute significantly to nutrient dense diets [195] and health promotion [196].

Such ancient wheat varieties are not only more nutritious and promote antioxidant protection, but some also lack the highly immuno-suppressive α-gliadin peptides—the major component of gluten that provokes gluten intolerance. These are encoded by the D-genome of wheat. Thus, species that lack the D-genome of wheat, such as einkorn, emmer, and durum, show lower reactivity compared to common wheat [197]. Work in Italy is currently focused on einkorn, the oldest form of wild wheat first domesticated 12,000 years ago by hunter-gatherers in Mesopotamia. Along with wild emmer, also known as the mother of all wheats, "einkorn is considered a catalyst of agriculture and the initiation of wheat's vast biodiversity" [198] (p. 22). Einkorn appears to either pose no [199] or fewer adverse reactions in Celiac patients compared to modern wheat [200]. Athletes who have been diagnosed with Celiac's disease, should consult their sports dietitian before trying einkorn since it may still have the potential to induce the Celiac's disease syndrome [201]. For a great review see Kucek, Veenstra, Amnuaycheewa, and Sorrells, (2015) [202].

Understanding nutritional differences among grain varieties also opens the dialogue on bread. While the choice of grain permits greater nutrient intake, fermentation using a sourdough starter has also been shown to increase bioavailability of nutrients such as iron. This is most likely due to a reduction in phytates [135]. Fermented bread decreases post-prandial glycemic response through organic acids that delay gastric emptying [203]. This, therefore, is a great low glycemic alternative to processed white bread for active individuals, especially at breakfast. Finally, sourdough fermented bread also appears to retain antioxidants better due to lower pH levels [204], which if baked with an antioxidant and protein-rich grain, such as einkorn or emmer [193], by far exceeds the nutrient density compared to bread made with modern wheat.

Studies also show that both germination (sprouting) and fermentation (e.g., sourdough baking) can break down gliadin, one of the gluten proteins known to increase reactivity. While still not safe for Celiac patients [205], there are fewer immunoreactive peptides in sprouted products [202]. As for fermentation, lactic acid bacteria degrade some of the gliadins but multiple microbes appear to be needed to effectively degrade the majority of gliadin [206]. In a study by Greco et al., (2011), 97% of gluten was degraded by fermentation [207]. However, there were still a few Celiac patients in the study who showed measurable villi atrophy compared to non-gluten control treatments. Thus, wheat sourdough fermentation, as compared to non-fermented flour, does not degrade gluten enough to prevent adverse responses in Celiac patients [208].

Taken together, there does not seem a clear relief for Celiac patients, from ancient or heritage wheat, whether sprouted, fermented, or not. However, research suggests that there may be wide variability among reactivity to gluten, depending on the type of grain and level of processing. In addition, Celiac's disease expression, while triggered by gliadin-induced antibodies, can also be quite variable. While Celiac's disease has become more prevalent, with about 1% of the general population being affected, only 10–20% of people appear to be aware of their condition and follow a strictly gluten-free diet [209]. Mild forms of Celiac's disease, however, have the potential to worsen with age, thus, management through a gluten-free diet is necessary to decrease severe complications, such as osteoporotic fractures and intestinal cancers [209].

Interestingly, there are also other clinical presentations that do not fully correspond with Celiac's disease but rather consist of new clinical syndromes, typically termed non-celiac gluten and/or non-celiac wheat sensitivity. Though controversial and under-studied, it is generally accepted that these syndromes exist, but in the absence of gluten-ingested, celiac-specific antibodies [210] or wheat allergies [192]. What ultimately triggers these syndromes is unclear, as it may not need to be gluten but could include other components of wheat, such as the low fermentable, poorly absorbed, short-chain carbohydrates (FODMAPs) [211], other proteins [212], or insecticides such as glyphosate [29,30].

Regardless of exact mechanism, variability in clinical symptoms from grain or wheat ingestion pose new opportunities for nutrition professionals, considering both, the recent changes in clinical presentations and the modernization of many plants, including wheat [192]. While challenging, this should provide new avenues for dietary management of those who prefer a gluten-free diet for performance enhancement or health promotion, in the absence of Celiac's disease, to trial various approaches [192,207,213,214], as opposed to eating a strictly gluten-free diet. A gluten-free diet per se, with a high amount of processed gluten-free foods, may not meet nutritional recommendations, and a gluten-free, vegan diet could pose serious negative health and performance effects (e.g., B-vitamin deficiency). It has also been suggested that individuals should choose grains and their processing wisely, as this may reduce the risk of developing Celiac's disease in those who may have hereditary risk [202]. As ancient and heritage grain production is sweeping through the United States as a long-awaited player in the local food movement, the grain chain, from farmer to baker to table, is filled with food literacy opportunities for athletes such as making bread together. After all, bread has been a staple around the world with thousands of traditional uses. Bread is also one of the primary carbohydrate choices for athletes in training and competition, and carbohydrate is the major source of calories for most humans [113], including athletes [215].

While ancient and heritage grains are making their way back to the grocery stores, their production remains relatively small. However, these grains are known to be more drought tolerant [198] and using grains in crop rotation or as cover crop can meaningfully contribute to farm diversification and sustainable agriculture [78]. Grain production may soon take a turn for the better and become more sustainable as scientists at the Land Institute in Salina, Kansas [216] will likely announce that perennial grains (long roots capture carbon, enhance soil quality, and help reduce erosion) may replace modern wheat, not only on the field but also in people's bread baskets.

3.5. Food Literacy and Food Citizenship in Sports and Exercise

There is much to relearn when it comes to food. Perhaps we have moved away too far from field, farm, and the kitchen to know where food comes from and when it is in season. We also have lost important life skills such as cooking. We have to relearn and teach these simple skills to rebuild the knowledge needed to establish a healthy relationship with food. This brings us to the topic of food literacy. Recently, Vidgen and Gallegos, 2014 defined food literacy as the following:

"Food literacy is the scaffolding that empowers individuals, households, communities or nations to protect diet quality through change and strengthen dietary resilience over time. It is composed of a collection of inter-related knowledge, skills and behaviors required to plan, manage, select, prepare and eat food to meet needs and determine intake. This can simply be translated as the tools needed for a healthy lifelong relationship with food" [217] (p. 54).

Academic programs that promote food literacy, through curricula that meet joint goals of health promotion and sustainable development, especially in the health professions, may allow for transformative experiences [74]. Such food literacy discourse has the ability to diffuse, with outcomes that promote food citizenship in young people, and therefore, future generations [218,219]. Food citizenship is the practice of engaging in food-related behaviors (defined narrowly and broadly) that support, rather than threaten, the democratic, socially and economically just, and environmentally sustainable food systems [220] (p. 271).

Athletes and their support staff should be introduced to the link between daily food choices, health, and sustainability. It is most likely the sports dietitian who will bring this topic to the table, and the best and least confrontational approach, may be through a sustainably sourced meal cooked together such as a "Team Dinner" or a fun food literacy event with multiple stations, competitive team work, and food-related prizes. Shopping at local food outlets, including the farmer's market, and cooking together might be other options to open the dialogue pertaining to sustainable quantity and quality of food, as discussed above. Eating practices and fueling strategies are a performance-determining factor; however, becoming a food citizen [221] with knowledge and skill to navigate through an ever more complex food web opens the narrow sports-performance focus of a young athlete and introduces areas such as environmental conservation. Thus, sport nutrition education should begin to integrate sustainable food topics and promote food citizenship and food literacy by an enabling, participatory approach when the timing is right and where opportunities arise.

3.5.1. Athletes to Farm

While sport nutrition is a broad field and athlete performance and health issues take precedent over sustainability efforts, the sports dietitian will need to find a good balance that allows for sustainability integration, without feeling constrained but rather enabled in promoting awareness, building knowledge, and enhancing skills around food, ultimately improving dietary habits of young people. Thus, going to a local farm and/or market to buy food is only the first stop in this refreshed sport nutrition curriculum. While athletes often crave for the latest in exotic products from far away (e.g., Acai berries), eating some of the unfamiliar and wild foods grown close to home, may not only be more nutritious, but will also come with a plethora of learning opportunities. To allow athletes to make a connection with their home environment through the farmers who grow their food, training plans may need to be flexible to allow for Community Supported Agriculture (CSA) share pick up, a farmer's market visit, or a farm-field training day, as this may offer invaluable experiential nutrition education. The opportunity for athletes to experience "local life" is short but is increasingly meaningful, as sport teams and elite athletes are in the spotlight at home. Engaging with the local community may bring personal and team-related benefits for farm-fresh food support that has the potential to strengthen athletes' community involvement and build a sense of place. Finally, investing in the community, through food procurement from local farms, may also set the precedent for a supportive environment should athletes get injured or to facilitate the transition from athletic to normalized life after the career is concluded.

Eating locally grown and raised food has many benefits, but it may not automatically be more environmentally sustainable. Nevertheless, the local food movement might ignite people's desire for better taste, connection to place and to the people in their community. Local food seems to attract people also because of its economic benefit to the community, and there is a general sense, despite the fact that local food often costs more, that it is more affordable [222]. Regardless, those having worked and experienced the local food movement cannot let it go, and while the urgency to become more food secure in this changing world calls for revolutionary action through more sustainable food production [11], engaging in local food mobilizes people on a deeply emotional level, often difficult to express for those who are in it [223], but likely the reason why people may identify it as a realistic way to change eating behavior [55]. Recent research also shows that those buying direct from the farmer think and act around food very differently, compared to those going to a chain grocery store to procure their food [221]. Thus, the local food system is engaging inter-personally and economically within a community and it also teaches about food, the seasons, biodiversity, flavors, nutrition, cooking, culture and tradition.

While not always the most sustainable, the local food system may be a vehicle that could direct people to healthier and more mindful eating. A recent study illustrates how the awareness of dietary choices and eating can meet joint goals of individual health, environmental sustainability, and food security [224]. Thus, the many facets of a local food system can act as living learning laboratory to practice mindfulness training, even in athletes and their teams, as they cultivate both eating for sport and eating for planet Earth.

Local food systems are defined as "collaborative effort in a particular place to build more locally based, self-reliant food systems and economics—one in which sustainable food production, processing, distribution and consumption is integrated to enhance the economic, environmental and social health of a particular place." [225] (p. 100).

If athletes receive food money, a resource factsheet with local food procurement options could begin the collaboration with local business. A factsheet could also promote best choices when shopping at grocery stores, how to identify what's locally produced, what's seasonal, which labels to observe (e.g., USDA Organic; Buy Local; Marine Stewardship Council, MSC or Aquaculture Stewardship Council, ASC; GMO Free Project; Humanely Raised, American Grassfed, Direct or Fair Trade), the list of the dirty dozen [226], and how to order in bulk online, including heritage/ancient grains. Identifying farm-team partnerships requires farm visits and direct communication with the farmers [227]. In addition, providing some community service at the farm with 1 or 2 workouts held at the farm per year, supporting planting, weeding, or harvesting, will facilitate access to local, farm-fresh food because a connection is built much to the delight of the small-scale farmer who feels supported by the local sports team. Teams may also obtain group discounts if ordering in bulk through local buying clubs, food hubs, or food cooperatives. With CSA shares, there is great flexibility should shares get temporarily suspended when athletes travel. It is also possible to obtain surplus food and getting parents involved to preserve this food for later. Preservation, including fermentation, will not only support nutrition programming, but could be applied at times of increased team stress when athletes' immune function is more susceptible to illness. Locally, seasonally, and organically grown produce is more nutritious [175,179,180,188,228] and fermentation (e.g., pre- and probiotics) may add immune [229,230] support in times when athletes need it. Check with local University Extension offices for safe guidelines on canning and fermentation.

3.5.2. Taste Education and Cooking

Taste education with athletes can be integrated at any time, combined with a general team talk (locally grown fruit, vegetables, or grains as tasters), fueling or recovery workshops (integrating seasonal fruit, yogurt, and honey), or even during a travel nutrition talk (cultural food tasting of the travel destination). Nutrition should no longer be taught without hands-on learning from farm to kitchen. Written or visual materials (e.g., posters) or recipes that integrate local producers, topics of food citizenship (e.g., farmer's market shopping), or health benefits of diet diversity (e.g., biodiversity of greens) will keep building awareness and return home economics to young people's lives. Edible nutrition education is not only fun, inspiring, and tasty but it also teaches young people important skills and it builds a lifelong healthy relationship with food—and that is food literacy [217]. In addition, working with a farm-to-training table curriculum in sports also provides an opportunity to highlight local producers, dairies, farmers, or bakers, the history of the place, and this brings meaning and relational values [231]. If time is tight, University nutrition programs may partner to support a revisited curriculum that integrates agriculture and culinary training. One such example is the Flying Carrot Food Literacy Truck [232]. This program has been led by graduate students in sport nutrition at UCCS for the past 5 years [233]. After initial inception, several food-related courses, internships, and service learning experiences within the Southern Colorado regional food system, including a campus farm with its farm-to-table café, Food Next Door [134], and local food literacy farmhouse, are now serving a vigorous on-farm and in-kitchen curriculum for undergraduate and graduate students at UCCS, some of whom are in sport nutrition.

3.5.3. Budgets, Planning, and Food Waste

Food literacy should also integrate the full circle of engaged eaters' choices, including the discussion of food waste. Athletes and their families may tap into rescued food programs if budgets are tight. Most cities today have food rescue programs and some cities and programs, such as the one known as P.O.W.W.O.W. by the Borderland Foodbank in Southern Arizona [234], have made it possible to access fresh food, at affordable price, that otherwise would go to landfill. Food waste at the consumer level originates especially due to consumers' aesthetic preferences and arbitrary sell-by dates [36] as well as simply by purchasing, cooking, preparing and serving too much [39]. Teaching athletes to purchase what they can eat, cook what they purchase and promoting safe preservation and freezing techniques, are all part of food literacy training. The sports dietitian can help with weekly planning, providing input with shopping and cooking, so that athletes learn when, what, and how much to cook and to plan their dietary strategies, as much as the coach plans their training schedule. Cooking and planning ahead has been identified as a critical strategy to reducing food waste on the consumer level [39]. When traveling, a little bit of research ahead of time will pay off. Food cooperatives often have restaurants and there are many "Pay-What-You-Can" non-profit community restaurants in the US that serve local and organic food, often rescued from what would have otherwise been wasted, and sold at very low price (or what the team can pay [235]). These types of food outlets, including food "waste" supermarkets, are becoming more available everywhere. Obviously, each such stop will add to nutrition education and athletes learn they can eat this way everywhere they go. For good restaurant, market, and café guides that serve local, sustainable, and organic food, see Slow Food USA or Edible Communities [236,237].

3.6. Timing of Sustainability Integration in Exercise and Sports

In this paper, we addressed the environmental impact of food choices, easy changes that can be made (e.g., eating less meat), and paying attention to the food value chain to obtain high quality food with zero waste strategies. We have also integrated the local food system as a great entry way to connect sustainability and health, leveraging co-benefits for both planet and people. Posing the question on when to integrate sustainability principles in sports nutrition may sound as if athletes and sport teams have a special status concerning the food of the future. The answer is, nobody does, and shifting to a low-carbon consumer culture is a necessity rather than a choice. However, there needs to be careful consideration when to launch or what to initiate within the economic boundaries of grass-root sports, where parents are the coaches and kids are running from A to Z with plastic wrappers in their hands, squeezing out their pre-game meal. Likewise, timing considerations on the elite level must involve everyone because the budgets will have to, at least in part, account for increased food costs, cooking and team dinners, and time to pick up fresh food at farmers' markets, farm stands or neighborhood stores.

The best timing to plan any new programs within the world of sports is usually as the season is coming to an end and early before the start of the next training cycle. This is especially true should extra resources be needed to support the program. Farm CSA shares cost between $500–$600 for 6–8 months or about $20–$30 weekly, with each share providing food for about 4 people. Team talks with edible tasters will either require planning and connecting with local producers for samples or more expensive transactions at the store or market. Thus, the more time is invested to form farm-to-sports partnerships, the better and more economical the outcome.

All athletes spend time training at home. This is the best time to teach shopping and cooking. Depending on the season, it is also the best time to introduce local food with farm and market visits. Even though athletes are still on the go every day while in training, there is the potential for community connections through the local food system. Thus, providing a platform for this to occur may create a new sense of purpose, external to the identity of being an athlete. Participating in the community may balance the lives of the elite and new friendships may arise with those who work the land, which may create awareness of earth stewardship and food citizenship.

Once a program launches it is difficult to hold it back and it will evolve on its own. This is especially true for the local food movement. It needs ignition, but once the web is being explored and experiences are made, there is no going back. It is a paradigm shift. It's a local food revolution [223].

Should sustainability be a topic while traveling? The answer is yes, because in many countries, sustainable food systems are still the norm. Thus, traveling to European and Eastern European countries is often an eye-opener. Taking athletes into the grocery stores or through a local market is food literacy away from home, and sports dietitians also increase their knowledge and skills when exploring foods abroad. While most travels abroad are hectic with little time, surprisingly, the Olympics may be the perfect place for food literacy. The local volunteers are a great resource for information and they provide access to local markets to purchase fresh food. Thus, even when traveling, there are multiple opportunities to broaden food experiences and teach important cultural food differences.

Finally, introducing sustainability in sport nutrition may also be timely for those who are injured. These athletes may have more time and interest to learn about whole, nutritious food and cooking that could enhance healing. In addition, introducing athletes to other areas outside of sport, such as agriculture or cooking, may distract the overly occupied mind, and help maintain a positive attitude during the recovery and return-to-play period.

Taken together, while the timing of sustainability integration must be carefully considered to bring change to nutrition programming for athletes, small steps can fit everywhere and they bring with them deliciousness, beauty, and inspiration to participate in the food chain from farm to kitchen and table. There should be no doubt that this is the future of how nutrition should be taught, also in sports.

3.7. Integration of Sustainability Practices as Collective Commitment in Sports

3.7.1. Team Sustainability

Integrating sustainability in the sport nutrition program benefits first the athlete. However, coaches and other members of the sport science team, including athletic trainer, sports medicine doctor, and psychologist all benefit. Because of the performance enhancing team approach and multi-disciplinary strategies, sustainability and food will also open the dialogue of sustainable practices in general. This may mean that the team develops a vision or even a policy for sustainable development, especially considering training venues at home, where more influence is possible. Starting with food and drink, this may mean the team implements a recycling, re-using, and composting strategy. It may mean the team bans bottled water and throw-away, take-out containers. And it may mean preferred vendors for training tables or team meetings come from local businesses, using sustainably and locally sourced food. Catering may be enhanced through the-less-but-better meat initiative in combination with highly nutritious grains and beans, seasonal vegetables and fresh fruit. Team commitments may also include coach and support staff's eating practices that are coherent with the underlying philosophy of eating for performance and health. Finally, taking on a team vision for a sustainable future may also inspire parents and families and this could be supported by social media and website resources. A great example of how sustainability can be part of every sporting venue is the Green Sports Alliance [238].

3.7.2. Institutional Sustainability

Whether it is at a high school, university, or national/regional/local sport center level, integrating sustainable food procurement into food service starts to open many opportunities. It allows for a new seasonal menu. Reducing meat through the protein flip and boosting vegetarian offerings, sparks creativity in chefs and curiosity in athletes. Sourcing locally brings in the story of the farmer, unknown diet diversity, and awareness related to the link between fresh food and health on an individual, community, and environmental level. If institutions have gardens or farms, there is potential to integrate edible education linked to the menu served, in addition to the invaluable seed--to-plate menu. However, change is always more challenging than we think. Thus, to initiate a new menu, it is crucial that athletes and coaches understand the rationale behind the change. If resistance develops, athletes could be integrated in various educational activities that incorporate their own food preferences, cooking competitions, or recipe contests. It is helpful for athletes to see protein numbers of a meal and over a day to reduce fear of not getting enough. From a health perspective, there are many opportunities when food service commits to a more sustainable menu, with procurement gradually shifting to seasonal, organic, local, pasture-fed, free-range, and sustainably produced, fished or farmed food.

3.7.3. Event Sustainability

Integrating sustainable food into sporting events is being done on many levels. Some examples include London 2012 [239] and Rio 2016 [240]. Both local organizing committees published their sustainable food visions and made procurement with sustainable agricultural standards a priority. Especially the Rio Games were impressive as to the portrayed commitment to environmental consciousness through sustainable sourcing, improving supply chains, managing packaging, and reducing waste. As previously discussed, Brazil is one of the few countries whose governmental guidelines have embraced sustainability [56]. Whether visions and guidelines are ultimately implemented at the international events is difficult to tell, as there has been no labeling that details sustainable sourcing. This has previously been noted and published by Pelly et al., 2014 based on a survey conducted by sports dietitians, representing various countries at the 2012 London Olympic Games [241]. While the international sport nutrition organization, Professionals in Nutrition for Exercise and Sport (PINES) [242] reviews the menus for each Olympic cycle, an on-site implementation phase could help improve both menu and labeling, with inclusion of sustainable sourcing. In addition, the athlete dining hall and the Olympic village present an enormous challenge to sustain environmental commitments, considering food waste, bottled beverages, and to-go meals. In the future, food service at the Olympic Games should promote sustainability more visibly, highlighting a country's food culture and offering athletes experiential learning opportunities that showcase regional food traditions, seasonality, world heritage, and the story of farmers. Tokyo 2020 would be an excellent host city to bring change to the athlete dining hall with greater transparency for sourcing, local food literacy, and hands-on learning (e.g., how to make tofu or soba). The Olympics are long and many athletes have downtime. Why not learn something about the host country's food culture, sustainability efforts, seasonality of food, and how traditional foods are produced? While currently implemented at the Youth Olympic Games, integrating the host country's food traditions could augment the cultural experience of athletes visiting the Olympic village dining hall.

4. Conclusions

Environmental impact of food production is high, especially when considering the GhG emissions, land, and water use of animal agriculture. Many governmental organizations are beginning to integrate sustainability into their dietary guidelines and are calling on consumers to eat less animal and more plant-based foods. Integrating health and sustainability creates co-benefits, as for the most part, sustainable eating also means healthful eating. Nutrition recommendations, for active and athletic individuals should also begin to integrate sustainability. Using innovative approaches, including experiential learning from farm to table, renews the relationship of food by rediscovering the broad meaning of food, building knowledge and skills in the kitchen, and sharing food around the table. Initiating sustainable practices in sport, including sustainable food procurement, opens many opportunities for athletes and their entourage to engage in local and regional food systems, and by curbing the appetite for meat, individuals, teams, institutions and organizers begin to contribute to a reduction in global warming from the food sector.

Acknowledgments: We would like to thank the contributions of the Sustainability, Wellness & Learning Initiative (SWELL) at the University of Colorado, Colorado Springs (UCCS) and the United States Olympic Committee's Food and Nutrition Services for providing menu examples.

Author Contributions: Nanna Meyer wrote this concept paper with the support of Co-author Alba Reguant-Closa. Both authors contributed substantially to this manuscript.

Conflicts of Interest: The authors declare no conflict of interest.

References

1. Gerber, P.J.; Steinfeld, H.; Henderson, B.; Mottet, A.; Opio, C.; Dijkman, J.; Falucci, A.; Tempio, G. *Tackling Climate Change Through Livestock—A Global Assessment of Emissions and Mitigation Opportunities*; The Food and Agriculture Organization (FAO): Rome, Italy, 2013.
2. Sutton, C.; Dibb, S. *Prime Cuts, Valuing the Meat We Eat*; World Wildlife Fund, Food Ethics Council: Godalming, UK, 2013.
3. The Food and Agriculture Organization. *The State of World Fisheries and Aquaculture*; FAO: Rome, Italy, 2014; Volume 2014.
4. The Food and Agriculture Organization. *Livestock's Long Shadow Environmental Issues and Options*; FAO: Rome, Italy, 2007.
5. Pan, A.; Sun, Q.; Bernstein, A.M.; Schulze, M.B.; Manson, J.E.; Stampfer, M.J.; Willett, W.C.; Hu, F.B. Red meat consumption and mortality. *Arch. Intern. Med.* **2012**, *172*, 555–563. [PubMed]
6. Richman, E.L.; Stampfer, M.J.; Paciorek, A.; Broering, J.M.; Carroll, P.R.; Chan, J.M. Intakes of meat, fish, poultry, and eggs and risk of prostate cancer progression. *Am. J. Clin. Nutr.* **2010**, *91*, 712–721. [CrossRef] [PubMed]
7. Intergovernmental Panel on Climate Change. *IPCC, 2014: Climate Change 2014: Mitigation of Climate Change. Contribution of Working Groups I, II and III to the Fifth Assessment Report of the Intergovernmental Panel on Climate Change*; Cambridge University Press: New York, NY, USA, 2014.
8. Gornall, J.; Betts, R.; Burke, E.; Clark, R.; Camp, J.; Willett, K.; Wiltshire, A. Implications of climate change for agricultural productivity in the early twenty-first century. *Philos. Trans. R. Soc. Lond. B Biol. Sci.* **2010**, *365*, 2973–2989. [CrossRef] [PubMed]

9. Naylor, R.L.; Battisti, D.S.; Vimont, D.J.; Falcon, W.P.; Burke, M.B. Assessing risks of climate variability and climate change for Indonesian rice agriculture. *Proc. Natl. Acad. Sci. USA* **2007**, *104*, 7752–7757. [CrossRef] [PubMed]

10. Hansen, J.; Sato, M.; Hearty, P.; Ruedy, R.; Kelley, M.; Masson-Delmotte, V.; Russell, G.; Tselioudis, G.; Cao, J.; Rignot, E.; et al. Ice melt, sea level rise and superstorms: Evidence from paleoclimate data, climate modeling, and modern observations that 2 °C global warming could be dangerous. *Atmos. Chem. Phys.* **2016**, *16*, 3761–3812. [CrossRef]

11. Rockström, J.; Williams, J.; Daily, G.; Noble, A.; Matthews, N.; Gordon, L.; Wetterstrand, H.; Declerck, F.; Shah, M.; Steduto, P.; et al. Sustainable intensification of agriculture for human prosperity and global sustainability. *Ambio* **2017**, *46*, 4–17. [CrossRef] [PubMed]

12. Smil, V. *Feeding the World: A Challenge for the 21st Century*, 1st ed.; Massachusetts Institute of Technology, MIT Press: Cambridge, MA, USA, 2000.

13. Tilman, D.; Clark, M. Global diets link environmental sustainability and human health. *Nature* **2014**, *515*, 518–522. [CrossRef] [PubMed]

14. Vermeulen, S.J.; Campbell, B.M.; Ingram, J.S.I. Climate change and food systems. *Annu. Rev. Environ. Resour.* **2012**, *37*, 195–222. [CrossRef]

15. Kibria, G.; Yousuf Haroon, A.; Nugegoda, D.; Rose, G. *Climate Change and Chemicals: Environmental and Biological Aspects*; New Indial Publishing: New Delhi, India, 2010.

16. Bajželj, B.; Richards, K.S.; Allwood, J.M.; Smith, P.; Dennis, J.S.; Curmi, E.; Gilligan, C.A. Importance of food-demand management for climate mitigation. *Nat. Clim. Chang.* **2014**, *4*, 924–929. [CrossRef]

17. Miranda, N.D.; Tuomisto, H.L.; McCulloch, M.D. Meta-analysis of greenhouse gas emissions from anaerobic digestion processes in dairy farms. *Environ. Sci. Technol.* **2015**, *49*, 5211–5219. [CrossRef] [PubMed]

18. Ripple, W.J.; Smith, P.; Haberl, H.; Montzka, S.A.; McAlpine, C.; Boucher, D.H. Ruminants, climate change and climate policy. *Nat. Clim. Chang.* **2014**, *4*, 2–5. [CrossRef]

19. Eshel, G.; Shepon, A.; Makov, T.; Milo, R. Land, irrigation water, greenhouse gas, and reactive nitrogen burdens of meat, eggs, and dairy production in the United States. *Proc. Natl. Acad. Sci. USA* **2014**, *111*, 11996–12001. [CrossRef] [PubMed]

20. Nemecek, T.; Dubois, D.; Huguenin-Elie, O.; Gaillard, G. Life cycle assessment of Swiss farming systems: I. Integrated and organic farming. *Agric. Syst.* **2011**, *104*, 217–232. [CrossRef]

21. Sabaté, J.; Sranacharoenpong, K.; Harwatt, H.; Wien, M.; Soret, S. The environmental cost of protein food choices. *Public Health Nutr.* **2014**, *18*, 1–7. [CrossRef] [PubMed]

22. Auestad, N.; Fulgoni, V.L. What current literature tells us about sustainable diets: emerging research linking dietary patterns, environmental sustainability, and economics. *Adv. Nutr.* **2015**, *6*, 19–36. [CrossRef] [PubMed]

23. Tilman, D. Global environmental impacts of agricultural expansion: The need for sustainable and efficient practices. *PNAS* **1999**, *96*, 5995–6000. [CrossRef] [PubMed]

24. Herrero, M.; Havlík, P.; Valin, H.; Notenbaert, A.; Rufino, M.C.; Thornton, P.K.; Blümmel, M.; Weiss, F.; Grace, D.; Obersteiner, M. Biomass use, production, feed efficiencies, and greenhouse gas emissions from global livestock systems. *Proc. Natl. Acad. Sci. USA* **2013**, *110*, 20888–20893. [CrossRef] [PubMed]

25. Fantke, P.; Jolliet, O. Life cycle human health impacts of 875 pesticides. *Int. J. Life Cycle Assess.* **2016**, *21*, 722–733. [CrossRef]

26. Guyton, K.Z.; Loomis, D.; Grosse, Y.; El Ghissassi, F.; Benbrahim-Tallaa, L.; Guha, N.; Scoccianti, C.; Mattock, H.; Straif, K.; Blair, A.; et al. Carcinogenicity of tetrachlorvinphos, parathion, malathion, diazinon, and glyphosate. *Lancet Oncol.* **2015**, *16*, 490–491. [CrossRef]

27. O'Kane, G. What is the real cost of our food? Implications for the environment, society and public health nutrition. *Public Health Nutr.* **2012**, *15*, 268–276. [CrossRef] [PubMed]

28. Viel, J.-F.; Warembourg, C.; Le Maner-Idrissi, G.; Lacroix, A.; Limon, G.; Rouget, F.; Monfort, C.; Durand, G.; Cordier, S.; Chevrier, C. Pyrethroid insecticide exposure and cognitive developmental disabilities in children: The PELAGIE mother-child cohort. *Environ. Int.* **2015**, *82*, 69–75. [CrossRef] [PubMed]

29. Samsel, A.; Seneff, S. Glyphosate, pathways to modern diseases II: Celiac sprue and gluten intolerance. *Interdiscip. Toxicol.* **2013**, *6*, 159–184. [CrossRef] [PubMed]

30. Samsel, A.; Seneff, S. Glyphosate's Suppression of cytochrome P450 enzymes and amino acid biosynthesis by the gut microbiome: Pathways to modern diseases. *Entropy* **2013**, *15*, 1416–1463. [CrossRef]

31. Raanan, R.; Harley, K.G.; Balmes, J.R.; Bradman, A.; Lipsett, M.; Eskenazi, B. Early-life exposure to organophosphate pesticides and pediatric respiratory symptoms in the CHAMACOS cohort. *Environ. Health Perspect.* **2015**, *123*, 179–185. [CrossRef] [PubMed]
32. Stein, L.J.; Gunier, R.B.; Harley, K.; Kogut, K.; Bradman, A.; Eskenazi, B. Early childhood adversity potentiates the adverse association between prenatal organophosphate pesticide exposure and child IQ: The CHAMACOS cohort. *Neurotoxicology* **2016**, *56*, 180–187. [CrossRef] [PubMed]
33. Bassett, A.; Gunther, A.; Mundy, P. A Breath of Fresh Air: The Truth about Pasture-Based Livestock Production and Environmental Sustainability. 2013. Available online: http://animalwelfareapproved. org/wp-content/uploads/2013/01/A-Breath-of-Fresh-Air-v1.pdf (accessed on March 7 2016).
34. Carlsson-Kanyama, A.; González, A.D. Potential contributions of food consumption patterns to climate change. *Am. J. Clin. Nutr.* **2009**, *89*, 1704S–1709S. [CrossRef] [PubMed]
35. Macdiarmid, J.I.; Kyle, J.; Horgan, G.W.; Loe, J.; Fyfe, C.; Johnstone, A.; McNeill, G. Clean fuel for the future: Can we contribute to reducing greenhouse gas emissions by eating a healthy diet? *Am. J. Clin. Nutr.* **2012**, *96*, 632–639. [CrossRef] [PubMed]
36. Gustavsson, J.; Cederberg, C.; Sonesson, U. *Global Food Losses and Food Waste—Extent, Causes and Prevention*; FAO: Rome, Italy, 2011.
37. The Food and Agriculture Organization. *Food Wastage Footprint Summary Report*; FAO: Rome, Italy, 2013.
38. Reynolds, L.P.; Wulster-Radcliffe, M.C.; Aaron, D.K.; Davis, T.A. Importance of animals in agricultural sustainability and food security. *J. Nutr.* **2015**, *145*, 1377–1379. [CrossRef] [PubMed]
39. Parfitt, J.; Barthel, M.; Macnaughton, S. Food waste within food supply chains: Quantification and potential for change to 2050. *Phil. Trans. R. Soc. B* **2010**, *365*, 3065–3081. [CrossRef] [PubMed]
40. Hall, K.D.; Guo, J.; Dore, M.; Chow, C.C. The progressive increase of food waste in america and its environmental impact. *PLoS ONE* **2009**, *4*, 9–14. [CrossRef] [PubMed]
41. Gunders, D. Wasted: How America Is Losing Up to 40 Percent of Its Food from Farm to Fork to Landfill. Available online: https://www.nrdc.org/sites/default/files/wasted-food-IP.pdf (accessed on 3 November 2016).
42. Jones, T.W. Using Contemporary Archaeology and Applied Anthropology to Understand Food Loss in the American Food System. Available online: http://www.ce.cmu.edu/~gdrg/readings/2006/12/19/Jones_ UsingContemporaryArchaeologyAndAppliedAnthropologyToUnderstandFoodLossInAmericanFoodSystem. pdf (accessed on 15 October 2016).
43. Konikow, L.F. Groundwater Depletion in the United States (1900–2008). Available online: http://pubs.usgs. gov/sir/2013/5079 (accessed on 11 June 2015).
44. Mekonnen, M.M.; Hoekstra, A.Y. A Global Assessment of the Water Footprint of Farm Animal Products. *Ecosystems* **2012**, *15*, 401–415. [CrossRef]
45. International Organization for Standarization (ISO). *Environmental management—Life Cycle Assessment—Principles and Framework*; ISO/TC 207; Environmental Management, Subcommittee SC5: Geneva, Switzerland, 2006.
46. Springmann, M.; Godfray, H.C.J.; Rayner, M.; Scarborough, P. Analysis and valuation of the health and climate change cobenefits of dietary change. *Proc. Natl. Acad. Sci. USA* **2016**, *113*, 4146–4151. [CrossRef] [PubMed]
47. Godfray, H.C.J.; Garnett, T. Food security and sustainable intensification. *Philos. Trans. R. Soc. B* **2014**. [CrossRef] [PubMed]
48. Donini, L.M.; Dernini, S.; Lairon, D.; Serra-Majem, L.; Amiot, M.-J.; del Balzo, V.; Giusti, A.-M.; Burlingame, B.; Belahsen, R.; Maiani, G.; et al. A consensus proposal for nutritional indicators to assess the sustainability of a healthy diet: the mediterranean diet as a case study. *Front. Nutr.* **2016**. [CrossRef] [PubMed]
49. Macdiarmid, J.I. Is a healthy diet an environmentally sustainable diet? *Proc. Nutr. Soc.* **2013**, *72*, 13–20. [CrossRef] [PubMed]
50. Hallström, E.; Carlsson-Kanyama, A.; Börjesson, P. Environmental impact of dietary change: A systematic review. *J. Clean. Prod.* **2015**, *91*, 1–11. [CrossRef]
51. Masset, G.; Vieux, F.; Verger, E.O.; Soler, L.G.; Touazi, D.; Darmon, N. Reducing energy intake and energy density for a sustainable diet: A study based on self-selected diets in French adults. *Am. J. Clin. Nutr.* **2014**, *99*, 1460–1469. [CrossRef] [PubMed]
52. Friel, S.; Dangour, A.D.; Garnett, T.; Lock, K.; Chalabi, Z.; Roberts, I.; Butler, A.; Butler, C.D.; Waage, J.; McMichael, A.J.; et al. Public health benefits of strategies to reduce greenhouse-gas emissions: Food and agriculture. *Lancet* **2009**, *374*, 2016–2025. [CrossRef]

53. Westhoek, H.; Lesschen, J.P.; Rood, T.; Wagner, S.; De Marco, A.; Murphy-Bokern, D.; Leip, A.; van Grinsven, H.; Sutton, M.A.; Oenema, O. Food choices, health and environment: Effects of cutting Europe's meat and dairy intake. *Glob. Environ. Chang.* **2014**, *26*, 196–205. [CrossRef]

54. Sabaté, J.; Harwatt, H.; Soret, S. Environmental nutrition: A new frontier for public health. *Am. J. Public Health* **2016**, *106*, 815–821. [CrossRef] [PubMed]

55. De Boer, J.; de Witt, A.; Aiking, H. Help the climate, change your diet: A cross-sectional study on how to involve consumers in a transition to a low-carbon society. *Appetite* **2016**, *98*, 19–27. [CrossRef] [PubMed]

56. The Food and Agriculture Organization. *Plates, Pyramids, Planets. Developments in National Healthy and Sustainable Dietary Guidelines: A State of Play Assessment*; FAO and the Food Climate Research Network at The University of Oxford (FCRN): Oxford, UK, 2016.

57. Hoekstra, A.Y. The hidden water resource use behind meat and dairy. *Anim. Front.* **2012**, *2*, 3–8. [CrossRef]

58. Rockström, J.; Steffen, W.; Noone, K.; Persson, Å.; Chapin, F.S.; Lambin, E.F.; Lenton, T.M.; Scheffer, M.; Folke, C.; Schellnhuber, H.J.; et al. A safe operating space for humanity. *Nature* **2009**, *461*, 472–475. [CrossRef] [PubMed]

59. Aleksandrowicz, L.; Green, R.; Joy, E.J.M.; Smith, P.; Haines, A. The impacts of dietary change on greenhouse gas emissions, land use, water use, and health: A systematic review. *PLoS ONE* **2016**, *11*, 1–16. [CrossRef] [PubMed]

60. Aiking, H. Protein production: Planet, profit, plus people? *Am. J. Clin. Nutr.* **2014**, *100*, 483–489. [CrossRef] [PubMed]

61. United States Department of Agriculture. Profiling Food Consumption in America. In *Agriculture Fact Book*; The Delano Max Wealth Institute, Limited Liability Company: Las Vegas, NV, USA, 2003; pp. 13–22.

62. Scarborough, P.; Appleby, P.N.; Mizdrak, A.; Briggs, A.D.M.; Travis, R.C.; Bradbury, K.E.; Key, T.J. Dietary greenhouse gas emissions of meat-eaters, fish-eaters, vegetarians and vegans in the UK. *Clim. Chang.* **2014**, *125*, 179–192. [CrossRef] [PubMed]

63. Macdiarmid, J.I.; Douglas, F.; Campbell, J. Eating like there's no tomorrow: Public awareness of the environmental impact of food and reluctance to eat less meat as part of a sustainable diet. *Appetite* **2016**, *96*, 487–493. [CrossRef] [PubMed]

64. DeLonge, M.S.; Owen, J.J.; Silver, W.L. *Greenhouse Gas Mitigation Opportunities in California Agriculture: Review of California Rangeland Emissions and Mitigation Potential. NI GGMOCA R 4*; Duke University: Durham, NC, USA, 2014.

65. Lagerberg Fogelberg, C. *Towards Environmentally Sound Dietary Guidelines*; Swedish National Food Agency's Dietary Guidelines, IDEON Agro Food: Uppsala, Sweden, 2013.

66. U.S. Department of Agriculture (USDA). *Agriculture Fact Book 2001–2002*; USDA: Raleigh, NC, USA, 2002.

67. U.S. Department of Agriculture (USDA). *Scientific Report of the 2015 Dietary Guidelines Advisory Committee*; USDA: Raleigh, NC, USA, 2015.

68. U.S. Department of Agriculture (USDA). *2015–2020 Dietary Guidelines for Americans*; USDA: Raleigh, NC, USA, 2015.

69. Saxe, H.; Jensen, J.D. Does the environmental gain of switching to the healthy New Nordic Diet outweigh the increased consumer cost? In Proceedings of the 9th International Conference Proceedings LCA of Food, San Francisco, CA, USA, 8–10 October 2014.

70. Van Dooren, C.; Aiking, H. Defining a nutritionally healthy, environmentally friendly, and culturally acceptable Low Lands Diet. *Int. J. Life Cycle Assess.* **2016**, *21*, 688–700. [CrossRef]

71. Public Health England; Welsh Government; Food Standards Scotland; Food Standards Agency in Northen Ireland. *Eat Well Guide*; Food Standards, Scotland: Aberdeen, Scottland, 2016.

72. Krebs-Smith, S.M.; Guenther, P.M.; Subar, A.F.; Kirkpatrick, S.I.; Dodd, K.W. Americans do not meet federal dietary recommendations. *J. Nutr.* **2010**, *140*, 1832–1838. [CrossRef] [PubMed]

73. Schösler, H.; Boer, J.; de Boersema, J.J. Can we cut out the meat of the dish? Constructing consumer-oriented pathways towards meat substitution. *Appetite* **2012**, *58*, 39–47.

74. Hekler, E.B.; Gardner, C.D.; Robinson, T.N. Effects of a College Course about Food and Society on Students' Eating Behaviors. *AMEPRE* **2010**, *38*, 543–547. [CrossRef] [PubMed]

75. The Culinary Institute of America; Harvard School of Public Health The Protein Flip. Available online: http://www.menusofchange.org/images/uploads/pdf/CIA_The_Protein_Flip_C_FINAL_6-17-15.pdf (accessed on 10 October 2016).

76. Meatless Mondays. Available online: www.meatlessmonday.com (accessed on 10 August 2016).
77. Brundtland, G. Report of the World Commision on Environement and Development: Our Common Future. *Oxf. Pap.* **1987**. [CrossRef]
78. Reganold, J.P.; Wachter, J.M. Organic agriculture in the twenty-first century. *Nat. Plants* **2016**, *2*, 15221. [CrossRef] [PubMed]
79. Batello, C.; Wade, L.; Cox, S.; Pogna, N.; Bozzini, A.; Choptiany, J. *Perennial Crops for Food Security: Proceedings of the FAO Expert Workshop*; FAO: Rome, Italy, 2014.
80. The Food And Agriculture Organization. *Sustainable Diets and Biodiversity*; FAO: Rome, Italy, 2010.
81. Kjærgård, B.; Land, B.; Bransholm Pedersen, K. Health and sustainability. *Health Promot. Int.* **2014**, *29*, 558–568. [CrossRef] [PubMed]
82. Micha, R.; Wallace, S.K.; Mozaffarian, D. Red and processed meat consumption and risk of incident coronary heart disease, stroke, and diabetes mellitus: A systematic review and meta-analysis. *Circulation* **2010**, *121*, 2271–2283. [CrossRef] [PubMed]
83. Huang, W.; Han, Y.; Xu, J.; Zhu, W.; Li, Z. Red and processed meat intake and risk of esophageal adenocarcinoma: A meta-analysis of observational studies. *Cancer Causes Control* **2013**, *24*, 193–201. [CrossRef] [PubMed]
84. Goldberg, A.M. Farm animal welfare and human health. *Curr. Environ. Heal. Rep.* **2016**, *3*, 313–321. [CrossRef] [PubMed]
85. Garnett, B.T. Plating up solutions. *Sci. Mag.* **2016**. [CrossRef] [PubMed]
86. Egli, V.; Oliver, M.; Tautolo, E.S. The development of a model of community garden benefits to wellbeing. *Prev. Med. Rep.* **2016**, *3*, 348–352. [CrossRef] [PubMed]
87. Pedersen, K.; Land, B.; Kjærgård, B. Duality of health promotion and sustainable development: Perspectives on food waste reduction strategies. *J. Transdiscipl. Environ. Stud.* **2015**, *14*, 5–18.
88. Hanlon, P.; Carlisle, S.; Hannah, M.; Lyon, A.; Reilly, D. A perspective on the future public health practitioner. *Perspect. Public Health* **2012**, *132*, 235–239. [CrossRef] [PubMed]
89. Personal Footprint. Available online: http://www.footprintnetwork.org/en/index.php/GFN/page/personal_footprint (accessed on 31 October 2016).
90. TrueSport: U.S. Anti-Doping Agency. Available online: http://www.usada.org/truesport/ (accessed on 28 July 2016).
91. Sundgot-Borgen, J.; Meyer, N.L.; Lohman, T.G.; Ackland, T.R.; Maughan, R.J.; Stewart, A.D.; Müller, W. How to minimise the health risks to athletes who compete in weight-sensitive sports review and position statement on behalf of the Ad Hoc Research Working Group on Body Composition, Health and Performance, under the auspices of the IOC Medical Commission. *Br. J. Sports Med.* **2013**, *47*, 1012–1022. [CrossRef] [PubMed]
92. Bratland-Sanda, S.; Sundgot-Borgen, J. Eating disorders in athletes: Overview of prevalence, risk factors and recommendations for prevention and treatment. *Eur. J. Sport Sci.* **2013**, *13*, 499–508. [CrossRef] [PubMed]
93. Parnell, J.A.; Wiens, K.P.; Erdman, K.A. Dietary intakes and supplement use in pre-adolescent and adolescent Canadian athletes. *Nutrients* **2016**, *8*, 526. [CrossRef] [PubMed]
94. Gillen, J.B.; Trommelen, J.; Wardenaar, F.C.; Brinkmans, N.Y.J.; Versteegen, J.J.; Jonvik, K.L.; Kapp, C.; de Vries, J.; van den Borne, J.J.G.C.; Gibala, M.J.; et al. Dietary protein intake and distribution patterns of well-trained dutch athletes. *Int. J. Sport Nutr. Exerc. Metab.* **2016**, *27*, 105–114. [CrossRef] [PubMed]
95. Juzwiak, C.R.; Amancio, O.M.S.; Vitalle, M.S.S.; Pinheiro, M.M.; Szejnfeld, V.L. Body composition and nutritional profile of male adolescent tennis players. *J. Sports Sci.* **2008**, *26*, 1209–1217. [CrossRef] [PubMed]
96. Spendlove, J.; Mitchell, L.; Gifford, J.; Hackett, D.; Slater, G.; Cobley, S.; O'Connor, H. Dietary intake of competitive bodybuilders. *Sports Med.* **2015**, *45*, 1041–1063. [CrossRef] [PubMed]
97. Thomas, D.T.; Erdman, K.A.; Burke, L.M. American College of Sports Medicine Joint Position Statement. Nutrition and Athletic Performance. *Med. Sci. Sports Exerc.* **2016**, *48*, 543–568. [PubMed]
98. Churchward-Venne, T.A.; Murphy, C.H.; Longland, T.M.; Phillips, S.M. Role of protein and amino acids in promoting lean mass accretion with resistance exercise and attenuating lean mass loss during energy deficit in humans. *Amino Acids.* **2013**, *45*, 231–240. [CrossRef] [PubMed]
99. Moore, D.R.; Churchward-Venne, T.A.; Witard, O.; Breen, L.; Burd, N.A.; Tipton, K.D.; Phillips, S.M. Protein ingestion to stimulate myofibrillar protein synthesis requires greater relative protein intakes in healthy older versus younger men. *J. Gerontol. A Biol. Sci. Med. Sci.* **2015**, *70*, 57–62. [CrossRef] [PubMed]

100. Atherton, P.J.; Etheridge, T.; Watt, P.W.; Wilkinson, D.; Selby, A.; Rankin, D.; Smith, K.; Rennie, M.J. Muscle full effect after oral protein: Time-dependent concordance and discordance between human muscle protein synthesis and mTORC1 signaling. *Am. J. Clin. Nutr.* **2010**, *92*, 1080–1088. [CrossRef] [PubMed]

101. Areta, J.L.; Burke, L.M.; Ross, M.L.; Camera, D.M.; West, D.W.D.; Broad, E.M.; Jeacocke, N.A.; Moore, D.R.; Stellingwerff, T.; Phillips, S.M.; et al. Timing and distribution of protein ingestion during prolonged recovery from resistance exercise alters myofibrillar protein synthesis. *J. Physiol.* **2013**, *591*, 2319–2331. [CrossRef] [PubMed]

102. Res, P.T.; Groen, B.; Pennings, B.; Beelen, M.; Wallis, G.A.; Gijsen, A.P.; Senden, J.M.G.; Van Loon, L.J.C. Protein ingestion before sleep improves postexercise overnight recovery. *Med. Sci. Sports Exerc.* **2012**, *44*, 1560–1569. [CrossRef] [PubMed]

103. Phillips, S.M.; Chevalier, S.; Leidy, H.J. Protein "requirements" beyond the RDA: Implications for optimizing health. *Appl. Physiol. Nutr. Metab.* **2016**, *572*, 1–8. [CrossRef] [PubMed]

104. Phillips, S.M. A brief review of higher dietary protein diets in weight loss: A focus on athletes. *Sport. Med.* **2014**, *44*, 149–153. [CrossRef] [PubMed]

105. Helms, E.R.; Zinn, C.; Rowlands, D.S.; Brown, S.R. A systematic review of dietary protein during caloric restriction in resistance trained lean athletes: A case for higher intakes. *Int. J. Sport Nutr. Exerc. Metab.* **2014**, *24*, 127–138. [CrossRef] [PubMed]

106. Helms, E.R.; Aragon, A.A.; Fitschen, P.J. Evidence-based recommendations for natural bodybuilding contest preparation: Nutrition and supplementation. *J. Int. Soc. Sports Nutr.* **2014**, *11*, 20. [CrossRef] [PubMed]

107. Arciero, P.J.; Miller, V.J.; Ward, E. Performance enhancing diets and the PRISE protocol to optimize athletic performance. *J. Nutr. Metab.* **2015**. [CrossRef] [PubMed]

108. Pelly, F.E.; Burkhart, S.J. Dietary regimens of athletes competing at the Delhi 2010 Commonwealth Games. *Int. J. Sport Nutr. Exerc. Metab.* **2014**, *24*, 28–36. [CrossRef] [PubMed]

109. Della Guardia, L.; Cavallaro, M.; Cena, H. The risks of self-made diets: The case of an amateur bodybuilder. *J. Int. Soc. Sports Nutr.* **2015**, *12*, 16. [CrossRef] [PubMed]

110. Manore, M.M.; Meyer, N.L.; Janice, T. *Sport Nutrition for Health and Performance*, 2nd ed.; Human Kinetics: Champaign, IL, USA, 2009.

111. Council for Agriculture Science & Technology. *Animal Agriculture and Global Food Supply*; Library of Congress Cataloging in Publication Data: Ames, IA, USA, 1999; Volume 135.

112. Food and Agriculture Organization Corporate Statistical Database (FAOSTAT). Food and Agriculture Data. Available online: http://www.fao.org/faostat/en/#home (accessed on 29 August 2016).

113. Institute of Medicine. Dietary Reference Intakes: The Essential Guide to Nutrient Requirements. Available online: www.iom.edu (accessed on 15 November 2016).

114. Daley, C.A.; Abbott, A.; Doyle, P.S.; Nader, G.A.; Larson, S. A review of fatty acid profiles and antioxidant content in grass-fed and grain-fed beef. *Nutr. J.* **2010**, *9*, 10. [CrossRef] [PubMed]

115. Tessari, P.; Lante, A.; Mosca, G. Essential amino acids: Master regulators of nutrition and environmental footprint? *Sci. Rep.* **2016**, *6*, 26074. [CrossRef] [PubMed]

116. Melina, V.; Craig, W.; Levin, S. Position of the Academy of Nutrition and Dietetics: Vegetarian Diets. *J. Acad. Nutr. Diet.* **2016**, *116*, 1970–1980. [CrossRef] [PubMed]

117. Van Huis, A.; Itterbeeck, J.; Van Klunder, H.; Mertens, E.; Halloran, A.; Muir, G.; Vantomme, P. *Edible Insects. Future Prospects for Food and Feed Security*; FAO: Rome, Italy, 2013; Volume 171.

118. Babault, N.; Païzis, C.; Deley, G.; Guérin-Deremaux, L.; Saniez, M.-H.; Lefranc-Millot, C.; Allaert, F.A. Pea proteins oral supplementation promotes muscle thickness gains during resistance training: A double-blind, randomized, placebo-controlled clinical trial vs. whey protein. *J. Int. Soc. Sports Nutr.* **2015**, *12*, 3. [CrossRef] [PubMed]

119. The Food and Agriculture Organization. Animal Production and Health Division. In *Greenhouse Gas Emissions from the Dairy Sector: A Life Cycle Assessment*; FAO: Rome, Italy, 2010.

120. Von Keyserlingk, M.A.G.; Martin, N.P.; Kebreab, E.; Knowlton, K.F.; Grant, R.J.; Stephenson, M.; Sniffen, C.J.; Harner, J.P.; Wright, A.D.; Smith, S.I. Invited review: Sustainability of the US dairy industry. *J. Dairy Sci.* **2013**, *96*, 5405–5425. [CrossRef] [PubMed]

121. Pilet, V.; Owens, S.; Rouyer, B.; Jachnik, P.; Valstar, M.; Scheepstra, J.; Jansen, J.; Krijger, A. *The World Dairy Situation 2010*; Bulletin 446/2010; International Dairy Federation (I.N.P.A): Brussels, Belgium, 2010; pp. 1–212.

122. Buttriss, J.L. The Eatwell Guide refreshed. *Nutr. Bull.* **2016**, *41*, 135–141. [CrossRef]

123. Vergé, X.P.C.; Maxime, D.; Dyer, J.A.; Desjardins, R.L.; Arcand, Y.; Vanderzaag, A. Carbon footprint of Canadian dairy products: Calculations and issues. *J. Dairy Sci.* **2013**, *96*, 6091–6104. [CrossRef] [PubMed]

124. McFarland, L.V. From yaks to yogurt: The history, development, and current use of probiotics. *Clin. Infect. Dis.* **2015**, *60*, S85–S90. [CrossRef] [PubMed]

125. Slow Food USA. Slow Meat. Available online: https://www.slowfoodusa.org/slow-meat (accessed on 6 July 2016).

126. Culinary Institute of America; Harvard School of Public Health. Protein Plays: Foodservice Strategies for Our Future. Available online: www.menusofchange.org (accessed on 16 November 2016).

127. Team USA Nutrition. Available online: http://www.teamusa.org/nutrition (accessed on 20 February 2016).

128. Reguant-Closa, A.; Harris, M.; Meyer, N. Validation of the athlete's plate quantitative analysis (Phase 1). *Int. J. Sport. Nutr. Exerc. Metab.* **2016**, *26*, S1–S15.

129. Reguant-Closa, A.; Judson, A.; Harris, M.; Moreman, T.; Meyer, N.L. Including sustainability principles into the Athlete's Plate Nutritional Educational Tool. In Proceedings of the 17th International Confederation of Dietetics Associations, Granada, Spain, 7–10 September 2016.

130. Drewnowski, A.; Fulgoni, V. Nutrient density: principles and evaluation tools. *Am. J. Clin. Nutr.* **2014**, *99*, 1223S-8S. [CrossRef] [PubMed]

131. Lobstein, T.; Davies, S. Defining and labelling "healthy" and "unhealthy" food. *Public Health Nutr.* **2009**, *12*, 331–340. [CrossRef] [PubMed]

132. Knapik, J.J.; Steelman, R.A.; Hoedebecke, S.S.; Austin, K.G.; Farina, E.K.; Lieberman, H.R. Prevalence of Dietary supplement use by athletes: Systematic review and meta-analysis. *Sports Med.* **2016**, *46*, 103–123. [CrossRef] [PubMed]

133. Judson, A.W.; Moreman, T.; Meyer, N.L. Integrating Sustainability into Sports Nutrition: The Protein Flip for Athlete's. 2016; Unpublished work.

134. University of Colorado, Colorado Springs (UCCS). Dining and Hospitality Services: Food Next Door. Available online: http://www.uccs.edu/diningservices/swell/food-next-door.html (accessed on 1 October 2016).

135. Scheers, N.; Rossander-Hulthen, L.; Torsdottir, I.; Sandberg, A.-S. Increased iron bioavailability from lactic-fermented vegetables is likely an effect of promoting the formation of ferric iron (Fe(3+)). *Eur. J. Nutr.* **2016**, *55*, 373–382. [CrossRef] [PubMed]

136. Bering, S.; Suchdev, S.; Sjøltov, L.; Berggren, A.; Tetens, I.; Bukhave, K. A lactic acid-fermented oat gruel increases non-haem iron absorption from a phytate-rich meal in healthy women of childbearing age. *Br. J. Nutr.* **2006**, *96*, 80–85. [CrossRef] [PubMed]

137. Hallberg, L.; Rossander, L. Absorption of iron from Western-type lunch and dinner meals. *Am. J. Clin. Nutr.* **1982**, *35*, 502–509. [PubMed]

138. Kwak, C.S.; Lee, M.S.; Oh, S.I.; Park, S.C. Discovery of novel sources of vitamin B 12 in traditional korean foods from nutritional surveys of centenarians. *Curr. Gerontol. Geriatr. Res.* **2010**, *2010*, 1–11. [CrossRef] [PubMed]

139. Nieman, D.C. Physical fitness and vegetarian diets: Is there a relation? *Am. J. Clin. Nutr.* **1999**, *70*, 570S–575S. [PubMed]

140. Barr, S.I.; Rideout, C.A. Nutritional considerations for vegetarian athletes. *Nutrition* **2004**, *20*, 696–703. [CrossRef] [PubMed]

141. Venderley, A.M.; Campbell, W.W. Vegetarian diets: Nutritional considerations for athletes. *Sports Med.* **2006**, *36*, 293–305. [CrossRef] [PubMed]

142. Dinu, M.; Abbate, R.; Gensini, G.F.; Casini, A.; Sofi, F. Vegetarian, vegan diets and multiple health outcomes: A systematic review with meta-analysis of observational studies. *Crit. Rev. Food Sci. Nutr.* **2016**. [CrossRef] [PubMed]

143. Craddock, J.C.; Probst, Y.C.; Peoples, G.E. Vegetarian and omnivorous nutrition—Comparing physical performance. *Int. J. Sport Nutr. Exerc. Metab.* **2016**, *26*, 212–220. [CrossRef] [PubMed]

144. Fisak, B.; Peterson, R.D.; Tantleff-Dunn, S.; Molnar, J.M. Challenging previous conceptions of vegetarianism and eating disorders. *Eat. Weight Disord.* **2006**, *11*, 195–200. [CrossRef] [PubMed]

145. Hamerschlag, K. *Meat Eaters Guide to Climate Change and Health*; Environmental Working Group: Washington, DC, USA, 2011; Volume 115.

146. Horgan, G.W.; Perrin, A.; Whybrow, S.; Macdiarmid, J.I. Achieving dietary recommendations and reducing greenhouse gas emissions: Modelling diets to minimise the change from current intakes. *Int. J. Behav. Nutr. Phys. Act.* **2016**, *13*, 46. [CrossRef] [PubMed]

147. Athlete's for Farming. Available online: https://athletesforfarming.com (accessed on 1 January 2016).

148. Mouillé, B.; Charrondière, U.R.; Burlingame, B.; Lutaladio, N. Nutrient Composition of the Potato: Interesting Varieties from Human Nutrition Perspective. Available online: http://www.fao.org/fileadmin/templates/food_composition/documents/upload/Poster_potato_nutrient_comp.pdf (accessed on 15 February 2016).

149. Burlingame, B.; Charrondiere, R.; Mouille, B. Food composition is fundamental to the cross-cutting initiative on biodiversity for food and nutrition. *J. Food Compos. Anal.* **2009**, *22*, 361–365. [CrossRef]

150. Burlingame, B.; Mouillé, B.; Charrondière, R. Nutrients, bioactive non-nutrients and anti-nutrients in potatoes. *J. Food Compos. Anal.* **2009**, *22*, 494–502. [CrossRef]

151. Pinela, J.; Barros, L.; Carvalho, A.M.; Ferreira, I.C. F.R. Nutritional composition and antioxidant activity of four tomato (*Lycopersicon esculentum* L.) farmer' varieties in Northeastern Portugal homegardens. *Food Chem. Toxicol.* **2012**, *50*, 829–834. [CrossRef] [PubMed]

152. Dickerson, G.W. Nutritional Analysis of New Mexico Blue Corn and Dent Corn Kernels. In *Guide H-223,Cooperative Extension Service, College of Agriculture and Home Economics*; New Mexico State University: Las Cruces, NM, USA, 2003; pp. 1–2.

153. Rivera, D.; Obón, C.; Heinrich, M.; Inocencio, C.; Verde, A.; Fajardo, J. Gathered Mediterranean Food Plants—Ethnobotanical Investigations and Historical Development. In *Local Mediterranean Food Plants and Nutraceuticals*; Karger: Basel, Switzerland, 2006; pp. 18–74.

154. Saxe, H.; Larsen, T.M.; Mogensen, L. The global warming potential of two healthy Nordic diets compared with the average Danish diet. *Clim. Chang.* **2013**. [CrossRef]

155. Van Dooren, C.; Marinussen, M.; Blonk, H.; Aiking, H.; Vellinga, P. Exploring dietary guidelines based on ecological and nutritional values: A comparison of six dietary patterns. *Food Policy* **2014**, *44*, 36–46. [CrossRef]

156. Marsh, B.; Curtius, M. Nutritional Weaklings in the Supermarket. Available online: http://www.nytimes.com/interactive/2013/05/26/sunday-review/26corn-ch.html?_r=1&ref=sunday& (accessed on 18 October 2016).

157. The Food And Agriculture Organization. International Network of Food Data Systems (INFOODS): Nutrition and Biodiversity. Available online: www.fao.org/infoods/infoods/food-biodiversity/en/ (accessed on 9 August 2016).

158. Bioversity International Annual Report, 2013. Available online: http://www.bioversityinternational.org/e-library/publications/detail/bioversity-international-annual-report-2013/ (accessed on 8 December 2016).

159. Storkey, J.; Meyer, S.; Still, K.S.; Leuschner, C. The impact of agricultural intensification and land-use change on the European arable flora. *Proc. R. Soc. Lond. B Biol. Sci.* **2012**, *279*, 1421–1429. [CrossRef] [PubMed]

160. Fanzo, J.; Hünter, D.; Borelli, T.; Mattei, F. *Diversifying Food and Diets: Using Agricultural Biodiversity to Improve Nutrition and Health (Issues in Agricultural Biodiversity)*; Routledge: Halewood, UK, 2013.

161. Antibiotic/Antimicrobial Resistance. Available online: https://www.cdc.gov/drugresistance/ (accessed on 30 December 2016).

162. Broom, D.M.; Galindo, F.A.; Murgueitio, E. Sustainable, efficient livestock production with high biodiversity and good welfare for animals. *Proc. R. Soc. B Biol. Sci.* **2013**. [CrossRef] [PubMed]

163. Calder, P.C. Omega-3 polyunsaturated fatty acids and inflammatory processes: Nutrition or pharmacology? *Br. J. Clin. Pharmacol.* **2013**, *75*, 645–662. [CrossRef] [PubMed]

164. The Food and Agriculture Organization/World Health Organization. *Report of the joint FAO/WHO Expert Consultation on the Risks and Benefits of Fish Consumption*; FAO: Rome, Italy; World Health Organization: Geneva, Switzerland, 2011; p. 50.

165. Mickleborough, T.D. Omega-3 polyunsaturated fatty acids in physical performance optimization. *Int. J. Sport Nutr. Exerc. Metab.* **2013**, *23*, 83–96. [CrossRef] [PubMed]

166. Usydus, Z.; Szlinder-Richert, J. Functional properties of fish and fish products: A review. *Int. J. Food Prop.* **2012**, *15*, 823–846. [CrossRef]

167. Nichols, P.D.; Glencross, B.; Petrie, J.R.; Singh, S.P. Readily available sources of long-chain omega-3 oils: Is farmed Australian seafood a better source of the good oil than wild-caught seafood? *Nutrients* **2014**, *6*, 1063–1079. [CrossRef] [PubMed]

168. Lundebye, A.; Lock, E.; Rasinger, J.D.; Jakob, O.; Hannisdal, R.; Karlsbakk, E.; Wennevik, V.; Madhun, A.S.; Madsen, L.; Gra, E.; et al. Lower levels of persistent organic pollutants, metals and the marine omega 3-fatty acid DHA in farmed compared to wild Atlantic salmon (Salmo salar). *Environ. Res.* **2017**, *155*, 49–59. [CrossRef] [PubMed]

169. Nøstbakken, O.J.; Hove, H.T.; Duinker, A.; Lundebye, A.-K.; Berntssen, M.H.G.; Hannisdal, R.; Lunestad, B.T.; Maage, A.; Madsen, L.; Torstensen, B.E.; et al. Contaminant levels in Norwegian farmed Atlantic salmon (Salmo salar) in the 13-year period from 1999 to 2011. *Environ. Int.* **2015**, *74*, 274–280. [CrossRef] [PubMed]

170. Seierstad, S.L.; Seljeflot, I.; Johansen, O.; Hansen, R.; Haugen, M.; Rosenlund, G.; Froyland, L.; Arnesen, H. Dietary intake of differently fed salmon; the influence on markers of human atherosclerosis. *Eur. J. Clin. Investig.* **2005**, *35*, 52–59. [CrossRef] [PubMed]

171. Sprague, M.; Dick, J.R.; Tocher, D.R. Impact of sustainable feeds on omega-3 long-chain fatty acid levels in farmed Atlantic salmon, 2006–2015. *Sci. Rep.* **2016**, *6*, 1–9. [CrossRef] [PubMed]

172. Rosenlund, G.; Torstensen, B.E.; Stubhaug, I.; Usman, N.; Sissener, N.H. Atlantic salmon require long-chain n-3 fatty acids for optimal growth throughout the seawater period. *J. Nutr. Sci.* **2016**, *5*, e19. [CrossRef] [PubMed]

173. National Oceanic and Atmospheric Administration Fisheries. Status of Stocks 2015. Annual Report to Congress on the Status of U.S. Fisheries. Available online: http://www.nmfs.noaa.gov/sfa/fisheries_eco/status_of_fisheries/archive/2015/2015_status_of_stocks_updated.pdf (accessed on 15 February 2017).

174. Fry, J.P.; Love, D.C.; MacDonald, G.K.; West, P.C.; Engstrom, P.M.; Nachman, K.E.; Lawrence, R.S. Environmental health impacts of feeding crops to farmed fish. *Environ. Int.* **2016**, *91*, 201–214. [CrossRef] [PubMed]

175. Palupi, E.; Jayanegara, A.; Ploeger, A.; Kahl, J. Comparison of nutritional quality between conventional and organic dairy products: A meta-analysis. *J. Sci. Food Agric.* **2012**, *92*, 2774–2781. [CrossRef] [PubMed]

176. Lucey, J.A. Raw Milk Consumption: Risks and Benefits. *Nutr. Today* **2015**, *50*, 189–193. [CrossRef] [PubMed]

177. Van Neerven, R.J.J.; Knol, E.F.; Heck, J.M.L.; Savelkoul, H.F.J. Which factors in raw cow's milk contribute to protection against allergies? *J. Allergy Clin. Immunol.* **2012**, *130*, 853–858. [CrossRef] [PubMed]

178. Worthington, V. Nutritional quality of organic versus conventional fruits, vegetables, and grains. *J. Altern. Complement. Med.* **2001**, *7*, 161–173. [CrossRef] [PubMed]

179. Barański, M.; Średnicka-Tober, D.; Volakakis, N.; Seal, C.; Sanderson, R.; Stewart, G.B.; Benbrook, C.; Biavati, B.; Markellou, E.; Giotis, C.; et al. Higher antioxidant and lower cadmium concentrations and lower incidence of pesticide residues in organically grown crops: A systematic literature review and meta-analyses. *Br. J. Nutr.* **2014**, *112*, 794–811. [CrossRef] [PubMed]

180. Di Renzo, L.; Di Pierro, D.; Bigioni, M.; Sodi, V.; Galvano, F.; Cianci, R.; La Fauci, L.; De Lorenzo, A. Is antioxidant plasma status in humans a consequence of the antioxidant food content influence? *Eur. Rev. Med. Pharmacol. Sci.* **2007**, *11*, 185–192. [PubMed]

181. Wunderlich, S.M.; Feldman, C.; Kane, S.; Hazhin, T. Nutritional quality of organic, conventional, and seasonally grown broccoli using vitamin C as a marker. *Int. J. Food Sci. Nutr.* **2008**, *59*, 34–45. [CrossRef] [PubMed]

182. Stein, M.M.; Hrusch, C.L.; Gozdz, J.; Igartua, C.; Pivniouk, V.; Murray, E.S.; Ledford, G.J.; Marques dos Santos, M.; Anderson, R.L.; Metwali, N.; et al. Innate Immunity and Asthma Risk in Amish and Hutterite Farm Children. *N. Engl. J. Med.* **2016**, *375*, 411–421. [CrossRef] [PubMed]

183. Jabr, F. Bread Is Broken. Available online: http://www.nytimes.com/2015/11/01/magazine/bread-is-broken.html (accessed on 17 October 2016).

184. Van den Broeck, H.; de Jong, H.C.; Salentijn, E.M.; Dekking, L.; Bosch, D.; Hamer, R.J.; Gilissen, L.J.; van der Meer, I.M.; Smulders, M.J. Presence of celiac disease epitopes in modern and old hexaploid wheat varieties: wheat breeding may have contributed to increased prevalence of celiac disease. *Theory Appl. Genet.* **2010**, *121*, 1527–1539. [CrossRef] [PubMed]

185. Lis, D.; Stellingwerff, T.; Shing, C.M.; Ahuja K, D.K.; Fell, J. Exploring the popularity, experiences and beliefs surrounding gluten-free diets in non-coeliac athletes. *Int. J. Sport Nutr. Exerc. Metab.* **2014**. [CrossRef]

186. Lis, D.; Stellingwerff, T.; Kitic, C.M.; Ahuja, K.D.K.; Fell, J. No effects of a short-term gluten-free diet on performance in nonceliac athletes. *Med. Sci. Sports Exerc.* **2015**, *47*, 2563–2570. [CrossRef] [PubMed]

187. Aune, D.; Keum, N.; Giovannucci, E.; Fadnes, L.T.; Boffetta, P.; Greenwood, D.C.; Tonstad, S.; Vatten, L.J.; Riboli, E.; Norat, T. Whole grain consumption and risk of cardiovascular disease, cancer, and all cause and cause specific mortality: Systematic review and dose-response meta-analysis of prospective studies. *BMJ* **2016**, *353*, i2716. [CrossRef] [PubMed]

188. Vaher, M.; Matso, K.; Levandi, T.; Helmja, K.; Kaljurand, M. Phenolic compounds and the antioxidant activity of the bran, flour and whole grain of different wheat varieties. *Procedia Chem.* **2010**, *2*, 76–82. [CrossRef]

189. Fan, M.S.; Zhao, F.J.; Poulton, P.R.; McGrath, S.P. Historical changes in the concentrations of selenium in soil and wheat grain from the Broadbalk experiment over the last 160 years. *Sci. Total Environ.* **2008**, *389*, 532–538. [CrossRef] [PubMed]

190. Dinelli, G.; Segura-Carretero, A.; Di Silvestro, R.; Marotti, I.; Arráez-Román, D.; Benedettelli, S.; Ghiselli, L.; Fernadez-Gutierrez, A. Profiles of phenolic compounds in modern and old common wheat varieties determined by liquid chromatography coupled with time-of-flight mass spectrometry. *J. Chromatogr. A* **2011**, *1218*, 7670–7681. [CrossRef] [PubMed]

191. Fan, M.S.; Zhao, F.J.; Fairweather-Tait, S.J.; Poulton, P.R.; Dunham, S.J.; McGrath, S.P. Evidence of decreasing mineral density in wheat grain over the last 160 years. *J. Trace Elem. Med. Biol.* **2008**, *22*, 315–324. [CrossRef] [PubMed]

192. De Lorgeril, M.; Salen, P. Gluten and wheat intolerance today: are modern wheat strains involved? *Int. J. Food Sci. Nutr.* **2014**, *65*, 963–7486. [CrossRef] [PubMed]

193. Hidalgo, A.; Brandolini, A.; Pompei, C.; Piscozzi, R. Carotenoids and tocols of einkorn wheat (*Triticum monococcum* ssp. *monococcum* L.). *J. Cereal Sci.* **2006**, *44*, 182–193. [CrossRef]

194. Lachman, J.; Orsák, M.; Pivec, V.; Jírů, K. Antioxidant activity of grain of einkorn (*Triticum mono-coccum* L.), emmer (*Triticum dicoccum* schuebl (schrank)) and spring wheat (*Triticum aestivum* L.) varieties. *Plant Soil Environ.* **2012**, *58*, 15–21.

195. Hussain, A.; Larsson, H.; Kuktaite, R.; Johansson, E. Mineral composition of organically grown wheat genotypes: Contribution to daily minerals intake. *Int. J. Environ. Res. Public Health* **2010**, *7*, 3442–3456. [CrossRef] [PubMed]

196. Sofi, F.; Whittaker, A.; Cesari, F.; Gori, A.M.; Fiorillo, C.; Becatti, M.; Marotti, I.; Dinelli, G.; Casini, A.; Abbate, R.; et al. Characterization of Khorasan wheat (Kamut) and impact of a replacement diet on cardiovascular risk factors: Cross-over dietary intervention study. *Eur. J. Clin. Nutr.* **2013**, *67*, 190–195. [CrossRef] [PubMed]

197. Molberg, O.; Uhlen, A.K.; Jensen, T.; Flaete, N.S.; Fleckenstein, B.; Arentz-Hansen, H.; Raki, M.; Lundin, K.E.A.; Sollid, L.M. Mapping of gluten T-cell epitopes in the bread wheat ancestors: Implications for celiac disease. *Gastroenterology* **2005**, *128*, 393–401. [CrossRef] [PubMed]

198. Rogosa, E. *Restoring Heritage Grains*; Chelsea Green Publishing: White River Junction, VT, USA, 2016.

199. Pizzuti, D.; Buda, A.; D'Odorico, A.; D'Incà, R.; Chiarelli, S.; Curioni, A.; Martines, D. Lack of intestinal mucosal toxicity of *Triticum monococcum* in celiac disease patients. *Scand. J. Gastroenterol.* **2006**, *41*, 1305–1311. [CrossRef] [PubMed]

200. Zanini, B.; Petroboni, B.; Not, T.; Di Toro, N.; Villanacci, V.; Lanzarotto, F.; Pogna, N.; Ricci, C.; Lanzini, A. Search for atoxic cereals: A single blind, cross-over study on the safety of a single dose of Triticum monococcum, in patients with celiac disease. *BMC Gastroenterol.* **2013**, *13*, 92. [CrossRef] [PubMed]

201. Vaccino, P.; Becker, H.-A.; Brandolini, A.; Salamini, F.; Kilian, B. A catalogue of Triticum monococcum genes encoding toxic and immunogenic peptides for celiac disease patients. *Mol. Genet. Genomics* **2009**, *281*, 289–300. [CrossRef] [PubMed]

202. Kucek, L.K.; Veenstra, L.D.; Amnuaycheewa, P.; Sorrells, M.E. A grounded guide to gluten: How modern genotypes and processing impact wheat sensitivity. *Compr. Rev. Food Sci. Food Saf.* **2015**, *14*, 285–302. [CrossRef]

203. Björck, I.; Elmståhl, H.L. The glycaemic index: Importance of dietary fibre and other food properties. *Proc. Nutr. Soc.* **2003**, *62*, 201–206. [CrossRef] [PubMed]

204. Lindenmeier, M.; Hofmann, T. Influence of baking conditions and precursor supplementation on the amounts of the antioxidant pronyl-L-lysine in bakery products. *J. Agric. Food Chem.* **2004**, *52*, 350–354. [CrossRef] [PubMed]

205. Stenman, S.M.; Venäläinen, J.I.; Lindfors, K.; Auriola, S.; Mauriala, T.; Kaukovirta-Norja, A.; Jantunen, A.; Laurila, K.; Qiao, S.-W.; Sollid, L.M.; et al. Enzymatic detoxification of gluten by germinating wheat proteases: Implications for new treatment of celiac disease. *Ann. Med.* **2009**, *41*, 390–400. [CrossRef] [PubMed]

206. Gallo, G.; De Angelis, M.; McSweeney, P.L.H.; Corbo, M.R.; Gobbetti, M. Partial purification and characterization of an X-prolyl dipeptidyl aminopeptidase from Lactobacillus sanfranciscensis CB1. *Food Chem.* **2005**, *91*, 535–544. [CrossRef]

207. Greco, L.; Gobbetti, M.; Auricchio, R.; Di Mase, R.; Landolfo, F.; Paparo, F.; Di Cagno, R.; De Angelis, M.; Rizzello, C.G.; Cassone, A.; et al. Safety for patients with celiac disease of baked goods made of wheat flour hydrolyzed during food processing. *Clin. Gastroenterol. Hepatol.* **2011**, *9*, 24–29. [CrossRef] [PubMed]

208. Engström, N.; Sandberg, A.S.; Scheers, N. Sourdough fermentation of wheat flour does not prevent the interaction of transglutaminase 2 with α2-gliadin or gluten. *Nutrients* **2015**, *7*, 2134–2144. [CrossRef] [PubMed]

209. Kurppa, K.; Collin, P.; Viljamaa, M.; Haimila, K.; Saavalainen, P.; Partanen, J.; Laurila, K.; Huhtala, H.; Paasikivi, K.; Mäki, M.; Kaukinen, K. Diagnosing mild enteropathy celiac disease: A randomized, controlled clinical study. *Gastroenterology* **2009**, *136*, 816–823. [CrossRef] [PubMed]

210. Catassi, C.; Bai, C.; Bonaz, B.; Bouma, G.; Calabrò, A.; Carroccio, A.; Castillejo, G.; Ciacci, C.; Cristofori, F.; Dolinsek, J.; et al. Non-celiac gluten sensitivity: The new frontier of gluten related disorders. *Nutrients* **2013**, *5*, 3839–3853. [CrossRef] [PubMed]

211. Biesiekierski, J.; Peters, S.; Newnham, E.; Rosella, O.; Muir, J.; Gibson, P. No effects of gluten in patients with self-reported non-celiac gluten sensitivity after dietary reduction of fermentable, poorly absorbed, short-chain carbohydartes. *Gastroenterology* **2013**, *145*, 320–328. [CrossRef] [PubMed]

212. Junker, Y.; Zeissig, S.; Kim, S.-J.; Barisani, D.; Wieser, H.; Leffler, D.A.; Zevallos, V.; Libermann, T.A.; Dillon, S.; Freitag, T.L.; et al. Wheat amylase trypsin inhibitors drive intestinal inflammation via activation of toll-like receptor 4. *J. Exp. Med.* **2012**, *209*, 2395–2408. [CrossRef] [PubMed]

213. Lis, D.; Ahuja, K.D.K.; Stellingwerff, T.; Kitic, C.M.; Fell, J. Case study: Utilizing a low FODMAP diet to combat exercise-induced gastrointestinal symptoms. *Int. J. Sport. Nutr. Exerc. Metab.* **2016**, *26*, 481–487. [CrossRef] [PubMed]

214. McKenzie, Y.; Bowyer, R.; Leach, H.; Guila, P.; Horobin, J.; O'Sullivan, N.; Pettit, C.; Reeves, L.; Seamark, L.; Williams, M.; et al. British Dietetic Association systematic review and evidence-based practice guidelines for the dietary management of irritable bowel syndrome in adults (2016 update). *J. Hum. Nutr. Diet.* **2016**, *29*, 549–575. [CrossRef] [PubMed]

215. Burke, L.M.; Hawley, J.A.; Wong, S.H.S.; Jeukendrup, A.E. Carbohydrates for training and competition. *J. Sports Sci.* **2011**, *29*, S17–S27. [CrossRef] [PubMed]

216. The Land Institute Kernza Grain: Toward a Perennial Agriculture. Available online: https://landinstitute.org/our-work/perennial-crops/kernza/ (accessed on 10 September 2016).

217. Vidgen, H.A.; Gallegos, D. Defining food literacy and its components. *Appetite* **2014**, *76*, 50–59. [CrossRef] [PubMed]

218. Gill, M.; Stott, R. Health professionals must act to tackle climate change. *Lancet* **2009**, *374*, 1953–1955. [CrossRef]

219. Wiek, A.; Withycombe, L.; Redman, C.L. Key competencies in sustainability: A reference framework for academic program development. *Sustain. Sci.* **2011**, *6*, 203–218. [CrossRef]

220. Wilkins, J. Eating right here: Moving from consumer to food citizen. Agriculture and Human values. *Agric. Hum. Values* **2005**, 22–269.

221. O'Kane, G. A moveable feast: Exploring barriers and enablers to food citizenship. *Appetite* **2016**, *105*, 674–687. [CrossRef] [PubMed]

222. Feldmann, C.; Hamm, U. Consumers' perceptions and preferences for local food: A review. *Food Qual. Prefer.* **2015**, *40*, 152–164. [CrossRef]

223. Brownlee, M. *The Local Food Revolution: How Humanity Will Feed Itself in Uncertain Times*; North Atlantic Books: Berkley, CA, USA, 2016.

224. Fung, T.T.; Long, M.W.; Hung, P.; Cheung, L.W.Y. An expanded model for mindful eating for health promotion and sustainability: Issues and challenges for dietetics practice. *J. Acad. Nutr. Diet.* **2016**, *116*, 1081–1086. [CrossRef] [PubMed]

225. Feenstra, G. Creating space for sustainable food systems: Lessons from the field. *Agric. Hum. Values* **2002**, *19*, 99–106. [CrossRef]

226. Environmental Working Group (WEG's) 2016 Shopper's Guide to Pesticides in Produce. Available online: https://www.ewg.org/foodnews/dirty_dozen_list.php (accessed on 16 August 2016).

227. Local Harvest. Available online: http://www.localharvest.org (accessed on 10 May 2016).

228. Bøhn, T.; Cuhra, M.; Traavik, T.; Sanden, M.; Fagan, J.; Primicerio, R. Compositional differences in soybeans on the market: Glyphosate accumulates in Roundup Ready GM soybeans. *Food Chem.* **2014**, *153*, 207–215. [CrossRef] [PubMed]

229. Shokryazdan, P.; Faseleh Jahromi, M.; Navidshad, B.; Liang, J.B. Effects of prebiotics on immune system and cytokine expression. *Med. Microbiol. Immunol.* **2017**, *206*, 1–9. [CrossRef] [PubMed]

230. Martinez, R.C.R.; Bedani, R.; Saad, S.M.I. Scientific evidence for health effects attributed to the consumption of probiotics and prebiotics: An update for current perspectives and future challenges. *Br. J. Nutr.* **2015**, *114*, 1993–2015. [CrossRef] [PubMed]

231. Chan, K.M.A.; Balvanera, P.; Benessaiah, K.; Chapman, M.; Díaz, S.; Gómez-Baggethun, E.; Gould, R.; Hannahs, N.; Jax, K.; Klain, S.; et al. Opinion: Why protect nature? Rethinking values and the environment. *Proc. Natl. Acad. Sci. USA* **2016**, *113*, 1462–1465. [CrossRef] [PubMed]

232. Meyer, N.L. The Meaning of Local Food in Education. Available online: http://www.localfoodshift.pub/the-meaning-of-local-food-in-education/ (accessed on 7 October 2016).

233. The Flying Carrot. Available online: http://www.uccs.edu/diningservices/swell/the-flying-carrot.html (accessed on 20 October 2016).

234. Borderlands Food Bank. Available online: http://www.borderlandfoodbank.org (accessed on 10 June 2016).

235. One World Café. Available online: http://oneworld-cafe.com/ (accessed on 28 September 2016).

236. Slow Food USA. Available online: www.slowfoodusa.com (accessed on 3 July 2016).

237. Edible Communities. Available online: http://www.ediblecommunities.com/ (accessed on 10 October 2016).

238. Green Sports Alliance. Leveraging the Cultural & Market Influence of Sports to Promote Healthy, Sustainable Communities Where We Live & Play. Available online: http://greensportsalliance.org/ (accessed on 18 August 2016).

239. Food Vision for the London 2012 Olympic Games and Paralympic Games. Available online: http://learninglegacy.independent.gov.uk/documents/pdfs/sustainability/cp-london-2012-food-vision.pdf (accessed on 18 November 2016).

240. Diagnostic Analysis for the Supply of Healthy and Sustainable Food for the 2016 Rio Olympic and Paralympic Games. Available online: www.riofoodvision.org (accessed on 7 June 2015).

241. Pelly, F.; Meyer, N.L.; Pearce, J.; Burkhart, S.J.; Burke, L.M. Evaluation of food provision and nutrition support at the London 2012 Olympic Games: The Opinion of sports nutrition experts. *Int. J. Sport Nutr. Exerc. Metab.* **2014**, *24*, 674–683. [CrossRef] [PubMed]

242. Professionals in Nutrition for Exercise and Sport. Available online: www.pinesnutrition.org (accessed on 7 March 2016).

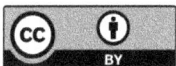

nutrients

MDPI

Article

Effects of Carbohydrate and Glutamine Supplementation on Oral Mucosa Immunity after Strenuous Exercise at High Altitude: A Double-Blind Randomized Trial

Aline Venticinque Caris [1], Edgar Tavares Da Silva [2], Samile Amorim Dos Santos [2], Sergio Tufik [2] and Ronaldo Vagner Thomatieli Dos Santos [2,*]

[1]   Department of Psychobiology, Universidade Federal de São Paulo, São Paulo 04032-020, Brazil;
      alinecaris@hotmail.com
[2]   Department of Bioscience, Universidade Federal de São Paulo, Santos 11015-020, Brazil;
      edgartavares@uol.com.br (E.T.D.S.); samile.unifesp@gmail.com (S.A.D.S.); sergiotufik@zipmail.com.br (S.T.)
*   Correspondence: ronaldo.thomatieli@unifesp.br; Tel./Fax: +55-133-870-3700

Received: 29 July 2016; Accepted: 6 March 2017; Published: 3 July 2017

Abstract: This study analyzed the effects of carbohydrate and glutamine supplementation on salivary immunity after exercise at a simulated altitude of 4500 m. Fifteen volunteers performed exercise of 70% of VO_{2peak} until exhaustion and were divided into three groups: hypoxia placebo, hypoxia 8% maltodextrin (200 mL/20 min), and hypoxia after six days glutamine (20 g/day) and 8% maltodextrin (200 mL/20 min). All procedures were randomized and double-blind. Saliva was collected at rest (basal), before exercise (pre-exercise), immediately after exercise (post-exercise), and two hours after exercise. Analysis of Variance (ANOVA) for repeated measures and Tukey post hoc test were performed. Statistical significance was set at $p < 0.05$. $SaO_2\%$ reduced when comparing baseline vs. pre-exercise, post-exercise, and after recovery for all three groups. There was also a reduction of $SaO_2\%$ in pre-exercise vs. post-exercise for the hypoxia group and an increase was observed in pre-exercise vs. recovery for both supplementation groups, and between post-exercise and for the three groups studied. There was an increase of salivary flow in post-exercise vs. recovery in Hypoxia + Carbohydrate group. Immunoglobulin A (IgA) decreased from baseline vs. post-exercise for Hypoxia + Glutamine group. Interleukin 10 (IL-10) increased from post-exercise vs. after recovery in Hypoxia + Carbohydrate group. Reduction of tumor necrosis factor alpha (TNF-α) was observed from baseline vs. post-exercise and after recovery for the Hypoxia + Carbohydrate group; a lower concentration was observed in pre-exercise vs. post-exercise and recovery. TNF-α had a reduction from baseline vs. post-exercise for both supplementation groups, and a lower secretion between baseline vs. recovery, and pre-exercise vs. post-exercise for Hypoxia + Carbohydrate group. Five hours of hypoxia and exercise did not change IgA. Carbohydrates, with greater efficiency than glutamine, induced anti-inflammatory responses.

Keywords: supplementation; carbohydrate; hypoxia; physical exercise; glutamine; high altitude; innate immune response; oral mucosal immunity

1. Introduction

Mucosal immunity, particularly in saliva, is considered the first line of defense against pathogens, because it contains numerous protective proteins. Some of these, such as salivary immunoglobulins (Igs), are involved in innate and adaptive immune responses [1]. In addition to Igs, there are also cytokines, such as interleukin (IL)-1ß, tumor necrosis factor (TNF)-α, and IL-6, that are used to assess the response to acute stress, stimulating immune cells, and modulating local inflammation [2,3].

Recent data suggest that exposure to hypoxia may modulate important aspects of innate immune responses [4], inflammation [5–7], and metabolism [8,9]. However, this issue has not been fully clarified, and only a few studies have been conducted under hypoxic conditions with the specific objective of investigating different immune/inflammatory parameters among humans [10].

It is known that exercise influences mucosal immunity, but the nature of this effect has not reached a consensus yet [11,12]. Some studies show that acute moderate-intensity exercise can result in a reduction of immunoglobulin A (IgA) concentration post-exercise; some do not describe any changes, while others report an increased concentration of IgA [13]. IgA is the most abundant protein in the antibacterial mucosal and it is considered the best indicator of oral mucosal immunity. Intense exercise causes a reduction in IgA levels [13] and increases inInterleukin-1 ß (IL-1ß), TNF-α, and IL-6 concentrations [2], resulting in poor performance of the immune function of the mucous membranes, increasing the incidence of upper respiratory tract infections (URTIs), and the emergence of other opportunistic diseases [14].

Thus, it is observed that exercise may modulate mucosal immunity under normal atmospheric pressure, but when exercise takes place in high altitude, it becomes a greater challenge for the body, since hypoxia and exercise are considered stressors that can act together. Evidence suggests that this combination may result in a more pronounced impact on the immune function of the oral mucosa and may trigger an intense immunosuppression [15,16].

On the other hand, studies have analyzed nutritional strategies that are efficient at sea level [17–20] to help mitigate the effects of exercise at altitude, providing better performance and prevention of infections [21].

When considering the anti-inflammatory effect of glutamine on stress factors, like exercise, harsh environments [21], and diseases (cancer, sepsis, burns, trauma) [22], this supplement can regress inflammation even during long-term exercises performed at sea level. Therefore, glutamine supplements have been shown to decrease the number of URTIs in athletes by promoting the production of IgA [23] and maintaining the balance of pro/anti-inflammatory markers [24].

On the other hand, carbohydrate supplements are used as a strategy to reduce the effects caused by the exercise on the immune system [25], and also contribute to improve performance. The intake of carbohydrate can significantly alter the immune response to intense exercise by attenuating the proliferation of lymphocytes, and by modulating cytokine pro/anti-inflammatory markers [26].

It has been shown that carbohydrate and glutamine supplements can be used isolated as a strategy to reverse the deteriorating mucosal immunity after strenuous exercise at sea level [23,27], however, the combined effect of both supplements is still not clarified.

In this context, we propose that the nutritional strategies used to prevent immune suppression after strenuous exercise at sea level can also be effective in hypoxic conditions. Thus, the objective of this study was to analyze the effect of carbohydrate and glutamine supplementation on oral mucosal immunity after exercise at a simulated altitude of 4500 m.

2. Methods

2.1. Experimental Design

This was a randomized, double-blind, placebo controlled crossover study and the sample size was determined using a statistics website from the Australian government [28]. After starting the clinical study, there were no changes in the methodology.

2.2. Participants

The sample of this study included 15 healthy male volunteers (women were not included in the sample to avoid the possible influences of female sex hormones) that were physically active (performing physical activity at least 3x/week for 90 min each session) with the following physiological and anthropometric characteristics: age: 26.4 ± 3.9 years old; body mass: 73.7 ± 8.7 kg;

height: 1.76 ± 0.02 m; Body Mass Index (BMI): 23.7 ± 2.5 kg/m^2; VO$_{2\text{peak}}$: 50.6 ± 5.4 mL/kg/min; maximum heart rate: 189.9 ± 8.2 beats per minute. Exclusion criteria were defined as: health problems; alterations in the electrocardiogram (ECG) at rest, stress and clinical evaluations, smoking, use of drugs, alcohol abuse, use of any medication that could interfere with the study results, and exposure to hypoxia during the previous six months. Figure 1 is a CONSORT flow diagram [29], explaining the stages of the randomized study. Initially, 60 volunteers were recruited to take part in the study, however 37 were eliminated based on the exclusion criteria. Of the 23 volunteers remaining, only 15 completed all the requirements.

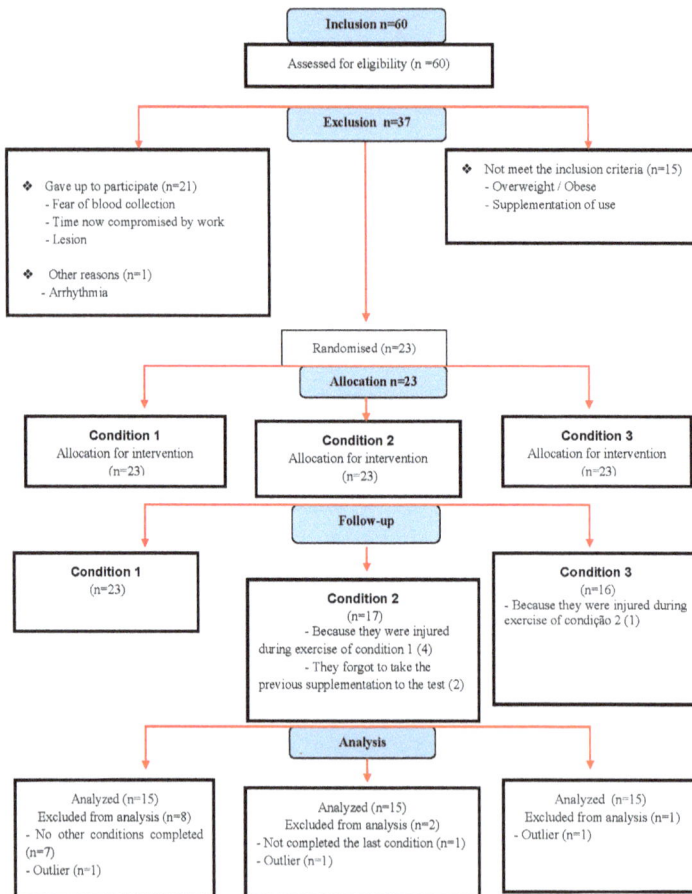

Figure 1. CONSORT flow diagram 2010.

Data were collected at the Interdisciplinary Laboratory for Exercise Physiology (LAIFE), Federal University of São Paulo (UNIFESP), São Paulo, between December 2014 and July 2015. The study procedures were approved by the Research Ethics Committee of the Federal University of São Paulo (Ethical approval code: 69 839/2014) on 4 March 2015 and are in accordance with the guidelines established by Resolution #466 of the Ministry of Health and the International Declaration of Helsinki.

2.3. Intervention

The participants came to the laboratory four times, with an interval of six days between each visit. During the first session, relevant information was presented, which consisted of objectives, procedures, guidelines for not taking supplements, and only low-intensity exercise. The participants were randomized into three groups [30] and were asked to sign a consent form. Next, they performed resting ECG, stress and cardiopulmonary exercise tests. The blinding process occurred in order to offer supplements and placebos that had the same characteristics of color, consistency, smell, taste, and presentation. An individual, oblivious of the study, was responsible for delivering the supplements to the participants every week, so the researches had no contact with the supplements. During the next three visits, the participants performed three random, blinded exercise sessions:

1. Group Hypoxia (Exercise + Altitude + Placebo): Participants consumed glutamine placebo supplements during the six days prior to the test (10 g corn starch + 10 g lactose), taken in the evening. During test day, they performed an exercise session at 70% of VO_{2peak} at a simulated altitude of 4500 m and were given a carbohydrate placebo supplement (Crystal Light®—Kraft Foods, Inc. strawberry, Chicago, IL, USA), 200 mL every 20 min during exercise and during recovery for two hours.

2. Group Hypoxia + CHO (Exercise + Altitude + Carbohydrate): Participants consumed glutamine placebo supplements during the six days prior to the test (10 g corn starch + 10 g lactose) taken in the evening. During test day, they performed an exercise session at 70% of VO_{2peak} at a simulated altitude of 4500 m, and were given carbohydrate supplements (Maltodextrin strawberry flavor—Probiótica®—Laboratories, Embu das Artes, São Paulo, Brazil), 200 mL at a concentration of 8% every 20 min during exercise and during recovery for two hours.

3. Group Hypoxia + GLN (Exercise + Altitude + Carbohydrate + Glutamine): Participants consumed 20 g of glutamine (Probiótica®—Laboratories, Embu das Artes, São Paulo, Brazil) in the six days prior to the test, between 8:00–10:00 p.m. During test day, they performed an exercise session at 70% of VO_{2peak} at a simulated altitude of 4500 m, and were given carbohydrate supplements (Maltodextrin strawberry flavor—Probiótica®—Laboratories, Embu das Artes, São Paulo, Brazil), 200 mL at a concentration of 8% every 20 min during exercise and during recovery for two hours.

For all exercise sessions, water intake was ad libitum. However, there was no control of the ingested volume.

Determination of VO_{2peak}

To determine the VO_{2peak} in normoxic conditions, a test was performed with progressive intensity on a treadmill (LifeFitness®- 9700HR, Rosemont, IL, USA) with an initial speed of 7 km/h and increase of 1 km/h every minute until exhaustion (defined as the incapacity to keep up with the speed of the treadmill for 15 s or until the volunteer requested to stop the test after being encouraged to continue [31]) The encouragement for the volunteers was similar in all tests and carried out by the same person. During the test, we used a fixed inclination of 1% to simulate the physical stress of field tests [32].

Heart rate was monitored with a Polar Vantage NV watch (*Polar®*, Sark Products, Waltham, MA, USA), blood pressure was monitored by sphygmomanometer and stethoscope, and perceived exertion by the Borg scale (6 to 20) [33]. The respiratory parameters were measured by a gas analyzer (Cosmed Quark PFT model, Albano Laziale, Rome, Italy), pulmonary function (FRC & DLCO, Albano Laziale, Rome, Italy) was analyzed using a facemask (Hans Rudolph Inc., Shawnee, KS, USA). All calibration procedures were performed according to the manufacturer's recommendations.

2.4. Altitude Simulation

A normobaric chamber was used (normobaric chamber CAT—Colorado Altitude Training™/CAT-12 Air Unit®, Lousiville, CO, USA) to simulate an altitude of 4500 m (changing carbon dioxide and oxygen concentrations (equivalent to a barometric pressure of 433 mmHg and a fraction of inspired oxygen of 13.5% O_2)).

2.5. Sessions of Exercise and Recovery

The participants spent the first two hours in the hypoxic chamber at rest and then began to exercise on a treadmill (LifeFitness®- 9700HR, Rosemont, IL, USA) with a fixed inclination of 1% and intensity of 70% of VO_{2peak} until exhaustion or up to one hour. After exercising, they remained in the chamber for two more hours for recovery. Each test was followed by six days of rest, which was considered long enough to eliminate the effects of hypoxia [34] and supplementation [24]. All exercise session were performed after an overnight of fasting to avoid possible influences of diet and to maintain a standardized metabolic condition. Testing began at 7:30 a.m. to avoid circadian influences.

2.6. Hemoglobin O_2 Saturation (SaO_2%)

During all tests, the SaO_2% was monitored by a pulse oximeter on the finger (FingerPulse®, MD300C202 model, Beijing, China) and assessed during four stages with saliva collection.

2.7. Saliva Collection

The saliva samples were collected using the Salivet method (cylindrical roller bearings that absorb saliva during the period of a minute) during four moments: immediately before entering the chamber (baseline), immediately before starting exercise (pre-exercise), immediately after exercise (post-exercise), and after two hours of recovery (after 2:00). After collection, the sample was put into a tube and centrifuged at a speed of $600 \times g$ for 20 min. Then, a clear fluid specimen was obtained and stored frozen ($-80\,^\circ$C) for analysis.

2.8. Determinants in Saliva

IgA was determined by immunoturbidimetric method using Kits from Labtest® (Lagoa Santa, MG, Brazil) and cytokines (TNF-α, IL-6, and IL-10) were determined using Milliplex Kits® (Darmstadt, Germany).

The flow rates of IgA, TNF-α, IL-6, and IL-10 were calculated by multiplying the concentration of each parameter by salivary flow (mL/min) as described by Usui et al. (2011) [2].

2.9. Statistical Analysis

Data normality was verified by the Shapiro-Wilk test. Descriptive analysis consisted of mean and standard error. ANOVA for repeated measures followed by post hoc Tukey test verified the interactions between groups and time, and Cohen's d was calculated to estimate effect size: 0.20–0.30 = small effect size; 0.40–0.70 = medium effect size, and $\geq$0.80 = large effect size. The software Statistics® 7.0 (StatSoft, Inc., Tulsa, OK, USA) was used for the statistical analyzes and the level of significance was set at $p < 0.05$.

3. Results

The results are presented in tables and figures. There was no significant difference between groups Hypoxia, Hypoxia + Carbohydrate, and Hypoxia + Glutamine for SaO_2% (F = 2.2, $p = 0.119$), as shown in Table 1. However, significant differences were observed regarding time (F = 248.5, $p < 0.001$). When comparing the moment of measurement, we found reduction of SaO_2% at baseline versus pre-exercise ($p < 0.001$) and baseline versus post-exercise ($p < 0.001$). Additionally, there was reduction at baseline in relation to after recovery for all three groups ($p < 0.01$). There was also a reduction of SaO_2% in pre-exercise versus post-exercise ($p < 0.001$) for the hypoxia group. However, an increase was observed in pre-exercise compared to recovery for both groups with supplements ($p < 0.001$), and between post-exercise and recovery for all groups ($p < 0.001$). There was significant difference in the interaction between the groups and time (F = 5.5, $p < 0.001$), with an increase in Hypoxia group compared to Hypoxia + Glutamine group in recovery ($p = 0.02$).

Table 1. O_2 saturation percent (SaO$_2$%).

		Condition		
		Hypoxia	**Hypoxia + CHO**	**Hypoxia + GLN**
	Basal	97.13 ± 0.27	97.13 ± 0.21	96.87 ± 0.24
SaO$_2$%	Pre-exercise	85.47 ± 1.35 [A]	82.40 ± 1.23 [A]	84.33 ± 1.01 [A]
	Post-exercise	79.67 ± 1.37 [AB]	81.47 ± 1.02 [A]	81.53 ± 1.43 [A]
	2 h after	85.40 ± 1.00 [AC]	89.33 ± 0.46 [ABC]	90.27 ± 0.55 [ABC*]

The results of SaO$_2$ (%) were described by mean ± Standard Error (SE). The interactions of group versus time was Analysis of Variance (ANOVA) for repeated measures followed by Post hoc of Tukey test. The level of significance was set at $p < 0.05$. $n = 15$ volunteers. [A] statistically significant in relation to basal. [B] statistically significant in relation to pre-exercise. [C] statistically significant in relation to post-exercise. * Statistically significant in relation to hypoxia condition. Hypoxia + CHO = Hypoxia + carbohydrate and hypoxia + GLN = hypoxia + glutamine.

Figure 2 shows results of time to exhaustion. There were no statistical differences regarding time to exhaustion between Hypoxia group (27.6 ± 5.46), Hypoxia + Carbohydrate group (29.2 ± 6.49), and Hypoxia + Glutamine group (23.66 ± 4.95).

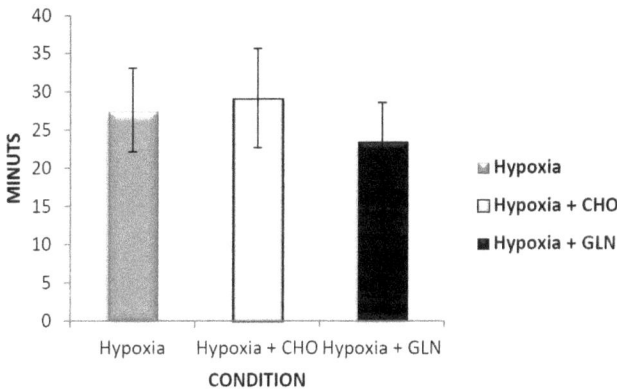

Figure 2. The results of time of exhaustion (min) was described by mean ± Standard Error (SE). The interaction of group versus time was analyzed by Analysis of Variance (ANOVA) for repeated measures followed by post hoc of Tukey test. The level of significance was set at $p < 0.05$. $n = 15$ volunteers. Hypoxia + CHO = Hypoxia + carbohydrate and hypoxia + GLN = hypoxia + glutamine.

Salivary flow (mL/min) results are presented in Table 2. No differences were observed between groups (F = 0.78, $p = 0.925$), but significant difference was found regarding time (F = 7.927, $p < 0.001$). There was an increase of salivary flow post-exercise versus recovery ($p < 0.001$) for the Hypoxia + Carbohydrate group. In the interaction of groups versus time, there was no significant difference (F = 0.863, $p = 0.524$).

Table 2. Salivary Flow.

		Condition		
		Hypoxia	Hypoxia + CHO	Hypoxia + GLN
SaO$_2$%	Basal	0.90 ± 0.11	0.89 ± 0.12	0.89 ± 0.09
	Pre-exercise	0.88 ± 0.11	0.81 ± 0.10	0.76 ± 0.08
	Post-exercise	0.75 ± 0.10	0.76 ± 0.11	0.79 ± 0.13
	2 h after	0.92 ± 0.11	1.04 ± 0.14 [C]	0.85 ± 0.10

The results of Salivary Flow (mL/min) were described by mean ± Standard Errros (SE). The interactions of group versus time was Analays of Variance (ANOVA) for repeated measures followed by Post hoc of Tukey test. The level of significance was set at $p < 0.05$. $n = 15$ volunteers. [C] statistically significant in relation to post-exercise. Hypoxia + CHO = Hypoxia + carbohydrate and hypoxia + GLN = hypoxia + glutamine.

Regarding immunity, we measured IgA and cytokines. The salivary concentration of IgA showed no difference between groups (F = 0.080, $p = 0.923$), time (F = 2.578, $p = 0.057$), and interaction (F = 1.133, $p = 0.347$). However, Cohen's effect size d for the concentration of salivary IgA of pre-exercise versus post-exercise was 0.9 and pre-exercise versus recovery was 2.27 for the Hypoxia group; for the Hypoxia + Carbohydrate group, pre-exercise versus recovery showed effect size d = 1.06, and baseline versus post-exercise d = 1.9. The Hypoxia + Glutamine group showed effect size d = 2.6 for baseline versus recovery (Table 3). The Cohen's effect size d > 0.08 is considered a high effect. IgA secretion rate presented no differences between groups (F = 0.074, $p = 0.929$). However, a significant difference was observed for time (F = 6.462, $p < 0.001$), and a reduction was found from baseline versus post-exercise ($p < 0.001$) for the group Hypoxia + Glutamine. The Hypoxia group showed a reduction of 22.5% post-exercise compared to baseline, with no statistical difference, but Cohen's effect size d of 1.58. There was no interaction of groups versus time (F = 1.262, $p = 0.280$) (Figure 3).

Table 3. IgA, IL-10, TNF-α e IL-6 Concentration

		Condition		
		Hypoxia	Hypoxia + CHO	Hypoxia + GLN
IgA	Basal	48.40 ± 2.07	46.47 ± 1.6	49.80 ± 2.27
	Pre-exercise	49.93 ± 2.21	50.47 ± 3.30	48.40 ± 1.67
	Post-exercise	47.33 ± 3.34	50.80 ± 3.88	45.60 ± 2.02
	2 h after	45.07 ± 1.25	46.73 ± 3.70	47.00 ± 2.60
IL-10	Basal	1.11 ± 0.15	1.22 ± 0.16	1.13 ± 0.17
	Pre-exercise	1.14 ± 0.17	1.27 ± 0.19	1.25 ± 0.20
	Post-exercise	1.08 ± 0.12	1.01 ± 0.13	1.02 ± 0.17
	2 h after	1.11 ± 0.16	1.22 ± 0.15	1.24 ± 0.15
TNF-α	Basal	2.06 ± 0.80	2.07 ± 0.69	3.69 ± 1.79
	Pre-exercise	2.18 ± 0.67	2.30 ± 0.80	2.74 ± 0.75
	Post-exercise	2.02 ± 0.98	1.54 ± 0.62 [AB]	3.06 ± 2.25
	2 h after	1.34 ± 0.44	1.12 ± 0.39 [AB]	2.03 ± 0.73
IL-6	Basal	1.05 ± 0.26	1.50 ± 0.68	1.42 ± 0.58
	Pre-exercise	0.93 ± 0.22	1.57 ± 0.51	1.92 ± 0.63
	Post-exercise	0.97 ± 0.30	1.15 ± 0.36	1.26 ± 0.48
	2 h after	0.82 ± 0.22	1.12 ± 0.37	1.06 ± 0.37

The results of concentration of Immunoglobulin A (IgA) (mg/dL), Interleukin-10 (IL-10), Tumoral Necrosis Factor-α (TNF-α) e Interleukin-6 (IL-6), in pg/mL were described by mean ± Standard Error (SE). The interactions of group versus time was Analysis of Variance (ANOVA) *for repeated measures* followed by *Post hoc of Tukey* test. The level of significance was set at $p < 0.05$. $n = 15$ volunteers. [A] statistically significant in relation to basal. [B] statistically significant in relation to pre-exercise. Hypoxia + CHO = Hypoxia + carbohydrate and hypoxia + GLN = hypoxia + glutamine.

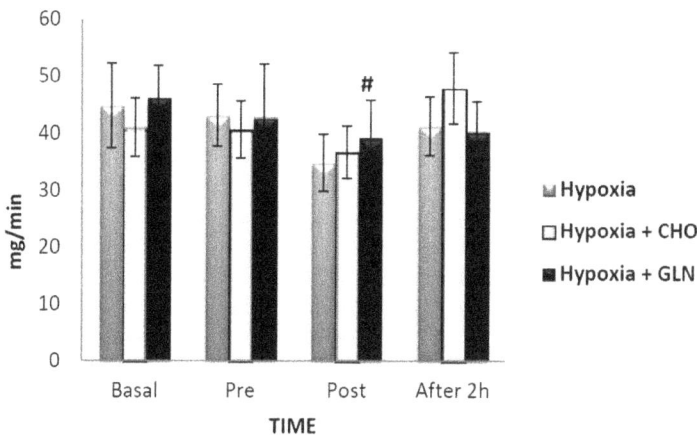

Figure 3. The results of secretory immunoglobulin A (IgA) (mg/min) was described by mean ± Standard Error (SE). The interaction of group versus time was analyzed by Analysis of Variance (ANOVA) for repeated measures followed by post hoc of Tukey test. The level of significance was set at $p < 0.05$. $n = 15$ volunteers. # Statistically significant in relation to basal. Hypoxia + CHO = Hypoxia + carbohydrate and hypoxia + GLN = hypoxia + glutamine.

Results related to pro- and anti-inflammatory cytokines are presented in Table 3. Regarding IL-10 concentration, there was no significant differences between groups ($F = 0.148$, $p = 0.863$), time ($F = 0.893$, $p = 0.447$), and interaction ($F = 0.487$, $p = 0.817$). Cohen's effect size d for all comparisons related to IL-10 was below 0.2. This is considered a small effect size.

Regarding the rate of saliva secretion with IL-10 (Figure 4), there were no significant differences between the three groups ($F = 0.170$, $p = 0.844$), but there was a significant difference in time ($F = 6.119$, $p < 0.001$). Among these differences, there was an increase between post-exercise versus recovery ($p < 0.001$) for Hypoxia + Carbohydrate group. There was no interaction for this parameter ($F = 0.589$, $p = 0.739$).

The salivary concentrations of TNF-α (Table 3) showed no difference between the three groups ($F = 0.48$, $p = 0.624$). Regarding time, a reduction was observed ($F = 15.88$, $p < 0.001$) from baseline versus post-exercise ($p = 0.001$) and after recovery ($p < 0.001$) for the Hypoxia + Carbohydrate group. Similarly, a lower concentration was observed in pre-exercise time versus post-exercise ($p < 0.001$) and recovery ($p < 0.001$). There was no interaction of groups versus time ($F = 1.61$, $p = 0.148$).

When considering the rate of saliva secretion of TNF-α (Figure 5), there was no significant difference between the three groups ($F = 0.33$, $p = 0.723$). However, there were differences in time for TNF-α secretion rate ($F = 14.63$, $p < 0.001$). Among these differences, we observed a reduction from baseline versus post-exercise ($p < 0.001$) for both supplemented groups, and a lower secretion of baseline compared to recovery ($p < 0.001$), and pre-exercise versus post-exercise ($p < 0.001$) for Hypoxia + Carbohydrate group. There was no interaction for this parameter ($F = 3.01$, $p = 0.408$).

Table 3 shows the salivary concentration of IL-6 and Figure 6 shows the salivary secretion rate of IL-6. Table 3 and Figure 4 showed no significant differences between groups ($F = 0.213$, $p = 0.809$) and ($F = 0.138$, $p = 0.872$), time ($F = 3.200$, $p = 0.02$) and ($F = 2.555$, $p = 0.05$), and interaction ($F = 0.726$, $p = 0.629$) and ($F = 0.600$, $p = 0.730$), respectively.

The ratio of salivary secretion rate of TNF-α/IL-10 is presented in Figure 7 and showed differences between groups ($F = 5.2$, $p < 0.001$), with an elevation of Hypoxia + Carbohydrate versus Hypoxia + Glutamine ($p = 0.01$). A significant difference was observed for time ($F = 608.0$, $p < 0.001$), and the reduction was found at baseline versus pre-exercise ($p < 0.001$), post-exercise ($p < 0.001$), and recovery ($p < 0.001$) in the group Hypoxia + Carbohydrate and Hypoxia + Glutamine. There was interaction of groups versus time ($F = 4.6$, $p = 0.001$), including an elevation between baseline in Hypoxia group compared to Hypoxia + Glutamine group ($p = 0.01$), and baseline in Hypoxia + Carbohydrate group compared to Hypoxia and Hypoxia + Glutamine group ($p = 0.01$).

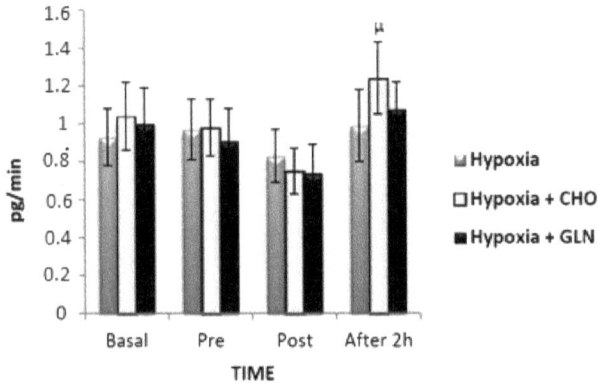

Figure 4. The results of interleukin (IL)-10 secretory (pg/min) was described by mean ± Standard Error (SE). The interaction of group versus time was analyzed by Analysis of Variance (ANOVA) for repeated measures followed by post hoc of Tukey test. The level of significance was set at $p < 0.05$. $n = 15$ volunteers. μ statistically significant in relation to post-exercise. Hypoxia + CHO = Hypoxia + carbohydrate and hypoxia + GLN = hypoxia + glutamine.

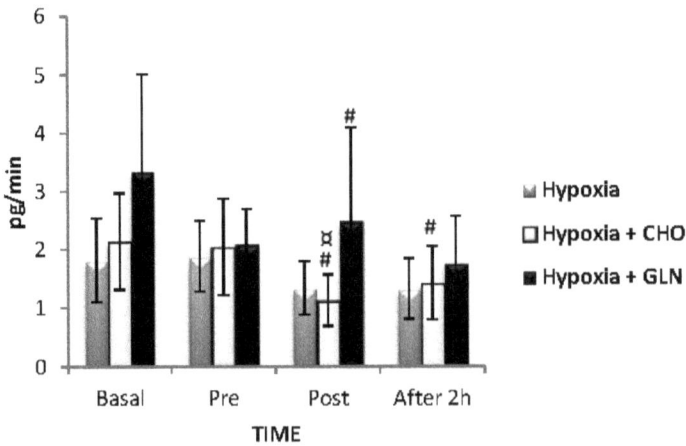

Figure 5. The results of tumor necrosis factor (TNF)-α secretory (pg/min) was described by mean ± Standard Error (SE). The interaction of group versus time was analyzed by Analysis of Variance (ANOVA) for repeated measures followed by post hoc of Tukey test. The level of significance was set at $p < 0.05$. $n = 15$ volunteers. # Different in relation toBasal. ¤ Statistically significant in relation to pre-exercise. Hypoxia + CHO = Hypoxia + carbohydrate and hypoxia + GLN = hypoxia + glutamine.

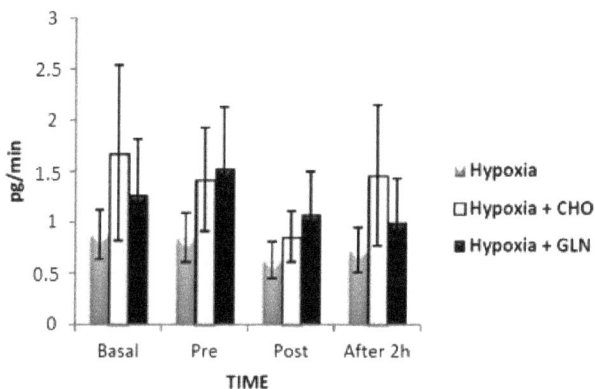

Figure 6. The results of IL-6 secretory (pg/min) was described by mean ± Standard Error (SE). The interaction of group versus time was analyzed by Analysis of Variance (ANOVA) for repeated measures followed by post hoc of Tukey test. The level of significance was set at $p < 0.05$. $n = 15$ volunteers. Hypoxia + CHO = Hypoxia + carbohydrate and hypoxia + GLN = hypoxia + glutamine.

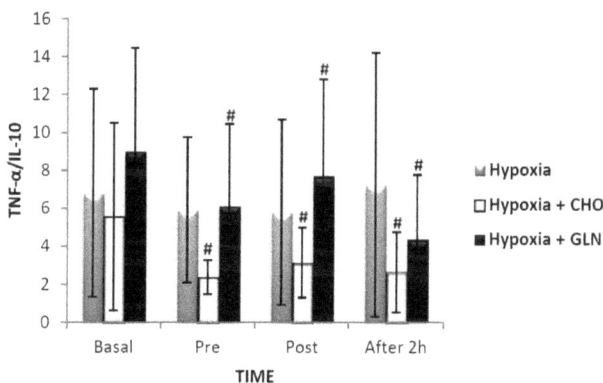

Figure 7. The results of salivary secretion rate of Tumor necrosis factor- α/Interleukin-10 (TNF-α/IL-10) was described by mean ± Standard Error (SE). The interaction of group versus time was analyzed by Analysis of Variance (ANOVA) for repeated measures followed by post hoc of Tukey test. The level of significance was set at $p < 0.05$. $n = 15$ volunteers. # Different in relation to Basal. Hypoxia + CHO = Hypoxia + carbohydrate and hypoxia + GLN = hypoxia + glutamine.

4. Discussion

The aim of this study was to analyze the effect of carbohydrate and glutamine supplementation on oral mucosal immunity after exercise at a simulated altitude of 4500 m. The main finding of this study was that strenuous exercise associated with hypoxia, with or without supplementation, did not change salivary IgA. Despite the decrease in the pro/anti-inflammatory balance, an anti-inflammatory response was found in the group with carbohydrate supplementation because of changes in IL-10 and TNF-α concentrations.

According to several studies conducted at sea level, carbohydrate and/or glutamine supplementation have shown to be effective on mitigating the stress effects of vigorous exercise on the immune system. Taking into consideration that the number of people that travel to places of high altitudes for tourism, work, and sports increases each year, it becomes of great importance to elucidate the effects of carbohydrate and/or glutamine supplementation in hypoxic environments on the oral mucosal immunity, which is considered a practical method to indicate stress. Therefore, in the future, new interventions may be proposed and designed to minimize the effects of hypoxia among athletes, travelers, workers, and people chronically exposed to high altitudes.

Regarding results involving $SaO_2\%$, the values at baseline were not significantly different for the groups, since they are in normal oxygen concentration. However, a reduction in $SaO_2\%$ was found after two hours of exposure for all groups, proving the efficiency of the hypoxia model used in this study and confirming the results found in the studies conducted by Tannheimer et al. [35], Mazzeo [14], and Pomidori et al. [36]. However, after two hours of recovery in hypoxia, $SaO_2\%$ increased almost immediately post-exercise, suggesting recovery. However, this was not enough time to restore the values to baseline levels.

The $SaO_2\%$ results of the Hypoxia + Carbohydrate group were similar to the group with no supplementation at baseline, but different after two hours of recovery with an increase in $SaO_2\%$ compared to pre-exercise and post-exercise. Such modifications are related to carbohydrate intake, increasing the concentration of CO_2 to a level that stimulates ventilation, thus enhancing blood oxygenation and reducing the desaturation of hypoxia [37,38]. The Hypoxia + Glutamine group showed similar changes compared to the Hypoxia group at baseline, although the results were different after two hours of recovery, showing an increase at pre-exercise, post-exercise, and hypoxic condition. The reasons for the restoration of $SaO_2\%$ in the Hypoxia + Glutamine group are not known, but it is suggested that the increased availability of plasma glutamine may interfere with the central synthesis of glutamate, an excitatory neurotransmitter that stimulates ventilation [39], and thus contribute to $SaO_2\%$ recovery.

Despite not evaluating plasma concentration of glutamine, a previous study with a similar protocol showed a 65.8% increase of glutamine post-exercise when compared to pre-exercise [24], reinforcing our hypothesis. Another fact to consider in the Hypoxia + Glutamine group is the combined action of the two supplements [40], contributing to increased ventilation in different pathways [37,39].

Pilardeau et al. [41] were the first to describe salivary flow in hypoxia; today it is known that salivary secretion can be affected by neural control of the autonomic nervous system, which indirectly regulates salivary flow and saliva composition [13]. The stress of intense exercise added to hypoxic environment stimulates the sympathetic nervous system, contracting blood vessels in salivary glands, which leads to a reduction in flow rate [27]. Our results are partly explained by these mechanisms, showing that salivary flow in hypoxic condition reduced 17% from baseline. However, the intake of both supplements appears to alleviate this effect, since the Hypoxia + Carbohydrate group showed a reduction of only 14% in salivary flow post-exercise compared to baseline. Interestingly, after two hours of recovery, supplementation with carbohydrates was able to promote a significant increase of 27% in flow compared to the end of the exercise. Bishop et al. [27] analyzed participants in normoxic conditions after two hours of riding a bicycle at 60% of VO_{2max} and found that consumption of carbohydrates (60 gL) increased salivary flow one hour after exercise, probably due to a reduction of sympathetic/parasympathetic balance [1].

The changes in salivary flow during and after exercise directly affect the concentration of salivary IgA [13,42], however, our results showed that the stimulation of salivary flow followed by the stress of exercise and hypoxia was not able to promote changes of total IgA concentration in any of the conditions. These results are similar to a study by Svendsen et al. [43] that analyzed participants exposed to hypobaric hypoxia conditions equivalent to 2000 m during 75 min of cycling at 70% VO_{2peak}. This finding may have occurred due to the high intensity of exercise and its immunosuppressive function, preventing the elevation of IgA [44], or because the reduced time of exposure to hypoxia was not enough to modify secretion of IgA [1].

The IgA secretion rate in the Hypoxic group was reduced by 22.5% post-exercise compared to baseline; statistically this reduction was not significant, but it can be physiologically important, since IgA is the most abundant protection protein in saliva [1]. The lower level of IgA secretion indicates a specific reduction in the synthesis and/or secretion of salivary IgA in response to stress created by intense exercise [18,45] coupled with hypoxia. When supplements were taken by the participants, this reduction was slightly smaller (i.e., 10.6% in the Hypoxia + Carbohydrate group and 15.5% in the Hypoxia + Glutamine group). Our findings are similar to the study conducted by Krzywkowski et al. [45], involving normoxia with glutamine supplementation (17.5 g), which showed the same tendency of exercise (two hours of bicycle exercise at 75% VO_{2max}) to reduce salivary IgA during and up to two hours after exercise.

The production of IgA in saliva may be mediated by several factors, such as stress hormones, nutritional factors, circadian cycle, hydration, alcohol intake, and also cytokines [1,2,13,46]. The effects of exercise on the production of cytokines in saliva are not well understood [2], especially in hypoxia [21]. Therefore, the present study was the first to investigate the effect of carbohydrate and glutamine supplementation on concentration of cytokines after exercise in hypoxic condition.

The concentration of IL-10 and its secretion rates were not different when comparing time for any of the groups. However, despite the secretion rate being slightly lower in post-exercise when compared to baseline, we found that supplementation with carbohydrates was able to increase IL-10 after two hours of recovery, showing that the anti-inflammatory role of carbohydrate [46] can also be observed in saliva, thereby contributing to the maintenance of homeostasis at this site and helping to preserve mucosal immune responses [47]. We found similar results in the Hypoxia + Glutamine group, suggesting that, despite the increase of IL-10 by approximately 25% post-exercise compared to baseline, glutamine supplementation was not able to modulate the pro/anti-inflammatory balance by modification of IL-10.

The concentration and rate of secretion of TNF-α did not change in the Hypoxia group, however, in normoxic conditions, an increase of TNF-α was found in saliva during and after intense exercise [2], and a reduction after one-hour of recovery [48]. When assessing the Hypoxia + Carbohydrate group, TNF-α decreased after exercise and recovery, suggesting that the increase of IL-10 in saliva, mediated by supplementation with carbohydrates, may be responsible for a decrease in TNF-α secretion rate, similar to what occurs in other tissues, and enhancing the anti-inflammatory role of carbohydrates. In fact, supplementation with carbohydrates was able to attenuate the inflammatory process promoted by exercise and hypoxia, and modulated the balance between pro- and anti-inflammatory cytokines in saliva, as in normoxic conditions [49].

Regarding glutamine supplementation, we observed a decrease in TNF-α secretion rate immediately after exercise, and the reduction was more evident at the end of the second hour of recovery. These results demonstrated the anti-inflammatory role of glutamine in saliva, which has been observed in other tissues, directing the pro-inflammatory/anti-inflammatory balance toward an anti-inflammatory response [21,22].

The salivary concentration and secretion rate of IL-6 did not change in any of the groups. There are no results in the literature showing the effect of exercise on salivary IL-6 in hypoxia. Our results contradict the findings of Usui et al. [2], who observed an increase of IL-6 levels in saliva in normoxic conditions during and after exercise at 75% of VO_{2max}, including 80 min post-exercise. Thus, we cannot suggest what mechanisms are responsible for regulating IL-6 in hypoxia, but they are probably different from those in normoxic condition (i.e., maintaining homeostasis of blood and hepatic glucose and stimulating the release of C Reactive Protein (CRP). We believe this finding is a reflection of the increased use of IL-6 in its hematopoietic purpose [50,51] because it causes almost immediate reduction of SaO_2% and deterioration of O_2 due to hypoxia.

5. Conclusions

We conclude that five hours in hypoxia associated with strenuous exercise was not enough to promote a change in salivary IgA. Supplementation with carbohydrates and glutamine produced changes in the pro/anti-inflammatory balance, stimulating an inflammatory response in oral mucosa.

However, our results should be interpreted with caution in regards to their generalizability because we only assessed male subjects.

Acknowledgments: All authors are grateful to the Conselho Nacional de Desenvolvimento Cientifico e Tecnológico (CNPq), Fundação de Amparo a Pesquisa do Estado de São Paulo (FAPESP) FAPESP: 2013/01324-4, Associação Fundo de Incentivo à Psicofarmacologia (AFIP) e à Prof.ª Dra. Marília Cerqueira Leite Seelaender from Biomedical Science Institute (ICB)—Universidade de São Paulo.

Author Contributions: Aline Venticinque Caris conceived and designed the experiments, analyzed the data, and wrote the paper; Edgar Tavares Da Silva and Samile Amorim Dos Santos performed the experiments; Sergio Tufik contributed reagents/materials/analysis tools; Ronaldo Vagner Thomatieli Dos Santos conceived and designed the experiments and wrote the paper.

Conflicts of Interest: The authors declare no conflict of interest.

References

1. Born, D.P.; Faiss, R.; Willis, S.J.; Strahler, J.; Millet, G.P.; Holmberg, H.C.; Sperlich, B. Circadian variation of salivary immunoglobin A, alpha-amylase activity and mood in response to repeated double-poling sprints in hypoxia. *Eur. J. Appl. Physiol.* **2016**, *116*, 1–10. [CrossRef] [PubMed]
2. Usui, T.; Yoshikawa, T.; Ueda, S.-Y.; Katsura, Y.; Orita, K.; Fujimoto, S. Effects of acute prolonged strenuous exercise on the salivary stress markers and inflammatory cytokines. *J. Phys. Fit. Sports Med.* **2012**, *1*, 1–8. [CrossRef]
3. Slavish, D.C.; Graham-Engeland, J.E.; Smyth, J.M.; Engeland, C.G. Salivary markers of inflammation in response to acute stress. *Brain Behav. Immunity* **2015**, *44*, 253–269. [CrossRef] [PubMed]
4. Mishra, K.P.; Ganju, L.; Singh, S.B. Hypoxia modulates innate immune factors: A review. *Int. Immunopharmacol.* **2015**, *28*, 425–428. [CrossRef] [PubMed]
5. Hartmann, G.; Tschöp, M.; Fischer, R.; Bidlingmaier, C.; Riepl, R.; Tschöp, K.; Hautmann, H.; Endres, S.; Toepfer, M. High altitude increases circulating interleukin-6, interleukin-1 receptor antagonist and C-reactive protein. *Cytokine* **2000**, *12*, 246–252. [CrossRef] [PubMed]
6. Hagobian, T.A.; Jacobs, K.A.; Subudhi, A.W.; Fattor, J.A.; Rock, P.B.; Muza, S.R.; Cymerman, A.; Friedlander, A.L. Cytokine responses at high altitude: Effects of exercise and antioxidants at 4300 m. *Med. Sci. Sports Exerc.* **2006**, *38*, 276–285. [CrossRef] [PubMed]
7. Koeppen, M.; Eckle, T.; Eltzschig, H.K. The hypoxia-inflammation link and potential drug targets. *Curr. Opin. Anaesthesiol.* **2011**, *24*, 363–369. [CrossRef] [PubMed]
8. Shay, J.E.; Celeste Simon, M. Hypoxia-inducible factors: Crosstalk between inflammation and metabolism. *Semin. Cell Dev. Biol.* **2012**, *23*, 389–394. [CrossRef] [PubMed]
9. McNamee, E.N.; Korns Johnson, D.; Homann, D.; Clambey, E.T. Hypoxia and hypoxia-inducible factors as regulators of T cell development, differentiation, and function. *Immunol. Res.* **2013**, *55*, 58–70. [CrossRef] [PubMed]
10. Mishra, K.P.; Ganju, L. Influence of high altitude exposure on the immune system: A review. *Immunol. Investig.* **2010**, *39*, 219–234. [CrossRef] [PubMed]
11. Kunz, H.; Bishop, N.C.; Spielmann, G.; Pistillo, M.; Reed, J.; Ograjsek, T.; Park, Y.; Mehta, S.K.; Pierson, D.L.; Simpson, R.J. Fitness level impacts salivary antimicrobial protein responses to a single bout of cycling exercise. *Eur. J. Appl. Physiol.* **2015**, *115*, 1015–1027. [CrossRef] [PubMed]
12. Rosa, L.; Teixeira, A.; Lira, F.; Tufik, S.; Mello, M.; Santos, R. Moderate acute exercise (70% VO$_{2peak}$) induces TGF-β, α-amylase and IgA in saliva during recovery. *Oral Dis.* **2014**, *20*, 186–190. [CrossRef] [PubMed]
13. Papacosta, E.; Nassis, G.P. Saliva as a tool for monitoring steroid, peptide and immune markers in sport and exercise science. *J. Sci. Med. Sport* **2011**, *14*, 424–434. [CrossRef] [PubMed]
14. Mazzeo, R.S. Altitude, exercise and immune function. *Exerc. Immunol. Rev.* **2005**, *11*, 6–16. [PubMed]
15. Shephard, R.J. Immune changes induced by exercise in an adverse environment. *Can. J. Physiol. Pharmacol.* **1998**, *76*, 539–546. [CrossRef] [PubMed]
16. Mazzeo, R.S. Physiological responses to exercise at altitude: An update. *Sports Med.* **2008**, *38*, 1–8. [CrossRef] [PubMed]
17. Castell, L.M.; Poortmans, J.R.; Newsholme, E.A. Does glutamine have a role in reducing infections in athletes? *Eur. J. Appl. Physiol. Occup. Physiol.* **1996**, *73*, 488–490. [CrossRef] [PubMed]

18. Castell, L.M.; Newsholme, E.A. The effects of oral glutamine supplementation on athletes after prolonged, exhaustive exercise. *Nutrition* **1997**, *13*, 738–742. [CrossRef]
19. Wong, S.H.; Williams, C.; Adams, N. Effects of ingesting a large volume of carbohydrate electrolyte solution on rehydration during recovery and subsequent exercise capacity. *Int. J. Sports Nutr.* **2000**, *10*, 375–393. [CrossRef]
20. Nieman, D.C.; Henson, D.A.; Smith, L.L.; Utter, A.C.; Vinci, D.M.; Davis, J.M.; Kaminsky, D.E.; Shute, M. Cytokine changes after a marathon race. *J. Appl. Physiol.* **2001**, *91*, 109–114. [PubMed]
21. Walsh, N.P.; Gleeson, M.; Pyne, D.B.; Nieman, D.C.; Dhabhar, F.S.; Shephard, R.J.; Oliver, S.J.; Bermon, S.; Kajeniene, A. Position statement. Part two: Maintaining immune health. *Exerc. Immunol. Rev.* **2011**, *17*, 64–103. [PubMed]
22. Bailey, N.; Clark, M.; Nordlund, M.; Shelton, M.; Farver, K. New paradigm in nutrition support: Using evidence to drive practice. *Crit. Care Nurs. Q.* **2012**, *35*, 255–267. [CrossRef] [PubMed]
23. Krieger, J.W.; Crowe, M.; Blank, S.E. Chronic glutamine supplementation increases nasal but not salivary IgA during 9 days of interval training. *J. Appl. Physiol.* **2004**, *97*, 585–591. [CrossRef] [PubMed]
24. Caris, A.V.; Lira, F.S.; de Mello, M.T.; Oyama, L.M.; dos Santos, R.V. Carbohydrate and glutamine supplementation modulates the Th1/Th2 balance after exercise performed at a simulated altitude of 4500 m. *Nutrition* **2014**, *30*, 1331–1336. [CrossRef] [PubMed]
25. Nieman, D.C. Immunonutrition support for athletes. *J. Nutr. Rev.* **2008**, *66*, 310–320. [CrossRef] [PubMed]
26. Carlson, L.A.; Kenefick, R.W.; Koch, A.J. Influence of carbohydrate ingestion on salivary immunoglobulin A following resistance exercise. *J. Int. Soc. Sports Nutr.* **2013**, *10*, 1–8. [CrossRef] [PubMed]
27. Bishop, N.C.; Blannin, A.K.; Armstrong, E.; Rickman, M.; Gleeson, M. Carbohydrate and fluid intake affect the saliva flow rate and IgA response to cycling. *Med. Sci. Sports Exerc.* **2000**, *32*, 2046–2051. [CrossRef] [PubMed]
28. National Statistical Service. Sample Size Calculator.Disponivel em. Available online: http://www.nss.gov.au/nss/home.nsf/pages/Sample+Size+Calculator+Description?OpenDocument (accessed on 2 April 2016).
29. Moher, D.; Hopewell, S.; Schulz, K.F.; Montori, V.; Gøtzsche, P.C.; Devereaux, P.J. CONSORT 2010 explanation and elaboration: Updated guidelines for reporting parallel group randomised trials. *Int. J. Surg.* **2012**, *10*, 28–55. [CrossRef] [PubMed]
30. Research Randomizer. Disponível em. Available online: https://www.randomizer.org/ (accessed on 2 February 2016).
31. Sassi, A.; Marcora, S.M.; Rampinini, E.; Mognoni, P.; Impellizzeri, F.M. Prediction of time to exhaustion from blood lactate response during submaximal exercise in competitive cyclists. *Eur. J. Appl. Physiol.* **2006**, *97*, 174–180. [CrossRef] [PubMed]
32. Jones, A.M.; Doust, J.H. A 1% treadmill grade most accurately reflects the energetic cost of outdoor running. *J. Sports Sci.* **1996**, *14*, 321–327. [CrossRef] [PubMed]
33. Borg, G.A. Psychophysical bases of perceived exertion. *Med. Sci. Sports Exerc.* **1982**, *14*, 377–381. [CrossRef] [PubMed]
34. Coppel, J.; Hennis, P.; Gilbert-Kawai, E.; Grocott, M.P. The physiological effects of hypobaric hypoxia versus normobaric hypoxia: A systematic review of crossover trials. *Extreme Physiol. Med.* **2015**, *4*, 2. [CrossRef] [PubMed]
35. Tannheimer, M.; Thomas, A.; Gerngross, H. Oxygen saturation course and altitude symptomatology during an expedition to broad peak (8047 m). *Int. J. Sports Med.* **2002**, *23*, 329–335. [CrossRef] [PubMed]
36. Pomidori, L.; Bonardi, D.; Campigotto, F.; Fasano, V.; Gennari, A.; Valli, G.; Palange, P.; Cogo, A. The hypoxic profile during trekking to the Pyramid Laboratory. *High Alt. Med. Biol.* **2009**, *10*, 233–237. [CrossRef] [PubMed]
37. Golja, P.; Flander, P.; Klemenc, M.; Maver, J.; Princi, T. Carbohydrate ingestion improves oxygen delivery in acute hypoxia. *High Alt. Med. Biol.* **2008**, *9*, 53–62. [CrossRef] [PubMed]
38. Charlot, K.; Pichon, A.; Richalet, J.P.; Chapelot, D. Effects of a high-carbohydrate versus high-protein meal on acute responses to hypoxia at rest and exercise. *Eur. J. Appl. Physiol.* **2013**, *113*, 691–702. [CrossRef] [PubMed]
39. Honda, Y.; Tani, H.; Masuda, A.; Kobayashi, T.; Nishino, T.; Kimura, H.; Masuyama, S.; Kuriyama, T. Effect of prior O_2 breathing on ventilatory response to sustained isocapnic hypoxia in adult humans. *J. Appl. Physiol.* **1996**, *81*, 1627–1632. [PubMed]

40. Favano, A.; Santos-Silva, P.R.; Nakano, E.Y.; Pedrinelli, A.; Hernandez, A.J.; Greve, J.M. Peptide glutamine supplementation for tolerance of intermittent exercise in soccer players. *Clinics* **2008**, *63*, 27–32. [CrossRef] [PubMed]

41. Pilardeau, P.; Richalet, J.P.; Bouissou, P.; Vaysse, J.; Larmignat, P.; Boom, A. Saliva flow and composition in humans exposed to acute altitude hypoxia. *Eur. J. Appl. Physiol. Occup. Physiol.* **1990**, *59*, 450–453. [CrossRef] [PubMed]

42. Allgrove, J.E.; Gomes, E.; Hough, J.; Gleeson, M. Effects of exercise intensity on salivary antimicrobial proteins and markers of stress in active men. *J. Sports Sci.* **2008**, *26*, 653–661. [CrossRef] [PubMed]

43. Svendsen, I.S.; Hem, E.; Gleeson, M. Effect of acute exercise and hypoxia on markers of systemic and mucosal immunity. *Eur. J. Appl. Physiol.* **2016**, *116*, 1219–1229. [CrossRef] [PubMed]

44. Bishop, N.C.; Gleeson, M. Acute and chronic effects of exercise on markers of mucosal immunity. *Front. Biosci.* **2009**, *14*, 4444–4456. [CrossRef]

45. Krzywkowski, K.; Petersen, E.W.; Ostrowski, K.; Link-Amster, H.; Boza, J.; Halkjaer-Kristensen, J.; Klarlund Pedersen, B. Effect of glutamine and protein supplementation on exercise-induced decreases in salivary IgA. *J. Appl. Physiol.* **2001**, *91*, 832–838. [PubMed]

46. Silva, R.P.; Natali, A.J.; Paula, S.O.; Locatelli, J.; Marins, J.C.B. Imunoglobulina A salivar (IgA-s) e exercício: Relevância do controle em atletas e implicações metodológicas. *Rev. Bras. Med. Esporte* **2009**, *15*, 459–466. [CrossRef]

47. Yamaoka, M.; Yamaguchi, S.; Okuyama, M.; Tomoike, H. Anti-inflammatory cytokine profile in human heart failure: Behavior of interleukin-10 in association with tumor necrosis factor-alpha. *Jpn. Circ. J.* **1999**, *63*, 951–956. [CrossRef] [PubMed]

48. Rahman, Z.A.; Abdullah, N.; Singh, R.; Sosroseno, W. Effect of acute exercise on the levels of salivary cortisol, tumor necrosis factor-alpha and nitric oxide. *J. Oral Sci.* **2010**, *52*, 133–136. [CrossRef] [PubMed]

49. Bishop, N.C.; Blannin, A.K.; Robson, P.J.; Walsh, N.P.; Gleeson, M. The effects of carbohydrate supplementation on immune responses to a soccer-specific exercise protocol. *J. Sports Sci.* **1999**, *17*, 787–796. [CrossRef] [PubMed]

50. Faquin, W.C.; Schneider, T.J.; Goldberg, M.A. Effect of inflammatory cytokines on hypoxia-induced erythropoietin production. *Blood* **1992**, *79*, 1987–1994. [PubMed]

51. Klausen, T.; Olsen, N.V.; Poulsen, T.D.; Richalet, J.P.; Pedersen, B.K. Hypoxemia increases serum interleukin-6 in humans. *Eur. J. Appl. Physiol. Occup. Physiol.* **1997**, *76*, 480–482. [CrossRef] [PubMed]

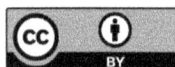

MDPI AG

St. Alban-Anlage 66

4052 Basel, Switzerland

Tel. +41 61 683 77 34

Fax +41 61 302 89 18

http://www.mdpi.com

Nutrients Editorial Office

E-mail: nutrients@mdpi.com

http://www.mdpi.com/journal/nutrients

www.ingramcontent.com/pod-product-compliance
Lightning Source LLC
Chambersburg PA
CBHW051701210326
41597CB00032B/5327